A MAN'S GUIDE TO HEALTHY AGING

A Johns Hopkins Press Health Book

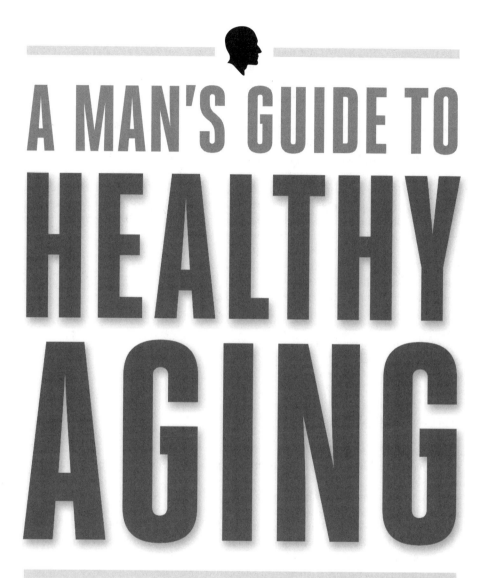

A MAN'S GUIDE TO
HEALTHY AGING

STAY SMART, STRONG, AND ACTIVE

EDWARD H. THOMPSON, JR., AND LENARD W. KAYE

The Johns Hopkins University Press
Baltimore

Note to the Reader. This book is not meant to substitute for medical care, and treatment should not be based solely on its contents. Instead, treatment must be developed in a dialogue between the individual and his physician. This book has been written to help with that dialogue. The author and publisher are not responsible for any adverse consequences resulting from the use of information in this book.

Drug dosage. The author and publisher have made reasonable efforts to determine that selection and dosage of drugs discussed in this text conform to the practices of the general medical community. The medications described do not necessarily have specific approval by the U.S. Food and Drug Administration for use in the diseases and dosages for which they are recommended. In view of ongoing research, changes in governmental regulations, and the constant flow of information relating to drug therapy and drug reactions, the reader is urged to check the package insert of each drug for any change in indications and dosage and for warnings or precautions. This is particularly important when the recommended agent is a new and/or infrequently used drug.

© 2013 The Johns Hopkins University Press
All rights reserved. Published 2013
Printed in the United States of America on acid-free paper
9 8 7 6 5 4 3 2

The Johns Hopkins University Press
2715 North Charles Street
Baltimore, Maryland 21218-4363
www.press.jhu.edu

Library of Congress Cataloging-in-Publication Data

Thompson, Edward H., Jr., 1945–
   A man's guide to healthy aging : stay smart, strong, and active / Edward H. Thompson, Jr., and Lenard W. Kaye.
       pages cm. — (A Johns Hopkins Press health book)
   Includes bibliographical references and index.
   ISBN 978-1-4214-1055-5 (hardcover : alk. paper) — ISBN 1-4214-1055-9 (hardcover : alk. paper)
— ISBN 978-1-4214-1056-2 (pbk. : alk. paper) — ISBN 1-4214-1056-7 (pbk. : alk. paper) —
ISBN 978-1-4214-1057-9 (electronic) — ISBN 1-4214-1057-5 (electronic)
   1. Men—Health and hygiene. 2. Older men—Health and hygiene. 3. Longevity.
I. Kaye, Lenard W. II. Title.
   RA777.8.T56 2013
   613'.04234—dc23   2012047831

A catalog record for this book is available from the British Library.

Figures 12.1, 12.4, 13.1, 14.1, 17.4, 18.2, and 18.3 and the figure on page 77 are by Jacqueline
    Schaffer.
Figure 17.1 is by Carlyn Iverson.

Special discounts are available for bulk purchases of this book. For more information, please contact Special Sales at 410-516-6936 or specialsales@press.jhu.edu.

The Johns Hopkins University Press uses environmentally friendly book materials, including recycled text paper that is composed of at least 30 percent post-consumer waste, whenever possible.

To Stephen Thompson and Natalie Thompson
and Ruth Mendala-Thompson
with love and gratitude

To Dyan Walsh with love and appreciation for
her sound advice, unflinching support,
and inordinate patience

Contents

PART IV. LIVING WITH OTHERS

Acknowledgments

This book began, as many projects in the health field do, as an "aha" moment. Early in an Aging and Health seminar taught at the University of Massachusetts Medical School, one of the distinguished lecturers asked the audience what differentiated women's myocardial infarct symptoms from men's, and there was a pervasive silence. People had not expected gender to affect symptoms. Nor did the gerontology and medical students know where to begin to find information about men's health when, in the same week, a geriatrician asked the audience how men report the experience with passing a kidney stone, if women equate it with labor pain. There was no ready sourcebook about men's health approximating the classic *Our Bodies, Ourselves* or its companion volume, *Ourselves Growing Older*. The project was born, and previously unrecognized for their early inspiration are Jeffrey Burl, Deborah Liss Fins, Jim Hamos, Mary Leonard, Lynn Li, Ira Ockene, Susan Rezen, Stephen Roizen, Gary Tanguay, Henry Wiesman, and Rosalie Wolf. Most inspirational was Betty Friedan's encouragement when the idea for this book was little more than "aha." We also want to warmly acknowledge Abraham Monk, Jordan Kosberg, Jeffrey Applegate, Gail Werrbach, Sandy Butler, Nancy Kelly, and Nancy Fishwick.

It is certainly difficult to know where to start when it comes to thanking all the people who have contributed to this book. Any significant project in the health field involves a large number of colleagues and assistants, and we are truly grateful to the many people who contributed to this major undertaking. First and foremost, we are deeply indebted to the colleagues identified in the "Contributors" section who worked closely with us to offer very thoughtful suggestions and develop smart, readable chapters. Their contributions made the manuscript into a vastly better book. Along the way many other undergraduate students, graduate students, and faculty colleagues also provided invaluable support, and we warmly thank them. Some who contributed especially helpful comments, opportunities to talk through issues, or information as the book developed include Meagan Fisher, Andy Futterman, Ann Marie Leshkowich, Kendal Nielsen, Ivy Pruitt, John Quaresima, Sara Stockman, and Samantha Surface. Thanks also are due to the many graduate and undergraduate students (too numerous to mention) who have focused their education on gerontological health and human services practice over the years at the College of the Holy Cross and the University of Maine, including those enrolled in the Hartford Partnership Program for Aging Education, the Program in Leadership in Rural Gerontological Practice, and the Interprofessional Graduate Certificate in Gerontology. Their inquisitive nature and unbridled enthusiasm for better understanding and responding to the challenges and opportunities of an aging society have been both extremely contagious and invigorating. Colleagues at the School of Social Work and the Center on Aging at the University of Maine have been powerful forces in refining Kaye's perspective on so many issues associated with contemporary aging and practice in the human services.

A number of people have read and commented on all or parts of this book. Two anonymous reviewers for the Johns Hopkins University Press read the manuscript and offered many suggestions. We appreciate their investment to make our work into a better book. Thompson's fall 2009 Men and Aging seminar students read earlier drafts of several chapters, providing invaluable critiques and recommendations for how their fathers would read and react to the information itself and its framing. Kaye's fall 2009 gerontology seminar students engaged in initial background research on a number of topics addressed in this book, and three of the brightest were eventually recruited to be contributors. We are especially indebted to the colleagues listed in the "Reviewers" section, who graciously accepted the invitation to read and critique a chapter. They brought their expertise and contributed immensely helpful comments to clarify ideas, assist with factual issues, and offer advice. Their influence on this book is tremendous.

This book has received generous assistance along the way from the College of the Holy Cross and the University of Maine, especially the Committee on Faculty Scholarship at Holy Cross for its financial assistance for some of the anatomical drawings and for the award of a Batchelor-Ford Faculty Fellowship to complete the book manuscript. Parts of the material within chapters were presented at annual meetings of the Gerontological Society of America, the American Sociological Association, the American Society on Aging, Social Work with and for Men, the Council on Social Work Education, the National Association of Area Agencies on Aging, and the American Assembly for Men in Nursing. We thank the participants at these different venues for their helpful comments.

Regarding the preparation of this book, we greatly appreciate the editorial suggestions made by people at the Johns Hopkins University Press, especially Jackie Wehmueller, executive editor, and Sara Cleary, acquisitions assistant, who provided guidance throughout the process, from contract, to a clear vision for the direction of the book, to the inevitable need for expert editing. As well, we are very thankful for Jeremy Horsefield's contribution as our copy editor.

We reserve our deepest gratitude for our families, who have stood alongside us throughout. Their ongoing encouragement is heartfelt, as are the countless hours they patiently spent listening, discussing ideas, and normalizing frets. We cannot overstate our gratitude.

PART I
MANAGING OUR LIVES

CHAPTER 1

Men's Health and Healthy Aging

Men who are getting older are redesigning later life to emphasize new vitality. When the baby boomers started to hit 50, then 60, their decisions and plans helped to reshape the nation's thinking about how "older men" are supposed to act. Most men in their late fifties and midsixties are sexually active, plan to launch themselves into new jobs or postretirement "encore" careers, are resilient and more frugal, and believe that their lives are better despite the Great Recession setbacks.[1] They also intend to contribute their valuable skills and experiences to their communities and to travel more. This group refuses to embrace the ageist stereotype of men who are "winding down," sitting on a porch or deck without an agenda. They feel healthier than their parents did when they turned 60, are captivated by the possibilities of their "longevity bonus," and intend to remain productive as they create an adventurous new life stage that begins in their sixties.[2] Think about it this way: men in their late sixties and seventies are proud of their age and do not worry much about what other people think of them and their less-than-perfect bodies.

> Well, I'm 77, and I can't climb on the roof any more. At first, I felt I had lost something, I don't know what, but it did affect me. Now, I couldn't care less about it. If I can't do it, then someone else will. That's my attitude to anything now, but it takes a bit getting used to.[3]

Becoming older means becoming smarter, wiser, and more mature; it also means beginning to do some of the things on our "bucket list."

The self-care needed to age well depends on how we think about ourselves and our future lives as older men. We can extend the quality of our everyday lives and our bodies' health by eating well, remaining active, taking some time for ourselves, and managing stress. We need to resist the negativity so common in anti-aging messages and stay engaged in our relationships with family, friends, and our communities.

The message in this book is for men, but it will also help women better understand their brothers, fathers, and husbands. Working to make the second half of men's lives physically and emotionally healthier than the first can pay enormous dividends. We explore the challenges and the pleasures of growing older and offer all kinds of information useful for middle-aged and older men. Everything in this book—from the realities of how aging changes our bodies to understanding wills and trusts, from caregiving to retirement decisions, from sexuality in later life to how much friends matter—is to provide you with information you need to live a healthier life for many years to come. There is much for everyone to learn about adult men's health and healthy aging experiences.

MODERN AGING: NO LONGER "PAST YOUR PRIME"

Aging is a natural part of life. The shrewd comedian George Burns said, "You can't help getting older, but you can help getting old." He was keenly aware that too many people confuse aging with getting old and are thus apprehensive about it. Throughout history, people have tried to delay aging. Attempts to discover a substance to rejuvenate the body and mind inspired Chinese alchemists, Egyptian prophets, and many explorers, past and present, to search the globe. Contemporary medicine also touts many different "fountain of youth" fixes, from a Botox treatment to eliminate wrinkles to testosterone replacement therapy to boost stamina.

In America's youth-obsessed culture, generations of men have been encouraged to view aging as a catastrophe that brings only problems.[4] Clichés such as "past your prime" and "over the hill" cast a dim light on getting older. The vanity drugs, or "cosmeceuticals," that advertise a "Repair" gel or "Age Defense" facial cream for men in their twenties and thirties start with the premise that aging is ugly and unnatural. It is vital to the quality of our lives to not get sucked into this damaging and false image of getting older. Aging is not the apocalypse that myths and media suggest. Aging is an ongoing process, commencing at birth and continuing throughout our existence—it is *not* a disease or a destination.

Ageism—a concept coined in 1969, 2 years after the Beatles released "When I'm Sixty-Four"—refers to a mind-set that stigmatizes people simply because of their chronologic age and results in discrimination.[5] At age 50, AARP (American Association of Retired Persons) automatically offers us membership. Their offer suggests that we have crossed over a threshold to be officially among those "getting older." At 62, the U.S. Forest Service will sell you a lifetime "Senior Pass" that permits access to any National Park. We also become eligible to receive a monthly Social Security check, though we are encouraged to wait until at least age 66 or 67. Less flattering ageist reminders are all around us—from images of aging in "humorous" birthday cards, to seating an older couple away from the active area of a restaurant where families with young children are gathered, to older guys not being invited to have a beer and burger with the younger people they work with.

Myths about our cognitive and physical decline are what perpetuate ageist attitudes. The myths are powerful. Following up on a study of how men and women viewed aging, Becca Levy, from Yale University's School of Public Health, found that 20 years later those who believed in ageist myths and stereotypes were in poorer health. Levy persuasively argues that "mind matters" and what you believe influences your health behavior—whether it is daily flossing and adding berries to your cereal, intentionally taking the stairs for the exercise, or just the opposite and falsely believing that getting older is filled with "senior moments" and rocking chairs.[6]

Rather than succumbing to ageist messages or the media depictions of the approaching elder "tsunami," which collectively suggests we are part of a destructive and needy force about to strike our communities, most midlife and older men are vital and productive. According to one 91-year-old Deer Isle (Maine) man who has worked with a garden club for more than 50 years to mow and trim brush at a memorial park:

> We just try to keep the place in order. I like to do it. I've just been somebody who's been willing to do it. I'm still willing. I've been active, I'm still active and I'm just tickled to death to be there doing something I think is useful.[7]

Challenging the stereotype of becoming an inevitable burden on others, we are and continue to be a valuable resource for our families and communities. As we strive to be physically, emotionally, and socially the best we can be, we can take advantage of the skills, wisdom, and capacities gained over a lifetime of experience. Not to do this would represent a terrible waste of personal possibilities and our abilities to give back.

Ironically, it is younger men and women who have the greatest fear of aging.[8] They have little firsthand experience and mostly media imagery as their guides. As we reach middle age, men actually are unafraid and have

Age is an accomplishment. It is more social than chronological or biological.

begun looking forward to becoming older, distinguished, judicious, and perhaps retired; we gear up to experience renewed productivity and purpose in life as an older man. Researchers find that as men turn 50, then 60, we experience greater certainty of who we are and feel more confident and powerful.[9] Is 60 the new 40, some people have asked? This already trite question is sociologically interesting: it reflects the fact that many more middle-aged and older men are living longer, staying healthier, and enjoying life more. They do not "feel their age," and becoming older is no longer viewed as "getting old."[10]

MEN'S HEALTH

There is optimistic news to report. Only 1 in every 25 men in the United States reached age 65 in the early 1900s.[11] Living to become an older man who will celebrate his seventieth birthday is now common enough to be taken for granted. Men's life expectancy of 46 years in the early 1900s has lengthened to, on average, 75 years,[12] mainly because of fewer early heart disease deaths, less dangerous jobs, and public health measures that include occupational safety and better foods. More than ever, men also are smarter about their health—and we're seeing real dividends. Most men who are 50 years old can now expect to live into their eighties; 65-year-olds can anticipate living another 20 years with few limitations.[13]

Despite these astounding changes, men's longevity improved at a slower rate throughout the twentieth century compared to women's.[14] Clinical and public health researchers have identified many biological forces that influence men's health and longevity, including hormones like testosterone and cortisol. No doubt all these "mother nature" factors partly explain why men report fewer aches and illness than women but die earlier. But biology is not destiny. Women outlived men only by 1 year a century ago, not the 5-year difference we now find (which is down from a 7-year difference of two decades ago). Both authors either have already outlived or expect to outlive their fathers' life spans. Researchers are convinced that, more than our genes, it is our lifestyle habits that chiefly determine our health, pace of aging, and longevity.[15] The takeaway message in this book is to take responsibility for your health right now in order to reap the reward of more independence later. Prevention works, and it is never too late to adopt new health habits. Most unhealthy habits are amenable to change. Two things alone—eating well and staying active—strengthen our body's ability to repair itself, improve mood, and even support healthy blood flow to the brain and, by the way, a natural erection.

While we were younger, most of us were unfamiliar with the positive health habits message. When we were doing what was expected of us *as young men*, we most often adopted attitudes, beliefs, and behaviors that, all too often, had an insidious effect on our health.[16] Boys and younger men continue to experience tremendous pressure to adopt unhealthy "masculine" practices that increase the risk of disease and injury—everything from "real men" eat red meat (daily), to "Hey, play through the pain," to "Why should I consult a doctor, I feel fine!" to "Smoking relaxes me."[17] When we were younger, we weren't urged to think about the foods we eat, the stresses we juggle, the actual number of beers or drinks occasionally downed, or how much exercise we really get.

Having an age, such as passing 50 or passing 60, means taking note of our bodies along four dimensions: activity and fitness, appearance, energy, and ailments.

Source: Laz, C. (2003). Age embodiment. *Journal of Aging Studies, 17,* 503-519.

Times have changed, and we have become more mature. Greater numbers of men are paying more attention to their bodies and overall well-being than ever before. Scan the health section of any newspaper: articles report on how adult men are looking for ways to improve health, usually with lifestyle adjustments. Watch the commercials during the evening news; most are geared toward middle-aged and older folks and advocate "healthy aging." Experts recognize that the pace of our body's intrinsic aging is heavily influenced by our attitudes and lifestyle habits, and we are choosing to live longer and healthier by adopting healthy habits. Adopting healthy habits may well be the most accessible fountain of youth. Medical experts estimate that maintaining just four healthy habits—not smoking, being physically active, eating well, and scheduling regular preventive medical visits—can delay the life-altering disabilities associated with many chronic illnesses for as much as 20 years.

MANAGING OUR HEALTH

Men's chosen lifestyle habits are only part of the issue. We also need reliable information and others' support. Knowing what are health risks and what behaviors are health promoting is critically important.[18] When men lack information on how their health-impairing habits affect them, they see no reason to make the effort to change a habit that they are used to and enjoy. Getting healthy and aging well are both about attitude and knowledge.[19] This sourcebook is filled with the most vital information you need to live well.

As important as it is for each man to take charge of his own health and wellness, no one can do it alone. A popular cliché is that it takes a

RECOMMENDED PHYSICALS AND SCREENING SCHEDULE

What you need	When
Basic physical exam: head-to-toe examination, review medical history, and discuss your health	Every year, age 50+
Blood tests and urinalysis: samples of urine and blood screened for diabetes, infections, hormone balance, and cholesterol levels	Every year, age 50+
Blood pressure check: screen for high blood pressure (hypertension), which causes heart disease and permanent damage to other organs if untreated	Every year, age 50+
EKG (electrocardiogram): measures the electrical activity of the heart and screens for changes since baseline and for abnormalities (e.g., arrhythmia)	Every 3–5 years, age 50+
DRE (digital rectal exam): a gloved finger inserted into the rectum screens for prostate cancer and for the lumps and hardening of colon cancer	Every year, age 40+
Tuberculosis test: an airborne bacterial infection screened by a simple skin test	Every 5 years, age 40+
Colonoscopy: a flexible fiber optic scope examines the rectum and wall of the colon for cancer and removes growths, called *polyps*, for examination in labs for cancer	Every 5–10 years, age 50+

community to raise a child; well, it also takes a community to facilitate men's health. Men need the support of family, employers, and health care providers. Men should not feel compelled to be "sturdy oaks" weathering all difficulties and troubles by themselves. We can "employ" medical providers for advice, regular physicals, and age-appropriate screenings; ask our family to support our decisions to change health habits; and ask our employers if we have access to wellness programs.

Mature men know that they can earn respect by standing out from the herd and making healthy choices. When it comes to smoking and reporting "I quit," or ordering a chicken Caesar salad for lunch (light on the dressing) rather than a 1,200 calorie, half-pound sirloin burger with fixings, the other guys we're with will nod their approval. There will be a few who are dumbstruck and throw a verbal dig that is intended to question your manhood. But we know that the real challenge isn't about a salad versus a burger; rather, it is being fit enough to still play tennis, swim, join in a game of tag with the grandkids, or carry our golf clubs into our late sixties and beyond.

In the pages that follow, you will not find directions to the elusive fountain of youth. Like the proverbial pot of gold at the end of the rainbow, the anti-aging advertisements that promise fountain of youth miracles are empty promises. What you will discover here is the next best thing—the most current thinking on how men can maximize their chances of living well and long, even when we wake up mornings with several nagging chronic problems such as stiff joints or an enlarged prostate. We offer you clear, understandable information that is based in sound science. This sourcebook provides you with the knowledge needed to understand men's healthy aging.

CHAPTER 2

Staying Active

with Elizabeth Conner

Flexing one's bicep has become a symbol of manliness in many cultures. In societies that equate being a man with strength and independence, the decline of muscle mass that accompanies physiological aging can be one of the most challenging aspects of growing older. Men are expected to be able to tote heavy objects. We are expected to be the physical and metaphorical "protector" of the household. But the fact is that our muscle mass begins to decline at a rate of about 1 percent per year starting around age 45. The gradual loss is intrinsic aging and called *sarcopenia*;[1] it is also determined by lack of exercise and protein deficiency. Fortunately, there are precautionary measures one can take to prevent, or significantly delay and barely notice, the natural erosion of muscle mass. Participating in regular exercise is crucial. Someone once said, "Regular physical activity is the closest thing there is to a miracle drug."

The relationship between physical activity (and exercise) and healthy aging is both complex and simple. The "complex" is the many ways that physical activity determines healthy aging, and this is examined in greater detail in the rest of the chapter. The "simple" is that along with eating well, physical activity in whatever form, whether a daily exercise routine or 60 minutes of walking while at work, is the line of defense that keeps us healthy and independent.[2]

Compared to men who are sedentary, being physically active greatly helps maintain our health and functional ability. The evidence is so strong that researchers and clinicians now advocate that all men—even sedentary 75-year-olds—engage in moderate physical activity (defined below) on a regular basis.[3] Because physical activity alters the pace at which our bodies age, you are never too old to gain a positive result from exercise. Simply by standing, you burn three times as many calories as you do sitting. Walking your dog in a grass field burns three times the calories as walking on a paved street. Studies have shown that regular exercise by middle-aged men can set back the clock 20 to 40 years when compared to men who are inactive.

Three reminders are important. First, many men want an instant fix to their now sedentary lifestyle and the weight gain that took years to accumulate. Add a pound a year from age 35 to 50, and odds are that you barely noticed the weight gain. You might not have even changed pant size and do not feel it necessary to carve out a half hour or more several times a week to "work out." You can also forget the empty promises of the paid programming on television that sell you a sculpted body in 60 days with their exercise equipment and special diets. While it might well be possible for three or four out of 100 men, odds are you won't be able to integrate their fitness plan of *intensely* working out every day for months and months and months. The real goal is to construct a healthy lifestyle of your own—one that includes physical activity, perhaps even an exercise routine, but one that fits your needs.

It's difficult to fully appreciate that maintaining moderate physical activity is for the long haul; it will make a noticeable difference 10 years from now, not next month. The objective is to change our lifestyle choices—engaging in regular physical activity versus continuing to be inactive. All adult men need to schedule active time and quiet time for ourselves within our daily routines and stick with the ways we find comfortable to stay active. We also need to manage the demands of physical activity on our bodies. Energy conservation is the way activities can be done to minimize fatigue, joint stress, and pain—such as a slow steady rate of work with frequent short rest breaks, planning your heavy activities to fit your own best times, and analyzing the work to be done in order to eliminate unnecessary steps. When we use our bodies efficiently, we can remain physically active well into our eighties and nineties.

Second, there is an aging myth that needs to be met head-on. Many people think that getting older is associated with a decline in physical activity. Is it? Reverse the cause and effect. Have you ever considered that inactivity may actually be a cause of much of our (early) physical aging? Inactivity in fact accelerates age-related changes in our muscles, joints, and endurance.

Third, there is no doubt that the age-related changes in our metabolism affect our bodies, and the decline in testosterone can make staying physically active more challenging as we get older.[4] However, staying active (and eating well) is the fountain of healthy aging—it slows the pace of intrinsic aging.[5]

Being physically active improves metabolism and reduces appetite, puts a brake on the falling off of testosterone, and fights off the natural erosion of muscles, bone density, and flexibility. Being active maintains cardiorespiratory fitness and heart health. It lowers the risk of developing Alzheimer's disease[6] and other serious health challenges, including later-life diabetes. Staying physically active keeps our mental functions sharper and promotes brain health. It also supports mental health—we feel better about ourselves, even when facing troubles.

PHYSICAL ACTIVITY VERSUS EXERCISE

For many of us, the prospect of running a 5K or playing in an over-50 basketball league sounds more like punishment than fun. Even thinking about exercise sometimes seems like an unpleasant chore because we simply find it difficult to fit it in when already working long hours. Whatever the case may be, there is an important distinction between being physically active and exercising. To clarify, exercise always involves physical activity, but physical activity does not have to be exercise, and it can still provide many of the same benefits.

When you think of exercise, picture what you did during a high school gym class or sports practice—jumping jacks, running (long distance or sprinting), or some kind of weight training. While the benefits of these activities are undeniable, they require a certain time commitment and physical capability. If you have the time, physicality, and, of course, willpower, by all means exercise on a regular basis—take a run or get on a bike. If you lack the stamina or strength but have the desire, start out slowly—take a walk and begin to own the feelings of being active.

Physical activity is less regimented than an exercise routine and can often be done without totally interrupting daily life. Physical activity is simply using your muscles and putting your body in motion. Examples include mowing the lawn (as long as it isn't a riding mower), taking the stairs rather than the elevator, washing your car, going for a walk in a park, and throwing the football with your grandson. In these examples, you are either doing chores, getting where you need to go, or enjoying your family while engaging in some cardiovascular activity. As with exercise, some types of physical activity are more beneficial than others. Taking out the trash does not give you a free pass for extra dessert. There are, however, alternatives that, when done regularly, can help keep you in shape and protect against ailments, such as high blood pressure and diabetes.

BENEFITS OF PHYSICAL ACTIVITY

Domain	Benefit	Comments
Health and fitness	↑ Moderate to large	Improves general health, and reduces risk of illness (e.g., cardiovascular disease)
Brain health	↑ Small to moderate	Improves your mental sharpness and insight
Mental health	↑ Small to moderate	Improves your spirits and gives you more positive outlook on life
Energy level	↑ Moderate to large	Increases your energy level and vitality
Functional capacity	↑ Moderate to large	Keeps you independent and improves your ability to more easily walk, carry groceries, and climb stairs
Pain	↓ Small to moderate	Improves flexibility and reduces pain and stiffness in your joints
Quality of life	↑ Moderate to large	Adds to a sense of well-being and your willingness to engage more fully in life

Physical Inactivity

The scientific evidence is clear: being sedentary is lethal. Physical activity means movement of the body that expends energy. Walking, climbing the stairs, and dancing the night away are examples of being active. Regular physical activity lowers blood pressure; helps maintain healthy bones, muscles, and joints; and promotes psychological well-being. Benefits also include a significant reduction in the risk of cardiovascular diseases, hypertension, obesity, diabetes, several cancers, and depression.

Despite the well-known benefits of being active, researchers find that the number of physically inactive men (who engage in less than a few occasions of 30 minutes of activity per week) has been increasing. One series of studies in the United Kingdom revealed that two-thirds of men didn't meet the minimal target for physical activity (30 minutes of moderately intense activity for 5 or more days a week), and there is a noticeable reduction of physical activity around the common retirement age, 65–74.[7] The patterns in the United States are similar.[8] The U.S. Department of Health and Human Services' Healthy People 2020 project, started in 2000, shows that 40 percent of adults engage in no leisure-time physical activity, and only 15 percent perform the recommended 30 minutes per day, 5 days a week of physical activity. The proportion of adult men engaging in no leisure-time physical activity has increased to nearly 50 percent, and the American Heart Association estimates that half of men age 65 and older are "sedentary," or physically inactive. These statistics are "red flags" warning us that too many men are not adopting healthy habits.

While aging and age-related changes in functional ability likely force a number of men into less activity, men do or do not participate in exercise or physical activity for many personal reasons. Men are often motivated to engage in physical activity because we feel enlivened and inspired by it. There is a robust association between self-perception/self-image and being physically active. Being active is an opportunity to perform or compete and gain validation and recognition. Throughout our lives we develop a sense of pride in our physicality, and physical activity is synonymous with showing that the body remains fit.

> I think as long as you exercise and can do as much as you can and the best that you can, then it's all you can do. I mean, even gardening. At least then you feel like your body is working. It feels like you have done something, and that makes you feel good.[9]

Most men who are physically active develop a routine or "habit" that includes physical activity. Rarely are we motivated to participate in types of physical activity and exercise because of the health benefits. Rather, we are physically active because of factors such as fun, enjoyment, camaraderie, and socializing with friends. The positive effect is the earned sense of achievement and the social support men gain from their participation in physical activity.

Barriers to physical activity range from the simple pragmatics of poor access, to time constraints and high costs, to complex issues relating to identity. Self-perception is terrifically important in motivating men to participate in any type of physical activity.[10] Some men do not want to walk alone, wary of the stigma of being thought of as loners, but runners and cyclists and swimmers often prefer being out by themselves to enjoy the solitude. The anxiety about not "fitting in" because of one's unfamiliarity and/or a lack of confidence about entering unfamiliar spaces such as a pool or the gym culture or the group that is line dancing are serious barriers leading to some men's lack of participation in physical activity. But the biggest barrier is the set of lifestyle habits already in place that make adding time for getting active a challenge.

YOUR LEVEL OF ACTIVITY

Excess body weight is chiefly a result of an imbalance between energy intake and energy expenditure. Physical activity is energy expenditure. When energy expenditure is equal to energy intake, your body weight will be maintained. If you are a bit overweight and keep your energy intake on par with your energy expenditure, you will remain a bit overweight. It is the proportion of calories eaten (energy intake) to the level of physical activity (energy expenditure) that determines our weight gain or loss.

Casual surveillance of the U.S. population reveals that many people seem overweight (and out of shape). Research shows that nearly three-fourths of men age 50 and older are carrying excess body weight.[11] The fact is, 4 out of 10 of those men are also "sedentary"—they take part in no exercise whatsoever. We have been told for years that inactivity and carrying extra weight can lead to unwanted and troubling health problems. But most adult men live with these risks. We have not yet reclaimed enough time for ourselves and used the time to be physically active. However, it's our physical activity decisions that will have greater impact than just changing our eating habits. The bulk of the weight gain in older men is also because of our body's slower metabolism, and in order to counteract this effect of intrinsic aging, men must crank up their metabolism by getting and staying active.

To identify your current level of physical activity (or energy expenditure), use these guidelines:

> *Sedentary.* You sit most of the day and find that you rarely move around, whether it is at work or at home. Your work has you sitting in a truck or in front of a computer; and when you're home, you cut the lawn with a tractor mower, are in front of the television, or are in a chair reading the newspaper. You are sedentary. This lifestyle is a serious risk to a man's health, especially as we get older, and it almost always leads to weight gain. You are not burning the calories you take in.

> *Light.* Light activity includes some movement, like sanding and painting a window, a teacher who moves about the classroom, gardening, or strolling around a few blocks while talking about the events of the day or walking your dog. Do you see yourself leaning on the cart while walking throughout a "big-box" store (such as BJs, Super Walmart, Costco), instead of walking upright and pushing the cart in front of you? While this is certainly better than being sedentary, and while it does begin to lower the risks of ill health, light activity will not combat the ordinary weight gain that comes with lower metabolism.

> *Moderate*. Moderate activity is generally the ideal and includes activities such as brisker walking, skiing, slow jogging, and swimming. Think about the UPS or FedEx driver who zips up in a truck, walks the package to the address, and walks back to the truck. The walking the driver does daily is more than most of us do. To achieve this preferred level of daily activity, we need some heart-pumping activities. You might consider a greater number of minutes of walking every day, pulling your golf clubs and walking the course rather than riding in a cart, hiking a mile uphill on a trail and comfortably walking back, or parking the car anywhere and walking at a good clip for a mile.

> *Heavy*. Heavy activity is similar to moderate, only revved up a bit. It builds strength and muscle tone, stronger bones, and stamina; improves blood chemistry (including high-density lipoprotein [HDL], the "good" cholesterol); and eats up calories. The people unloading and loading 20–40 UPS or FedEx trucks each shift are doing the heavy work. So too are men who run a couple miles daily, ride a bike at a good clip, or continue to play a sport. If you find yourself physically able to engage in more strenuous activities like these, go for it. If not, moderate exercise will certainly benefit your health.

We need to remain realistic about our fitness and take into consideration our age and body type. If you have health limitations, you are advised to slowly increase your levels of physical activity. Resist wanting the electric scooter that advertisers urge you to purchase to make you more mobile. A scooter might make zipping around a grocery store seem convenient, but it is another means to being sedentary. If your current activity level is sedentary or light, the goal is to be more rather than less active.

If you are fit enough to meet the recommendation of 30 minutes of moderately intense physical activity a day for 5 or more days a week, yet not this active, you need a plan. Adding 150 minutes of "exercise" per week may sound overwhelming at first, but this time can be spread out into 10- or 15-minute intervals. Studies show that just 10 minutes of cardio activity provides cardiovascular benefits. So if either time or endurance is a problem, break up your exercise routine into shorter intervals. As you begin to integrate being physically active, and as your endurance builds, challenge yourself to exercise more often and for longer periods of time—you'll be surprised at the results. But be realistic. Plan to take *small* steps toward improving your fitness, and reward yourself when you reach them (but not with two added beers).

One older man recommended that you buy yourself a pedometer (step counter) and wear it during your waking hours for a few days to track your

CDC Fitness Recommendations

The Centers for Disease Control and Prevention now urges two types of fitness recommendations for men age 65 and over:

1. Moderately intense activity

   - 2 hours and 30 minutes of moderate-intensity aerobic activity every week
   - and on 2 or more of these days, engage in muscle-strengthening activities to keep from losing muscle as you age;

2. Vigorous activity

   - 1 hour and 15 minutes weekly of vigorous-intensity aerobic activity (e.g., jogging or running)
   - and muscle-strengthening activities on 2 or more days a week that work major muscle groups (legs, hips, back, abdomen, chest, shoulders, and arms).

physical activity. His comment: "This is your life." A pedometer, about the size of a pager and worn on the waistband, measures and counts the motion of the hips. This device can be purchased for as little as $10. After a couple of days of recording what you normally do, if you are already within the recommended physical activity levels, great. If not, you now know and the question becomes, are you ready? The goal of healthy aging is to increase our physical activity, beginning with the number of steps taken daily. If you set a personal goal to increase your steps and wear the pedometer, you will likely find that you've added 1,000 or more steps within a few weeks. You become conscious of walking and start walking more.

For the three-fourths of the men who are already overweight, fitness goals ought to include strategies for both greater energy expenditure and less calorie intake. Weight loss needs to be gradual, and you'll want to consider a target date—what is a reasonable amount of time to reach that desired weight loss? So if you want to drop 10 pounds, many people recommend that whatever target date you choose, double the timetable. You'll be more likely to be successful. If you think you can achieve your 10-pound target in 4 months, plan on at least 8. Honestly, it takes time to integrate the "exercise" (better yet, fitness) plan into one's lifestyle and change one's metabolism, much less modify eating habits. It probably took you several years to add the pounds.

Whatever your current level, can you increase your daily physical activity by 3–5 minutes? If so, within 4–8 weeks you would be accumulating 10–15 minutes of added activity. Look at the pattern, not the dailies.

You did 5 minutes one day, and you know you're up from where you started, even if below the recommended amount. But keep at it. Slowly work up to 5 additional minutes of accumulated activity. As you become more active, try to enjoy it. This feeling may takes weeks or months, but 6 months forward and looking back, you've changed your life. As the old adage says, hindsight is 20/20.

For men without health limitations, you are among the men who are advised to participate in 30 minutes of moderately intense physical activity for 5 or more days a week, totaling at least 2.5 hours per week. Moderately intense activity is good "cardio" activity because it gets you breathing harder and your heart beating faster. How do you know if what you are doing is moderately intense activity? It will make you breathe harder and your heart beat faster. As long as you're doing this activity for at least 10 minutes at a time, you're tallying the minutes. The daily amount of physical activity can be accumulated in 10-minute stints—walk at a good pace (outdoors or indoors) during a morning break and again at the lunch break, and you've chipped away at the *minimum* daily recommendation.

Getting Serious

Moderate physical activity has major health benefits, yet it is the more vigorous exercise that has the added benefits. A minute of vigorous exercise is about the same as 2 minutes of a moderately intense form of activity— jogging (not even running) a minute and walking a minute tally to 3 minutes. Do this pattern five times and you've mixed together 5 minutes of

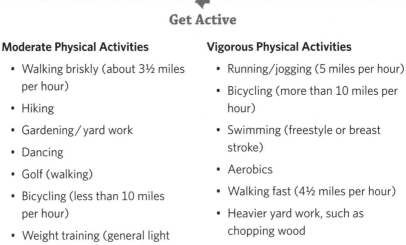

Get Active

Moderate Physical Activities

- Walking briskly (about 3½ miles per hour)
- Hiking
- Gardening / yard work
- Dancing
- Golf (walking)
- Bicycling (less than 10 miles per hour)
- Weight training (general light workout)

Vigorous Physical Activities

- Running/jogging (5 miles per hour)
- Bicycling (more than 10 miles per hour)
- Swimming (freestyle or breast stroke)
- Aerobics
- Walking fast (4½ miles per hour)
- Heavier yard work, such as chopping wood
- Tennis or basketball (competitive)

BURNING CALORIES

Activities	Calories burned per hour	
	150 lb man	**190 lb man**
Lying down or sleeping	80	85
Standing	140	150
Bicycling, <8 mph, leisure	280	340
Bicycling, >15 mph	800	1,000
Calisthenics (push-ups, sit-ups), vigorous effort	550	690
Cleaning, light/moderate effort	220	275
Dancing, ballroom, square	375	460
Fishing, general	280	340
Fishing in stream, in waders	420	515
Golf, using a cart	240	300
Golf, pulling clubs	350	430
Hiking, cross-country	420	510
Kayaking or canoeing	325	400
Lawn mowing	350	475
Raking lawn	280	340
Rowing, moderate effort	590	730
Running, jogging 5 mph (12 minute mile)	560	690
Running, 8 mph (7½ minute mile)	880	1070
Sex (for an hour)	315	450
Shoveling snow, by hand	420	515
Skiing	490	600
Stretching, yoga	280	340
Swimming laps, leisurely	420	515
Swimming laps, freestyle, light/moderate effort	560	690
Swimming, breaststroke	700	860
Tai chi	280	340
Tennis, doubles	420	515
Tennis, singles	560	690
Walking, moderate pace (2½–3 mph)	240	300
Walking, faster pace (3½–4 mph)	280	345
Walking, uphill	420	510
Walking, upstairs	560	690

vigorous and 5 minutes of moderately intense exercise, which fulfills the daily minimum recommendation. If you can and do engage in vigorous exercise for 30 minutes, three times a week, this will yield noticeable cardiovascular fitness.

A long-term commitment to activity is required for building muscle and for weight loss. As we get older, it will take longer to lose the fat (remember—our metabolism slows, and it is metabolism that burns the calories). Because of this, it is recommended that we engage in longer periods of moderately intense physical activity in order to burn calories and to achieve measurable weight loss over a number of months. As tough as it seems to carve out time from our other greedy commitments, we need to crank up our energy expenditure. The current recommendation is that by age 60 we also find ways to engage in resistant exercises (e.g., using weights; stepping on and off a plastic step stool) if we want to combat natural muscle loss. Despite people's best intentions to lose weight and maintain muscle mass, however, the majority of adult men do not engage in the minimum recommended level of physical activity.[12]

EXERCISE OPTIONS

If you've ever walked into a gym, what are the odds of seeing a 75-year-old working with free weights? Slim you think, because older men did not grow up in a culture that encouraged most men to use a gym. Gyms were for boxing. Nowadays, you are more likely to find two old men working out together. Most health insurance plans provide a partial reimbursement for the cost of joining a fitness center. The healthy aging culture has changed the meaning of "working out," and there are many types of fitness centers and sport clubs available. Here are a few options to keep you physically active, and each will bring about healthy changes for your body:

Swimming is a great form of exercise because it is easy on your joints and is still a great cardiovascular workout. Recreational swimming is a good way to reduce stress and relax while getting a full-body workout. Doing laps will help build and maintain muscle mass in your legs, shoulders, arms, and abs, as well as increase your endurance. You can swim using a kickboard, and to avoid boredom, people usually switch up the routine by trying different strokes or, if available, swimming in the ocean or a quarry as opposed to a pool. Don't worry about how you look in a baggy swimsuit; most men over 50 look less than perfect. You're there for yourself; use the goggles and feel the freedom.

Walking, not strolling slowly along, has aerobic benefits. Two types of walking contribute to long-term improvements in cardiorespiratory fitness.[13] One is moderate intensity, high frequency—walking at a pace that makes you breathe a little bit harder than usual but you are able to keep up a full conversation, and doing this five to seven times a week for 30-minute sessions. The other is high intensity, low frequency—walking at a faster pace three to four times a week for 30 minutes, where you are able to speak only in short sentences and are huffing and puffing a bit.

The *elliptical* and *rowing machines* found in nearly all "workout" rooms in hotels, gyms, YMCAs, and school athletic facilities are other good choices because they tend to be low intensity—meaning that you are not pounding on your feet and knees. These machines are smart choices because they are easily adjustable to your physical needs. If you are just starting to exercise, for example, you can have no resistance and a low incline, whereas more experienced users can crank up the resistance to make for a more intense workout.

Bicycling, or *cycling*, is a great alternative to running because it gets you feeling independent and is a little more relaxing while also a fantastic workout. It not only enables you to enjoy scenic places but also goes a long way to ensuring your overall fitness, especially heart health. Biking is an especially valuable option for people just getting back into an exercise routine, because it is easy to adjust your level of difficulty—with both the gears on the bike and your chosen paths. For men who are carrying added weight, cycling can prove to be very beneficial, for it helps in getting rid of the increased waistline. Check out local parks for bike routes in warm weather, or try a stationary bike in the winter and time yourself by watching a half hour of television. You can convert your own bike into a stationary bike at a modest cost. The best part about this activity is that you can find cycling a delightful experience, without even realizing that it is doing good things for your body.

Playing *tennis* is an awesome way to exercise[14] and be with friends. It is a sport that will certainly increase your cardiovascular endurance and strengthen muscles. You typically burn more calories playing tennis than you will by swimming and biking. It is an exercise that involves "anaerobic" fitness—meaning that you are engaged in short, intense bursts of activity followed by periods of rest, and this helps muscles use oxygen more efficiently. If you don't have a tennis partner, find a court with a wall and make it your 20- to 30-minute partner. This is the way many racquetball and handball players warm up or practice. Most elementary and middle schools also have hardtop surfaces running up to a solid wall that will not be damaged by your tennis ball.

Strength training and muscle strengthening become more important as we get older, because of our lower levels of testosterone and declines in muscle mass. Strength training involves pushing yourself to a point where you feel the "burn." One example of doing a simple workout is to use a solid four-leg chair and slowly lower yourself, but do not actually sit. Instead, just before your butt touches the chair, slowly stand up, and repeat this up to eight times. This exercise works multiple muscle groups (legs, hips, back, abdomen). Then, do at least 20 push-ups from a wall (or the floor). This simple indoor exercise plan works a range of different muscle groups, and you will notice the benefits after 6 months. You'll find that it takes increasingly longer workout sessions to feel the "burn."

SHOULD YOU SEE A PHYSICIAN BEFORE YOU EXERCISE?

Whatever we do for physical activity, not injuring ourselves is the number one goal. In competitive over-50 sport leagues, the rule of thumb is, "Do not hurt yourself. Playing is more important than sitting."

If you find yourself generally healthy—you do not have any life-threatening illnesses, your body doesn't have any unusual aches or pains, and you feel capable—it is unlikely that you need to consult a physician before you start working out. That being said, seeing a doctor is never a bad idea, especially if you have specific goals in mind or have any kind of history of medical problems.

The time when you should certainly see a doctor is if you have any pre-existing illnesses, especially ones related to your heart. As important as exercise is, there are some circumstances where it can be harmful, especially if you push yourself too hard and your heart is unable to handle the challenge. Seeing a doctor will establish first and foremost whether you should be exercising at all and, secondly, what exercises are appropriate given your health.

Whether you are in peak condition or just starting out, if you experience dizziness, shortness of breath without overexertion, chest pain/discomfort, or anything else that doesn't seem right with your body, stop working out! Speak with a doctor. It may seem like nothing, but avoiding medical attention when it *could* be needed can make easily resolvable problems much more serious and significant.

MUSCLE FATIGUE AND MINOR INJURIES

As much as exercise and diet are essential to strengthening and maintaining muscle, did you also know that *resting* muscles is considered equally important? During taxing physical activity, muscle fibers are routinely damaged. The damage is temporary, if the muscles have adequate time to rest and recover. Because it takes longer for our muscles to recover from laborious work as we age, it is important to pace ourselves. It is equally important that our diet provide the nutrients that the body needs to repair and rebuild these muscle groups before we again tax them.

Most experts suggest 48 hours of recovery time in order for a particular muscle group to fully repair after resistance training or some other muscle-taxing activity. This is the reasoning for only 3–4 days weekly of high-intensity exercising. However, this does not mean that you should only exercise every 3 days. By rotating which muscle groups you use during a particular routine, you can isolate certain muscle groups while letting the others repair and rest. Adding variety to your exercise routines will ensure that your muscle groups have enough time to recover and keep your routine exciting.

Caution: Snow Shoveling

Heart attacks, back strain, and muscle soreness are just a few of the problems associated with shoveling snow. Snow shoveling is very demanding on the body. What makes shoveling more dangerous than other average tasks around the house is the temperature. Your heart rate and blood pressure increase during strenuous activity. Add the body's natural response when exposed to the cold—constricting arteries and narrowing blood vessels—and you have a perfect storm for a heart attack. If you shovel for 30 minutes, you'll burn 200–250 calories.

In order to minimize the frequency and effect of the injuries, follow the principles of the PRICE (protection, rest, ice, compression, and elevation) method of treating minor injuries. Not surprisingly, the first step is *protection*. If you know that a certain body part is hurt or weak, do not overuse the muscle and, if possible, use a wrap or brace during exercise to give the area more support and minimize your risk of injury. There are all types of knee, ankle, wrist, and elbow protective "wraps" commercially available. In addition, you'll likely need sunglasses if you are rowing; swimming goggles if you are heading to a quarry or pool; new shoes that have the needed support inside for any walking, running, or hiking; or protective gloves and eyewear for other activities. Notice how professional golfers always have hats or caps to protect their eyes, as well as a driving glove; that glove isn't just to grip the club, it's to prevent soreness. Men planning on cycling will surely need a helmet and a brightly colored shirt/jacket to make them visible to motorists.

After you have a muscle, bone, or joint injury, you need to take some time off from your physical activities to allow your body to recover. Once you do sustain an injury, *rest* the body part, and do not resume activity until it is healed. *Icing* (not heating) the injured body part for 15 minutes helps to reduce tissue swelling and inflammation around the injured area. Ice should be put on an injury as soon as possible, and putting ice on early helps the injury heal faster. It's best to wrap a plastic bag of ice in a thin towel before icing the injury. If ice is not available, use a bag of frozen vegetables. Applying some type of *compression* wrap or bandage also may be needed to help reduce inflammation. Lastly, *elevate* the injured part above the level of your heart, so as to prevent blood from pooling at the affected area.

The probability of becoming injured, as well as the recovery time that minor injuries necessitate, seems to increase with age. Any type of taxing physical activity increases the risk of sustaining a nagging injury and can prolong recovery time. If you find that a minor injury is interfering with your exercise routine, incorporate a different activity that uses other muscles. This way, you can stay on track with your fitness program, without stressing the injured body parts. For example, if you sustained a shoulder injury while playing tennis, try riding the stationary bike or swimming using a kickboard. If your injury was caused by resistance training in a gym, take a break from the weights and just stick to cardio until you're healed. Men who are just beginning to develop a physical activity plan need to pay attention to how their body is "talking back"—to distinguish between feeling the "burn" and symptoms of developing injuries.

EXERCISE AFTER 70?

"What's the point?" you ask. You might just be surprised. Throughout our lifetime, it is always easy to find excuses not to be physically active and stay fit. Work, family, social events, and hobbies all frequently take precedence over time we need for exercise, which is so easily thrown on the back burner if it is not as enjoyable as other activities. Perhaps the most important barrier to physical activity is a belief that it is too late, or that in order to get the benefits you seek, you must exercise vigorously every day like an athlete. The tendency to believe this myth increases with the lack of physical activity, to the point where taking a walk seems harder and harder to do.

Almost all older men can benefit from additional physical activity. Men who start working out at age 70 can increase their life span by 12 percent— that's right, *starting* to work out at 70 can add 8 years or more of independence. The men age 70 and older who were studied in clinical trials were not the ones who did a triathlon until the age of 60, nor were they "ex-athletes" who have forever been into fitness. They were average men, maybe like you, who were able to optimize their aging and lives.[15] Becoming active even after age 70, without previously being in shape, sharply increases our odds of remaining functionally independent and not becoming frail. Getting active, no matter your age, increases the length and the quality of your life. We always have something to gain by putting our body in motion, and odds are we will find several companions and enjoy the social time together, too.

Staying Active after 70

A 71-year-old man who has moderately well-controlled hypertension and osteo-arthritis of both knees and the right hip is active in two bowling leagues and enjoys walking, but both activities are becoming limited by pain in his knees.

His physicians recommended that he will benefit from increasing his level of activity and incorporating resistance training into his exercise routine. The man began cross training with non-weight-bearing activities of swimming and biking three times per week. He was encouraged to wear good athletic shoes and may benefit from bracing and nonsteroidal anti-inflammatory medication (e.g., ibuprofen).

Source: Nied, R. J., & Franklin, B. (2002). Promoting and prescribing exercise for the elderly. *American Family Physician, 65,* 419–427.

"FRINGE BENEFITS" OF EXERCISE

In addition to promoting physical well-being, numerous studies report that exercise and other health-conscious behaviors are closely linked to a positive body image and self-evaluation and to a more optimistic outlook on life in general. This positive self-image is partly due to the physical results of being healthy and feeling "fit," and partly due to feelings of satisfaction that result from the exercise itself. We develop a sense of self-efficacy through exercise, which promotes overall mental and physical health.

Why? As you exercise, your body releases "feel-good" brain chemicals called *endorphins*. They are released from the pituitary glands to parts of your brain during physical activity and serve to elevate your mood. As neurotransmitters, endorphins lead to feelings of euphoria and the so-called runner's high. Researchers find that endorphins also act as natural pain relievers. Not only will exercise improve your physical health, but it positively affects your emotional well-being as well.

CHAPTER 3

Eating Well and Less

with Elizabeth Kayajian

Eating is a great opportunity to give yourself a breather, whether the time is spent nightly with family, among friends while watching a ball game, or alone with a good book. Food is one type of "social glue,"[1] since most of the time eating occurs with others and is symbolic of togetherness. Having an enjoyable meal involving personal favorites or traditional foods and sampling the cuisines of other cultures can be the day's pleasure. However, it is important to acknowledge that eating is much more than a way to take a break, get together, or relax. The food eaten is part of the larger picture of our health. When it comes to men's health and healthy aging, good nutrition is a first line of defense in keeping men independent and well.

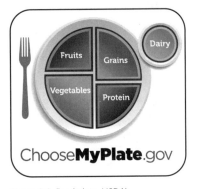

Figure 3.1. Food plate. USDA's ChooseMyPlate.gov.

Generally speaking, an adult male's body requires similar nutritional intake as it did when younger, in terms of protein, vitamin C, and proper hydration. But there are certain nutritional changes that come with age, such as a greater need for fiber, the importance of managing cholesterol levels, and the value of foods fortified with vitamin B12, such as fortified cereals. By age 50, there is also a need for more protein and fewer calories. The average 50-year-old man who is "lightly active" (exercises 1–3 days per week) needs just 2,200–2,300 calories per day; a "moderately active" man needs 2,500. At age 70, that man would typically need 200 fewer calories. Properly taking care of ourselves requires some knowledge about basic nutrients and vitamins and minerals.

FOUR COMMANDMENTS OF EATING WELL

For most men food choice becomes routine. Personal preferences become established after decades of eating, which results in the nutritional aspects of eating going unnoticed. "Nutrition"means little in most men's lives. Comfortable with their dietary status quo,[2] most men are a bit resistant to change, especially if they're long-term partnered or never married.[3] Many men view healthy eating as something for the nutritionally vulnerable, and they seem to think that only men who have serious health problems need to pay attention to diet.[4] The word *nutrition* is often tied to an ugly word: *dieting*. Dieting is never fun—the constant "eat this, don't eat that," counting carbs or grams of fat, and inevitable feelings of deprivation are exhausting. And diets are hard (if not impossible) to maintain. Even more, the act of dieting is almost exclusively seen as a "female thing"[5] and something men let fall by the "weigh" side (pardon the pun). As one 54-year-old suggests,

> the men don't seem to worry that they are overweight, whereas the women are more inclined towards the sort of vanity of being overweight, y'know. Most of the men that I know . . . were doing it (dieting) for some sort of medical reason . . . something pushed them into it.[6]

If we put healthy eating under a spotlight, it simply means to choose a mix of foods that give your body the nutrients it needs. It also means consuming the right foods for the number of calories we consume. A disturbing fact is that most men do not eat well—for example, barely 20 percent of men eat the recommended minimum amount of fruit and vegetables, and more than half eat more than the recommendations for calorie intake set by Healthy People 2010.[7]

There are four commandments, or core values, of eating well.

1. A basic rule most adult men identify with is that nutrition equals dieting and dieting is something feminine. It is important to realize that nutrition should not be understood as a diet, which you go on and eventually (read "inevitably") go off. Instead, eating well and nutritiously can be a lifestyle where no foods are off-limits and there is flexibility to fit your individual likes and dislikes. Do you hate butternut squash? Don't eat it; choose a different vegetable. Love steak? Have it, but not every day. In fact, eliminate the word *diet* from your vocabulary—it serves only as a mental hurdle, keeping you from a healthy life. Be sensible—enjoy all foods, just don't overdo it.

2. While eating well may initially result in some weight loss (intentionally or otherwise), refrain from thinking of eating nutritiously as being a means to looking fit. Though losing some weight is often the result of eating well and can do wonders for our self-esteem, there are so many other

benefits to healthy eating that extend far beyond vanity. Eating well keeps you energized, helps build and maintain muscle mass, and fights off illness. It is not a stretch to say that eating well can help you live a longer, more satisfying life. Being mindful of nutrition will help you reach certain goals, whether it's teaching your granddaughter how to throw a baseball or avoiding that seasonal cold.

Hunger versus Appetite

Appetite is the desire to eat based on the pleasure derived from foods and from eating. It is appetite that must be managed.

Your body's physical response to the need for food is hunger. If you skip breakfast, by lunchtime it is not surprising if you are hungry. Your body wants nutrients. Common symptoms of hunger are weakness, dizziness, hunger pains, nausea, and loss of concentration. If you are day trading and skip a meal, the effect of a loss of concentration could be missing a trade window.

What Is a "Healthy Diet"?

It emphasizes fruits, vegetables, whole grains, and fat-free or low-fat milk and dairy products; includes lean meats, poultry, fish, beans, eggs, and nuts; and is low in saturated fats, trans fats, cholesterol, salt (sodium), and added sugars.

---

3. Eating well means just that—to *eat*. Unfortunately, eating well is too often thought of as going without and restricting food intake. Undereating can be just as bad as overeating—your body is not meant to run on empty or on full. There are many reasons for why men may experience a loss of appetite (e.g., the side effects from certain medications), but it is absolutely necessary to get certain vitamins, minerals, and food groups into our bodies regularly to remain healthy and to fight off an illness. If you find yourself skipping meals, losing your appetite, or unable to keep food down, there could be a medical reason for it. If you are bored with food choices, be adventurous—expand your tastes to enjoy a variety of foods. As Americans, we have lots of choices.

4. Eat smaller portions, especially as you get older. Eating "three squares" regularly is crucial to good health, and so too is not eating too much. Food is everywhere, and too much is usually available, served, and eaten. We ought to enjoy our meals, but just smaller portions than what has become too customary for restaurants to serve or what we think we need. When eating out, you might share an entrée and/or take home the leftovers. You do not need to eat it all at one sitting. The Clean Plate self-congratulatory award is not the attitude wanted any more. Older

bodies need fewer calories. Focus on smaller portions and eating the same amount at each meal—not a light lunch and a massive dinner. You can make small changes in what and how much you eat. Small steps over time work better than giant leaps and crashing.

NUTRITION 101: A GOOD FOOD PLAN

There is constantly conflicting information about how to eat healthy—Should I eat real butter or use margarine? Should I be taking supplemental vitamins and fish oil pills? Should I stay away from fat all together? How many carbs are too many? Am I getting enough protein? With experts providing differing advice and too little time to pay enough attention to "food groups," most men stop listening.

Nutrients are not that complicated. There are only six classes of them: carbohydrates, fats, proteins, vitamins, minerals, and water. To make it even simpler: water, minerals, and vitamins don't provide calories. To eat well, it's best to choose a mix of nutrient-dense foods, which means foods that are high in nutrients but low in calories.

Researchers at the Harvard Medical School and the School of Public Health identified two major dietary patterns. One they called "Western," which is characterized by higher consumption of red meat, processed meat, French fries, high-fat dairy products, refined grains, and sweets and desserts. It is quite high in calorie intake. They labeled the other "prudent," because it was characterized by higher consumption of vegetables, fruit, fish, poultry, and whole grains.[8] It is the prudent nutrient-dense, low-calorie food choices that prove to be healthy, and the Western "fat and meat" pattern that is dangerous.[9]

Depending on your lifestyle, you can make choices and form new habits that conform to what nutritionists and physicians agree are smart eating decisions. Eight rules of thumb:

1. *Stay away from refined sugars.* Refined sugars are a little tricky to identify because nutritional labels do not say "refined sugars." Instead, they are disguised as high fructose corn syrup or corn sweeteners. Refined sugars are most frequently talked about as "sweets" (cookies, ice cream, donuts), but they are found in more inconspicuous places too, like ketchup, salad dressings, soups, cold cuts, and even crackers. The best way to keep your refined sugar intake in check is to read the labels and know what to look for—if one of the first few ingredients listed is one of the words ending in "ose," such as fructose or maltose, try to stay away from it. If you are hankering for something sweet, skip the glazed donut and try to stick to natural forms of sugar like fruit (fructose).

2. *Eat complex carbohydrates.* Carbohydrates are made out of units of sugar, ranging from a single unit to millions. Complex carbohydrates are just that—complex, meaning that they are made from three or more units of sugar linked together. Because of their complexity, they take longer to digest and work their way into your system. What does this mean for you? Essentially, complex carbs provide longer-lasting energy that will be sustained over time, rather than the quick spurt that comes with simple carbs. Examples of complex carbs are whole grain breads for sandwiches, a bagel or whole grain cereals for breakfast, spaghetti, fruit, and root vegetables such as carrots and potatoes.

3. *Rely on lean protein.* There are so many ways to get protein, but some foods carry with them high caloric and fat content, so make them an occasional choice. Red meat, whole milk, and cheddar cheese are all examples of great sources of protein that have the nutritional downfall of their fat. It is okay to eat these in moderation, not only in frequency but in amount. Two servings of red meat a week is enough, and this recommendation challenges "Western" choices. A better basis for the lean protein foods is to choose grilled chicken and fish, roast turkey, sushi, and black beans. Salmon is nature's heart medicine. A toasted peanut butter sandwich (with no more than 6 tablespoons) is also okay. If you are not allergic to peanuts, the monounsaturated fats in peanut butter may lower your risks for heart disease and diabetes.

A small (not more than a half pound) broiled porterhouse steak is a great source of protein—about 40 grams worth. But it also delivers three-fourths of the recommended daily fat intake. Had you selected a salmon dinner, you would have the same amount of protein and one-third the fat. Eggs also are an excellent, inexpensive source of lean protein, packed with nutrients and a mere 75 calories. Even though eggs contain dietary cholesterol, dietary cholesterol isn't the same type of harmful cholesterol within saturated fat. A small omelet with spinach and mushrooms, or a breakfast of eggs and whole wheat toast (but skip the bacon), provides the lean protein and fiber and fills your stomach longer, reducing the likelihood that you will eat larger lunches. Research shows that for men with normal cholesterol metabolism, it's not dietary cholesterol that clogs arteries, but foods high in saturated and hydrogenated fats.

4. *Not saturated but unsaturated fat.* Food contains fat; that's nature's way. Most foods contain several kinds of fat. Not surprisingly, fats are loaded with calories and provide too little protein or carbohydrates. This is why fats should be eaten only sparingly. Some people are led to believe that fat is universally bad, but in fact some fat in your meal plan is necessary

to insulate your body, protect your organs, and keep your skin and hair healthy. The key is to pick the right fats, which are unsaturated (whether polyunsaturated or monounsaturated). These include the oily fishes (tuna, salmon, trout, sardines packed *in water*); olive, peanut, and canola oil; raw nuts (peanuts, almonds, cashews); avocadoes and olives; and beans (garbanzo, kidney). Fats to avoid are those that are saturated and tend to raise "bad" cholesterol levels. These include some tasty favorites like cookies, steak, and chips. There are also some lesser-known culprits such as whole milk, butter, cheddar cheese, and poultry with skin. You can reduce your intake of saturated fat by selecting leaner cuts of meat and trimming the fat off, skipping fried food as much as you can, and opting for low-fat or fat-free dairy.

5. *Easy on the salt.* Sodium is not bad for you. It is a mineral that is important for our bodies, but in small doses—so small, in fact, that it is almost impossible to be sodium deficient. Most men tend to have no idea how much sodium is in the foods we eat, and many men will often add table salt (sodium chloride) for flavor. The problem is that a high-sodium diet puts us at serious risk of developing high blood pressure, which can easily escalate into more lethal heart disease problems. Sodium holds fluid in the body, causing the heart to work harder. Packaged processed foods, salty snacks, and canned vegetables all add unnecessary sodium, so try to eat them in moderation. If food is bland, try adding pepper or even hot sauce, which helps kick up your metabolism.

American Heart Association Recommendation

Aim to eat less than 1,500 mg of sodium per day (1 teaspoon salt = 2,300 mg sodium).

6. *Fiber, fiber, fiber.* The reason why fiber is such an important part of a healthy eating plan for adult men is because it helps prevent constipation and keep your bowels moving. This may sound like a laughable issue, but constipation is more serious than simply feeling bloated and uncomfortable. If you aren't "moving," your body is probably storing unwanted waste that may lead to more serious problems, such as colon and rectal cancer. To get more fiber, stick to complex carbohydrates and stay away from refined foods—opt for whole wheat toast, not "just" toast.

7. *Vegetables.* Growing up, we all heard someone say, "Eat your vegetables." As adults, we ought to eat a minimum of three and preferably five servings of fresh or cooked vegetables daily. It is hard to argue against the health benefits of vegetables. Skip the potatoes and their carbohydrates. Choose other vegetables, green, yellow, and orange ones, and the deeper in color the better. Dark green leafy choices such as spinach and dark green and red lettuce are packed with vitamins, minerals, and antioxidants.

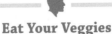

Eat Your Veggies

Can you get your veggies without *really* getting your veggies?

You've seen the advertisements for drinks like V8 that provide servings of vegetables, and sometimes fruit, in a painless liquid form. Does this alternative seem too easy? In a lot of ways, it is. There is no substitute for getting fresh (and especially raw) fruits and vegetables into your system—you reap the benefits and soak up the most nutrients from the real deal.

Vegetable juice drinks also tend to have too much sodium; stick to real fruits and veggies. These drinks are not all bad—they certainly are a step up from soda and other "fruit" juices that provide no nutritional value at all. They should *not*, however, be relied on as your only source of vegetables.

8. *Hydration.* Ever feel lethargic for no apparent reason? Can't seem to get rid of that terrible headache, even after you've had your daily dose of caffeine? Find yourself bound up, despite eating plenty of fiber? In a given day, we should aim for two liters of water: eight glasses, or four of the "standard" 16.9-ounce bottles. If you exercise or are physically active, you should plan on drinking even more water, and this does not mean sugary sports drinks. They may taste good, but they will not hydrate as well and will add sugar to your diet that is unneeded.

TERRIBLE EATING HABITS

Most of us choose what we eat, and out of habit we might choose to eat the wrong foods in the wrong amounts and are not even aware of it. The result is that most adult men end up overweight—nearly 75 percent of men age 50 and older already are.[10]

Habit #1

Overeating is perhaps the worst eating habit. It is self-perpetuating, with injurious health consequences. Overeating as little as once or twice a week slowly adds pounds, the bigger body sends the "feed me" message, and then men feed again. Yes, overeating typically means to "feed" or binge, rather than to eat. Insert food, chew, swallow, fill up, and eventually stop. You ignore the discomfort of your full stomach and continue to stuff bite after bite down the hatch. This habit contributes to chronic diseases such as diabetes, heart disease, and cancer.

Overweight men approach food differently and overeat more frequently.

A recent study of the habits of people at all-you-can-eat Chinese buffet restaurants observed the height, weight, sex, age, and behavior of hundreds of patrons. Trained observers recorded the various seating, serving, and eating behaviors and compared these to their estimates of the patrons' body mass index (BMI). Overweight people made the food more convenient to eat and ate in excess. Instead of looking over the buffet and deciding what they wanted, they seized a plate and started filling it. They used larger plates. They chose seats closer to and facing the buffet, looking over what to select next while they ate. Those with a BMI in the healthy range sat farther away, often with their backs to the display of food, more often talked throughout the meal, and more often chose to eat with chopsticks rather than a fork. They chewed each bite longer and ate less. They ate a dinner, rather than binging.[11]

Overeating or "feeding" is also the result of the size of available portions. Unlimited food at a buffet, having "seconds" immediately instead of waiting a bit for the brain to recognize a pleasant feeling of fullness, the American way of restaurants and fast-food drive-thrus serving many more calories than we need, or going for a large dessert just after a lunch or dinner—each contributes to (regular) overeating.

When we're famished, we've waited too long to eat. So we wolf down anything and everything available. We were justifiably hungry. Nonetheless, to avoid the binging and overeating, it is best to eat timely and more often. We eat less when our stomachs are not "on empty" and growling. And, when eating, we enjoy the tastes and eat less. Drink water with and after every meal; this will make you fuller and help prevent overeating. Eat slowly and drink water, and you will be satisfied with less food. And, always eat (a little) dessert. Sweets such as a cookie or small portion of low-fat ice cream signal to your brain that the meal is over. Without the sweets, you might not feel satisfied, and an hour or two later you will be foraging in the kitchen for something.

Age and Metabolism

Ever wonder why weight tends to creep up as we age, even though you eat the same things? It's because our metabolism slows down as we get older. That's why that extra piece of pizza or extra beer that never made a difference now ends up on your stomach.

Add just one pound a year, and in 30 years you are 30 pounds heavier. To avoid the bulge, it is important to either increase physical activity or reduce calories. If exercise is not your thing, certainly don't reach for that extra piece of pizza. But try changing your routine to include more exercise.

Habit #2

Eating too fast is the little brother to overeating. If you have a lot on your mind, are angry or frustrated, or are stressed about time, chances are you will become a speed eater. An invisible starter gun is fired, and many of us then pound the food down; this is especially true whenever we are preoccupied and/or our negative emotions and stress levels are cranked up. Ever grabbed a bite to go while on a long drive and barely remember eating, because you were speed eating while concentrating on driving? Ever had lunch "in the office" and your lunch hour shrunk to 10 minutes or less? When we eat with others and participate in conversation, we eat much more slowly and healthily.

When we eat too fast, more is eaten. This is because it takes time for the stomach to send a feeling-of-fullness message to the brain. This is especially an issue when your habit of wolfing food quickly is presented with an opportunity to have appetizers or finger foods. You likely eat faster (and more) when the food eaten requires no utensils. Sandwiches, finger foods, and snacks take less time to finish than food that requires fork and knife. Next time you are on a long drive, add 30 minutes to the drive by getting out and enjoying the pit stop. Next lunch time, choose to "dine" with friends instead of quickly fueling up; conversation slows your eating. Both choices make you more conscious of how fast you finish compared to the people around you.

Habit #3

The foods we choose. The habit of nearly always choosing to eat meat and not vegetables and fruit is deeply rooted in most men's biographies. When researchers survey people's preferences, they find the same thing over and over: men are much more likely to be poultry and meat eaters—preferring beef, enjoying chicken and pork, and more willing to eat shrimp and oysters—and do not eat enough fruits and vegetables. Most men also have not ever tried a "diet" and do not know the nutritional value of what is eaten.

You don't have to look too deeply into American culture to observe that the grill is a "man's stove." Whenever our fathers and uncles barbequed, their grilling rarely prepared anything but meat. "Sides" were cooked indoors by our mothers and aunts, and maybe not eaten. Meat was good enough, and lots of it was filling. Now, because grills are bigger, men sometimes add vegetables to go with the hot dogs or porterhouse steaks.

Habit #4

Mindless munching. Do you find yourself sitting in front of a computer at work, mindlessly snacking on cookies or a bag of trail mix? Do you turn on the TV and then a few minutes later grab something to munch on, perhaps a bag of (fried) chips? Most men don't think about what they're eating, or why—they're focused on the next bite and/or whatever else they're doing.

Your munching ritual is emotional hunger, and you comfort yourself with food as the TV tries to entertain you or the computer stresses you. Your concentration is somewhere else and you mindlessly eat, emptying half or more of the bag of chips. The habit of spaced-out eating while working or watching TV, or munching on a tin of peanuts while reading a newspaper or book, is a sure source of trouble. It is too easy to overindulge.

Mindless eating is a habit more than being hungry, and it is a symptom of unhealthy eating. If at home, it's likely that your munching habit is a way to wind down from a stressful day. Whatever the reason, the habit adds calories. Do yourself a favor: if you like munching, change your habit into mindful munching and decide beforehand what to eat. Munch on grapes or carrots with a glass of cold water. The water helps fill you and is good for you, and often we are misreading being thirsty for being hungry. The grapes or carrots replace calorie-dense food. Also consider raisins, celery, popcorn, and whole-grain cereals.

Habit #5

Eating convenient food. The reason junk food is called "junk" is simple: junk foods are rarely nutritious, usually filled with fats and chemicals, and loaded with unnecessary calories. Junk foods offer a convenient escape, and they're easy to purchase, carry, and consume. We are a fast-food nation. Whether the junk food comes from the grocery store or a fast-food drive-thru, the food selected isn't nutritious. The bad habits result from the convenience of feeding and not thinking about what we eat.

Men typically prefer "junk" snack foods. All they provide are empty calories and a distraction. The food additives and colors (mostly chemicals) are intended to enhance appearance, flavor, and texture. The (un)conscious ritual of selecting the Oreos, a tin of potato sticks, or a bag of orange-dyed Cheetos to nibble makes it easy to overindulge. The containers are huge. Similarly, the decision to go for a convenient, high-calorie fast-food lunch is linked to memories of how high-fat foods are tasty. And junk food, whatever the type, is habit forming, nearly addictive. It adds weight and is very expensive over the course of a year.

CREATING HEALTHIER LUNCHTIME ALTERNATIVES

How to Optimize a Sandwich's Potential

Sandwiches are the quintessential lunch item—they are quick to make, are easy to eat, and keep you full until dinner. What is more, when made properly, they can be nutritious and healthy, providing servings of protein, calcium, and vegetables. Not all sandwiches, though, are created equally, and while some may be a healthy choice, others are loaded with saturated fats and processed sugar. To craft a sandwich that is as healthy as it is delicious, follow these few simple tips:

> *Bread.* The best bread option is whole grain. It also can be carbohydrate conscious, like a wheat wrap or pita, and nutritionally dense, like multigrain bread that gives you lots of nutrients for your caloric buck. Generally speaking, stay away from white bread (which averages 100 calories a slice and 300 grams of sodium). If you're in the mood for a sub sandwich, ask if there is a whole wheat option. If you are really trying to cut back and reduce your weight, try using one piece of bread and having an open-face sandwich.

> *Meat.* Prepackaged, sliced cold cuts such as bologna or olive loaf are not the best choice nutritionally, but most *deli* meats tend to be healthier options because they have less fat, nitrates, and sodium. The best is turkey, which has 6–10 grams of protein per 2 ounces (or a couple of slices) and is extremely low in fats. If you are more of a red meat lover, roast beef is also a good option because it is low in sodium and high in protein. Ham is more of a mixed bag—it is low in calories and fat but it is extremely high in sodium, so if you choose ham, take its heavy salt content into consideration when choosing cheese and condiments. While these options are all sound, stay away from salami and bologna—both are full of fat and sodium.

> *Cheese.* In general, cheese tends to be full of fat, but some are far better than others. Mozzarella, for example, has a good balance between fats and proteins and is satiating, so it will keep you full. The same can be said for Swiss, which is low in sodium and complementary to almost any sandwich meat. Other cheeses, however, should be eaten more in moderation, like sharp cheddar and pepper jack, which are loaded with sodium and saturated fat. The cheese to regularly avoid, though, is American, which is entirely processed. It has some protein and calcium, yet a slice of American cheese (white or yellow) has over 20 percent of the recommended daily intake of saturated fat. If you are trying to be really good, skip the cheese altogether.

> *Condiments.* The best condiments are not the most obvious ones. Hummus, for example, is a flavorful addition to a sandwich. It has a texture similar to mayonnaise that many people like and is much better for you. Guacamole is another great option that is full of healthy fats, as is pesto, which also has monounsaturated fats and healthful

antioxidants, which help prevent cancer. Poor options include sodium-laden Italian dressing; ranch dressing, which is full of fat; and mayonnaise, because a small serving size of 2 tablespoons often has 180–200 calories—the equivalent of a Krispy Kreme donut.

> *Vegetables.* Always include vegetables on your sandwich—lettuce, tomatoes, onions, cucumber, bean sprouts, mushrooms, and even peppers. If you do not like biting into a huge piece of onion or pepper, try chopping the vegetables, which will give you the same great flavor but in a less abrasive way. A piece of lettuce on your sandwich has nearly zero calories, yet it is very high in vitamins A, B6, and C, as well as iron and magnesium.

Snacks

We snack when we're hungry; we snack when we're bored; we snack when we're watching a movie or while reading a book. Snacking can actually be good for you—if you eat one or two small snacks in between meals, it can curb hunger so you aren't ravenous when you sit down for a meal and don't overeat. Snacking on nutritious food can keep your energy level high and your mind alert without taking up a lot of your time. The problem is that there are too few healthy options compared to the many unhealthful snacks from which to choose. Grocery stores have entire aisles set aside for unhealthy snacks. There are a few strategies that you can use to make sure your snack choices are worth it:

The best snacks are 100–150 calories. Keeping them within this range ensures that you don't blow your entire day's recommended caloric intake on an in-between nosh. Snack, don't feed. Popcorn without the salt or (fake) butter and a bottle of water are filling and enjoyable. Snack on some multigrain cereal with almonds, rather than chips; they're priced about the same.

Fruit and vegetables are always a great snack. A strawberry smoothie made with natural fruit is loaded with nutrients. You can eat celery sticks until you're stuffed, and you've mostly consumed water, minerals, and vitamins.

Particularly if you are snacking to hold you over until your next meal, it's important to have a little bit of (good) fat and some protein in your snack—peanut butter on a slice of wheat toast is good, but packaged peanut butter crackers aren't. Mozzarella cheese sticks or hummus and pita chips are great options.

If you are really hankering for chips, eat the baked alternatives. A number of manufacturers of Mexican corn chips and potato chips offer this healthier option. Also, put the amount you're going to eat into a bowl, and put the bag away.

MODERATION, AND WHAT COUNTS AS A SERVING

The new climate in healthy eating (and drinking) is to have what you like, but in moderation. But what does *moderation* mean? Typically, it means two things. One is to have what you want, but not every day. Let yourself order the small steak with mashed potatoes and dessert to follow—it's fine every once in a while. The other meaning of moderation refers to the *amount* you are eating (and drinking). Whether it be your favorite steak or sandwich, size counts. Be mindful of the quantity you're eating; this might take some getting used to. The supersizing of food served at restaurants and packaged at grocery stores isn't moderation. Maybe you rarely have ice cream, but that doesn't justify eating an entire pint or ordering a medium (or large) chocolate chip Blizzard from Dairy Queen when a small one is a satisfying option, providing 550 rather than 950 or more calories. Recognize that the 500+ calories from the small Blizzard is almost one-quarter of the total recommended daily calorie intake.

When eating at a restaurant or ordering out, keep in mind the adage "beware of fried things and the three Bs: butter, breading, and bacon." Many *entrees* offer fried options, calorie-rich creamy pasta sauces (pasta carbonara, fettuccini alfredo), or things cooked in butter (chicken marsala, New England clam chowder). Moreover, a lot of the *appetizers* (fried calamari, breaded mushrooms) have more calories than you'll have in the rest of the meal. Typically, we underestimate how much we've eaten. Consider an order of breaded and fried onion rings. An ordinary serving size of eight or nine rings provides at least 270 calories and 15.5 grams of fat, or one-quarter of the total fat recommended for the day; the "Blooming Onion" served at Outback Steakhouse averages 2,200 calories, without the added calories from the dipping sauce.

You can learn techniques to help yourself recognize just how much food you can expect in a *healthy* serving size. Here's one way to gauge serving sizes: half of the food on each plate ought to be vegetables and fruit, so even in moderation, a steak and potatoes dinner with a small salad on the side shouldn't be your regular diet. What's needed is more balance and less quantity. How much is recommended, and what counts as a serving?

Maintaining Healthy Weight

For a 60-year-old, 6-foot, 170-lb man to maintain current weight, he needs to consume no more than the following:

Calories	2,524 cal
Carbohydrates (55%)	1,339 cal = 347 g
Proteins (15%)	379 cal = 95 g
Fats (30%)	757 cal = 84 g

Source: http://calculators.hpathy.com/calories-need.asp.

SERVING SIZE FOR VARIOUS FOODS

Food	What it contains	Approximate size
Porterhouse steak, 6 oz	570 calories, 32.5 g fat	Palms of two hands clasped together
Tenderloin steak, 4 oz	240 calories, 11.4 g fat	Palm of one hand
Chicken, breast quarter	300 calories, 12 g fat	Palm of one hand
Pork chop, medium, 5½ oz	215 calories, 12.5 g fat	Palm of one hand
Burger, ¼ lb (without bun and condiments)	460 calories, 23 g fat	Deck of cards
Fish, 3 oz (grilled or baked)	125 calories, 1.3 g fat	Checkbook
Spaghetti or linguini, ½ cup	100 calories, 1 g fat	Size of fist
Lasagna with meat, 8 oz	525 calories, 15.5 g fat	Two hockey pucks
Cheesecake, one slice	250 calories, 18 g fat	Width of two fingers
Apple pie, one slice	410 calories, 19 g fat	Width of three fingers
Ice cream, 1 cup	290 calories, 16 g fat	Baseball
Blue cheese dressing	154 calories, 16 g fat	Golf ball
Butter, 1 teaspoon	34 calories, 4 g fat	Tip of thumb

Reading the Label

Most people really never read the "Nutrition Facts" label on most food products. We might occasionally skim one. Take a look at the Nutrition Facts for a medium-sized bag of plain, salted potato chips (figure 3.2). The information commonly presented by the manufacturer is for "one serving," not the whole bag. But how many guys eat just one serving? The point is that a single bag of chips contains more than 1,200 calories, 45–65 percent of what a mature man ought to consume in a day, and half the sodium (salt) that is daily recommended. The entire bag provides a little protein, about the same as you'll find in one-third (a couple of bites) of a lean beef burger. But it contains 131 percent of the daily value of fat. The Food and Drug Administration (FDA) has required that saturated fats and cholesterol be listed on food labels since the mid-1990s, chiefly because saturated (and

Nutrition Facts

Serving Size 1 bag 8 oz 227 g (227 g)

Amount Per Serving	
Calories 1242	Calories from Fat 749

	% Daily Value*
Total Fat 85g	131%
Saturated Fat 25g	124%
Trans Fat	
Cholesterol 0mg	0%
Sodium 1192mg	50%
Total Carbohydrate 113g	38%
Dietary Fiber 10g	40%
Sugars 1g	
Protein 15g	

Vitamin A 0%	Vitamin C 70%
Calcium 5%	Iron 20%

*Percent Daily Values are based on a 2,000 calorie diet. Your daily values may be higher or lower depending on your calorie needs.

Figure 3.2. Sample Nutrition Facts label (potato chips)

trans) fats raise cholesterol in the blood, which is a cause of heart disease—the most lethal disease for men.

Nutrition Facts labels found on packaging are based on a 2,000- or 2,500-calorie-per-day diet and break down the "facts" (Percent Daily Values) in terms of servings. The serving size is not the recommended serving; it is just a convenient way of showing the "facts." It is unlikely to have any relevance to the size of the serving you choose to eat. Odds are you will not eat just one "serving," whether it is whole grain cereal or those tasty but unhealthy potato chips. If you eat more than the serving size listed, do some simple math. Compute the nutrients you're getting based on the amount of food you eat. If, for example, you pour two "servings" of cereal into a bowl, you can estimate the nutrients eaten by doubling the amounts listed.

Recommended Daily Servings

Grains (bread, cereal, rice, pasta) are divided into whole grains and refined grains, and at least half of all grains should be whole grains. Six servings per day are recommended. Each of the following is a 1 oz serving:

- 1 slice of bread; ½ English muffin
- ½ cup cooked cereal, rice, or pasta
- 2 small (3") pancakes, or 1 larger 4" pancake
- a 6" corn tortilla

Common portions:

- 1 large bagel = four servings
- Blueberry muffin = three servings

Vegetables also are grouped: dark green, red and orange, beans and peas, starchy (corn, potatoes), and "other" (e.g., artichokes, avocado, sprouts, cucumbers, celery, onions, mushrooms, iceberg lettuce). At least five ½ cup servings of vegetables per day are recommended. Each of the following is a ½ cup serving:

- ½ cup cooked, green vegetable
- 1 cup raw, leafy green vegetable
- 1 medium carrot (or 6 baby carrots)
- 1 raw whole tomato
- 1 small ear of corn (about 6" long)
- ½ cup tomato juice

Fruit: At minimum four ½ cup servings per day are recommended, and each of the following is a serving:

- 1 small orange, apple, peach, or half of a large one
- 1 banana (6″ long) or 1 large plum
- ½ medium-sized grapefruit
- ½ cup fruit juice (orange, pineapple, grapefruit)
- ½ cup halved or sliced fruit (strawberries)

Dairy (milk, yogurt, cheese) maintains muscles as much as protein. A serving = a cup, and you are recommended to have at least three servings daily. Each of the following is a serving:

- a half-pint container of milk, or a glass of milk
- an 8 oz container of yogurt with fruit or nuts
- 1½ oz hard cheese

Protein (all meat, seafood, dry beans, nuts, eggs): The recommendation for men age 50 and older is 5½ oz daily, and each of the following is equivalent to 1 oz:

- 1 tbsp peanut butter
- 1 egg
- ½ cup split pea soup
- 1 oz of any meat, poultry, or seafood

Common portions:

- 1 small chicken breast half = 3 oz
- 1 small hamburger = 2–3 oz
- 1 small steak = 3–4 oz
- 1 egg = 1 oz

Drink This, Not That

It is easy to forget that drinks (alcoholic and nonalcoholic alike) can add weight. This forgetfulness can often turn itself into the extra 5, 10, or 15 pounds that tend to creep up across a decade, especially if you are not physically active. Even healthy-sounding drinks like Vitamin Water pack a powerful caloric punch, particularly when not compensated by cutting back elsewhere or exercising. If you find yourself in this slow weight gain predicament, it is important to know exactly what is in those drinks you are enjoying. Below are examples of popular drink choices that are not nutritiously smart and some alternatives that can be used in replacement.

1. *Beer* is a classic go-to drink in a social situation because it is dependable and tasty. But it is full of empty calories, meaning that there is no nutritional benefit. Even more, as you drink, you are more likely to eat, especially if you are with others. Any 12-ounce beer you order is undoubtedly pushing 150 calories. Two Sierra Nevada India Pale Ales have as many calories as a Big Mac. So, if you are drinking just one, go ahead and enjoy the tasty full-bodied beer. If not, *instead, drink*: light beer, the options for which are far less caloric, especially if your plan is to have several beers. Michelob Ultra, Miller Lite, Bud Light, Amstel Light, and Heineken Light are all beers that are less than 100 calories; recently, even lower-calorie beers have been introduced (such as MGD 64, Bud Select 55). Their alcohol content is half that of a full-bodied beer.

2. *Soda* is a poor beverage choice to make on a consistent basis. Nutritionists often say that soda is filled with sugar and little else. In other words, there are virtually no redeeming qualities to soda. The natural sugar in soda and artificial sugar in diet soda may actually make you want to eat and drink more. If you think you are being healthier by drinking diet soda, think again. There is evidence that when our gut "tastes" the sweetness of natural sugars, there is an increased feeling of fullness, but the artificial sweetener in diet cola has minimal effects on appetite.[12] In short, keep the soda (regular and diet) intake to a minimum. *Instead, drink*: tonic—you still get the appealing fizz of soda (or "pop," for those who are from the Midwest).

Give It a Rest

Whether you had a poor night's sleep or simply a busy day, it is common to start dragging your feet by the middle of the afternoon. The most common fix to snap out of it is to get some caffeine. While a cup of coffee or caffeinated soda will certainly act as a temporary quick fix, a better option is to actually indulge your drowsy eyes and *take a break, or nap.* A scheduled 15- to 20-minute afternoon break will help keep you energized much longer than cola, coffee, or tea. If possible, try planning on your break at the same time each day and approximately 8 hours after you wake up. You maximize the value of the rest.

3. *Coffee* itself is not a problem. The caffeine in coffee is an antioxidant,[13] and researchers think that coffee consumption may reduce the risks of age-related decline in cognitive function and the risks of cancer. When served black, coffee has no calories. Coffee beans + water = virtually calorie free. But many people do not drink their coffee black and prefer it instead with cream and sugar. With the availability of a latte on every corner, whether Starbucks, McDonald's, or Dunkin' Donuts, people are drinking far more calories than they realize. Consider a tall (read "small") caffè mocha: even without the whipped cream or a shot of flavored syrup, you are getting a whopping 300–400 calories for one drink. *Instead, drink*: regular coffee, and try to limit how many cups you have a day. If you opt to have several cups, try to replace your cream with lower-fat milk or do with less or no sugar.

4. *Vitamin Water* sounds healthy (hydration and vitamins in one tasty drink), but it comes with a hidden cost. One bottle has 32 grams (two mountainous tablespoons) of sugar, which is far more than a drink that is technically considered water should have. Moreover, your body can only absorb so many vitamins, so if you eat a balanced diet or you regularly take a multivitamin, chances are a vitamin-fortified drink is providing no additional benefit. Most adult men are deficient only in their vitamin D3 intake and do need supplements, which are inexpensive and reduce the risk of non-skin cancers.[14] Otherwise, most men already consume more than the Recommended Dietary Allowance (RDA) of most vitamins and minerals. *Instead, drink*: good old-fashioned water. It is the best way to hydrate, and with zero calories, it is hard to beat. If plain water is too boring, try seltzer (sometimes called sparkling water—which is carbonated water with no calories) or an 8-ounce bottle of Gatorade's G2, which contains only 75 calories but enough salts to help the body balance electrolytes; in addition, Vitamin Water does have a less "fattening" line, called Vitamin Water 10.

5. *Wine* sometimes hits the spot—after a day at work, or when socializing with friends, or when reading a good book in the winter. Calorically speaking, white and red wines are pretty comparable—give or take 100 calories per glass. However, red wine has antioxidants, which are heart healthy and help prevent against a number of cancers. In contrast, white wine only has the empty calories, though (very) good taste, so if you are in the mood to relax with some wine, opt for a glass of red.

PROTEIN, CARBOHYDRATES, AND FATS: WHY YOU NEED THEM

Most everyone knows that meat and nuts are sources of protein, breads and pasta are a type of carbohydrate, and butter contains a significant amount of fat. But what does this mean? What do different foods do for your body? Understanding why your body needs certain foods (and could do without others) is an essential aspect to eating well. Our bodies are for life and must be properly managed in order to remain functional and active.

Protein. Critical to every cell in your body, no other nutrient is as involved in keeping you alive and healthy. Important for muscles and the maintenance and repair of tissue, protein is especially important for men with an active or stressful lifestyle. Protein does a lot of work behind the scenes—it is crucial for building new cells and sending messages from one cell to the next—and it allows you to function in the world. Extra bonus: if you eat a *lean* protein-rich meal (chicken, fish, shellfish, ground sirloin, eggs), you will feel fuller longer than if you eat strictly carbohydrates and fat.

Carbohydrates. If (immediate) energy is what you are looking for, carbohydrates should be your go-to food. Whether to keep going during a long outdoor project, before a bike ride, or just to get you through a long day, eating carbohydrate-rich food will protect your body and mind. Carbohydrates also help keep your cholesterol and blood pressure in check. Choose good (or the complex) carbs. The easily digested carbohydrates from white bread, white rice, pastries, and sugared sodas are not as healthy.

Fat. Too often thought to be synonymous with "bad," fat does have a place in eating well. Fat transports important vitamins (A, D, and E) throughout your body. In addition to the work of carbohydrates, fat also serves as a source of energy and can be stored in your body for later use, which brings us to why fat can be bad. If this stored energy resource goes untapped, the fat turns into rolls on your body.

VITAMINS AND MINERALS: WHY YOU NEED THEM

Vitamins and minerals are essential for the body to function well and contribute to the prevention of a number of diseases. Always getting a cold? Have trouble seeing or night blindness? Tingling in the fingers and toes? Nails brittle? Getting leg and toe cramps more frequently? "Hitting the wall" and feeling fatigued earlier and/or more often than you used to? Vitamin and/or mineral deficiencies may be the cause.

Minerals are vital for our bodies to remain healthy and are found in all cells. They act as catalysts for many biological reactions, including the transmission of messages through the nervous system. Our bodies use minerals to regulate body fluids, heartbeat, and sleep; activate enzymes; make glucose for energy; maintain metabolism and proper digestion; and avoid constipation.

There are two kinds of minerals: macrominerals and trace minerals. Macrominerals are the minerals found and needed in larger amounts—calcium, phosphorus, sodium, magnesium, potassium, chloride, and sulfur. We have and need just small amounts of the other minerals—iron, manganese, copper, iodine, zinc, cobalt, fluoride, and selenium. Though they're called "trace," they are not insignificant. Iron, for example, is important in the formation of hemoglobin, the oxygen-carrying factor in red blood cells; without it your body could not produce DNA. Both the "Western" and "prudent" diets typically provide all the minerals men need. Still, some individuals on limited budgets or fixed incomes may be at risk of having low iron or zinc intakes because good food sources of both, such as beef, seafood, and fresh green leafy vegetables, are expensive.

We need all the minerals, but neither too much nor in too small amounts.

If mineral levels are overabundant in the body, they may facilitate negative effects in the body. High sodium levels, for example, elevate blood pressure. Though we have more calcium in our body than all other minerals, it is probably not enough. The body absorbs calcium and stores it in the bones and teeth to keep them strong, and it is found throughout the body in blood, muscles, and the fluid between cells. As we age, calcium is one of the minerals we again need in greater quantity, much like when we were kids. It helps make our muscles and blood vessels contract and expand as needed, and it is needed to counteract the effects of intrinsic aging on bone loss.

Do you still drink milk? It does taste good, and men ought to have the equivalent of a glass of milk daily. Did you know that high-protein diets (often common among men) increase the body's demand for calcium? In addition, because there is a continuous loss of bone calcium as we get older, men age 50 and older are recommended to get the amount of calcium (1,200 milligrams per day) our bodies need through calcium-rich food like milk, broccoli, beans, and almonds. If you think that you are not getting enough calcium through food, talk to someone about calcium supplements. This will reduce the risk of arthritis, periodontal disease, leg cramps, and troubles sleeping.

There are two types of vitamins: water soluble (B and C) and fat soluble (A, D, E, and K). Because the water-soluble vitamins cannot be stored in the body, we need to acquire them daily from our drinks and food. You probably remember the grade school stories of fifteenth-century explorers stocking up their ships with citrus fruits to assure people sufficient vitamin C. It is best to achieve the recommended level of daily intake of water-soluble vitamins through a healthy diet—or, eating well, and not drinking too much alcohol. Alcohol interferes with the nutritional process by affecting digestion, storage, and use of nutrients. For example, drinking reduces the effectiveness of the vitamins consumed, and people who regularly drink should make sure they try to eat well. A daily multivitamin is a great nutrition insurance policy.

Vitamin dosage is measured in weight and in International Units (IU).

Water-Soluble Vitamins

Vitamin B (the *big* three Bs: B6-pryidoxine, B12-cobalamin, and folate-folic acid; and the *common* Bs: B1-thiamine, B2-riboflavin, B3-niacin, B5-pantothenic acid, and B7-biotin)

> The definition of a healthy daily intake of B vitamins isn't set in stone, though there are "dietary reference intakes" that change every 5 years or so. The recommended daily need: B6—2 milligrams; B12—3 to 6 micrograms; folate—400 to 800 micrograms.

> Sources: meat, poultry, fish, asparagus, spinach, broccoli, avocado, bananas, milk, eggs, yogurt, nuts, sunflower seeds, whole grain cereals, pasta, and tomato juice. All men over the age of 50 should strive to meet their RDA by eating foods fortified with vitamin B12, such as fortified cereals, or by taking vitamin B supplements.

> Why you need them: important for digestion and making energy from food, for red blood cell metabolism and repairing other cells, and in aiding the immune and nervous systems.

Vitamin C

> There isn't reliable evidence that megadoses of vitamin C improve health, though a megadose might relieve symptoms at the onset of a cold. Generally, the recommended daily need is about 90 milligrams a day; one large orange is equivalent to 70 milligrams. But smokers need more.

> Sources: citrus fruits, broccoli, and tomatoes.

> Why you need it: crucial to maintaining healthy gum tissue and preventing periodontal disease, as well as maintaining healthy bones and aiding in the absorption of iron.

Fat-Soluble Vitamins

Vitamin A

> Recommended daily need: 900 micrograms (equivalent to 3,000 IU).

> Sources: many breakfast cereals, juice, sweet potatoes, carrots, spinach, and apricots.

> Why you need it: important for vision and the immune system.

Vitamin D

> Recommended daily intake of vitamin D up to age 50 is 5 micrograms (200 IU), 10 micrograms (400 IU) between the ages of 51 and 70, and 15 micrograms (600 IU) after age 70. But intakes much higher are optimal. There are upper limits, although this is not a vitamin most men can get too much of. Men tend to have lower levels of vitamin D when living in places where the sun is out less (e.g., Boston; Portland, Oregon; or Portland, Maine), being indoors most of the day, or being dark skinned.

> Sources: sunlight; very few foods provide vitamin D, but "fatty" fish do, such as salmon, shrimp, and tuna; milk fortified with the vitamin.

> Why you need it: helps maintain bone density, allows you to absorb needed calcium and phosphorus, and helps increase muscle strength.

Vitamin E

> Recommended daily need: bare minimum is 15 milligrams (20–25 IU), yet researchers suggest that men's intake ought to be near 200 IUs per day to prevent heart disease. Most multivitamins contain around 30 IUs.

> Sources: sunflower seeds, oil-based salad dressings, dark leafy greens, peanut butter, and wheat germ.

> Why you need it: antioxidant (which helps prevent cancer), reduces risk of heart disease.

Vitamin K

> Recommended daily need: 120 micrograms.

> Sources: leafy green vegetables, soybeans, cabbage, and cauliflower.

> Why you need it: significantly helps protect against blood clots.

ANOREXIA: WORRISOME PROBLEM FOR A FEW

Although a high proportion of middle-aged and older men are overweight, a concern among a smaller number of older men is a decline in food intake and the loss of motivation to eat. Anorexia is too often thought of as a disorder of adolescent girls, but it can and does occur among older men. Perhaps one in eight men age 65 and older already have daily diets of 1,000 calories or less, which puts them at risk of undernutrition.[15] As much as our appetite is prone to fluctuate throughout our lives, it may dangerously diminish later in life and manifest into what is known as "anorexia of aging." Signs of anorexia are having no interest in food, maybe even a refusal to eat, and becoming 15 percent or more below one's healthy weight.

The root of the problem for why an older man may become malnourished is physiological—as we age, our senses of taste and smell diminish, and appetite naturally decreases because food remains in our stomach longer. Declines in taste and smell begin around age 60. Appetite decreases for many reasons. Sometimes, appetite is related to over-the-counter and prescribed medications we take; some medications suppress interest in eating, and some can deplete nutrients. Other times, illness triggers little interest in eating, and with age we are more likely to live with multiple chronic illnesses. Weight loss is also associated with heavy alcohol drinking. When both tastes and testosterone diminish and we are using appetite-suppressing medications (or alcohol as a self-medication), it is more difficult for an older man to maintain a hearty appetite.

Share a Meal

If you live alone yet prefer being around others or are looking to make new friends, having a meal together is a great way to get to know people and create new bonds. There are plenty of places where you can enjoy an affordable meal and the company of others.

Senior citizen centers. Though meal programs differ for each center, many provide one or more daily meals for citizens over 60, and some are free, asking only for donations. Whether you go by yourself or with a friend, it's a great way to meet new people. For more information, check out your local phone book or the Internet.

Veteran meals. Veteran meals tend to be more of an annual or semiannual occurrence, but they present a great opportunity to get back in touch with old friends or meet others who have had similar experiences. Check the newspaper for announcements.

Rotary clubs. Rotary clubs frequently sponsor occasional dinners with favorites like spaghetti or roasted turkey, while also hosting dinners on holidays such as Valentine's Day and the Fourth of July. Being part of a club can be a good way to get out of the house and be part of a group of like-minded people.

Community centers. Many communities host meals, whether for a holiday or just for fun, which are a good way to get to know your neighbors. Community center dinners are great options for families and singles alike, regardless of age.

The chief social factor that affects how we eat is social isolation. In addition, psychological considerations play a part in disinterest in eating. Depression is more prevalent among men in later life than earlier. With shrinking social networks or a new chronic illness, it makes sense that older men are at greater risk of becoming depressed. Depression often causes a loss of appetite. It is important to note that the development of anorexia of aging is multi-determined, which is to say that there is no one clean-cut cause or treatment. For example, a man might be depressed because he has cardiovascular disease, causing a diminished interest in eating, but the drugs to treat his illness speed up his metabolism and he burns off what little nutrients he eats. Talk to your doctor about why your appetite is fading and try to figure out a plan that best suits your personal needs.

FOOD IN LATER LIFE: SHIFTING ROLES AND RELATIONSHIPS

Eating together is a central part of the daily routine for men in long-term relationships. Researchers affirm that companionship is core to the worth of a good meal.[16] At the same time, eating itself is also very important. Men are likely to skip meals when they are temporarily or newly alone. The same multinational study revealed that changes in men's relationships present food issues. When managing the transition from worker to retiree or dealing with the loss of a wife or partner, men's eating behavior is affected. Our basic preference is for a long-established way of doing things—rituals and habits. Change disrupts. Recently retired men may skip lunch. Newly alone men who've become widowers are thrust into an uncomfortable experience of preparing meals just for themselves.[17] The challenge becomes to build new routines. Some men tackle food preparation as a new hobby, rather than a domestic chore. For others, their strategy is getting someone else to prepare the food, enabling them to maintain their customary pattern of being cooked for and served.

CHAPTER 4

Psychology of Healthy Aging

with Clifford M. Singer

George Vaillant, a psychiatrist who has studied men's aging, notes that "aging well" may seem like an oxymoron.[1] But he recognizes that aging is a complex process of adaptation and development as much as decline. We have all seen older men coping with severe challenges with inspiring grace. What accounts for some men's remarkable ability to maintain a sense of calmness through adversity? What psychological characteristics contribute to satisfying adaptations to old age? What are the psychological challenges for men as we age? In this chapter we'll begin with an overview of brain aging, since that is intimately related to a man's behavior, thinking, and feelings. The next focus is on the psychology of aging, including an overview of personality development and a look at the major themes affecting men's emotions in middle and old age. A review of the major mental disorders of late life follows, and we end with some strategies for successful adaptation by men as they grow older.

NEUROLOGY OF AGING

Brain Development

It has long been thought that aging brings a steady, determined decline in all aspects of brain function. As is often the case, reliable data are inconsistent with widely held assumptions. At about age 30, when the myelination (or insulating) of the brain's long communication tracts is finally complete and the frontal lobes are fully formed, our brain structure is mature. Contrary to folk wisdom, once the brain is mature, there is no gradual decline in the number of brain cells (neurons). Brain researchers have learned that if we do not have a disease that causes neurons to die, then nearly all of the neurons remain healthy until we die.[2] What does change as we get older is the thinning of the fatty sheath (or myelin) coating of the nerve axons (or the white matter)[3] and shrinking of the synapses between brain cells, as well as some shrinkage of neuron size (or the gray matter).[4] These changes slow the flow of information from one area of the cerebral cortex to another. The result is a slowing of instance processing speed and of memory recall, which begins in the fourth decade of life with healthy aging. The change is only measurable in milliseconds. In fact, the performance decrement is so subtle at first that it is obvious only at the highest levels of performance demands, such as in Olympic and professional athletes and, famously, among physicists. The history of science is populated by figures having their "blockbuster" insights as young adults.

Here's the good news about brain aging. The old beliefs were that the brain is a static organ, unresponsive to events, with a fixed structure and with cell populations that are unable to repair or reproduce. These beliefs are now dead, pushed aside by the findings of brain research. There has been a torrent of evidence coming from modern neuroscience that the brain can grow and adapt in late life. The growth of new brain cells, the formation of new synaptic connections between those brain cells, and the acquisition of new knowledge and skills are common in older adults. True, these processes are slower and not as effortless as in youth, but they do occur. The mechanisms that promote adaptability and growth in the human brain are not as strong in older adults. Learning requires more repetition and practice. Functional imaging studies demonstrate that the brain has to work harder in older adults to achieve the learning performance of young adults. Memorization tasks cause the brains of middle-aged and older adults to recruit more help from the frontal lobes, bringing greater awareness and focus to learning efforts. This process is sometimes referred to as "top-down processing," as it is reliant on the frontal lobes or "higher brain centers." Even when brain injuries occur, there is slower healing and less complete recovery in older adults than young people, but improvement and repair do occur. In experiments with research animals, experiences and novel situations have been found to stimulate neuronal growth in the old as in the young.[5] The growth and adaptation of brain cell circuits to stress, injury, and new demands is called *neuroplasticity*.[6]

There is an equivalent to neuroplasticity in the body. Called *myoplasticity*, it is the ability of muscles to adapt and respond to stress, injury, and new demands. The fact is that our muscle strength and endurance are less at 50 than at 20. The adaptation of muscles to stress and workload, as in weight lifting, takes more time and may not yield the same large, hard muscle mass as years before. This doesn't mean that older muscles don't respond well to exercise and performance demands. Even modest increases in demand result in improved strength and performance in 90-year-olds. The same is true of our aging brain.

In old age, our brain still responds to increased demands. It just does so less swiftly than at age 30 and with less potential peak performance. Once this is understood and accepted, we can come to terms with the changes in memory and attention that accompany aging (see chapter 13 for more details). With patience, persistence, and mindfulness, we can achieve high levels of intellectual and creative activity. Knowing this, you may be less likely to shy away from mental challenges that may be frustrating at first but even more satisfying in the end. The satisfaction of achievement, in this case, is even sweeter with the awareness that the effort itself provokes growth and renewal in the brain.[7]

MEN'S EGO

We live in a culture where the masculinity code tells us to strive to be the "big wheel" and, if need be, "give 'em hell."[8] We are competitive. We learn to crave power and status, thinking that this is the way we attract fame, ensure the survival of our offspring, and secure the essentials of life. In adolescence, our competitiveness may be expressed through sports and academics or played out in more direct ways through attempts to stand out in social situations or through physical aggression and violent confrontation. As adults, the workplace is our coliseum.

The need to maintain a stable sense of identity often faces new challenges as we transition through our middle ages and early older adult years. Sometimes the challenge comes from a sudden and unexpected event, such as an injury, a disabling illness to a partner or wife, or being laid off from a job we expected to have the rest of our life. Sometimes it comes gradually as we begin to recognize the aging of our bodies. We may notice that young women no longer glance our way as we pass. Our first experiences with erectile dysfunction (ED) or long intervals before our next feelings of arousal raise fears that sex will never again be fun for us or satisfying for our partners. Young people, men and women, suddenly seem so full of enthusiasm, energy, quick wit, and the latest knowledge of the field, and they are suddenly your colleagues or even your supervisors. Your children may be grown and appear to be less dependent on your skills or wisdom. Your spouse or partner may be achieving success in his or her career and earn more than you do. You may even feel a little more vulnerable and have a keen awareness that you cannot always control events. These are heavy things for us to cope with.

The saving grace for many of us is that we move away from trying to be the big wheel. As we age, wisdom, increasing confidence, and the way the natural decline in reproductive hormones affects our body tend to move us toward new masculinity plateaus. If things go well, we may become more compassionate and collaborative. Those of us who allow ourselves to grow emotionally become secure enough to acknowledge our shortcomings and wise enough to depend on others to help compensate for them. We even become more accepting of flaws in others. The end result is that the drive to compete quite commonly declines in the hierarchy of personal goals as the typical man ages. In fact, researchers in Oregon have found that risk-taking behavior and the desire to enter into competition to achieve bigger payoffs appear to peak in the fifties and then begin to decline (especially for men).[9] Of course, for the hard-driving elite, it may be a different story.

Milestones of Development

Erik Erikson, a mid-twentieth-century psychoanalyst, conceived of human psychological development as sequential chapters of life, each unfolding under the influence of biology and culture. His stages of development, beginning in infancy, are dependent on the successful negotiation of the major developmental task of the previous stage.[10] For example, the task of forming a stable sense of who we are and how we behave as (young) men is the major psychological milestone of adolescence (ages 12–20); Erikson did acknowledge that working through each stage may take years longer for many people. He referred to the tensions during this period of life as "identity versus role confusion," and he thought that the formation of a predictable, consistent identity is essential for the successful negotiation of the stage of "intimacy versus isolation." People, and perhaps men in particular, can create and tolerate intimate relationships only when they feel confident in their own identity and self-worth. In order for us to give love, we must feel worthy to receive it in turn.

To succeed in adult relationships, he argued, we must feel comfortable with the reciprocity of relationships, being willing to rely on others as they rely on us. This is not so easy for men who are apprehensive to ask for help from others or who do not even know what they need from others. There may be denial of needs and exaggerated expressions of independence. Men may feel excessively burdened by meeting the most basic needs of a partner and seek escape by addictive behavior, such as drinking, overworking, compulsive exercise, or spending long hours on the Internet. Of course, everyone needs alone time away from family and friends. Those who can't negotiate the balance of intimacy and isolation may become too detached from others, increasing their risk of depression and health problems later in life.

In the sequence of psychological stages that Erikson conceived, the capacity for intimate relationships sets the stage for adulthood (ages 35–65). This "middle" period of life pivots on what Erikson called "generativity versus stagnation." He believed that in adulthood men will strive to build a legacy, something of lasting value for the benefit of the next generation. Without this sense of purpose, we may feel stagnant or "go through the motions" without really caring about outcomes or having a sense that what we do matters. It is during this phase that most men strive to create financial stability for themselves and their loved ones, raise children, mentor young colleagues, and achieve what they hope to achieve in life. We also grow to be more forgiving of ourselves and others in the effort to get along. We may learn to take fewer risks because there are more people counting on us and what we provide, emotionally and materially.

Men of all ages can be preoccupied with thoughts of strength and success, failure and mortality, but these themes reemerge as among the strongest late in life. Erikson called this life stage "integrity versus despair." The terms refer to the psychic struggle of later life, in which we must come to terms with the life we have lived, for better or worse. By "integrity," Erikson meant coming to feel that our life has followed a story line true to a person's heart and values: a feeling that life has been worthwhile and fulfilling, and we come to accept without fear that death will occur probably in the not-too-distant future. "Despair," of course, is the opposite pole. It could be a belief that not much good has come from your life and there is little to be done about it at this point. Such feelings can leave us mired in regret and paralyzed by demoralization. Or there could be isolation and bitterness from a grim perception that the world is changing for the worse and we can either passively resign to "let the fools have it their way" or fall into a paranoid state in which others are seen as different, dangerous, or just inferior. Of course, we all know people at both extremes of "integrity versus despair," and we certainly know whom we'd rather invite over for Thanksgiving dinner.

Erikson's model provides a useful framework for thinking about the changing challenges of life as we age, and it is supported by research. Various studies indicate that there are certain competencies most relevant at different life stages, and good outcomes are dependent on achieving those milestones in our lives. For middle-aged and older men, the quality of our lives is said to hinge on generativity versus stagnation and integrity versus despair. Erikson also believed that there is value in the ability to balance the various developmental challenges over our lifetime. Balancing is a skill that allows us to deal with the apparent paradox that exists between developmental challenges (e.g., integrity versus despair). Learning to balance challenges effectively reflects what Erickson called wisdom. Of course, many people consider this model oversimplified and culture specific. As Erikson even cautioned, any attempt to define discrete developmental stages can't be taken too literally since our lives do not follow linear trajectories.[11]

Relationships

The psychology of men's aging will influence any relationship that spans the years of middle and old age. The identity issues and lifestyle changes surrounding retirement and "empty nesting" can challenge men and their partners. These later life stages usually mean that more time is spent together and there are fewer distractions from the marital relationship. This may be an opportunity to regain intimacy and friendship. Many long-term relationships and marriages thrive when the children are grown and work demands lessen. Two people can again focus on their own and their partner's needs and their relationship. There may be a sense of reacquaintance between two partners, or even learning new things about each other. But if your relationship is empty or dysfunctional, there will be increased stress. If partners do not share interests, they may live "parallel" lives, each pursuing their own interests, activities, and friends. Such relationships would not be fulfilling for some people, but they can meet the needs of more independent sorts, particularly if they find mutual satisfaction in family gatherings or a few shared friendships. Divorce is not unusual at this stage of life, when partners confront the realities of a relationship held together by forces outside of themselves.

When two men are partnered, these issues may be amplified by each partner's struggles with similar identity challenges. As men see themselves or their partners aging and losing "sex appeal," impulses to reexperience youthful exuberance may expresses themselves through affairs with younger partners, second or third marriages with a partner half their age, or attempts to stop the time clock with plastic surgery, hair coloring, cosmetic dermatology, and the like. Whereas attempts to look more youthful may have healthy origins, attempts to actually be healthy through diet and lifestyle changes will yield greater happiness in the end. Moreover, to accept a partner's aging, men are challenged to find "beauty within" their partner—to adjust notions of beauty to accommodate aging faces and bodies and the elegance not found in simpler features of youth.

If you think of your main contribution to a relationship, marriage, or family as bringing in the money, midlife unemployment or forced retirement can be especially stressful for your ego above and beyond the very real financial stresses these events bring. If your partner relies on your strength and mechanical skills around the house, physical or mental disability can deprive you of an important source of your self-esteem within the relationship. People in these situations run the risk of losing their sense of purpose in life, which can be very demoralizing and lead to the unmasking of self-doubt and insecurity.

Luckily, most men and their partners adapt. For instance, you may assume more kitchen responsibilities and revel in praise for your newly developed cooking skills. Or, you may start a new hobby, such as landscape painting or furniture making. These new talents redefine you within the family or neighborhood as the "artist in residence." Those of us who are fortunate enough to have grandchildren can find new life in experiencing this still-uncharted relationship. Less happily, men may transition into being a caregiver for a spouse with a terminal or chronic disease. Although this experience imposes enormous physical and emotional burden, there can be a sense of fulfillment that brings forth the most loving and generous aspects of ourselves.

Meeting the challenges to late-life relationships with partners and spouses may yield enormous benefits. Experience, common sense, and research studies tell us that happiness is based on successful relationships. Social isolation and stressful relationships are associated with poor health, alcohol abuse, and premature death. It is telling that there is a gender difference in the willingness of people to remarry following divorce or widowerhood in later life. A higher percentage of men than women choose to remarry, and the period of time remaining single is shorter for men. Of course, this may just be due to the fact that it is easier for men to remarry later in life because there are more available women than men. But there are clearly other factors. The majority of men have spent little time living alone since they were young adults, and it is more stressful being alone. There is overwhelming evidence that good marriages and positive relationships sustain men's lives.[12]

Parenting

People in the United States are increasingly mobile. We voluntarily move hundreds or thousands of miles for a job, an education, love, or warmer weather. The disruption created by such moves in our social lives can have unforeseen consequences, because for many of us our daily connections to people who matter are fewer as we grow older. There are certainly ways for those of us who have never had children, who have lost our children, or whose children and grandchildren live far away to meet the need to feel included. One way men can feel appreciated is by contributing to the welfare of younger non-kin through teaching, foster care, and other volunteer work. Men can also maintain family ties at a distance through phone calls, video chats, social networking sites, e-mail, texting, and travel. Indeed, many men who are parents or grandparents appreciate the peacefulness of distance and the convenience of electronic communications such as Skyping.

Work

One of the most challenging aspects of aging for many men is the transition from work to retirement. For some men work is a means to an end; it is a source of income to support the family and finance our true interests, such as sports, travel, and hobbies. If they are financially able, retirement isn't a loss. For other men, work is an end in itself, and success in our career may be the major source of our identity and self-esteem. These men may delay retirement or avoid it altogether. Even so, for the majority of men, retirement, once entered, ends up being maneuvered successfully, with minor if any enduring negative effects on their self-esteem, the quality of their personal relationships, or their physical and mental health. Seemingly quite resilient and adaptive, the majority of men don't let leaving their day-to-day involvement in their work community, minor disabilities, reduced income, or even widowerhood impact their satisfaction with life and self-esteem in significant ways. Only significant disability that directly impacts our ability to function independently on a daily basis has been repeatedly shown as strongly related to declines in our personal sense of worth and well-being.[13]

Self-esteem is the idea that you matter and that you are "good enough." If you do not think that this is the case, your self-esteem has room to improve.

There are data to suggest that men who stay active in their occupations later in life are healthier and live longer than those who retire early.[14] Of course, such findings may be explained, at least in part, by the obvious reality that healthier men are able to work more years. Nevertheless, a sense of purpose is essential to happiness, and people who devote their lives to their work may face a struggle to find that same sense of purpose outside the workplace. Men who have cultivated interests, volunteer activities, and friendships outside of work fare much better with retirement. Researchers find that men's self-esteem can peak at or near retirement age; further, men with better education, income, health and employment status, and happy marriages report higher levels of self-esteem as they age,[15] until physical health affects independence.[16] Without new interests or postretirement involvement, our self-esteem and overall psychological health are threatened. There is compelling evidence that working after retiring postpones poor health outcomes and improves psychological health.[17]

Even those men who stay on in the workplace will face challenges to self-esteem as they experience erosion of influence or work skills. We have all seen the sad image of the aged business owner who refuses to let go and allow the next generation to take over the reins. Although without doubt these men may have true wisdom and sound judgment, they may not realize that the best mentors keep a distance and allow younger colleagues to gain confidence in their own abilities. The inability to let go and welcome the challenge that comes with life transitions is the "stagnation" that Erikson was referring to, in contrast to the "generativity" of true mentorship. As difficult as it may be, those of us who move on and develop new interests in late life are all the better for it.

Sex

Serum testosterone levels begin to decline at around 40 years of age and do so at a rate of about 1 percent per year, so that, on average, men 75 years of age have lost about one-third of the testosterone levels they likely had as young men.[18] As in all things, levels of testosterone are highly variable from one person to the next, but it is estimated that 20 percent of men in the 60–80 age group have below-normal levels. Many of these men will experience low libido and erectile dysfunction (ED). Although testosterone replacement can help with libido, it often does not affect ED. Mild to moderate ED is experienced by 52 percent of men over 40. Of these, fewer than 10 percent will have low testosterone levels.[19] There are many men therefore who experience normal or mildly reduced libido and some degree of ED, situations that also negatively affect self-esteem, confidence, and the quality of sexual relationships. Fortunately, many men adapt to these changes without much trouble. If you are married or partnered, remember that your spouse may also be experiencing similar changes and having to deal with fluctuating levels of sexual desire. Explorations of physical intimacy not dependent on erections may be very satisfying and fun. Medications and techniques to enhance erectile function can be used to the satisfaction of both partners. Many men report an appreciation for feeling a sense of freedom from intrusive thoughts of sex and welcome the greater appreciation of the nonsexual elements of their relationships with women.

Health

Illness and disability are difficult for anybody to adjust to, but they may be more troubling for men. A man's ego can be very reliant on projecting an image of strength and independence. Health issues of greatest concern to men include ailments that risk compromising independence and quality of life.[20] As a result, for some men illness represents weakness. Dependency on others during illness can also threaten a man's need to be independent and feel self-sufficient. A consistent research finding is that men's self-ratings of their health tend to take their lifestyle and mortality risks into account, and in fact men's self-ratings of health are better predictors of their mortality.[21]

Mortality

Not only does positive self-esteem reflect our health status, but it can improve our health. Men participating in health surveys and rating their health as "poor," "fair," or sometimes just "good" have a significantly higher risk of mortality than those who considered their health "excellent."[22] The point is that our sense of our health is a strong predictor of our acquired mortality risk. Men in good health know it and feel better about themselves, which is a good reason to eat well and stay active. Equally impressive, positive self-perceptions about growing older actually improve our health and increase longevity.[23] Perception is powerful.

Anxiety about aging and dying (called "death anxiety") may challenge your self-esteem and can be activated by initial experiences of serious health conditions in yourself or your contemporaries. Many of us remember the first time we heard of someone our age dying of a heart attack. "I'm too young to start losing friends to heart disease" is a common thought. Little wonder that when heart disease (or any other disabling chronic illness) is first experienced, there is a higher risk of developing depression after the event, though sometimes not until months afterward. Rather than letting their family and close friends know about the struggles and anxieties they are facing, most men keep it all to themselves. This "suffer silently" strategy of internalizing stress increases our risk for depression and suicide.

Men are four times as likely as women to actually take their own lives, and almost three-quarters of men who commit suicide have seen a physician within a few weeks of killing themselves. They actually sought help but probably never asked aloud for the help they so wanted. Perhaps they were seeking relief from pain and sleeplessness—but guys do not talk directly about that stuff. It is also easy to imagine a scenario where the man anticipated positive news but left the physician's office with a feeling of hopelessness regarding a newly diagnosed medical condition that may mean he will never have the same life he had come to expect. Whatever the circumstances of that final doctor visit, men, *on average*, do not adapt as well as women to declining physical capacity, and they are more likely to keep their vulnerable inner lives hidden. The traditions of men's vulnerabilities being hidden from public display may be one reason older men, especially white men, have the highest suicide rates of any age group in our society. The suicide may not be a reaction to actual pain or disability, but to meaning of the diagnosis. One of the most challenging things for men with a life-threatening chronic illness is to maintain a sense of purpose in life—to be able to contribute and not be dependent on others.

A man ending his own life by choice could be interpreted as his final insistence on control of personal destiny. Viewed in this way, suicide in the face of an unacceptable quality of life may be an act of empowerment and maintaining dignity. By comparison, men who choose to face chronic illness and their disability with some form of acceptance are equally powerful, representing "grace under pressure." These men continue with life, perhaps because they find pleasures in the smallest corners of life.

Loss and Grief

Faced with spousal or partner loss, men experience an array of emotions, including anger, shock (especially if the death is unexpected), profound sadness, numbness, and feelings of dismemberment.[24] They exhibit intense feelings of restlessness, impatience, frustration, wanting to give up, and sleep deprivation, as well as increases in anxiety, drinking, and smoking and decreases in appetite, all of which are now considered to be behaviors that mask their understandable underlying depression.

Widowerhood is not a well-charted territory, but it is well known that men's experiences pose serious challenges to their identities. For many men, the loneliness and emptiness experienced reflect a loss of the taken-for-granted security that being married and being a husband (or partner) provided. Many men undergoing spousal loss regard themselves as independent and as a resilient "sturdy oak" in the face of emotional challenges.[25] Yet most men are absolutely unaware of how socially and emotionally dependent they are on their wife/partner. Their marital relationship provided them with a sense of normalcy, stability, and having succeeded as a man. These emotional responses are not unlike those of grieving fathers who must live with the loss of a child.

No matter what type of loss, men tend to control their emotions. Some men express their emotions more openly than others. But they typically hold back and cry less openly. Widowers, more often than not, will channel their energy into active coping and problem-solving strategies like work, physical activity, or addressing disruptions in the household. At other times they may prefer to be alone with their thoughts, reflecting their quiet ways to cope with their new situation. Men usually express their feelings of grief in solitary ways, but this should not be construed as any less intense than a woman's grief. These patterns suggest that while some responses may be more typical, any one widower's experience can be somewhat unique as well.

Not surprisingly, adaptation to loss varies from individual to individual. The most difficult times are usually the first 6 months to a year, yet some men adapt more quickly. Some methods associated with more successful adaptation include keeping busy with meaningful activity (such as work), having adequate support and ability to do things with others or to share feelings, and a sense of retaining control.

PSYCHOLOGICAL DISORDERS

Men's Depression

Is there a clinical entity called "Depression" that exists somewhere within a person, much like a cancer tumor can be located within the body? No, not at all. There is increasing evidence that there is no coherent entity we can call depression.[26] It's not whether you have "it." Rather, men can be more or less depressed, ranging from debilitating severe depression to just "feeling down." Signs and symptoms of depression include doubting our own confidence in our decision making, feeling as if we are "hitting the wall" way too often, feeling apart from things even when with people, being no longer interested in succeeding, and saying that we prefer quiet time when in fact we just do not want to engage ourselves in social activities.[27] Men who strongly adhere to the masculine norms to be in control of their destiny and are quiet about their feelings will most often mask their depression through grouchiness and heavier drinking.

Striving to remain respected, a middle-aged or older man ultimately will find the generation behind him rising up. At first he might add more hours

When Silence Hurts

Partners of depressed men often express fear that naming the man's condition will only make matters worse. It is better just to "get on with it" and "not dwell on the negatives." But when we minimize a man's depression, for fear of shaming him, we collude with the cultural expectations of masculinity in a terrible way. We send a message that the man who is struggling should not expect help. He must be "self-reliant."

Source: Real, T. (1998). *I don't want to talk about it: Overcoming the secret legacy of male depression.* New York: Simon & Schuster, p. 38.

to keep up; consequently, his sleep may become restless, his easygoing demeanor turns edgy, and his unflappable disposition percolates into irritability. His emotional responses and behavior suggest he is experiencing depression, but he and his partner are more likely to label his mood as irritation or anger. He isn't likely to turn to friends to talk; instead, he keeps his distress to himself and uses swearing, a sport, alcohol, or pounding a wall or the steering wheel as a response to being distressed. He isn't likely to cry; he's more likely to yell. And his loved ones will rarely acknowledge his pain directly.

Clinicians working with men who have mental health troubles have increasingly argued that there is collusion in Western societies that covers up the depression men feel.[28] Men's depression becomes "masked" when men follow masculinity norms and convert their worries and sad mood into somatic symptoms such as digestive disturbances or the fatigue and muscle tension that accompanies negative mood and/or anxiety. Somaticizing is what men (are supposed to) do, and it is not surprising that men are three times more likely to complain about gastrointestinal symptoms but three times less likely to seek help for "depression" than women. Depressed men have learned not to reveal sad feelings. A man might cry, but in a private place where others never witness the sadness and pain.

Hundreds of studies indicate that adult men are half as likely as women to divulge their depression in ways that correspond to the symptoms physicians expect. Even when men disclose their suffering to family members, they are still twice as reluctant to seek a professional's help for their depression.[29] Unfortunately, men's unrecognized and untreated depression ruthlessly increases suffering and adds to the risk of death from many causes—in particular death from cardiovascular disease and suicide. The chart provides an overview of the signs and symptoms of men's depression.

In addition, Western cultures normalize men's heavier drinking as "self-medication." The message heard is that men are expected to manage their feelings by themselves. Even the 1990s Seagram's VO advertising slogan "It's what men do" encouraged men to think of having a few drinks. Equally disturbing, older men are expected to "slow down," and signs of their depression such as fatigue, sleepiness, and a decrease in mental agility will be misinterpreted as age related. Depression-related symptoms coexist with other medical illnesses and disabilities, often causing doctors and family to misread men's depression as evidence of medical problems. The result, all too often, is that what we *feel* is never investigated.

A lingering emptiness or sadness isn't normal no matter what your age, and when we misread depression, effective treatment gets delayed, if even provided. Too few people appreciate that depression is perhaps the most frequent cause of suffering among middle-aged and older men. Too

DEPRESSION-RELATED SYMPTOMS IN OLDER MEN

Emotional/mood symptoms	Cognitive symptoms	Physical/behavioral symptoms
Sadness	Hopelessness	Low energy and initiative
Irritability	Excessive guilt	Altered sleep
Anxiety	Slowed thinking	Altered appetite
Apathy	Reduced motivation	Self-neglect
Chronic anger	Memory impairment	Decreased immunity
Lack of pleasure from usually enjoyable activities	Thoughts of death and suicide	Increased cardiac mortality risk

few people recognize that depression need not have "the big D"; rather, it is a persistent negative mood (whether anger or sadness) that undermines quality of life.

Depression in Later Life

Most older men have at one time or another been temporarily immobilized by depression. By age 65 it is estimated that about one-half of all men in the United States have experienced at least one depressive episode lasting 2 weeks or more. Their unshakable depressed mood or markedly diminished interests in most of their normal activities are key signs of clinical depression.[30] Furthermore, statistical patterns reveal that *on average* one in seven men age 60 and older will be living with a major depressive disorder and his suffering will remain untreated. Current estimates tell us that 16–18 percent of men age 60 and older are depressed, but these estimates fail to accurately count the true prevalence of depression, because only one-half of the middle-aged and older men with *severe* symptoms ever seek help from their physician or will be pushed toward a physician by a family member. This leaves about half of men living with depression undiagnosed and untreated.[31]

When these symptoms are present most of the time for a period of at least 2 weeks, major depression is likely the cause. You may not experience all of these symptoms. Older men may not experience low mood or sadness, for example, or changes in sleep patterns and appetite. These symptoms may come and go, but many could be present at least in mild if not severe form. The symptoms listed are not exactly those within the diagnostic criteria for major depression as presented in the *Diagnostic and Statistical Manual of Mental Disorders (DSM)*, but they nevertheless are depression-related symptoms that strongly warrant our attention, especially for older men.

Etiology of Depression

To understand depression, remember that all of our thoughts and feelings are generated by the electrochemical processes within the brain and affected by brain health. It is also essential to remember that although the mind is the brain's creation, it is also its master. The brain is a dynamic organ that responds to the thoughts and feelings we create. Our thoughts and experiences shape the brain through what is called *neuroplastic response*. Joyful experiences, secure relationships, fulfilling work, lifelong learning, and intellectual activity systematically structure the brain to reduce our risk of both depression and dementia in old age. By contrast, threatening and painful experiences actually alter brain structure and function and increase our risk for depression later in life.

Many people think that you can always "think" or "will" your way out of depression. This is true to a degree. Psychotherapy, spiritual practice, enjoyable activities and hobbies, art, music, friendships, and close family ties all can help your recovery from depression and reduce the risk of relapse.[32] However, once depression becomes severe enough, our thinking becomes impaired because our brain structure has changed. Medical and mental health professionals call this state "major depression." You might have heard it referred to as "clinical depression" because of the need for clinical intervention.

In major depression, brain function is impaired by changes in the structure of a fatty sheath (or myelin) coating of the nerve axons (the white matter) and the synapses between brain cells (the gray matter). Physical functions such as sleep, appetite, immune response, and metabolism become deregulated. There is ample evidence that major depression accelerates physical and cognitive decline. The longer the depression stays, the harder it can be to come out of it. Complicating this, certain age-related diseases of the brain such as a stroke or Parkinson's disease affect mood and the expression of emotions (affect). When major depression is associated with brain disorders, it can be especially severe and recovery tends to be less than optimal, with residual symptoms and high risk of relapse.[33]

Depression can have organic roots as much as it is based on social experiences. Many of the medications older men take can cause or worsen their depression, as noted in the insert. Major depression and some other mood disorders, such as bipolar disorder, also tend to run in families. Genetic risk factors have been identified. Having a parent with a mood disorder such as major depression increases your own risk for several reasons, including genes and early life experiences. Having a parent with bipolar disorder, with intense "highs" and "lows" in their life history, is an even greater risk factor for a man's mood disorder. The natural history of depression is highly variable, and the condition may spontaneously remit within weeks or months. The longer a man remains in a depressed state, the higher the risk of him developing chronic symptoms of depression. In depressed men, the stress hormone cortisol may continue to be secreted even though the levels of the hormone are already high in their body. Once the depression disappears, cortisol levels return to normal.

The duration and severity of depressions are predictive of relapse risk. The more time you remain in a depressed state, the higher your risk of developing a recurrent illness with little or no connection to life events. There may not be any obvious "cause" for becoming depressed once you have developed this form of depressive illness. "I don't know why I'm feeling so out of it" is a common thought. In other cases, men may assume that the cause is a current stressor they are experiencing even though that stress may be something they could easily cope with when they are feeling well. Treatment of depression with medication, talking therapies, and cognitive and behavioral therapies can be helpful for most men. Milder depressions frequently run their course and spontaneously remit or resolve with positive life changes and implementing new and more positive health and lifestyle habits.

Although depression can be severely disabling, most men manage to endure repeated episodes of it and lead productive, inspiring lives. Abraham Lincoln is one of the most well known of these men, but the list is long. At least one Lincoln biographer has speculated that despite the suffering and paralysis of depression, the experience of illness may bring emotional depth and compassion that enhances a person's other attributes of greatness which are then expressed when the depression is in remission.[34]

Medications That Can Cause or Worsen Depression

- Blood pressure medication (clonidine)
- Beta blockers (e.g., Lopressor, Inderal)
- Sleeping pills
- Tranquilizers (e.g., Valium, Xanax, Halcion)
- Calcium-channel blockers
- Medication for Parkinson's disease
- Ulcer medication (e.g., Zantac, Tagamet)
- Heart drugs containing reserpine
- Steroids (e.g., cortisone, prednisone)
- High-cholesterol drugs (e.g., Lipitor, Zocor)
- Painkillers and arthritis drugs

Source: Helpguide.org (2011). *Depression in older adults and the elderly: Recognizing the signs and getting help.* http://helpguide.org/mental/depression_elderly.htm.

Other Syndromes

There are three "cousins" of depression which men need to be aware of. Dysthymia is chronic, long-term sadness, sometimes called a chronic type of minor depression. It may begin in childhood and become a defining feature of a man's personality. It can also develop over time as a result of repeated loss, disappointment, loneliness, and hardship. Typically, a man with dysthymia will feel little sense of joy or optimism. He may respond warmly to pleasant events, compared to a person with major depression, but his feelings of happiness are fleeting. The physical and cognitive symptoms of depression, such as changes in appetite, sleep, or energy or a deep sense of despair, are not usually present. If they do occur, major depression may have developed.[35]

Moods Related to Depression

Bereavement and grieving

Dysthymia

Demoralization

Apathy

Demoralization is another cousin, but it is purely situational and lacks the intensity of depression. If you are a demoralized person, you have given up trying to improve a difficult situation. "Burnout" is one form of demoralization (see chapter 5). As men age, they may lose zest for life, interest in work, or passion in their marriage. They "sleep walk" through life and feel as if nothing they do really matters. Men who are depressed are often demoralized too.

Apathy is yet another syndrome that can look a lot like depression. Apathy is a state of uncaring indifference. There is a profound lack of motivation, similar to the absence of goal-directed behavior among men with damage to the frontal lobes of the brain. Apathy in older men is usually associated with cognitive impairment caused by cardiovascular and brain diseases. The brain diseases that produce apathy also result in dementia. Alzheimer's disease, the most common cause of dementia in men, produces apathy that is progressively more severe and disabling in that men will lose the desire to do things even before the disease affects their cognitive ability to do them.

Should You Consider Taking an Antidepressant?

While medications can help relieve the various symptoms of depression, they should not be seen as a cure. Furthermore, it is important to know that they come with risks—both physical and psychological. It is essential that you weigh the advantages and disadvantages of taking antidepressants, so that you can make an informed decision about whether a particular medication is right for you.

Bereavement and grieving are common in late life as we experience the loss of loved ones and friends. Bereavement may look and feel similar to depression and can certainly affect a person's health and function, but it is not depression. Loss of appetite, difficulty sleeping, problems with concentration and memory, and an overwhelming sense of loneliness and despair are symptoms that bereavement and depression have in common. However, grieving as a result of a loved one's death has a clear cause, and it typically lessens gradually over several months. Sometimes, with the loss of a child, spouse, or partner, the grieving may persist indefinitely under the surface. It is when excessive guilt, hopelessness, impaired function, or suicidal thoughts persist after several months of grieving that you should seek special help.

Other Major Mental Illnesses in Later Life

Anxiety is the most common symptom of psychological depression; however, in *generalized anxiety disorder* there is a high level of anxiety almost all the time, regardless of circumstance. Phobias and posttraumatic stress disorders are examples of anxiety disorders in which overwhelming fear or panic can be triggered more by perceived than actual danger. A social anxiety disorder is a condition in which someone becomes anxious and extremely self-conscious around other people, particularly strangers, and stays in the backdrop of social situations or avoids them altogether. Obsessive-compulsive disorder can be a disabling form of anxiety disorder in which any disruption of routine, ritual, or order becomes intolerable. These conditions typically begin early in life. Anxiety disorders beginning in late life, however, are usually due to depression, medical disorders, neurologic diseases, or medications. Escalating or new-onset alcohol abuse can indicate a newly developing or worsening anxiety disorder or depression.

Bipolar disorder is a distinctive mood disorder affecting about 2 percent of the adult population,[36] and its onset occurs earlier in men than in women.[37] It is characterized by discrete periods of depression followed by excessive energy, intense and dramatic reactions to events, rapid and excessive speech, decreased need for sleep, getting involved in many new and unrealistic ventures, impulsive behavior such as overspending and sexual indiscretions, driving too fast, and disinhibited behavior that may be uncharacteristically offensive or arrogant. When elevated, men may be euphoric, but often with much irritability. In severe form, exaggerated beliefs and grandiose delusions can form. The "manic" episodes may occur several times a year or may be experienced only once or twice in a man's lifetime. Debilitating depressions also typically occur in bipolar disorder. The frequency of episodes may increase as men age.

Bipolar disorder tends to present in young adulthood but may develop before that. However, it is often diagnosed for the first time in middle age or old age, and in these cases symptoms have usually been present years before the diagnosis. Less severe forms of the illness are much more common, with the low- and high-energy periods having symptoms with much less severity. Both severe and milder forms of the "bipolar spectrum" can show seasonality, with high-energy times (mania or the less severe hypomania) coming in spring and fall. Treatment of these cyclical mood disorders relies primarily on "mood-stabilizing" medications, and in most cases people do well. Nonmedical treatments are very helpful as well. Counseling, sleep hygiene, managing stress, and proper diet can be helpful. If a person does not stick with treatment, the social consequences can be devastating and include divorce, loss of career, bankruptcy, substance abuse, and legal problems. This illness has an increased risk for cognitive impairment and possibly dementia.[38]

Schizophrenia is a chronic mental illness that manifests in abnormal thinking and sensory perceptions. The delusional thinking can include auditory hallucinations, and the disorder may cause major disability through impaired executive functions such as muted motivation, poor judgment and insight, and underdeveloped interpersonal skills. Schizophrenia usually develops in adolescence or young adulthood and is more common in men. The onset of schizophrenic-like symptoms among older men is often due to medical issues, neurological problems, or severe mood disorders. Men with schizophrenia from the baby-boom generation have additional health problems because of their high rates of cigarette smoking and neglect of physical health care. They grow older in poorer health and with fewer financial and social resources. Many middle-aged and older men with schizophrenia are winding up in nursing homes, which may provide food, warmth, basic care, human contact, and safety but leave much to be desired in terms of cost to society and quality of life for the person with the illness.

Attention deficit disorder (ADD) is typically considered a disorder of childhood, and many people do "grow out of it" as they enter adulthood. The progressive development of the brain's frontal lobes through adolescence and young adulthood allows better focus and impulse control. It is the motor restlessness or extraneous movements ("hyperactivity") common to the condition that prompt the name *attention deficit hyperactivity disorder* (ADHD). Restlessness is not always a sign, and it can be suppressed through growth and development of the frontal regions of the brain. However, inattention, forgetfulness, impulsive behavior, and poor organizational skills may affect a man's occupational and social functioning during his entire life. Chronic lateness, procrastination, impulsive decision making, and disorganization take their toll on relationships and careers. Many men with ADD or ADHD may not have the diagnosis or realize the severity of their problem until mid- to late adulthood.

ADD and ADHD represent an extreme on the spectrum of individual differences in ability to focus, organize, and prioritize. When adult men with ADD or ADHD come to realize that they have the disorder, they can change their lives for the better, especially with effective treatment. You can use stimulant medications, such as methylphenidate or dextroamphetamine, and psychotherapy and life coaching to help simplify and prioritize are also very helpful.

PSYCHOLOGICAL ADAPTATION TO LATER LIFE

If you are adapting well to later life, you are likely to be balanced and flexible in your thinking and attitudes, make decisions that are based more on reality and less on fear, may be less anxious and therefore more even-tempered, may be less competitive and more nurturing, and may be more generous with your time in teaching and helping others. If this sounds like you, you can expect that others will more likely view you as being wise, because you maintain active social roles as a mentor or leader. Of course, underlying these idealized traits of later-life maturity are states of mind that may take decades to master. To better understand the mental attitudes that facilitate adaptation to old age, we conclude by examining three concepts.

The Concept of Impermanence

Change is inevitable; human relationships and living circumstances rarely last a lifetime. The Buddhist concept of impermanence is useful to consider: acceptance of change and the transient nature of life's circumstances can lead to greater appreciation of the present moment and ability to adapt. When we embrace the inevitable—our changing health, the loss of someone or something we cherish—we are more likely to take full advantage of what we have. For a man to appreciate the finality of life is to understand how precious every day is in whatever form, for there is always something to be savored. As we age, we may be more apt to appreciate a day without pain, or another day with a spouse recently diagnosed with cancer. With time, we learn many lessons of impermanence. Studies of men's aging indicate that healthy adaptation to impermanence is influenced by how well a man applies these lessons, and it does seem that older men learn to avoid situations that distress them or make them sad.[39] When we fully accept mortality and the transient nature of being, we will be better prepared for whatever may come. For example, if you live long enough or develop certain disabilities, you will likely have to give up driving. For men who are city dwellers or those with family nearby, this transition may be barely noticed. For men living independently in rural and suburban settings for whom driving is crucial to remaining independent, being able to adapt to the loss of driving privileges requires a willingness to change habits. Spending time with others, especially friends, as you accept rides may make you wonder why you didn't share trips to the grocery store, club, and church earlier. If we anticipate changes and can be psychologically ready for them, the transitions will be accomplished with a lower risk of depression.

The Concept of Ego Flexibility

Acceptance of change will better enable you to "roll with the punches" and tolerate the fickle nature of fate. Conversely, the more reliant you are on things staying as they are, the more you are at risk of depression if you lose the person to whom you are most attached or move from the place with which you most identify. A man's ego (or sense of self) must conform to unfolding realities, even if they are unexpected. Winning a large sum of money in a lottery or later-life grandparenthood can be as stressful and identity changing as selling the home your children grew up in. Men who score high on measures of adaptability and "ego flexibility" are at lower risk of depression as they age. They are able to adjust to changes with less disruption to their happiness, pride, and sense of purpose in life. Older men who have been able to develop flexibility are able to maintain a more positive perspective.[40]

The Concept of Ego Continuity

Although the ability to adapt to circumstances of life is important to aging well, there is another side to this. It is also important for men to maintain some continuity of ego (or sense of identity). Your values, ties to family and friends, long-time possessions, and unique life story can be critical to happiness. In therapy groups of older adults, a popular activity is to promote life review and reminiscence. The creation of a coherent life story can restore a man's feeling of comfort and improve his morale by encouraging recognition that there has been much consistency in his beliefs and behavior through the years.

As we age, we transition to many new life chapters—from retirement, to living with chronic disabilities, to leaving behind a community to move to better climates or be closer to children and grandchildren. In these cases, we must be strong enough to maintain our sense of self among the new realities of life. Maintaining hobbies, becoming closer to our spouse or

Memory Boxes

In some long-term care facilities, there are often "memory boxes" hanging outside the doorways of the residents' rooms. The memory boxes generally contain photographs and mementos evocative of different periods in the residents' past. These displays can help people with dementia remember themselves and help ground them among the disjointed, confusing experiences of their daily lives.

No less important, they give the paid caregivers an extended view of the residents' lives, allowing them to see that the disoriented, forgetful person under their care was once a star of the high school football team, a gifted musician, a loving husband, a skilled carpenter, a scholar of history, a captain of the local police force, or a favorite uncle. These fragments of our life stories are woven into an identity that men can carry into old age as refuge from the sometime disruptive effect of widowerhood and loss of friends, home, and health.

partner, staying in touch with friends, or maintaining some connection to our work or recreational interests can all be very comforting during periods of transition.

SUMMARY

The transitions through middle age and into later life present many challenges to men. Few people will negotiate these years without some unexpected and unwanted changes. Yet, we have within us the capacity to meet these challenges and thrive in the last decades of our lives. Even in late life, our bodies, brains, and spirit retain the ability to change and evolve in ways that can bring us contentment and increased receptivity and deep appreciation for those moments of real joy that may come at any time.

CHAPTER 5

Men's Stress and Health

Stress was originally an engineering term referring to the pressure of an external force against a resisting body. Stories about social stress now far outnumber reports about surface wind stress. The causes of social stress, although they vary depending on a person's age, financial resources, and friends, are all cultural and social—and they can be as powerful as a natural force like the wind.[1]

By the mid-1950s, medical sociologists and health psychologists were routinely calling attention to the pressures men experienced: at work and as breadwinners, as husbands and fathers, and when facing retirement. The researchers first recognized that stress affects heart health, and now we know that chronic psychological stress or even an accumulation of negative and positive life disruptions weakens the immune system,[2] depresses mood,[3] elevates cortisol, and causes early-onset hypertension and cardiovascular disease.[4]

To begin, let's think of stress in three distinct ways. One, some degree of stress keeps us engaged and challenged. It increases arousal and alertness, enhances performance, and can lead to physiological toughness.[5] Similar to the way aerobic exercise toughens our body, seeking challenges and coping effectively with social stress are psychologically toughening and result in better health. Some positive life events (e.g., a promotion, the end of paying college tuitions) and even some unpleasant experiences (e.g., having a dentist repair a cracked tooth, preparing for your second colonoscopy) may be stressful but do not cause harm. By contrast, it is when our stress piles up that the fulcrum tips and stress becomes dangerous. Whenever the

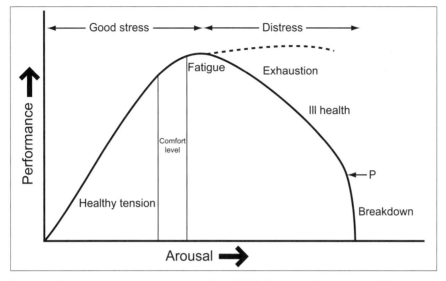

Figure 5.1. The stress response curve. From P. G. Nixon (1976). The human function curve. With special reference to cardiovascular disorders: Part I. *Practitioner, 217*, 765–770. P. G. Nixon (1976). The human function curve. With special reference to cardiovascular disorders: Part II. *Practitioner, 217*, 935–944.

number of stressors or amount of pressure exceeds our personal thresholds and defies our coping capacity, the level of arousal exhausts the body's ability to recover and clouds thinking (see stress response chart). Too much stress becomes damaging. In this sense, stress isn't an abstract concept or merely a restless state of mind. It is something real, measurable, and often dangerous—killing brain cells and challenging our heart's functional ability to the point of death.

Two, external stress needs to be distinguished from internal distress. External *stressors* (the events) include economic downturns, workplace demands, a grumpy neighbor, an empty marriage, arguments, a driveway full of snow, noise levels, or in-law troubles. By contrast, internal *distress* (our own particular response) is the effect the stressors have on us personally. It is the perceptible feeling of tension, frustration, or anxiety. External stress is as influential to our overall physiological and psychological health as our genetics.[6]

Three, stress is an individual experience. We all feel it and have to deal with it in our own way. Two men will cope with the same stress differently. In addition, what can be stressful for someone at one time may not be stressful for the same person at another time. Stress exists when we (even unconsciously) appraise a situation as taxing, a threat, and exceeding our coping resources.[7] Most men are not able to always recognize when stressors affect their lives—as men, we are encouraged to normalize the innumerable demands and inevitable setbacks, worries, and pressures regularly bearing down on us. It is what men do. However, these nearly ignored stresses can quietly chip away at the integrity of our body and our emotional resiliency. This chapter examines the physiology of stress, the known effects of stress on men's physical health and personal well-being, and strategies that best contribute to our ability to manage stress.

MASCULINITY AND STRESS

Most American men share a "masculine consciousness." Whatever our ethnic/racial heritage, social class, or politics, as men, we commonly live with the cultural expectations that define what a "man" should be. This imagined "man" has qualities such as toughness, independence, personal control, physical and sexual competence, assertiveness, being successful at all costs, and not being anything like the "ladies." Although the image of what a man is supposed to be will not be identical for a roomful of men, we all make judgments about ourselves and others based on a masculinity ideology.

> Tension is who you think you should be. Relaxation is who you are.
>
> —A Chinese proverb

Stress often arises when you believe that you are not living up to masculinity standards, or whenever a situation is interpreted as requiring "unmanly" behavior.[8]

> I asked the woman desk clerk who was in her mid-50s to find the hotel manager, and this perky little thing came up who was barely 30. I explained again that the room they assigned me wasn't what I asked for. I reserved a non-smoking room. The manager testily commented that there was no other available room; the hotel was full. It was nearly 11 p.m. and I didn't have the energy to go find another hotel. So, I bit my tongue, accepted my fate, knowing that I was going to have to pay for a smelly room for the night. As I walked back to the elevator, I could feel my blood pressure pounding in my neck! (Dave, 59-year-old man)

Stress was experienced because Dave confronted conflicting expectations and because "the man" in Dave's consciousness whispered "you wimp." He was caught between separate stressors—to fight a battle at 11 p.m. for his pride versus to stay the night in the unwanted room and not argue with the night-shift clerk.

Every one of us knows that we will fall short of the flawless manhood standard, and almost every day we find ourselves faced with contradictory expectations similar to what Dave faced. Unlike the ideal man who never experiences losses in independence, power, sexuality, and self-reliance, real men do. We are also oftentimes without a "wing man" and live with the risk of a loss of social contacts and the backing they provide.

STRESSES OF MIDDLE-AGED AND OLDER MEN

Men's hormonal reactions to stress, especially our secretion of testosterone while under stress and our lesser amounts of oxytocin, which boosts sociability, team up to sustain our festering distress for longer periods of time.[9] Fortunately, aging seems to defuse some of our physiological reaction: as we get older, we secrete less testosterone, engage in fewer "fight-or-flight" hormonal responses, and have a greater desire to tend and befriend than argue.[10]

But middle-aged and older men face distinct forms of social stress because of our age and gender. As we get older, we live with more life changes, and change—both good and bad—is stressful. Too many changes in a short period of time can overtax someone's ability to cope or adapt, leaving him more vulnerable to infection, injury, or disease.[11] As we get older, we encounter stresses more common to later life, such as leaving the workplace, living on a retirement income, the death of friends, or living with our aging body and medically related limitations. We can become overwhelmed by the "pileup" of these life changes. In the mid-1960s, a team of stress researchers identified a series of life events that are regarded as most stressful (see chart),[12] and it's not surprising that the more grave stressors are what men (and women) run up against as we get older. For example, the "readjustment" necessary when we face a "life event" such as a wife's or partner's serious illness is more likely to occur as we are aging and might occur about the time men are experiencing what it means to retire. Depending on how you interpret retirement (e.g., an end of a career, or escape from drudgery to choice), this "life event" and facing a personal illness can add up to be almost as stressful as bereavement, which is recognized as one of life's most heartbreaking, stressful experiences (see chart). Those life events that are negative and out of your control are much more predictive of distress than are positive, controllable life changes.[13]

Middle-aged and older men also face a whole new set of stresses caused by the ageism in our society. We are misperceived as healthier than

Life Events and Their Stress Rating

100	Death of a spouse or partner
73	Divorce
63	Death of close family member
53	Personal injury or illness
47	Fired at work
45	Retirement
44	Change in family member's health
39	Sexual difficulties
38	Change in financial status
37	Death of a close friend
35	Change in number of arguments with spouse
29	Son or daughter leaving home
26	Spouse stops work
20	Change in residence
18	Change in social activities
16	Change in sleeping habits

Source: Holmes, T. H., & Rahe, R. H. (1967). The social readjustment rating scale. *Journal of Psychosomatic Research, 11,* 213-218.

same-age women, even though men take more sick days than women and die earlier.[14] The misperception is especially dangerous when it comes to our psychological health. It is said that men's psychological well-being isn't as challenged as women's when our bodies age. All of these misperceptions become expectations that urge every man to continue to hide behind a mask of "I'm okay" and not admit to having fears and worries about getting older. They discourage others from asking, "How do you *feel*?"

IS STRESS A POISON?

Your new neighbor moves in with two barking dogs. Your daughter who lives alone and out of state calls to tell you she is headed to the ER because she is experiencing severe chest pain. Which ER? What's going on? These distinct stressors share one simple fact—stress is an attention getter, even if you are not consciously aware that stress is affecting you. Stress is greater when you are uncertain and do not understand what is going on. Stress is based on our (sometimes unconscious) appraisal of the situation as outside our control and as threatening. Cumulatively, stressors can become a slow poison that undermines our physical and psychological health.

STRESS AND PHYSIOLOGICAL HEALTH

How is stress poisonous? External stressors do not directly cause ill health, as might be the case when a deer tick bites and infects someone with Lyme disease. Rather, much as coastal winds affect the posture of some trees more than others, stress brings about bodily adaptations that prove to be more corrosive for some men than others. It all begins in our location on the social gradient and in the central nervous system and brain.

The social gradient reveals the social inequalities within our nation, or people's access to resources such as employment, health insurance, retirement income, housing, and diet quality.[15] Men who are lower on the totem pole and have fewer opportunities and resources to lessen the day-to-day psychological strain are at higher risk of stress-related health problems. Men with greater resources more often feel in control and are more able to defend themselves from stress.

Men who experience racial discrimination, for instance, live with more stress and have poor psychological well-being.[16] Men with more wealth have more resources for managing their (lesser) daily stresses. This stands to reason. Being white, having better employment opportunities, and earning higher incomes buffer many stressors. Even animal studies have found that the risk of stress is related to a social hierarchy—the "bottom tier" males in baboon troops are much less relaxed than the dominant males, largely because they are repeatedly challenged by the dominant males. Their stress hormones are not able to return to normal levels, and they are more likely to suffer from cardiovascular disorders such as atherosclerosis and hypertension.[17] People who feel that they cannot control their fate are much more likely to live with the ill effects of stress.[18]

Two neuroendocrine systems are specific to the stress-health connection. About the time of the Great Depression and thus only a generation after Darwin's theory of evolution, a Harvard physiologist (Walter Cannon) persuasively argued that the human organism is, similar to all other organisms, continuously adapting to its environment—whether the environmental "demands" are forces like the weather or what people *perceive* as personal challenges.[19] He theorized that the body seeks balance, or homeostasis. Using his analogy, when the weather is hot, the body sweats to allow evaporation to help cool the skin. When we have an infection, antibodies are produced to fight the germs. And when we encounter an external threat, our bodies engage in a fight-or-flight (or stress) response that mobilizes us for the perceived emergency.

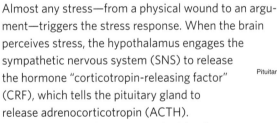

The Stress Response

Almost any stress—from a physical wound to an argument—triggers the stress response. When the brain perceives stress, the hypothalamus engages the sympathetic nervous system (SNS) to release the hormone "corticotropin-releasing factor" (CRF), which tells the pituitary gland to release adrenocorticotropin (ACTH).

The flooding of ACTH into the bloodstream, along with direct signals from the brain sent through the autonomic nervous system, stimulates the adrenal glands to secrete the stress hormones cortisol and epinephrine (adrenaline) into the bloodstream.

Cortisol and epinephrine help provide more energy and oxygen. They stimulate the heart, the brain, and other muscles and organs to amplify the body's response.

When the brain perceives that the stress has ended, hormones are returned to their baseline.

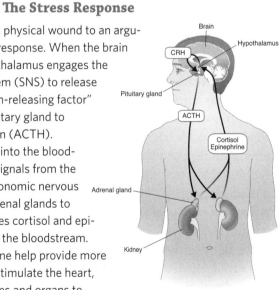

Physiology of stress response

The fight-or-flight response is defensive and self-protective. It is a biochemical reflex, just as antibodies are a defensive response to an infection. Imagine that you are trudging uphill in the dark in late November to the parking lot where your car is parked, and as you are climbing the walkway you hear the rattling of dog tags. Though it may seem like you *heard* the tags rattling barely milliseconds earlier and then envisioned milliseconds later the likelihood of a dog rapidly running at you, in fact when we experience a perceived threat the brain and body interact well before we are consciously aware. The perceived threat of a rushing dog triggers the immune, nervous, and neuroendocrine systems to prepare the body for the possible attack. What occurs, according to Hans Selye,[20] is that the brain and the endocrine system synchronize, immediately setting about a host of physiological responses—the hypothalamus at the base of the brain triggers the secretion of an array of hormones into the blood, including adrenaline and cortisol; glucose, simple proteins, and fats pour out of fat cells and muscles for a rapid mobilization of energy; heart rate increases to speed the transportation of nutrients and oxygen; and both the brain and the pituitary release endorphins and enkephalins, which are opiate-like hormones designed to limit the impending pain. All of this occurs in order to ensure our survival. It's primitive, instinctive. While these amazing physiological processes worked well for our prehistoric ancestors who came face to face with predators, they're not as useful in our postmodern world. Very rarely in our normal lives do we need to respond in prehistoric programmed ways to every perceived challenge, as if every stress required an immediate, intense physical effort to survive.

Yet that is what our bodies do, day after day. Put on a heart monitor with a digital readout and watch your heart rate climb multiple times as you slug your way through the accordion of highway speedups and brake slamming during rush hour. When you awake from a claustrophobic dream with a shortness of breath or grit your teeth when a telemarketer interrupts dinner, your neuroendocrine systems have secreted hormones, taken control of heart activity, and regulated many other body functions to weather the challenge.

The problem is that, with the way that it is hardwired, the brain doesn't distinguish one threat from another: a (perceived) threat is simply a threat, and the fight-or-flight reflex is activated. When *any* threat is presented, the brain signals the alert and the body mobilizes defensive reactions. The health-related problem isn't complicated—the human body has a finite reserve of adaptive energy. When you live with the chronic stress that usually involves too many demands and too little personal control, or when you face a prolonged accumulation of many disruptions (your car is towed because the "Do not park here on game day" sign is posted 10 feet higher than other signs, the impound yard is closed and you must rent a hotel room to wait it out, your briefcase is locked in the trunk, you end up late for work on Monday, etc.), your brain keeps the body in full-scale mobilization. This "survival" response actually ends up with the body at war with itself. The stress response becomes more damaging than the original stressors.

Here's the good news: initially in animal studies and later in human studies, researchers have demonstrated that when we are repeatedly exposed to certain stressors, we can become a bit immune to these stressors. We develop stress tolerance. As we learn to distinguish among challenges (e.g., a baby crying versus screaming), our brain is *conditioned* to recognize these stressors as ordinary.[21] The intense arousal isn't required. Similarly, whenever we encounter a challenging task in situations where we have high levels of personal control,[22] these "manageable" stress situations do not require energy-demanding responses. In both cases, only some of the stress hormones are released—the catecholamines (epinephrine, norepinephrine, and dopamine) are released and your heart rate and blood pressure increase, but cortisol levels are not elevated.

A word of caution: even though stress tolerance can be acquired and is desirable, learning to appraise stressors and manage stressful situations does not mean that our body's responsiveness to even normal stress is devoid of long-term ill effects. Recall the times you came home from an ordinary day at work and found yourself unexpectedly napping; your body was trying to recover from the pileup of the many ordinary, challenging, and stressful workday demands. Even when managing little stressors, the brain repeatedly triggers our primitive neurophysiological stress response. The brain is only conditioned not to *over*react. The body does not work as hard with these normal stressors, compared to what occurs when we face novel threatening situations. In addition, as we become older, our epinephrine (also known as adrenaline) and norepinephrine (also known as noradrenaline) levels are greater in a normal "resting state"; in other words, when older men encounter a stressful situation, hormone levels rise higher than they did in middle age and younger, and it takes older men longer to physiologically recover from the stress response.

Stress Consequences

Stress has become a major factor affecting men's health. The tension and emotional strain of day-to-day living have been linked to heart disease, high blood pressure, migraine headaches, diabetes, cancer, and a weakened immune response to disease.

AROUSAL AND PHYSICAL HEALTH RISKS

Some of the hormones associated with the stress response, notably epinephrine and cortisol, purposively raise blood pressure and cholesterol levels to help us physiologically survive immediate threats, but they end up putting us at much greater risk for everything from colds to an accelerated rate of cancer cell growth.

The stress-related mind-body response is most malevolent to our heart and cardiovascular system, increasing our risk of hypertension, myocardial infarction, and stroke. The hormone epinephrine that is flooded into the bloodstream causes fatty nutrients to form, and the long-term result is a thickening of the artery walls and narrowing of the blood vessels, or "hardening of the arteries." The secretion of epinephrine and norepinephrine also contributes to elevated blood lipid levels and increased blood clotting. Think in terms of the primitive stress response as cardiovascular reactivity: the frequent and large increases in blood pressure and heart rate strain the muscle integrity of blood vessels and the heart.

The relaxed heart rate for a middle-aged man is around 60–70 beats per minute. Moderate stress can raise the pulse rate to 100, and when we are facing more severe stress, the pulse rate can rise to 160–200 beats per minute. The work situation of air traffic controllers sharply increases their blood pressure, and a 20-year follow-up study revealed that these men had a long-term risk of hypertension (where the systolic blood pressure regularly exceeds 160).[23] Many other workplaces silently contribute to men's health problems and earlier death.[24] The effect of prolonged stress is compounded when we are unable to get the amount of sleep we need and/or when there is a paucity of supportive friends to help us diminish the ill effects of stressful situations. Fortunately, as we get older, we have had more experience with managing most stressful situations and do not experience the same degree of physiological reactivity.

Biomedical research supports the warning that the pileup of stress increases our susceptibility to infections. The immune system produces two types of white blood cells (lymphocytes) to promote immunities, the T-cell and B-cell. T-cells are created by the thymus gland to fight bacterial and some viral infections. Every time the stress hormone cortisol suppresses immune function, it depresses T-cell functioning and can promote long-term, persistent inflammation. Stress shuts down digestion (you might notice dry mouth and a lack of saliva) at the same time it impairs immune function, giving the *Helicobacter pylori* bacteria that contribute to ulcers an opportunity to flourish.[25] These physiological responses also prove advantageous for some kinds of cancer.[26]

Prolonged exposure to stress also seems to increase our risk of diabetes and memory problems. Health researchers find that when you're stressed out, there is a risk of weight gain because elevated cortisol levels slow metabolism.[27] Diabetes is a metabolic disorder linked to the metabolic syndrome[28] and its cluster of risk factors (e.g., abdominal obesity, low

Physical Signs and Symptoms of Stress for Men

- Clenched jaws and grinding teeth
- Shallow breathing; shortness of breath
- Increased perspiration
- High blood pressure
- Chest pain
- Overeating and/or frequent snacking
- Diminished (sometimes, increased) sex drive
- Erectile difficulties

- Muscle tightening, back and neck pain
- Fatigue and exhaustion
- Headaches
- Nausea, maybe dizziness
- Tight, dry, or a feeling of a lump in your throat
- Digestive disturbances; indigestion, constipation, and/or diarrhea

concentrations of high-density lipoproteins [HDLs], or "good" cholesterol). The stress hormone cortisol is an insulin antagonist that elevates blood glucose levels, severely challenging the well-being of men who live with undiagnosed diabetes. In addition, when cortisol continually enters the brain, it seems to damage hippocampal formation and our memory.[29] Ever experienced momentary forgetfulness when distressed? That is a symptom of the stress–(ill) health connection. In sum, stress is like a poison that can affect our immune, cardiovascular, digestive, and neurological systems. It is a real killer.

STRESS AND PSYCHOLOGICAL HEALTH

When stress is unchecked, it can erode our psychological health and quality of life. For instance, you might think that more frequent raiding of the refrigerator and a modest uptake in calories is quite benign, if not harmless. You might also think that nagging shoulder muscle tightness is just a sign of a lack of good sleep or your occasional circadian-type low-energy dip. Each of these experiences is surely related to your energy level and sleep, but they are also warnings of the buildup of psychological distress that you may be ignoring.

If you are like most men, you probably pay little attention to your emotional health. This is partly because men do not have an "emotional pulse." Unlike women, we've been encouraged to ignore feelings, and men learn to distract themselves from their moods by engaging in physical and task-oriented activities. Men usually respond to emotional distress by not thinking about it, whereas women are more likely to mull over the problem. What's more, we learn to interpret negative *feelings* in somatic terms. We end up bottling up and squirreling away the psychological stress in our muscles, arteries, and gut. This is called *somaticizing* the stress: converting distress into headaches, muscle tension in the neck and shoulders, digestive disturbances, or an abdominal gut-wrenching pain. Behind the mask of being in control often lurks grumpiness and anger, and since we are not often penalized for it, we express our distress in a manner that Hollywood depicts as "manly," such as uncorking into a "Mel Gibson rant," slinging cutting remarks and in the process wounding people you live or work with. Stress-related psychological difficulties can escalate into burnout, one of many clinical anxiety disorders, or posttraumatic stress.

Psychological Signs and Symptoms of Stress

- Mood swings
- Irritability, anger
- Restless anxiety, inability to relax
- Anxious, racing thoughts
- Feeling overwhelmed
- Inability to concentrate
- Insomnia or fitful sleep
- Worry

- Lack of confidence
- Loss of interest in sex
- Dissatisfaction with work, friends
- Sense of loneliness and isolation
- Depression
- Sadness
- Preference for solitude rather than being with others

BURNOUT

Prolonged stress can result in stress exhaustion or burnout. In burnout our emotions are blunted, whereas when stressed our emotions are heightened and reactive. Should the unremitting stress of daily hassles at work or at home have you feeling overextended and completely worn out, as if the tank is empty, you may be burnt out. When this happens, the littlest everyday problems seem insurmountable, and it's difficult to rally enough energy to really care—let alone do something. Your emotional resources are depleted. You feel demoralized.

Burnout differs from depression in that burnout typically involves stresses linked to a particular situation, such as your work and workplace or your home life, whereas depression globally affects a person's life. Burnout is defined by three dimensions: overwhelming exhaustion, feelings of cynicism, and a sense of ineffectiveness. It can occur when men are the 24/7 caregivers for an ill wife; when there are unrealistic expectations at work and you must always be "on," and the workplace is ripe with the politics and power struggles that make it hard to get excited about your work; or when the distinction between being at work and time away from work becomes very blurred because you are required to make yourself available, perhaps always carrying a beeper.

Burnout isn't just a state of mind. There is an excess of circulating glucose in the bloodstream triggered by chronic stress, and this blocks insulin production and inhibits the body from converting fats into needed energy. Chronic stress literally drains you. The feeling of being overloaded and physical exhaustion become a double-barrel assault on your health. Your immune system suffers, making you increasingly susceptible to viruses. We all have run up against stress exhaustion at one time or another—we crash. But the men who regularly suffer stress exhaustion are also aware of the unrelenting demands and unsupportive environment around them. It's not uncommon to experience appetite disruption, sleep problems, restless anxiety, and irritability.

Contrary to common sense, burnout is not a recognized clinical psychological disorder. Despite being similar to both depression and anxiety disorders, burnout is much more common—there are estimates that suggest that half of all physicians, teachers and professors, police officers, technical personnel in hospital settings, and ministers have experienced burnout.[30] A common denominator to the types of work that result in greater burnout is "people work" and the expectation to either display or suppress emotions on the job;[31] for example, ER physicians and nurses can become blunted and unable to be emotionally empathic.

Signs and Symptoms of Burnout

- Emotionally worn down
- Exhaustion, headaches, and trouble sleeping
- Negativity—being more cynical, irritable, impatient
- You lack the energy to be productive
- Self-doubt, and feeling unappreciated

- Lack of any positive feelings
- Feeling overwhelmed, foggy thinking
- Feeling disillusioned about work, life
- You drink to feel better, or just not feel
- Feelings of incompetence
- Lack of achievement

Men facing burnout immediately benefit by becoming more physically active, seeking better sleep, and reevaluating their nutrition in order to eat well. Sounds simple, but men often find it difficult to enact all of these positive changes. It is important to try to alter the daily schedule, reward yourself once completing a task with a well-earned coffee break, and take mini-vacations to escape the rituals. You need to give yourself the "Atta-boy" congratulations you deserve. Soaking in a hot tub, having a massage, and/or getting acupuncture to relieve nagging muscle tension caused by stress, as well as taking up one of the strategies of meditation (see below in treatment for anxiety), are all invaluable ways to manage burnout, once it's noticed.

ANXIETY

Anxiety is a normal reaction, and it is not the same thing as fear. As a mood or feeling, anxiety refers to the apprehensiveness, nervousness, restlessness, and tension we experience when faced with stressful situations. Anxiety is situational and related to a lack of mastery—ever hesitate to jump off a high diving board? Anxiety symptoms are similar to the signs of fear and may include trembling, headaches, sweating, elevated blood pressure, and changes in heart rate. But the ill ease of anxiety is when we do not feel in control of a situation. Anxiety can also arise from social changes that we do not control yet experience, such as an economic recession, and a poor diet, particularly low levels of vitamin B12.

All of us worry and feel anxious at times about our health, money, or family problems. It is when you are preoccupied about things, when you continue to ruminate, and when you feel a lack of confidence to manage the challenge that your anxiety level is no longer "normal." Anxiety disorders have the same physical and emotional symptoms as commonplace anxieties, but the symptoms are more severe, debilitating, and/or intrusive. Regrettably, anxiety disorders are understudied conditions in older adults. From what we know, about 10 percent of adult men meet the criteria for an anxiety disorder in any one year.[32] Adult men with a generalized anxiety disorder (GAD) experience almost constant, exaggerated worry and apprehension, even when there is little to provoke the feelings. Most people who experience the hyperarousal that distinguishes an anxiety disorder began dealing with the symptoms long before becoming middle-aged adults.

Adult men may experience a disturbing event, such as a terrible flight during a violent thunderstorm or witnessing a car hit a motorcycle and hurl the rider, and then begin to live with anxiety symptoms whenever there is a forecast for a pending thunderstorm or they see a driver tailgating. These

Signs and Symptoms of Anxiety

- Twitching or trembling
- Muscle tension, headaches
- Restlessness or feeling keyed up or on edge
- Dry mouth, trouble swallowing
- Rapid breathing; rapid or irregular heart rate
- Emotional flipping (marked mood swings)

- Emotional numbness
- Irritability, loss of temper
- Sleeping difficulties, weird dreams
- Decreased concentration
- Nausea, lack of appetite
- Avoidance behavior

"new-onset" anxiety problems are not uncommon among middle-aged and older men, but they are rarely treated. For instance, men who have been recently told that they have a heart condition may start to worry and fret, much more than their physician expected. They overcompensate and become "cardiac invalids." Their anxiety percolates, and it can become debilitating. Anxiety disorders are observed among men approaching retirement or just after retirement, or when their own sexual functioning declines. The clinical reality is that most cases of anxiety disorder in later life remain undetected and untreated.[33]

Treatment

There isn't one treatment that's best. There are many strategies to treat anxiety, and not all of them will be proper for you. In fact, what might be effective treatment for some men won't be for others. You will need to think about yourself and your willingness to manage your anxiety and, with the advice of others, decide what options can work for you. Unlike depending on pharmaceuticals, holistic approaches to treating anxiety combine several effective methods, starting with changes in your diet and lifestyle. Typically, you take up regular exercise, find time every day for relaxation, use herbal-based or prescription medicine, and, often, undergo psychological therapy for anxiety to help you reprogram your mind and stress reaction.

Regular exercise. The recommendation for staying healthy in mind and body is 30 minutes of regular exercise every day. The way exercise affects the mind and body is detailed in chapter 3, but for right now the message is simple: regular exercise releases the stress stored in our muscles, floods the brain with "good feeling" hormones, and encourages less fitful sleep;

as a result, fewer symptoms of anxiety will occur. Exercise is vital in every treatment plan.

Relaxation exercise. Some men can benefit from a number of very good relaxation exercises. These mind-body treatments teach you breathing strategies and movements to help relax your body and balance your body chemistry. Many of the exercises are Asian in origin, such as qigong, which could involve meditative training and visualization on specific ideas, sounds, images, concepts, or breathing patterns, and Tai Chi, which involves dynamic training, including special movements. Yoga combines physical postures, breathing exercises, and meditation and is one of the top relaxation practices.

Psychological treatment. Perhaps the most common, well-established, and highly effective anxiety therapy is *cognitive behavioral therapy* (CBT). It focuses on identifying, understanding, and changing your thinking and behavior. More often than not, benefits are seen quickly, sometimes within a month, other times within 12–16 weeks. In CBT, you are actively involved in your healing and have a sense of mastery. CBT can be used with or without drugs. But it is our belief, based on research, that CBT is better than turning to pharmaceuticals.

Medication. Treating anxiety with medication is generally safe and effective, though medication will not cure an anxiety disorder. It can keep the anxiety under control. Use of antianxiety and antidepressant medication necessitates a physician visit and a prescription for the medication. You will need to talk with your doctor about what's going on in order to receive the right medication and correct dosage and to minimize the danger of unwanted side effects. High-potency benzodiazepines (such as clonazepam and alprazolam) are successful in combating anxiety and have few side effects (other than drowsiness). At times, selective serotonin reuptake inhibitors (SSRIs—citalopram, escitalopram, fluoxetine, paroxetine, and sertraline) are prescribed because they relieve symptoms by blocking the reabsorption of serotonin within brain cells. This leaves more serotonin available, which improves positive mood. There are also serotonin-norepinephrine reuptake inhibitors (SNRIs—venlafaxine and duloxetine) to increase levels of the neurotransmitters serotonin and norepinephrine.

POSTTRAUMATIC STRESS

Exposure to trauma is not a rare event, and it is estimated that more than half of all American men have been exposed to at least one traumatic event in the course of their lives.[34] Exposure can lead to depression and posttraumatic stress symptoms well after the event. Unlike most stress-related disorders, posttraumatic distress does not feature anxiety as a primary presenting symptom. Four types of symptoms are characteristic: reexperiencing, avoidance, numbing, and hyperarousal. Originally a diagnostic category for only war trauma, our understanding of posttraumatic stress disorder (PTSD) has improved since 1980, when it was first introduced in the *Diagnostic and Statistical Manual of Mental Disorders (DSM)*.

Most men experiencing a traumatic event recover within a reasonable amount of time and do not develop posttraumatic stress. Traumatic events typically involve several stimuli, including sights, sounds, and smells. An awful car accident, for instance, is etched in slow-motion visual memory, the wrenching sounds of the crash, the rusty to metallic smell of blood, and the oddly, near-rational rhythm of EMTs taking over and transporting the injured person to medical care. Combat-related trauma is similarly coded in memory with all its chaos of voices, explosions, weather, smells, and visual images.

Posttraumatic stress and PTSD are now applied to men who suffer from a wide variety of noncombat-related traumas. Each involves a threat to the integrity of the self. A terrifying, triggering event buried in our biographies may involve a physical assault, living through a life-threatening myocardial infarction or a natural disaster such as a flash flood, a major injury arising from a motor vehicle accident, or witnessing a violent death.

Brief History of PTSD

The definition of PTSD has broadened since psychologists began treating Vietnam War veterans. Combat-related PTSD is thought to be a present-day version of "battle fatigue" and "shell shock," which is psychological breakdown found to occur during the stresses of war. As early as the Civil War, some men were described as having the condition "nostalgia" and were reassigned to less stressful duties. During World War I, soldiers were thought to suffer from the proximity of exploding shells, hence the "shell shock" label. Their posttraumatic stress was thought to be organic, related to the concussion of the exploding shells. By World War II, clinical experts now assumed that trauma wasn't organic and any soldier could break down under the trauma of war. "Battle-fatigued" men were temporarily reassigned to rest, and by the Korean War, the men were removed from the front line and given their R & R in Japan. The post-Vietnam era began to recognize the longevity of the symptoms of war trauma, even if the men (and women) had been asymptomatic for years.

Source: Karner, T. X. (2008). Post-traumatic stress disorder and older men: If only time healed all wounds. *Generations, 32* (1), 82–87.

Whenever painful symptoms fundamentally undercut ordinary life, recovering from the trauma may take considerable time. In some cases there occurs an extended "latency" period where the man is asymptomatic for months or years. Men who do not psychologically recuperate will repeatedly relive their trauma and can progressively become more distressed. These men are living with a PTSD, which researchers estimate affects 5 percent of American men.[35]

For men with PTSD, the traumatic event remains vivid and disabling, sometimes for decades or a lifetime. It is a dominating experience and retains its power to call to mind the terror, dread, or grief through daytime intrusive memories and nightmares. The intrusive thoughts and memories seem to be responsible for why men with PTSD continue to be owned by the trauma well after it occurred. Some men will relive the triggering event with all its disturbing visual and auditory recollections. Other men may experience sleep problems, depression, feeling numb and empty, or being easily startled. It is not uncommon for men with PTSD to lose interest in

Symptoms of PTSD

Reexperiencing Symptoms

- Frequent memories or upsetting thoughts
- Having recurring nightmares
- Flashbacks; feeling the event recur

- Feeling strong distress when reminded of the event
- Experiencing a surge in heart rate or sweating

Avoidance Symptoms

- Making effort to avoid discussion of the event
- Avoiding places and people you associate with the event
- Trouble remembering details of the event

- Losing interest in important activities
- Not having positive feelings, such as happiness

Hyperarousal Symptoms

- Disrupted sleep or trouble falling asleep
- Feeling more irritable and angry

- Having difficulty concentrating
- Feeling constantly on guard
- Jumpy, easily startled

Source: Blake, D. D., Weathers, F. W., Nagy, L. M., et al. (1990). A clinician rating scale for assessing current and lifetime PTSD: The CAPS-I. *Behavior Therapist, 13,* 187–188.

being with people they used to enjoy or have trouble feeling affectionate. Their "psychic numbing" is a coping strategy to try to obliterate the trauma-based memories and feelings. They may lose interest in most things.

Do you think you have PTSD? Use the following four questions as an assessment: have you ever had any experience that was so frightening, horrible, or upsetting that, in the past month, you

1. have had nightmares about it or thought about it when you did not want to?

2. tried hard not to think about it or went out of your way to avoid situations that reminded you of it?

3. were constantly on guard, watchful, or easily startled?

4. felt numb or detached from others, activities, or your surroundings?

If you answer "yes" to any three items, you should think about seeing a professional.[36] Talk to a physician or mental health professional or religious leader. If you are a veteran, contact your local VA hospital or vet center. Do not hesitate to tell a close friend and family member that you think you have PTSD. The treatments currently available for men with PTSD are CBT, bright light therapy, individual and group dynamic psychotherapy, and medication.

WHAT PROTECTS US FROM STRESS?

Distress varies by our availability of friends and social support and the comparisons we make between ourselves and other men. The way we compare ourselves to others affects our level of distress. In terms of the social comparisons we make, imagine a ladder and you standing on one of the rungs. Men who routinely look upward and compare themselves to others above them often feel distressed and "trapped," rather than confident and hopeful. A fairly wealthy white man may be dissatisfied and distressed with his station in life, if he perceives those around him as more successful. Thinking that someone else is better off than you provides two pieces of negative information: you are not as well off as many others, and it is possible for you to get worse.[37] This man's cortisol level would lessen if he used a comparison group similar to his own "station" in life. For example, an older Latino who earns a modest income and judges the adequacy of his financial health by comparing himself to his friends, neighbors, and close relatives is likely to feel satisfied with life. Even though his financial health is ranked lower on the totem pole than many other men, his comparisons were his equals. Furthermore, when we see others as less fortunate and genuinely feel compassion or reach out to volunteer support, we interact with other supportive people and receive validation, which leads to more stress resilience.[38]

The coping strategies men often draw on backfire and fuel rather than mitigate stress. When a "typical guy" has a bad day, he doesn't want to talk about it. He is not interested in reaching out to friends for support. Rather than dealing with stress by "tending and befriending,"[39] the typical guy internalizes the stress. He may decide to be by himself or brood. At the end of a stressful day, have you been brooding about things and then gotten frustrated with little things, like water from the sink splashing on your shirt or the phone ringing a third time in a row and interrupting your rest? Brooding and choosing to "shut down" are corrosive.

What protects us, however, are friends and lovers. Men's go-to stress absorber is support from a woman.[40] When men reach out to another man for support, our distress is not often reduced enough. Perhaps the reason is the way men communicate with one another—trading stories about our stressed-out days. It can be difficult for heterosexual or gay men to diffuse their pent-up stress if one-upmanship conversations keep the stress hormones elevated. But getting together with other men is most often a relaxing time-out and helps avoid the brooding. Stressed out? Go "hang out" with friends. Friends reduce the damaging effects of the stress hormone cortisol by distracting us, often making us laugh, and keeping us active. Don't stop returning e-mails, calling your buddies, or going out with your group when you are feeling stressed. Friend therapy is protective. If you want to expand your friend group, take a class, join a gym or club, attend a church or temple, or volunteer.

MANAGING STRESS

Men with good emotional health have an ability to bounce back from stress and misfortune. This ability is called *resilience*. They remain flexible and positive in bad times as well as good. The good news is that there are many steps you can take to build your resilience and your overall emotional health. But you are going to have to overcome some of the beliefs and practices we acquire as a result of growing up as men. For example, men tend to distract themselves from their mood by engaging in physical or instrumental activities; while these activities are stress reducing, they are "downstream" strategies for dealing with stress after the body and mind are knarred.

Upstream management strategies are best, and there are four essential ways of managing stress. First, keep your body healthy so that the stress you experience doesn't take an added toll on your heart and brain. Exercising regularly not only improves your physical health but also floods the body with endorphins (your body's "feel good" chemicals) and reduces the stress hormone cortisol.

Second, try to prevent the unnecessary buildup of the stresses. Here are a pair of examples: prioritize things and unplug yourself. If you're like other men, your life is overscheduled and demanding. Your objective is to learn to prioritize what you have to do and to have reasonable expectations that better assure achievable goals. It's not reasonable to always be the go-to guy and do everything others might expect. Become someone who understands triage—determine the most important of the tasks on your plate and methodically complete those first, and then move on to the next tier of tasks that are not as vital. The last tier is what you decide to ignore. Because we have become way too accessible as a result of e-mail and cell phones, we too often forget that these devices can become others' leashes to dictate our time. You need to build into your day some quiet time. Frankly, it's okay not to answer your phone every time it rings or to wait to respond to an e-mail. Set aside a block of time each day to return phone calls and answer e-mails, rather than being on a leash that anyone can tug.

Third, do things that help you relax. You might set aside a half hour during the day—whether it is your lunch time or a break you've built into your work schedule—for quiet time; this half-hour window is yours to meditate, play solitaire, read a chapter in a novel, or take a 20-minute nap. As "girly" as it might first *feel*, try to meditate. In fact, take a health-related course on how to use 15–20 minutes a day for quiet contemplation, breathing, and clearing your mind. This promotes less stress and better sleep. Most employers' health care benefit packages include "wellness programs" and a range of non-pharmaceutical strategies to help you relax which you can take advantage of for minimal cost.

Fourth, stay connected. The goal is to keep in touch with the people who make up your support network—family, friends, neighbors, coworkers—and especially stay connected with anyone who makes you feel relaxed and happy. For some men, it is their faith that is nourishing and provides a sense of coherence. For other men, their friendships and activities with other guys are what's nourishing: nickel-and-dime poker nights, a regular Tuesday night dinner with a few friends (which you had to initiate and get established), or breakfast one morning a week with neighborhood friends before everybody breaks away for their separate days. Set up regular time with your friends and family. When life gets hectic, it's too easy to let these relationships go unattended. Avoid the downside of "letting things go" and becoming solitary.

CHAPTER 6

Social Health

VITAL RELATIONSHIPS

Social health initially may seem to be an odd "supplement" to men's health, but it's crucial. It's the third leg of a three-legged stool, the other two being physical and psychological health. Before World War I, when biology (and religion) ruled people's thinking, physical health captured the nation's attention. In the United States, public health efforts to provide clean water, sanitation, and universal medical care dominated the agenda. After World War I, psychological health emerged as equally important. Most people continue to think that men's health means just their physical and psychological well-being. However, in 1947 the World Health Organization recognized that "health" extends beyond our physical and psychological status to also involve our social (and spiritual) lives. Social health refers to the degree to which each of us is "communal" and connected; it recognizes our "social animal" character and capacity to thrive in social settings.[1] At issue is the quality of our personal relationships and the fact that our involvement in them affects our own well-being and the welfare of others.[2] More than having vital relationships (e.g., contacts with friends, relatives, and coworkers; membership in different groups and participation in group activities), social health boils down to feeling cared for, respected, even loved, and not feeling socially isolated and/or emotionally lonely. Having a protective network of family, friends, and acquaintances buffers and lessens life stress. When there's a *sense* of community, the feeling men experience is a mixture of personal recognition, mutual trust, and respect for their autonomy and time.

By far the most important contributors to men's social health and overall well-being are personal relationships. In them, we become sons, friends, fathers, brothers, lovers, and husbands. Without them, we are vulnerable. Our personal relationships anchor us, providing our identities and an existential home—a sense of belonging. As the English poet John Donne wisely said, "No man is an island, entire of itself; every man is a piece of the continent, a part of the main." The strength of Donne's observation is reflected in the hundreds of sociological studies covering more than a century, and they show how much our overall health benefits from the quality of our personal relationships. In healthy relationships we prosper; without them, we wilt socially, psychologically, and physically. Not surprisingly, even fictional heroes are not presented as solitary men. Even the Lone Ranger had his "wing man" Tonto, a Native American, who called the Lone Ranger "kemo sabe," which means "trusted friend," and together they did well.

As part of the three-legged "health" stool, research has established how social health assists in improving other forms of health. Think of the three legs of the stool being interconnected rather than standing alone. The scientific literature is very clear: social contact and committed relationships actually promote physical and emotional health. Married and partnered men who are well integrated into their communities experience less illness and recover faster from infirmities—heart attacks, hip replacements, even the flu.[3] Put simply, they live longer and healthier. By contrast, social isolation has been shown to be a risk factor for multiple chronic illnesses and earlier death, and this risk is independent of unhealthy practices such as smoking or being physically inactive. More than a century ago, Emile Durkheim, a French sociologist, defined social health by the degree of social integration each of us has within our relationships and communities, and he found that suicide rates were predictably higher in societies where people were not actively involved in social activities or did not feel socially integrated.[4] He's still right. More than any other group, death from suicide is greatest among older white men, and their suicide rates increase with age and physical illness. Among widowers, the suicide rate is high for men who have few people to confide in, men who may be arguing with family or friends, and men who are struggling with depression.[5] The fact is that we are social animals who need to be with others. Men who are alone, and even men who are with others yet feel disconnected or unimportant, may retreat. Why? There is no clear answer. But we must recognize that among white North Americans and white Europeans, the masculinity expectations men are expected to live by strongly emphasize self-reliance, avoiding dependencies, and biting the bullet. On the other hand, African American,

Hispanic/Latino, and Asian men follow a code that affirms "leaning on others," especially family and close friends, when times are trying.

As we reach middle age and grow older, we experience the changing character of our personal relationships—becoming parents-in-law and no longer able to deny that we are empty nesters, becoming "grandpas," perhaps becoming widowers and dating again. These transitions inevitably impact every man's vitality, sense of himself, and quality of life. The impact can be positive or negative depending on our adaptability (our ability to roll with the punches). The quality of our lives also depends on our social health—forging lasting bonds with lovers, friends, and family that are elastic enough to weather maturing and challenges. As we mull over retirement, for example, we need new relationships that defend our authenticity after more than half our lives having been defined in the labor force.

> A friend is someone you can go to and share secrets. A friend means someone I can depend on, someone that is like an extended member of my family.
>
> —52-year-old African American man
>
> Source: Grief, G. L. (2009). Understanding older men and their male friendships: A comparison of African American and white men. *Journal of Gerontological Social Work, 52*, 618–632, p. 624.

Not surprisingly, married heterosexual men largely depend on their partner as their anchor—their best friend, social planner, and kin keeper.[6] Matters of intimacy and sexuality associated with "marriage-type" relationships—whether marriage itself or the long-term, cohabiting relationships that resemble being married—are addressed in a previous chapter. Sexual health, which is a key concern of the century-old American Social Health Association, is discussed in a later chapter. In this chapter we call attention to men's social health—our personal relationships and experiences within them.

FRIENDSHIPS

The old adage about "don't put all your eggs in one basket" certainly applies to men and their friendships. Beyond the intimacies we develop with partners and our children, men need to have friends. Many men, in fact, have a lot of people they have friendly relations with at work, in the neighborhood, and while playing darts, golf, or softball. We have few "best friends." For instance, have you mentioned to someone your "best friend" from high school or college—you know, the buddy you haven't been in touch with in nearly 35 years? Have you received an e-mail from a friend you worked closely with a few years back, yet it's actually the first time you two have "spoken" in nearly 3 years? Thinking about or talking with an old friend once every few months or years might not seem to be evidence of a friendship, yet why not?

There's been a legacy of viewing friendship from a feminine stance, which leads people to think that men have less serious and meaningful friendships, compared to women. But are men's friendships (and friendly relations) deficient simply because they lack the frequent checking in, or are they just different from women's? Most of our friendships with other men are not intense: no daily phone calls or "How are you feeling?" questions when your friend hasn't been ill. Why ask about his feelings? That's something he'll bring up if he wants to.

Men are not looking for a confidant when they are friends with a man, but a companion. We "do things" with friends. We maintain what one social psychologist called side-by-side friendships[7]—whether it's playing poker once a month on a Friday night; getting together annually for an adventure-packed weekend of hiking, white-water rafting, and fly-fishing;[8] taking in a few football games during the season; or taking a morning walk 4 days a week with a walking buddy. Our conversations may be about sports or how to go about repairing a wall or rebuilding a bookcase; we may also covertly talk about what we are feeling. Even widowers involved in a grief support group prefer just being among men going through the same life-rattling experience rather than coming together to talk about their feelings.[9] Men maintain a distinct type of intimacy—close enough to one another for razzing, joking, teasing.[10] Advertisers know this: in beer ads men are almost always talking and joking in groups.[11] When men stop to talk with a friend, the conversations are short and not complicated: "How you doing? [Fine. You?] Good. Marjorie enjoying being a grandmother? [Yeah. She also loves coming home at night without the little guy.] Ha. Bet you are glad she comes home rather than stays with the little guy. . . ."

Sarah Matthews, a sociologist who studies gendered friendships, found that men's ways of "doing friendship" had different styles. One style is the "independent," where the men do not identify any specific person as a friend, even though they are not isolated people. Rather, their circumstances determine their handful of associates—when they were in high school, when they worked or lived in a particular place, whether they've moved into a retirement community. During each phase of their lives, they have situational friends with whom they enjoy doing things, and they comfortably report they do not have really close friends.

> I got a lot of friends, too, but I don't say they're friends that I would depend upon. . . . I'm my own man. That's what I want to be. . . . Do I have friends now? I have people that I know.

By comparison, some men develop an "acquisitive" style and move through their lives collecting a variety of friendships, allowing circumstances and phases of life to create new pools of friendly relationships. However, they commit themselves to maintaining contact with their friends once the friendships are made:

> Oh, gosh, sometimes it's hard to draw the line between acquaintances and friends, but there must have been, I'd say, fifty or so of them, anyway, that I considered good friends, played cards with, just a lot of companionship.[12]

At first glance, these friendship styles seem similar—the men "collect" associates in a social convoy[13] as they move through their lives. And they are. Their subtle difference is that the "independents" model the masculinity script more strongly, which makes it okay that they consider their wives their best friend and "friendships" with others to revolve around doing things together, when together. Thankfully, neither of these styles is necessarily going to leave men socially isolated or threaten their social health.

The lesson to be drawn is that it is advisable for mature men to continue to break away from the masculinity directive that dominated their earlier lives and to reach out and make connections. The masculinity ideal of comradery and brotherhood is incredibly functional when we are involved in many networks. But when we get older, our networks may shrink. This is something that happens as life changes (e.g., change of residence, poorer health). We let go of peripheral relationships and concentrate on core relationships.[14] A recent study finds that the younger groups (ages 55–64) of mature men do not shrink their friendship networks as quickly as the older men.[15] Their convoys of work and neighborhood friends have continued through the transitions of retiring and even relocating, providing indispensable support and anchoring their past identities with the present.

What all this suggests is that it may not be a bad idea to call a buddy to ask his opinion about something, such as your upcoming retirement—guys are comfortable giving advice, when asked to focus on a task. To maintain good relationships and to make new friends, extend yourself. Get involved in activities where you will meet other people who already share a common interest of yours. Find or organize a breakfast club, where a half dozen or so guys get together in the morning over coffee to talk sports, politics, and news stories. Start hosting a Friday night dinner at your place, or pull together other couples and start having an every-other-Friday rotating dinner gathering, even potluck. Join a dart league; go to a public golf course, join a threesome, and invite them to play again next week; invite someone to become a walking buddy and walk 30 minutes daily, chatting away, even if it's just about the weather. As we get older and old friends are more difficult to maintain due to retirements, moving, and deaths, we need to meet new buddies as much as we need to maintain the rewarding relations with the long-time friends and family members who are most meaningful.

BROTHERS AND SISTERS

The sibling relationship is one of the longest relationships in people's lives, often spanning an entire lifetime. Although there is a cultural norm that we should be involved in our brothers' and sisters' lives, in fact in contemporary American and most European societies, whether men feel connected to their siblings is up to them. For most adult men, the research evidence is that we do consider our relationship with siblings as very important and we feel close to our sibling(s).[16] Being a brother is a relationship you work at, and our sibling relationships are more unique as we get older. Our sisters and brothers actively influence our sense of continuity and of who we have become. Other than our children and partners, they are our primary family. The solidarity and emotional closeness we maintain with brothers and sisters increase with age for most men. As we get older and live with the death of parents, siblings preserve our sense of belonging.

At first glance, pairs of brothers (brother-brother) may seem not to be as emotionally close as those of sisters (sister-sister). This is partly because emotional closeness is often viewed through a lens that misinterprets what men feel. Brothers tend to express affection differently than sisters. Similar to men's friendships, a brother's intimate expression toward his siblings is often made covertly—doing things together, enjoying one another's company. This is consistent with Dylan Thomas's observation: "It snowed last year too: I made a snowman and my brother knocked it down and I knocked my brother down and then we had tea."[17] Men who have positive relationships with siblings regularly report that getting together or talking on the phone with their siblings decreases feelings of loneliness, validates their biographies and experiences, and builds a sense of security.

BEING A GRANDPA

Not long ago, grandfatherhood was regarded as the last stage (or phase) of a man's family life cycle, and the transition to becoming a grandfather was something that occurred in middle age, not old age. But grandfathers were peripheral figures, since their need to continue to be breadwinners was a barrier to active grandparenting. But times and expectations have changed. Men born after World War II matured in a climate that has progressively expected us to be engaged, nurturing fathers, not just "providers," and as grandfathers we do not want to be remote figures. The majority of men view grandfathering as an opportunity to be actively involved in their families. Contemporary grandfathers welcome the opportunity but tread lightly. They feel that it is important to balance "being there," in terms of providing practical and emotional support for their grandchildren, with not interfering.[18] And distance no longer stops many grandfathers from "being there." As one 67-year-old commented, "I do texting and I can do emails and I have got Skype so I can see the baby—she brings the baby and I can see it on the web cam."[19]

When Paul McCartney was born in 1942, the life expectancy of a British or American man was, on average, younger than age 64, leaving most children McCartney's age little time with their grandfathers. Men's life expectancy and overall health, however, have improved so much over the past half century that nearly all mature men can expect to become grandfathers, and many even great-grandfathers. Studies find that by age 65, men who have children also have grandchildren 95 percent of the time. In 2006, at age 64, Sir Paul appeared on the cover of *AARP The Magazine*, and he already had three grandchildren. If you are 50, you are 2 years shy of when a *majority* of men in England and the United States first became a grandfather. Brett Favre (NFL quarterback) at age 40 in 2010, Jim Carrey (comedian) at age 47 in 2010, Steven Tyler (of Aerosmith) at age 54 in 2004, Harrison Ford (actor) at age 51 in 1993—the list goes on and on, to include perhaps you and most of your friends.

No longer is "grandparenting" a synonym for grandmothers. Being a peripheral, nearly invisible grandfather isn't good enough anymore. Men want to be an influential, very present, engaged "grandpa" or "papa,"[20] and because we live on average 15 years longer than earlier generations, we have many years to develop special bonds with our grandchildren. How we are individually as grandfathers is certainly fashioned by the cultural norms that are part of our regional, race, and ethnic traditions. We are also influenced by our fathers and grandfathers in how to be a "grandpa," or perhaps as often how not to be. But no longer is there a stereotypical grandfather, nor are there correct grandfathering styles we ought to follow.

What Can I Offer My Grandchild(ren)?

As is true for all close relationships, those between grandfathers and grandchildren require work to find an acceptable balance between not interfering and enjoying one another—between separateness and connectedness. For men who are not the primary caregivers of their grandchildren, we have the opportunity to know our grandchildren in a different way than we got to know our children. Freed from the parenting responsibility, we can be (and usually are) more open and laid-back when interacting with our grandchildren. This is reciprocated by the grandchildren, because they also feel open to ask questions, seek advice, and share information about their lives. Grandchildren tell grandfathers their dreams and wishes; they remind us of how fun it is to try new things and inspire us to be youthful. Developmental psychologists have argued that men become more nurturing as they get older, and through the development of relationships with grandchildren the tough image of masculinity softens. Being a grandfather can become a particularly rewarding experience—giving our grandchildren wanted affection, sharing experiences and stories, providing unconditional support, and demonstrating important values. We get back, too: we watch the grandchildren come back for more stories, advice, and a listening ear when they need it.

Loved Being a Grandpa?

Have your grandchildren grown up? Consider being a volunteer grandfather. The mentoring, caring experience of being an older man involved with surrogate grandchildren can be wonderful. There are plenty of children across the United States who could use the affection, support, and guidance of an older man with experiences, stories, and time.

One luxury of being a grandpa is "just being there"—simply being interested in what your grandchildren like, and listening to them as they tell you what is going on in their lives. This may entail being around one another when doing everyday activities such as cooking breakfast, playing in the yard, putting stickers in memory books, or accepting a challenge to a one-on-one game of basketball or chess. Following their cue, you are capable of passing down skills, rituals, and activities. These are often most memorable for your grandchildren—when you built a six-hole putt-putt golf course in the front lawn using old coffee cans, had them help you cook your mom's spaghetti sauce recipe, built a (snow) fort, took them to a farm and had the farmer show them what (raw) freshly picked corn tastes like, or showed them how to have a *real* pillow fight. No matter what you do together, the satisfaction comes from just knowing that you are creating memories that your grandchildren will treasure for their entire lives.

When not the primary caregiver or the weekday babysitter, nearly half of grandfathers see a grandchild once a week. Even if your grandchildren live too far away to make it feasible to see them on a weekly basis, there are ways to maintain a relationship. You might write personalized letters, send e-mails and/or videos (even "dumb" ones of a chipmunk in the backyard), call them, or send off-the-wall, inexpensive gifts to let them know that you are thinking about them. College students love weird grandfather gifts arriving at random. Given the volume of junk mail and spam e-mail, a mailed note is worth more than the stamp. Send care packages to match upcoming events in their lives—at the beginning of summer send them some sunscreen, funky sunglasses, and ingredients for s'mores. You don't have to buy plane tickets to Disneyland to make a memory or to enjoy "being with" them (even when not physically close).

Today many grandfathers live more than 200 miles from their grandchildren. Put simply, we've got to be creative about ways of "seeing" our grandchildren, and there are many ways for us long-distance grandpas to stay active with our grandchildren. Technology has made things easier. If you haven't tried web chatting via Skype, it is very easy and free and gives you face time with them, without hopping on a plane; if they are still young, you can "Skype" a bedtime story to them. If they're older, you can challenge them to online games of Scrabble, which can take days to complete, or have them join you in a fantasy sports league and together draft and trade players. Another strategy is to create a private account on Facebook or a private family website that only allows access to grandchildren, aunts, uncles, sisters, brothers, in-laws, and other family members and encourages them to post messages and pictures—to be "in" one another's lives.

It's Not All Fun and Games

Inevitably, there may be some difficulties encountered. For one, it's likely you are not the only grandpa. Kin keeping favors maternal grandfathers—you will likely have more opportunities to be a grandpa to your daughter's children. On average, your son's children are more likely to see their mom's father, the other grandpa. Statistically, by the time our children are age 18, more than one-third have a step-grandparent, and this is more often the consequence of divorce and remarriage in the grandparent than parent generation.[21] It also occurs when your divorced child remarries and you acquire step-grandchildren. It is possible that you will not get along "peachy" with some of the other grandpas because, similar to most things in our lives, guy-to-guy relationships have an element of competition. You may think that other grandparents' religious beliefs are too different from yours, or that they get to spend too much time with the grandkids because they live closer. What's important is to have your own close relationship with your grandchildren and trust that your values and beliefs will be recognized and appreciated.

Also common in recent generations, with half of first marriages ending in divorce, men will have to deal with complex families that include ex-spouses and their new partners at family gatherings. Family gatherings are not a time to take up old wars and hurts. The grandchildren will not want to spend (any) time with relatives who are constantly bickering.

Grandfathers have been and continue to be the "family go-to guys," being available in times of need. It's quite common for grandfathers to feel responsible for providing economic support to their children and grandchildren. You might get a call from a granddaughter who is away at college and got into a minor fender bender. The insurance policy carries a $1,000 deductible, the damage is $1,100, and she's totally against calling her mom and dad. She asks you to help.

If you are within driving distance, you are going to be called on to help out with the grandchildren. Our married children are typically in two-earner families of their own, busy with jobs, meetings, after-school activities, and errands. If they are lucky to have you around to "watch the kids" or be the taxi for soccer practice, you are going to be asked for help, especially if you've retired. It is difficult to say "no." But it is important to set reasonable expectations of how much and what type of support you can offer, even though there will be times you want to give more. Most grandfathers are still working and have their own responsibilities and commitments. All cautions aside, it is still a big deal hearing a grandchild say, "Hi, Grandpa. Thanks." The argument in favor of assuming the active sitter or chauffeur role is that your involvement will almost certainly be of great value to both your children and your grandchildren. But we cannot overlook our personal needs, including downtime.

The connections we make with our grandchildren go through stages, and we shouldn't assume that being a closely involved grandpa will always be good for grandchildren. As teens, they pull away from all adults; researchers[22] find that younger teens more frequently participate in a variety of recreational activities with grandparents and express positive feelings about spending leisure time with grandparents than older teens. As grandparents, we are valued primarily because we provide affection and reassurance of worth. They may pull away from frequent calls and visits, but we can easily cement the bond with an e-mail or card that expresses our love. Once our grandchildren start their marriages and families, we become great-grandpa and more likely occupy less central roles in their lives.

Primary Caregivers

The U.S. Census reported that 2.7 million grandparents were raising their grandchildren in their home in 2009 and were responsible for the grandchildren's most basic needs. Nearly 1 million were grandfathers.

Source: U.S. Bureau of the Census (2011, Aug. 26). Facts for features: Grandparents as caregivers. Washington, DC: U.S. Census Bureau. CB11-FF.17.

PARTNERS UNCOUPLING

No longer is the "package deal"[23] for a heterosexual man to establish a career, marry, purchase a home, be a father, and die earlier than his (first) wife. Within one generation the motto "one marriage for a lifetime" was replaced by "marriage, divorce, remarriage."[24] Barely more than half the men who married at the end of the 1970s celebrated their twentieth wedding anniversary with their first wife, and that pattern has not changed. Divorcing after decades of marriage is certainly less common than divorcing early in marriage, but it is not rare. One study calculated that fewer than 10 percent of men were older than 50 when they divorced in 1990, but things changed: 20 years later at least one in four men had passed his fiftieth birthday at the time of his divorce.[25]

Is it that men (and women) want more from marriage than they already have (e.g., a new sex life, a soul mate, not a wife)? The stereotypical Hollywood representation of men and divorce is the man "trading in" his old wife for a younger model and entering middle age invigorated. This image is nowhere near reality. Most midlife and later-life divorces (roughly two-thirds) are not initiated by the men.[26] Even when men from the boomer and more recent generations want intimacy in their partnerships and believe that it's better to go it alone than to settle for less,[27] they know that the uncoupling transition is going to be troublesome. Diane Vaughan, a sociologist who studied the divorce process, found that, parallel to the process of coupling, the same dramatic process occurs in reverse during uncoupling.[28] Partners must restructure their life as a couple into two single lives. Uncoupling affects each partner's psychological well-being, social support, social involvement, and economics. It disrupts our core identity and challenges our sense of the future. It is, frankly, life altering. Uncoupling men often feel they are not in control of their lives, particularly if the divorce is not what they want, and they sense that it is equally disruptive for their children, friends, and other kin. Yet the often-unspoken longing for a happier life and the relief to be freed from a difficult, unsatisfying marriage eventually trump the challenge.

After-marriage difficulties are common for men. What slams them most is their disrupted relationships with children and grandchildren. Not long after the divorce, there also is a profound sense of ambivalence—relief, mixed with an empty feeling and periodic depression, and then the bipolar excitement and fear of being single again. Most often, after a short time of relishing the opportunities of personal freedom, men's loss of a day-to-day partner inevitably creates periods of acute loneliness and recognition of being socially isolated. Postdivorce stresses go beyond missing having a ready partner; we lose a sense of ourselves, especially if the divorce was

Statistics on Marriage

A recent Census Bureau snapshot of the nation shows that nearly 15 percent of men age 50–64 and 11 percent of men over 65 are *currently* divorced, and most of these men are not averse to either dating again or remarriage. When the 2010 Census was counted, "married" was defined two ways— those men who stayed in their first marriage, and the men who were remarried following either divorce or the death of a spouse.

Source: Howden, L. M., & Meyer, J. A. (2011). Age and sex in the United States: 2010. Table A1: Marital status of people 15 years and older, by age, sex, personal earnings, race, and Hispanic origin. Washington, DC: U.S. Census Bureau.

not something we wanted. With time, wounds can become more distant memories if men recouple (discussed below) and rebuild family time with their children and grandchildren. For the nearly 30 percent of men who do not remarry,[29] the psychological distress doesn't abate easily and lingering feelings of depression are not uncommon.

BEING A WIDOWER

For far too long, bereavement and widowhood have been discussed as largely a women's issue, and perhaps rightly so because population aging isn't gender-neutral. In nearly all nations, it is women who are more likely to survive the death of their husbands, reflecting the health axiom that "men die sooner even if women get sicker." At the beginning of the twenty-first century, for example, of the nearly 14 million ever-widowed persons living in the United States, fewer than 4 million were men.[30] But is it fair to view widowhood as merely a women's issue? Think again—there are more widowers in the United States than all the people in Oregon or Kentucky.

Stepping away from the demographics, too little is known about the experiences of widowers. The widowers who participated in the late-1960s Harvard Bereavement Study equated the loss of their wife with a loss of their anchor and soul mate—their source of support and comfort. They felt "dismembered" and experienced the death of their wife as a loss of protection, strength, and reassurance that left many of them disoriented. These men quietly talked more about the loss of an intimate partner than the holes in parenting or their need to become head of housekeeping. At about the same time as the Harvard study, a British study discovered that widowers' deaths followed sooner than would have been expected after the men lost their wife, which is now called the risk of men's "broken heart."[31]

> First, my wife passed away. We had been married 44 years, a very happy marriage and . . . I couldn't accept it. I remained alone. The children were very good and supportive. They came and everything, but [short silence] it just wasn't right. It was awful, I lost a tremendous amount of weight and you could say I was on the verge of depression [silence] and after a while, after a year or two, friends . . . offered to introduce me to a woman and I said no, I can't accept this, I'm not ready for it, so the situation continued [short silence] until I met Malka. (age 77, cohabitating 6 years)[32]

Recent studies confirm that the widower effect puts men at risk for social isolation and various adverse psychological consequences, except in cases where the wife dies of Alzheimer's disease or Parkinson's disease.

Apparently, these widowers' "anticipatory grief" and relief from seeing their wives suffer better prepared them to be widowers without the accompanying *sudden* emptiness. But for all widowers, emptiness is a factor. Since older men's social networks shrink by circumstance and by choice, and since most men rely on their wives to coordinate social activities, they are caught off guard by being alone.

Recently, two research teams—one in the United States and one in the United Kingdom—studied widowers' experiences. Moore and Stratton,[33] the U.S. researchers, unexpectedly found that widowers' resilience was commonplace, yet some men were even more resilient than others. What distinguished the more resilient widowers was that they consciously changed their lives. Even when there was a continuing "hole in their lives," these men took control and sought social support. Bennett,[34] the lead U.K. researcher, examined the strategic ways widowers managed their profound emotional pain. She recognizes that the emotional consequences of partner loss—feeling knocked over and frequent crying—run contrary to the "no sissy stuff" and "the sturdy oak" masculinity norms. What she learned was that even though many of the men could not maintain the mask of masculinity—"Well there's hardly a day goes by without having a good cry"—these men chose to suffer quietly. Most of the widowers avoided talking about their loss and consciously began to hook up with friends—both male and female—to escape their loneliness. Some widowers remarry, particularly if the men are younger, and other widowers may couple again but choose not to remarry.[35]

COUPLING AGAIN

Demographic data in both the United States and United Kingdom indicate that previously married men are very likely to partner again, though divorced men are not in a hurry[36] and widowed men are even less so.[37] Their social life swings away from being couple oriented, yet both widowers and divorced men readily admit that they miss the companionship that had been a "natural" part of their everyday lives. Research supports the conclusion that most men would prefer being in (re)partnered relationships rather than alone. Men rely on their live-in partners for a sense of wholeness, and being partnered provides men with health-enhancing emotional intimacy. Widowers often talk about the death of their wife as part of their self being severed.[38] While divorced men often find that the grass seemed greener when they were married, they equate divorce with being lonely.[39] As one 53-year-old divorced man said, "I was lost after the divorce, terrified of being alone, and not just crying but sobbing."

The motive for a new romantic relationship is not to replace the man's former partner, but to rebuild a day-to-day sense of being a couple and to help erase the social isolation and emotional emptiness at dinnertime and when waking up alone in bed. Here two older men express their desire to find another partner:[40]

> 'Cause I didn't like being on my own. This being on my own, I found it very difficult. . . . I was back at work and I enjoyed my work . . . but I would come home at night. I was going stir crazy, so I thought "I've got to meet someone and start getting out again." And that's why I did that [contacted a dating agency]. . . . I can live on my own, I can do everything, I can cook and everything. But I like company. . . . I thought, there's other people out there like me, so why not two people to be happy? (age 65)

> The trouble about being on your own is, it doesn't matter how busy you are, at times, you are very lonely. And certainly if the right person came along, I would be only too pleased to get married. Just like that. (age 76)

Very little is known about men's (re)partnering experiences. We know that social norms are shifting, and older men are no longer expected to just sit home and be granddads. The message from reliable research is that getting a divorce or becoming a widower is more than an "ending." Being single again most often means dating and getting involved in new relationships. Many single-again mature men are interested in a new long-term partner. One national study of widowers found that 6 months after their wives had died, 17 percent of men who were older than 65 had dated.[41] After 18 months of being a widower, more than one-third (37%) were interested in dating and nearly one-quarter (23%) reported having gone on a date. Another nationally representative survey of men aged 57–85 who were without a regular partner found that 22 percent had been sexually active in the previous year.[42]

Looking back a generation, the principal option was remarriage. Remarriage is still the "norm," since three-quarters (78%) of men remarry after a divorce and one in eight (12%) after becoming a widower.[43] It may be the accepted form of recoupling, especially among men who have a more conservative or religious background, but getting remarried isn't the only way to recouple. Changing times have spawned alternatives, from "just dating," to cohabitation, to what is called "living-apart-together" relationships[44]—where partners maintain separate households and finances and share living quarters on an intermittent (e.g., several days a week or on weekends) basis. Not everybody wants another marriage, but most men want an engaging companion, whether for going to dinners or as a vacation partner. Many single-again men, and especially older widowers, have a "special friend" and date with or without physical intimacy. "I know many elderly people who start a relationship, simply for the sake of companionship. Most of them drink a cup of coffee together, share meals . . . to avoid feeling lonely. Weekends are awful for people who live alone" [age 80]. When single-again heterosexual men opt for a special-woman relationship, it is companionship and intimacy that take precedence. Issues of shared finances, a common household, and inheriting stepchildren are held in check. Whether age 50 or 70, men with a woman friend do not want to go through the trouble of convincing their children that their new partner is not a replacement for their mother. They also value their independence too much to get married again. They feel that it is preferable to date, maybe even live with another partner, but not to "start over again" with marriage.

Repartnering isn't only about companionship. An American Association of Retired Persons (AARP) survey reported that 68 percent of boomer men rank sexual activity as a critical part of a good relationship, and two-thirds reported that physical intimacy was important to their overall quality of life.[45] Single-again heterosexual men who choose to get "back in the game" and pursue new, sexually intimate relationships are advantaged in terms of finding women to date. By the time men reach their sixties, there are nearly three times as many women who are interested in dating as there were when the men were in their twenties, irrespective of race/ethnicity. Furthermore, men are no longer limited to their immediate community and the "old-fashioned way" of going through friends, neighbors, and relatives to find potential dates. They have the Internet. The Pew Research Center study reported that social networking among Internet users age 50 and older nearly doubled—from 22 percent to 42 percent—in one year, between 2009 and 2010.[46] Middle-aged and older men are renewing social contacts by e-mailing family, friends, and even high school lovers;[47] joining social media networks such as LinkedIn, Facebook, and Twitter; and using online dating sites geared to singles at least age 50 (e.g., www.maturesingles only.com or www.BabyBoomerPeopleMeet.com).

Internet daters are eager to meet the right person, but not desperate to meet just anyone. Internet-based social network and "matchmaker" sites allow you to view the profile of a potential date and gain helpful information about the person's interests, personality, and relationship goals. Most of the time, you can see a picture (your own profile and picture are also "screened" by the organization overseeing the site). You can use all this information to essentially weed out people you are not interested in and then "hook up" with those you are. What single-again men seem to want from a potential partner is little baggage from prior relationships, fitness and physical attractiveness, and a compatible attitude about romance and sexual intimacy, as well as not being in a rush to partner long-term.[48]

Your House or Hers, or Both?

For a good proportion of single-again men, living together isn't immediately on the radar, even if they are romantically involved. If a man has a life that he likes and interests he wants to pursue, perhaps he doesn't want to sacrifice those priorities to be someone else's soul mate. Most mature men are (or were) homeowners, and to remarry usually obliges either the man or his new partner to sell their home. For some men, moving in to his partner's place or having his partner move into his home boils down to a loss of residential independence and unwanted changes in household habits. Especially among widowers, relocating is an added, unwanted transition many men are just not interested in making.[49] A study of French widowers reports that many of the men wanted a safety valve—a place to go back to if things didn't work out with a new relationship:

> We get on fine together. But we've each kept our own home. . . . Because . . . well, you never know . . . we can pass away . . . and, we wouldn't want the one that's left to be out on the streets. Well, after all, there's children on both sides. . . . It's best to look ahead, all the same.[50] [widower, age 87]

For men who want more than a weekly dinner date or vacation partner, there are options that forego the weight of married life. When tired of "just dating," single-again men may choose to cohabit under one roof with a partner or alternate living at their home and their partner's. Both cohabitation and "living apart together" are on the rise, especially among older white widowers and younger, single-again African American men. Technically, cohabitation is when a couple live together in one household as if married, and this is something middle-aged and older divorced men opt for more than widowers. Most of the time when a couple cohabits, they begin with frequent "stay-overs" and eventually move under one roof to maintain a single residence.

By comparison, living-apart-together relationships offer opportunities to combine the benefits of being single with those of being partners. One study[51] estimated that by the late 1990s these living-apart relationships outnumbered cohabiting relationships nearly two to one. The "living-apart-together" label challenges the long-standing assumption of most Western thinking that two people must live in the same household to be considered a (monogamous) couple. But this invisible option is catching on. Already established in their lives, mature men have their own routines and commitments and are often loath to change much. And that's okay. So are many potential partners loathe to give up their autonomy. Boomer-generation men grew up during times more accepting of "alternative relationships," and they may enter their later adult years not wanting to walk down the aisle again. Both the men and their partners have their own possessions, financial arrangements, retirement incomes, children (and grandchildren), and even night-owl versus morning-person preferences. These would-be stumbling blocks are erased with the option of living apart together.

So too is the perception of greediness. A key reason a man and his partner both prefer to keep living in their own home is that their home holds good memories of an earlier life; another reason is that the man can continue his relationships with his children and grandchildren without challenging their place memories of "home." Still another is the nagging unease about complicating the inheritance we pass down—are stepchildren included or excluded? Does his new partner's financial well-being take precedence over his children's and grandchildren's?

Why (Re)couple? The Benefits

Close, committed relationships—whether our first marriage, remarriage, or living apart together—provide us with a sense of ontological security. A close relationship is therapeutic, for it gives us an opportunity to take off the Superman mask of always being invulnerable. We are allowed to stop performing, if only temporarily. Inside committed relationships—marriage, gay partnerships, and even close dating friendships—we come to judge ourselves and others less severely than is typically possible in men's public world, which constantly involves one-upmanship competition. We "soften" a bit. We feel better about ourselves and our lives, experience fewer stress hormones, and are happier.

Ironically, the benefits of a close, committed relationship weren't always self-evident when we were younger and establishing ourselves in the workplace and as husbands and fathers. These career and family "distractions" from being a full-fledged partner ease as we move into our sixties—when workplace challenges are usually ritualized, children have moved away, and tuition payments are history. When men "recouple," either by actually repartnering after divorce or becoming a widower, or by consciously renewing the glue that makes up the "we" in a long-term, first marriage, the pleasures of being within and part of a relationship are heightened.

Sociological studies show that married and partnered men benefit in many ways from their personal relationships, compared to "single" men. For one thing, the social lives of men in committed relationships involve greater interaction with friends and relatives than when single, making the former less likely to feel socially isolated. For another, their health is better. While the processes (or reasons) that provide greater immunity to ill health for married and partnered men are not completely understood, the risk of social isolation can be as dangerous to our survival as obesity and metabolic syndrome, high blood pressure, and a too-sedentary lifestyle.[52] The takeaway message is simple: being alone in widowerhood or divorce increases our risks of loneliness and poorer health, but being with a partner is usually helpful in increasing well-being.

SOCIAL HEALTH AMONG GAY MEN

Everything already discussed applies to both gay and heterosexual men, yet middle-aged and older gay men live with distinct inequalities that affect their social health. Using conservative estimates, there are well over 2 million gay men over the age of 60 in the United States,[53] which is equivalent to twice the population of Rhode Island and four times the population of Wyoming. Despite these numbers, gay men face unique social challenges because of antigay prejudices and discriminatory policies. The majority of older gay men lived through an era in which being openly gay was taboo. Everyone was presumed to be heterosexual. In the 1930s, 1940s, and 1950s when men now considered "old" were growing up, the open homosexual was queer—he was different, unusual, bullied, and stigmatized. Most gay and bisexual men did not publically or even privately identify themselves as nonheterosexuals; they kept their same-sex attraction hidden. To avoid being publically shamed, particularly in ethnic minority communities, and to be considered ordinary and masculine, gay men embodied heterosexual masculinity, including the kinesthetic movements that depict "being manly."

Living as if heterosexual, some gay men married in their midtwenties and had children and hid their sexual identity for years, even from themselves, only coming to identify themselves as gay in midlife and making the transition to gay life after unexpectedly becoming a widower or after a midlife divorce. Having children was common: as of 2000, for example, the households of more than one-fifth of middle-aged and older gay men who are living with a gay partner include their children.[54]

Other older gay men chose to remain unmarried and most often lived alone. These men were forced to navigate carefully the workplace and family gatherings as simply unmarried, and they proved to be resilient. Studies reveal that these older gay men are as well adjusted as the heterosexual men their age, and some are even more hardy.[55] They developed "crisis competence" and ways of living outside the institutional supports available to their heterosexual peers. They invented welcoming, gay-friendly communities and built networks of friends that became chosen families.[56] The following exchange between two men participating in one study's focus group conversation shows the importance of friendship:

> John, age 64. [The most important people in my life are] friends of long-standing who are, I would say, mostly gay, but not all.

> Jim, age 71. Yes, yes, I would agree with that, I think the older you get the more important friends are, and true friends. As far as I'm concerned that can mean gay and heterosexual people.[57]

Do not conclude that solo living always equals unpartnered. Gay men also participate in living-apart-together relationships with their partners because living together would have called attention to their sexual orientation during discriminatory times. Living apart together is also chosen to maintain an independent stance in terms of financial resources and, for some of the men, to assuage their children's and grandchildren's worries.

Also, don't think everything is all peachy because middle-aged and older gay men are resilient. The men find that both the heterosexual community and broader gay community aren't attentive to their aging-related needs and worries. The gay community is mostly geared toward the younger, unpartnered generation of men who are not as wary of being openly gay. Younger gays are put off by the older men and their aging bodies and stories,[58] and they haven't had to take up caregiving for an adult friend with AIDS or a family member with life-ending illness, whereas at least one in four gay boomers has already been a caregiver, more often to a parent or sibling than a partner or friend.[59] Many middle-aged and older gay men find it difficult to be old in the gay community; they know that they are perceived as less attractive and less masculine.

Gay men's experiences have deflated their confidence that health care professionals will treat them with dignity and respect should they become sick or disabled.[60] It is a very real social health problem. A study[61] of gay elders discovered that they felt particularly vulnerable about being bullied, abused, or neglected by the home health care aide, visiting nurses, and other providers they might be dependent on for medical care. As one person reported, "I'm afraid to have a stranger in my home, someone who may be very anti-gay, and then what if they find out about my life and now they're in my home regularly, and could somehow take advantage or mistreat me?" This man's worries are not unwarranted. There are many discriminatory policies and practices that refuse to treat gay partners as spouses when it comes to medical insurance, hospital visitation, Social Security and retirement pensions, and housing needs.[62] As one exasperated older man commented in a letter to the editor in the *Plain Dealer*:

> Jim, my partner of 32 years, and I were married in Toronto. . . . Over the years, we have faced opposition from family members, been damned to hell by our religions and have been denied opportunities in housing and employment. . . . It was with dismay that I learned from a representative of New York Life Insurance that the life annuity that I will begin to receive . . . will not continue for Jim upon my demise. When asked why . . . I was informed that the federal government prohibits Jim from receiving my benefits because the government does not recognize our marriage.[63]

Given the current lack of legal protection for gay couples, it is critically important that older gay men complete wills, a medical power of attorney, and a living will to spell out their long-term care housing preferences and end-of-life wishes.

COMMUNITY PARTICIPATION AND CIVIC ENGAGEMENT

Active engagement in your community and in society is unquestionably associated with better health and well-being. At a basic level, any amount of activity, even low levels, is more beneficial to our bodies and minds than lack of involvement. We're engaged. We *feel* involved and productive, and this feeling of well-being rolls over to reduce stress hormones that regularly kick in as a result of boredom and marginalization. When you are a member of a social, educational, fraternal, or religious group, you are interacting with people who mostly share your basic beliefs, and you recognize that your involvement serves as a vital resource for others. Imagine, for example, the middle-aged man who no longer wants to coach his daughters' soccer teams but who turns to helping his town's recreation department find funding to build a set of new, irrigated soccer fields, or the 66-year-old retired man who volunteers to drive cancer patients to and from their chemotherapy treatments, or who chooses to read detective fiction to an elder whose eyesight is failing to allow his spouse or partner to have a few hours respite.

Your volunteerism and civic engagement wouldn't be out of the ordinary. In a nation that one sociologist recently characterized as "Bowling Alone"[64] because the quantity and quality of social connections between people have eroded as people have disengaged from their communities, isn't it ironic that one-third of the baby boomers in their late forties and fifties and one-quarter of people age 65 and older volunteer?[65] More than men from European ancestry, African American men have a long, rich history and legacy of civic engagement, whether through their churches or formal organizations such as the Masons or the Order of the Eastern Star. What's holding others back? Basically, neither an organization nor someone in our social network has asked us to help.

Middle-aged and older men find new meaning in their volunteer work and the opportunity to improve their communities. If you no longer want to be bowling alone, there are countless organizations available for you to develop new social connections, purpose, and productive engagement.

PART II

MIND AND BODY

CHAPTER 7

Sleep

A NECESSITY OF LIFE

with Kristen Sutherland

Sleep helps keep our bodies healthy and our minds functioning. Although it may seem to be a relatively mundane part of life, without doubt good sleep is one of the most important aspects of our health. It is as important as eating right and staying active. The average man spends nearly a third of his life sleeping—and he needs that sleep. That's about 25 years, based on a life span of 77 years. Even the devoted sports fan will only spend about 20 percent as much of his time following the ups and downs of his beloved teams as he will sleeping. What, really, is so special about sleep that we spend so much of our lives doing it?

The simple answer is, without *good* sleep you would not function adequately enough to even stay awake to watch the highlights of last Sunday's top NFL plays, catch up on an episode of your favorite television series, or remember what you watched. Obtaining sufficient amounts of quality sleep is an absolute necessity for your health. Not sleeping long enough and not sleeping well enough (or having poor nighttime sleep) are associated with a host of health concerns.

Even though it seems simple, there are some important things to understand about sleep, including what is called *sleep architecture* and its normal age-related changes, how sleep affects our health, the possibility of developing sleep problems, and ways to improve the quality of our sleep. Even though prior to the 1990s most sleep research was done on men, it can be a challenge to find information specific to sleep and men's health. This might be the case because women have and tend to express more complaints about sleeping problems than men, and thus their concerns have been getting more attention.[1] The following sections contain helpful information about sleep with special attention given to how men experience sleep.

THE BASICS: WHAT AND WHY

It is important to understand the basics: what sleep is, why we sleep, and what happens while we sleep. Although there is a lot going on physiologically during sleep, the definition of sleep is actually relatively simple. It speaks more to the lack of what is happening rather than what is happening. Sleep is "a natural periodic state of rest for the mind and body, in which the eyes usually close and consciousness is completely or partially lost, so that there is a decrease in bodily movement and responsiveness to external stimuli."[2] While definitions of sleep can vary considerably, the same basic principles are described universally: it is normal, recurring, and nearly devoid of typical conscious actions such as thinking. But when we sleep, our brains and bodies are far more active than people usually recognize, although the sleeper shows relatively little movement, has minimal sensitivity to sounds and smells, and is ordinarily lying down. In fact, a brain's neurons are just as active during sleep as when a person is awake.

Sleep Differences between Men and Women

Men suffer from insomnia at half the rate that women do, yet men are twice as likely to have their slumber spoiled by sleep apnea, which is characterized by brief episodes of restricted breathing.

Sources: National Center on Sleep Disorders Research (NCSDR); National Heart, Lung, and Blood Institute (NHLBI); National Institutes of Health (NIH).

An interesting aspect of sleep is the process by which the body goes from being awake to slumber and then wakes again. It is more involved than just falling asleep until the alarm clock goes off, but it does have something to do with another kind of clock. One of our biological clocks, known as a circadian rhythm, is truly what controls the sleep-wake cycle. We feel sleepier depending on where we are in our 24-hour circadian cycle. During sleep, we also repeatedly cycle through stages of sleep. If you watch someone who is sleeping, you will notice that they initially slip into a phase of quiet sleep with regular, deep breathing. Later, after roughly 90 minutes, the normal sleeper enters the dreaming sleep phase, which includes muscle twitching and eye movement under the eyelids.

Interestingly, circadian rhythms are found in all living organisms, although they perform a different function for grass than for ants or humans. In mammals the information collected to regulate circadian rhythms is located in our "internal clock," or the two clusters of cells called the suprachiasmatic nuclei (SCN) within the hypothalamus.[3] Basically self-regulating, our internal clock responds to several cues, especially light and melatonin. When our eyes are closed and visual input no longer stimulates nerve cells, brain activity slows. As we move into deeper sleep, fewer centers within the brain stay active. The absence of light taken in through your eyes is interpreted by the SCN. This information is sent to the pineal gland, which has been called the "third eye" and works to produce important hormones, including melatonin. Secreted when there is decreased light, melatonin (discussed more later) decreases body temperature and lulls us to sleep.[4] Neurotransmitters also have a role in regulating this cycle. Adenosine, for example, acts like a natural tranquilizer and contributes to the feeling of drowsiness; it has been found to build up during consciousness and then slowly breaks down during sleep.

Full agreement as to why humans sleep in the rhythms we do has still not been reached. Multiple theories suggest an evolutionary foundation. The basis of these theories consists of the observation that animals sleep in response to environmental cues and ultimately to stay alive. Animals with fewer natural predators and fewer environmental stressors sleep more than those with more predators and stress. Rest must come when there is less danger so that the animal has adequate energy to escape or defend (the primitive fight-or-flight response). Similarly, physiological theories propose that the body needs a period of rest to heal, and supporting evidence shows that sleep in fact repairs and strengthens our immune and nervous systems, muscles, and much more. Psychological theories argue that sleep occurs because the brain is overloaded; during sleep, we deal with the emotional matters in our lives while dreaming, and the brain is able to sort through acquired memories, discard or store them, and prepare for newly learned information. Therefore, an explanation for why you had to look at the new 10-digit phone number three times to dial it could be, "You know I have not been sleeping well and because of that I have not been able to process those darn numbers." You could also use your poor sleep as an excuse when your partner or spouse asks why you forgot what was said a few hours earlier about putting your dirty socks in the laundry. None of the theories, however, explain our sleep-wake balance, or why our homeostatic balance influences the timing of sleep.

One very effective model of sleep homeostasis proposes two internal processes.[5] One is sleep pressure, which increases with time awake and then decreases during sleep. It is assumed that we have a "sleep homeostat," or internal gauge, that computes our need for sleep based on the time we are awake. Unlike "night owls" who usually wake at 10:00 a.m. and are alert later into nighttime, morning persons who start their day at 5:00 a.m. feel sleepy earlier because they become sensitive to sleep pressure in early evening. The other process is our 24-hour circadian rhythm, which parallels our body's core temperature.

SLEEP STAGES

Throughout an average sleep cycle, a normal sleeper alternates between two very different states, non-rapid eye movement (NREM) and rapid eye movement (REM) sleep. The NREM state actually consists of four stages of sleep, while the REM state only has one, for a total of five stages. These stages get longer each time they are repeated during the course of a night's sleep.

When first falling asleep, you enter stage 1, or transitional sleep, for about 5 minutes. In this stage you lose awareness of your surroundings, but environmental stimuli can still easily awaken you. Once aroused, it may feel like you had not even fallen asleep. In this stage our eye movements, muscle and brain activity, and breathing slow down. People dozing off while sitting may experience sudden muscle contractions preceded by a sensation of falling. Throughout the sleep cycle, each time you return to stage 1 after the initial time you will not be as vulnerable to stimuli.

Established sleep begins in stage 2. Here the body prepares for deep sleep: eye movement stills, heart rate and breathing slow down, and body temperature decreases. Brain waves become slower, yet occasional surges in brain activity occur; these bursts of the brain's electrical rhythms are referred to as "sleep spindles." Stage 3 marks the beginning of deep sleep. When brain activity is charted on an electroencephalogram (EEG), the brain mostly shows signs of long, slow waves during this stage. Stage 4 is the deepest sleep, also marked by these long, slow (or delta) waves. During deep sleep, the sleeper is difficult to arouse, and when awoken, he may be disoriented for the first few seconds. In deep sleep the body repairs and regenerates tissues (partially due to the release of human growth hormone [hGH], as mentioned below), builds bone and muscle, and appears to strengthen the immune system.

Once through stage 4 of NREM sleep, you begin REM. This fifth and final stage was named REM because of the significant amount of eye movement that occurs behind our closed eyelids. Breathing during REM also becomes more rapid, irregular, and shallow. Brain waves increase to levels experienced while an individual is awake. Despite all this activity, our body barely moves because most of our muscles are nearly paralyzed. It is believed that we can thank REM sleep, not deep sleep, for feeling rested and refreshed. In studies where research participants were deprived of REM, they were tired and had emotional changes such as increased irritability, suspiciousness, and social withdrawal. Approximately 80 percent of your dreaming occurs during REM sleep. If awoken during REM sleep, you may easily recall dreams and initially be quite alert. Usually, REM sleep occurs 90 minutes after sleep onset and typically lasts 10 minutes; each recurring REM stage lengthens, and the final one may last up to an hour.

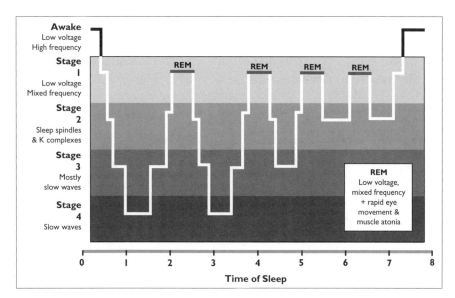

Figure 7.1. Sleep cycle

We can be certain that sleep is a resting state in a healthy sleep-wake cycle. However, a lot gets done while we are drooling on our pillow. Memories are not stored as they were initially encoded; rather, sleep is necessary for memory consolidation. Brain waves during certain periods of sleep are as large and fast as they are when we are conscious. One theory is that our mind is sorting through information gathered while awake and our awake experiences are processed while dreaming. Sleep plays a major role in this process, probably due to the neurochemical environment observed during the night.[6] When we sleep, certain hormones are released into our body to do a variety of jobs. Two important hormones—hGH and melatonin—are released either mostly or entirely during sleep. Melatonin, hGH, and sleep (or the quality of it) are interlinked, and people who get enough sleep are usually energetic, are in a good mood, and have better immunity.

Human Growth Hormone

Produced naturally during sleep, with increased amounts released during deep sleep, hGH is considered the fountain of youth as far as hormones are concerned. Human growth hormone is produced by the pituitary gland inside the brain, and how much is produced is dependent on the amount of slow brain wave sleep we get.[7] A night of active dreaming (or frequent REM sleep) produces less hGH, which helps explain why you get out of bed feeling unrefreshed. A buildup of "sleep debt," where we have prolonged periods of too little sleep or too much unrestful sleep, can threaten our health. No matter how macho it might be in popular culture to disregard sleep,[8] reduced sleep limits the amount of hGH released, which reduces the beneficial effects that it has on a man's body. Aging also reduces the amount of hGH, as much as 80 percent, which makes quality sleep an especially important issue as we get older.

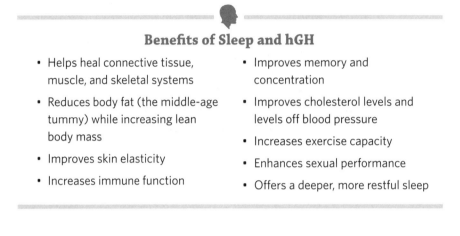

Benefits of Sleep and hGH

- Helps heal connective tissue, muscle, and skeletal systems
- Reduces body fat (the middle-age tummy) while increasing lean body mass
- Improves skin elasticity
- Increases immune function

- Improves memory and concentration
- Improves cholesterol levels and levels off blood pressure
- Increases exercise capacity
- Enhances sexual performance
- Offers a deeper, more restful sleep

Melatonin

A natural antioxidant, melatonin is made only in the dark. The pineal gland, which is deep inside the brain and signals the release of this hormone, activates when the environment is dark and can stay active for about 12 hours. Even if it is nighttime, if you are in a brightly lit place, the gland will not start releasing melatonin. It is even beneficial to lower the lights in your home when you are nearing the time you would like to go to sleep; this will activate the pineal gland and increase drowsiness.

Getting enough sleep to release enough melatonin is also important because this hormone helps coordinate our body's physiological rhythms and reset the circadian clock. It is interesting, however, how the pineal gland can be manipulated to release melatonin for men who face jet lag or working nights. Melatonin supplements are available over the counter and predominately used among men whose job changes from working days to working nights. Also, some research suggests that, like hGH, the natural production of melatonin may decrease with age, leaving older men with less antioxidant protection against stress-related disorders or "sundowning"—increased confusion in the afternoon and evening. Very preliminary research suggests that melatonin (and melatonin supplements) may help fight one of the most common malignancies men face—prostate cancer.[9]

> A good laugh and a long sleep are the best cures in the doctor's book.
>
> —An Irish proverb

HOW MUCH SLEEP SHOULD I BE GETTING?

A good sleep is recuperative and removes the feelings of fatigue. According to the National Sleep Foundation, adults should get, *on average*, between 7 and 9 hours of sleep per night. However, sources also say that the amount of desirable sleep is best determined individually, similar to individuals' preference for the timing of their sleep and waking activities (or what sleep researchers call "diurnal preference"). There are substantial individual differences in the patterns of sleep/wake activity and energy levels among men, and these seem to be governed by our internal circadian and sleep drive.[10] To understand your unique sleep needs, it may be useful to track how much sleep you get on a given night and then keep a record of how you feel throughout the following day. Think about how much sleep is not enough for you; on the days you feel drowsy by midafternoon, how much sleep did you get the night before? When you are sleep deprived, you also can become irritable and struggle with concentrating; have you noticed these symptoms? Whether you are a "long sleeper" or prefer to rise early, mentally chart your moods to assess how much sleep you truly need. Obtaining sufficient amounts of quality sleep is an absolute necessity for your good health. You can use this simple sleep-wake diary to log your sleep for a week.

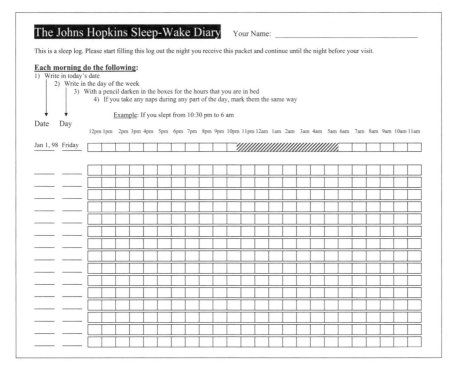

Figure 7.2. Sleep-Wake Diary. Courtesy of Johns Hopkins Pulmonary and Critical Care Medicine.

Sleep needs barely change over a man's lifetime. Adolescents actually need more sleep than adults, yet once we are in our twenties our sleep need remains roughly 8 hours. There is evidence, however, that as we get older changes in sleep are related to our decreased "ability" to sleep soundly for 8 hours. Older men may sleep only 6 hours a night and then get an additional 1–2 hours during daytime naps. Many men come to live with a reduction in their maximal capacity for sleep, because of work-related stress and how their nighttime sleep tends to become more fragmented.[11] As a result, the need for quality sleep among adult men is often unmet because of more frequent nighttime awakenings and other sleep disturbances.

Sleep patterns of older men also change, in some cases significantly. Basically, we are "diurnal" creatures—we prefer to remain awake during the day and to sleep at night. But the ability to have a restful sleep at night can be challenged as we grow older. As adults, it may take us longer to fall asleep, we sleep less, and we get less deep, slow-wave sleep than children and adolescents. You may find your sleep pattern disrupted by a chronic illness and the mediation needed to be healthy, the need to urinate several times during the night, or nighttime awakening that results from sleep-disordered breathing (discussed below). Because of your increasing daytime sleepiness, you may find yourself turning in earlier and find that your timing is more and more aligned with when the sun goes down, which may be as early as 5:00 p.m. in northern parts of the United States. These changes are probably beneficial; recent research suggests that morning-type people are healthier, more alert, and happier than "owls" who stay up late.[12]

The amount and timing of sleep are determined by many factors, including time awake, circadian rhythms, and social demands. A healthy sleep pattern can be difficult if not impossible to maintain if your work involves being awake during traditional evening hours. The sleep schedule maintained by night shift workers is completely the reverse of what their bodies are telling them to do. Trying to sleep on a schedule that is at odds with our natural, light-based circadian rhythm can be challenging. Establishing an "off-time" sleep pattern, with the external disturbances and noise more typical of the daylight hours, can be very difficult. Night shift workers more commonly report feelings of drowsiness than their daytime counterparts; men using "red-eye" flights rather than staying over an added night are forfeiting their healthy sleep and, by consequence, resistance to daily stress. Not surprisingly, accidents are also known to increase among sleep-deprived men.

SLEEP PROBLEMS AND DISORDERS

Very few men (or women for that matter) can say they enjoy good sleep night after night. Usually, if we are able to relax and not fixate on our lack of sleep, our bodies will force us to catch up with the sleep we need at some point. But if you start worrying about it, you will likely stress out and be even less able to sleep. If you find yourself waking up in the middle of the night and are unable to get back to sleep, don't turn on the light or TV. Instead, create a state of mind that is likely to allow you to fall back to sleep, rather than encourage you to wake up and worry about why you are awake. Do your best not to mull over upcoming project deadlines or meetings. With a little time lying in the dark, you will probably fall back asleep before you know it.

Unfortunately, some sleep difficulties are not so easily resolved. Although it is a myth that you will automatically have trouble sleeping when you get older, in general men's sleep difficulties increase with age. Aging is associated with changes in sleep amount, sleep quality, and specific sleep pathologies and disorders. Sleep problems may be caused by external stress, medical conditions, or a sleep disorder, and the American Academy of Sleep Medicine includes over 70 disorders in the International Classification of Sleep Disorders manual.[13] This section will discuss some of the more common sleep problems and disorders men may have as they age.

Signs of a Sleep Disorder

- Taking more than 30 minutes each night to fall asleep
- Waking several times each night and having trouble falling back to sleep
- Waking too early in the morning
- Feeling sleepy during the day, taking frequent naps, or falling asleep at odd times during the day
- Your bed partner says that you snore loudly, snort, gasp, make choking sounds, or stop breathing for short periods
- Having tingling, creeping sensations in your legs when you are trying to fall asleep
- Your bed partner notices that your legs (or arms) jerk often during sleep
- You feel as though you cannot move when you first wake up

Jet Lag

If you have flown coast to coast, you have likely experienced jet lag. It is usually a temporary sleep disorder that occurs among people who travel by jet across three or more time zones. Jet lag results from the slow adjustment of our body's circadian clock to the destination time, so that daily rhythms at your new destination are out of sync with the internal cycle of sleep and wakefulness. Interestingly, there is evidence to suggest that older adults are less likely to suffer from severe jet lag than younger persons.[14]

Insomnia

Nearly everyone has had a night of poor sleep, and these often occur at a time when stresses pile up. Typically, bad sleep nights, as unrestful and troubling as they can be, are few in number and pose little cause for alarm. In the 2011 National Sleep Foundation's Sleep in America annual poll, about 75 percent of people reported having had at least one symptom of a sleep problem for a few nights a week within the past year. The symptoms they report include having difficulty falling asleep, waking a lot throughout the night, prolonged periods of wakefulness during the sleep period, and waking too early and not being able to fall back asleep.[15]

Some men, however, face sleep disruptions that are not short-term. The same National Sleep Foundation study also reported that about one-half of the participants had experienced insomnia at least a few nights a week for a few weeks or a month within the past year, and one-third said they experienced at least one symptom every night or almost every night. Because insomnia seems to be a common sleep problem, and because the term *insomnia* is defined in a variety of ways, it continues to be misunderstood and underdiagnosed by both the general public and clinicians. Basically, it refers to difficulty sleeping and is distinguished by the symptoms listed above. Insomnia is the most common sleep problem and is reported more by older adults.[16] Estimates of its prevalence suggest that one-third of adults experience insomnia symptoms regularly enough to be troubled and 10 percent experience daytime impairment or distress as a result of their insomnia.[17] With or without the daytime impairment (such as midafternoon exhaustion and becoming inattentive), once insomnia becomes personally troubling, it is also clinically significant and worth bringing to the attention of your health care provider. If your insomnia lasts for 3 or more months, clinicians refer to what you are experiencing as *chronic insomnia*.

Most cases of insomnia are caused by an existing health problem or another sleep problem, yet unraveling the knot of reasons that likely play a part in why you have insomnia is complicated. Your insomnia could be "simply" the result of the emotional issues surrounding a significant life event (e.g., your daughter's wedding, your retirement) or caused by some combination of emotional stress, a physical disorder, alcohol, the self-criticism that typically intensifies about the time we fall asleep or in the early morning hours as we are waking up, and your advancing age. Some normal physiological changes that come with aging which contribute to insomnia are sleep apnea, leg cramps (discussed below), and the need to urinate. Men with heart disease, hypertension, diabetes, stomach ulcers, and arthritis are twice as likely to also cope with insomnia. Insomnia also arises when our circadian clocks are off cycle, as is common when stress increases our cortisol levels.

Can't get your body to fall back or spring forward? Worried a lot? Forgot to get to bed on time, or simply was not able to get to bed due to work or family obligations? Many insomnia issues may arise as a result of these straightforward reasons. However, bad sleep habits (or poor sleep hygiene) can cause and perpetuate insomnia as much as health problems. Deciding what sleep-related habits to change largely depends on your personal routines. In addition, review the medications you are taking—allergy and pain medications can often cause insomnia. Other "drugs" that promote insomnia include caffeinated foods and beverages using coffee and cocoa beans or cola nuts (coffee, hot chocolate, chocolate cake, cola drinks), as well as alcohol.

It is our belief, based on research, that insomnia is best managed by changing your behaviors and routines. Cognitive behavioral treatments are more effective in the long run than sleep-promoting medication. In fact, you may purchase an over-the-counter sleep-aid medication, begin taking it, and come to believe that the sleeping medication is necessary for sleep; however, in clinical studies comparing men using a placebo with men using a sleep medication, the placebo effects in treating insomnia are remarkably long-term.[18] It is the belief that the pill is helping with a good night's sleep that is most effective. Review the sleep hygiene tips in the boxed insert and the behavioral strategies discussed later to manage sleep deprivation.

Sleep Hygiene Tips

- Do the best you can to set a consistent sleep schedule; go to bed at the same time every night, and get up at the same time every morning, even if you feel tired.

- Make sure your bedroom is a quiet, dark, cool, and relaxing environment. Could the bedroom be made darker or cooler?

- Turn the TV and radio off.

- It is a myth that alcohol helps you sleep. For a few hours after consumption, alcohol has the opposite effect—it is a stimulant.

- Avoid large meals before bedtime, especially heavy, spicy, or sugary foods.

- Create a presleep ritual—a shower, or a cup of herbal tea. It can be anything that is calming and relaxing.

- Exercise, but not before bed. Regular exercise can help deepen sleep, but exercise too close to going to bed will increase your core body temperature, making it difficult to fall asleep.

Obstructive Sleep Apnea

The most common type of sleep-related breathing disorder among men is obstructive sleep apnea (OSA).[19] This occurs when the tissue in the back of the throat collapses during sleep, thus blocking your airway. This is a common disorder because as you sleep the muscles inside the throat relax and gravity causes the tissues to hang. The blockage can happen several to several hundred times in one night. Each time your airway is blocked it may last 10–20 seconds, or even up to a minute. Being overweight increases the chances of OSA because there is more fatty tissue in the throat area.

The interrupted breathing creates a lack of oxygen in the brain. These pauses in breathing cause the brain to arouse the sleeper for a split second to breathe again, yet the sleeper is not aroused to the point of becoming fully awake. Due to this, you may not even know you have a sleep problem. One clue that you are struggling with sleep apnea is that you have chronic fatigue during the day since your sleep was disturbed throughout the night. Another clue is snoring, yet you can have apnea without snoring.

Snoring is generally caused by a partial blockage of the airway during sleep. It tends to worsen with age. Normal snoring is not necessarily bad, but it may be annoying to your bed partner and could predict health trouble down the road. If you have been regularly told that you are a loud snorer and that your sleep is marked with gasps and snorts, then this is more concerning. You likely have OSA; the Wisconsin Sleep Cohort Study showed that 24 percent of men have sleep apnea.[20] Be sure to consult a health care provider if gaps and snorts are typically the way you snore. If you do not know, ask your partner or video-record yourself when going to bed. Being very temporarily embarrassed by discovering how you snore is going to be much less troubling than living with chronic fatigue and your partner's preference for you to sleep in a different room.

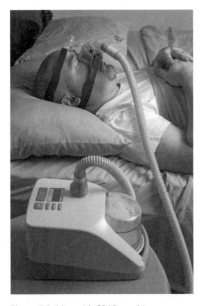

Figure 7.3. Man with CPAP machine. Courtesy of Amy Walters / Shutterstock.com.

Another sign of OSA may be frequent trips, two or more, to use the bathroom in the middle of the night. Why does this have anything to do with OSA? When you stop breathing, oxygen levels in your blood decrease, your heart pumps harder, and your blood pressure increases. After a while, fluids build up, which triggers the need to relieve the pressure, causing the need to urinate. Using the bathroom often also may be a sign of an enlarged prostate or high blood sugar, but in that case having to urinate would happen throughout the day and night.

If OSA continues without treatment, it has been shown to lead to increased risk of heart disease, high blood pressure, diabetes, and mood disorders. Losing weight, sleeping on your side, or raising the front end of the bed a couple inches does help some sleepers. However, severe OSA requires medical treatment. Although a number of surgical options remain available to help people who suffer from severe cases of OSA, nonsurgical treatments are now more often recommended. One possible nonsurgical treatment is continuous positive airway pressure (CPAP), which is a mask worn over the nose that provides a gentle and steady flow of air. The CPAP maintains an open airway and prevents pauses in breathing. Considered to be among the most effective treatments for OSA, it does require commitment on your part to use the CPAP machine correctly and consistently. Another treatment involves wearing an oral appliance, much like a mouth guard, that opens and sets your lower jaw slightly forward. Surgery is usually used only after trying other less invasive options.

Movement and Sleep Behavior Disorders

Restless leg syndrome (RLS) and periodic limb movement disorder (PLMD) are two movement disorders known to make it more difficult for people to fall asleep. Both of these conditions cause people to move their legs when they sleep, leading to poor sleep, insomnia, and drowsiness during the day. Often, both conditions can occur in the same person. Usually experienced when lying down, people with RLS are subjected to uncomfortable feelings in their legs such as tingling, crawling sensations, or pins and needles that are alleviated by moving the leg. Of course, symptoms like these can make it difficult to fall asleep and stay asleep. In the case of PLMD, people may extend their large toe, flex the ankle, or jerk and kick their legs every 20–40 seconds during the early NREM stages of the typical 90-minute sleep cycles. As you might guess, this can be very disruptive not only for the person who has this disorder but for his bed partner as well. One study found that roughly 40 percent of older adults have at least a mild form of PLMD.[21] RLS is also relatively common, affecting more than 15 percent of older men.

A less common sleep disorder called *REM sleep behavior disorder* (RBD) causes excessive movement and potentially violent behavior during REM sleep. Typically in REM sleep, our muscles are virtually paralyzed, but older men with RBD attempt to act out their dreams or nightmares and are unaware of the fact that they are in bed. RBD can be treated with medication, so if your partner says that when you sleep you sometimes violently move about, consult your physician. Recent studies have shown an association between RBD and an increased risk of developing Parkinson's.[22]

Narcolepsy

Narcolepsy is a chronic neurological condition where the brain cannot effectively regulate the wake-sleep cycle. Narcolepsy usually becomes evident between the ages of 12 and 20 and can last a lifetime. It results in "sleep attacks" causing you to suddenly fall asleep. The pressure for sleep episodes can strike at any time—when you are eating, talking, at a meeting, walking, or even driving. This condition rarely improves without treatment, but there is medication available. A sleep specialist is in the best position to make an informed diagnosis. If you have not experienced sleep attacks prior to midlife, it is unlikely that this will suddenly surface as an issue when you grow older. But if you find yourself so tired that you can fall asleep at any moment, do not delay having a conversation with your doctor. Your fatigue and sleepiness can be signaling a treatable health problem.

SLEEP DEPRIVATION

All sleep problems reduce needed good restful sleep. The multiple negative effects of sleep deprivation are highlighted in figure 7.4 and should drive home the point that adequate sleep is a central prerequisite to a healthy body as you grow older. Insufficient sleepers are twice as likely as other men to be unable to have sex, three times as likely to not work well or efficiently, and four times less likely to be able to exercise or engage in leisure activities.[23] This is just the tip of the iceberg. Although sleep does not seem

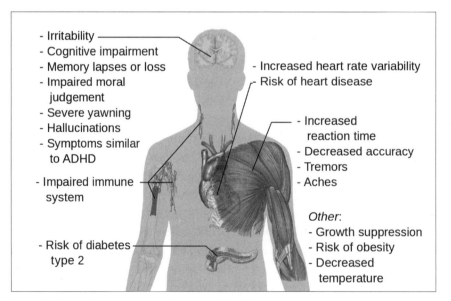

Figure 7.4. Effects of sleep deprivation. Courtesy of Mikael Haggstrom.

like something you should have on your to-do list, it should actually be at the top. Whether your sleep problems can be explained by simple bad habits or are interwoven with various other health and sleep issues, making relatively small adjustments can improve your quality of life significantly.

The Epworth Sleepiness Scale is used to determine the level of daytime sleepiness.[24] A score of 10 or more is considered sleepy. A score of 18 or more is very sleepy. If you score 10 or more on this test, you should consider whether you are obtaining adequate sleep, need to improve your sleep hygiene, and/or need to see a sleep specialist. These issues should be discussed with your personal physician. Use the following scale to choose the most appropriate number for each situation: 0 = would *never* doze or sleep; 1 = *slight* chance of dozing or sleeping; 2 = *moderate* chance of dozing or sleeping; 3 = *high* chance of dozing or sleeping.

EPWORTH SLEEPINESS SCALE

Situation	Chance of dozing or sleeping
Watching TV	_____
Sitting inactive in a public place	_____
Being a passenger in a motor vehicle for an hour or more	_____
Lying down in the afternoon	_____
Sitting and reading	_____
Sitting and talking to someone	_____
Sitting quietly after lunch (no alcohol)	_____
Stopped for a few minutes in traffic while driving	_____
Total score (add the scores up)	_____

WHAT TO DO ABOUT POOR SLEEP

Sleep is a complicated topic owing to all the different circumstances that play into it. However, there are many actions you can take to improve your sleep. Several were mentioned above as different sleep disorders were considered. There are additional resources worth knowing about.

Sleep Medications

Watch a half hour of the nightly national news, and you will very likely see at least one commercial for sleep medication. A simple web search for sleep aids kicks back an overwhelming amount of information. There are almost too many "aids" to comprehend. All have funny names, and all work a little differently for slightly different problems. It is noteworthy that many of these aids come with warning after warning. If not taken correctly, they will either not work, not work well, or do you harm. Also, as men age, our body processes medications differently than it did 10 years earlier, and sleep medications often affect men[25] differently than women. Some of the most common pharmacotherapy for insomnia for older adults includes Ambien, Sonata, Restoril, Zoloft, Sarafem, and Remeron.[26] All of these require a prescription. There are also many over-the-counter drugs available. The best advice is to consider nonpharmacological approaches and to see a doctor, especially when you find that sleep problems impact the quality of your daily life.

Behavioral Techniques

The American Academy of Sleep Medicine has identified a variety of treatment approaches for both short-term and chronic sleep disorders. In addition to better sleep hygiene and thus counteracting behaviors that interfere with sleep, one of the treatment approaches listed below also might be the best solution to your sleep problem.

Bright light therapy is used to help treat sleep disruptions that result from a problem with the circadian clock and, recently, for men struggling with posttraumatic stress disorder (PTSD). An out-of-sync internal circadian clock can be caused by jet lag or the advanced sleep phase syndrome, where the sleep-wake cycle is advanced in relation to clock time and results in gripping evening sleepiness. Bright light therapy consists of "setting" the circadian clock by exposure to artificial light to either stay awake or wake early. It also appears to reduce the severity of PTSD symptoms in combat veterans, as well as improve sleep and mood.[27]

Cognitive behavioral therapy (CBT) methods teach us how to change actions or thoughts that hurt our ability to sleep well. One approach to ending insomnia is to unlearn incorrect beliefs (such as that a "nightcap" will make me sleep well) and adopt helpful behaviors. They will help you develop habits that promote a healthy pattern of sleep without compounding your problems by unnecessarily taking a sleep medication that interacts with one of your prescriptions and causes harm. Sleep needs differ by individual, and you can best identify your needs by charting your hours of sleep, morning sleepiness, and midafternoon alertness. Can you get by on 6 or 7 hours of sleep, or do you need more?

Melatonin, as a nutritional supplement, is most effective in the treatment of certain circadian rhythm sleep disorders. These include jet lag, shift work, and delayed sleep phase.

Napping has been proven to help reduce sleep-related problems. Naturally, the body calls for a nap during the day when we hit the midafternoon slump. In one study, short naps after lunchtime improved reported sleep problems among a group of older adults. It also improved mental health, including mood and mental functioning.[28] Other studies also support taking short naps.

Tai Chi, a Chinese martial art practiced for both its defense training and its health benefits, also has proven its effectiveness in increasing self-reported sleep quality and reducing daytime sleepiness in older adults. In a 6-month study of men and women age 60–92, half were placed into a low-impact exercise program while the other group took part in Tai Chi. In the end, those in the Tai Chi program had improved their sleep quality, sleep-onset latency, sleep duration, and sleep efficiency and reduced sleep disturbances. The improvement in all of the areas was also greater than the results for the exercise group, including getting an average of more than 48 minutes more sleep per night.[29]

THE LATEST THINKING ON SLEEP

According to a 2010 National Sleep Foundation poll, as many as one in five men get less than 6 hours of sleep per night, and only about 40 percent of Americans will say that they usually are able to get a good night's sleep. Given that adult men need 7–9 hours of sleep on a regular basis, these statistics should be a reason for concern. Lack of sleep increases our risk for high blood pressure, diabetes, obesity, a compromised immune system, and increased levels of anxiety and stress. Beyond the tried-and-true strategies of keeping your bedroom cool, reducing your caffeine intake, and doing something you find relaxing before turning in for the night, there are several additional recommendations that are supported by recent research. Consider the following:

> ❯ Regular aerobic exercise appears to increase the quality of sleep for insomniacs. A Northwestern University study found that people who exercised for 40 minutes, four times a week, for 16 weeks reported improvements in sleep quality and less daytime sleepiness. It also resulted in fewer depressive symptoms.[30]

> Napping too much can negatively impact your sleep schedule. Research has found that napping is more common as men get older; however, frequently napping during the daytime can result in sleeping less at night and not sleeping as soundly.[31] Establishing a consistent routine for going to bed and waking each day appears to strengthen your circadian rhythms, the internal clock regulating sleep-wake cycles. Bottom line: take a nap if you need to during the day, but not too close to your normal bedtime and not for longer than 20 minutes at a time.

> We know that both aerobic and strength training exercise does a body good and helps you sleep better and longer. But we are also learning that different people will benefit most from exercising at particular times of the day. Consider keeping a sleep diary to determine when exercising during the day will most likely promote a restful sleep.[32]

CHAPTER 8

Appearances

OUR BODIES, HEAD TO TOE

Our bodies are symbolic. Think back to when you were starting high school. Did you think it was a put-down if someone said, "Kid, you are skinny" (or chubby)? For high schoolers 40 and 50 years ago, it was better to have weight than to need to gain it. Two bodily standards—muscles and fitness—still seem to define the idealized male body, as is evident on the covers of men's health and fashion magazines. In the popular culture, as long as a man maintains sufficient fitness and isn't thin or way too heavy, his body helps affirm his masculinity. Not everyone might think that this is true, yet our bodies are what others see and draw on to form their first impressions about us.

How much the age-related changes in our bodies affect our self-esteem is unclear.[1] Sometimes men report dissatisfaction with their bodies and sometimes not.[2] Only a small part of men's comfort with themselves actually rests on their body's size and shape.[3] Almost the entirety of the image we have of *ourselves* is rooted in what we do—being independent, self-reliant, able-bodied, and capable. The way our body changes with aging is commonly framed in words such as "I'm in pretty good shape for my age," even if the man's appearance suggests otherwise. Meet a weathered-face man in his late sixties who uses a cane, and he might confidently tell you that he doesn't feel old. You think he looks it. What you do not know is that he has been using a cane for 30 years, ever since his horse stumbled and threw him in a steeple chase, requiring several surgically implanted pins in his leg. Because he still works outdoors with horses—he is a trainer of racehorses—his skin has a distinctive weathered look. His physical appearance is consistent with his livelihood and age, and his body image is consistent with his resilience and functional ability.

BODY IMAGE

Body image was traditionally considered a "woman's thing." This is not to say that appearance is irrelevant to men; it is as much a part of our self-image as it is for women. Men are not apathetic about looking good. Body image is how a man feels about his appearance—his eyebrows, his weight, his mustache, his skinny legs—in the context of both cultural norms and the peers he uses for comparison. Even simple things matter: think about the way you feel about your appearance when you know that you need to get a haircut and then after it is cut. Having a positive body image means feeling satisfied with the way we look, appreciating our body for its capabilities, and accepting its imperfections. Psychological in nature, our body image is forever changing, responding to the social norms of what is attractive and "manly" for our age. We were not born critiquing our own looks; rather, we judge our body based on masculinity and age norms. We are socialized to judge our male bodies in terms of wholeness, and physical strength and being fit—enough to carry the ladder, rake leaves, lift a grandchild—continue to define the cultural ideal for men.

The Person in the Mirror

Have you had "the talk" with the person in the mirror and thought, "You really are getting older"? The next day you receive an invitation to attend your high school's thirtieth, fortieth, or fiftieth reunion. Do you smile and think, "This ought to be fun," or do you wince?

AGING AND APPEARANCE

In the rest of this chapter we examine from head to toe a variety of ways our appearance changes with aging. Typically, men's proportion of body fat doubles between ages 25 and 75, since our metabolism slows down and our bodies need fewer calories than we usually take in and burn up. The leathery look is often evident on our hands and faces, and less hair develops as skin cells decrease in size.

As you got within shouting distance of being middle-aged, you probably noticed many ways your appearance was changing. We do notice and keep track of our aging. Men can list matter-of-factly a number of physical traits when asked about their age-related changing appearance—wrinkles, thinning hair and balding, "age spots," stooped shoulders and hunching, thinning skin on our hands, a distinct belly, and skinnier legs with varicose veins. Even if some of the changes set off silent alarms, most bodily changes likely bring out little more than nodding recognition. Australian researchers reported that the older men they studied were less satisfied with their appearance but were not making much of an effort to improve self-presentation by using skin creams or polymers to make their thinning hair look thicker.[4] What's good to know is that our long-term partners also are less bothered with our changing appearance and are more interested in us maintaining a healthy body.[5]

HAIR LOSS AND BALDNESS

Men consider a full head of thick hair as more important to their virility and attractiveness than their weight.[6] After centuries of powerful men wearing wigs and/or growing long hair, men were persuaded to believe that as we lose our hair we become less powerful, less masculine, and less attractive.[7] Recall the biblical story of Samson losing his strength and being socially castrated after his hair was cut.

But the facts are that by the time we are age 50, one-half of all men reveal moderate to extensive hair loss and some baldness.[8] What causes the scalp hair loss that leads to baldness? Let's begin with what does not cause baldness. In general, rarely is it caused by disease, nor is poor diet or strong shampoo an important factor. When we lose our hair, we tend to lose it because it's our destiny. Men's hair loss is caused by a combination of genetics and age-related changes in our hormones. Clinically referred to as *androgenic alopecia*, the "andro" refers to the androgen hormones (testosterone and dihydrotestosterone [DHT]), and the "genic" refers to the male gene necessary for baldness to occur. Each hair follicle is genetically programmed when to quit producing new hairs *if* we are genetically predisposed for a receding hairline and/or baldness. Our genetic inheritance makes about half of us prone to what is called male pattern hair loss (MPHL).[9] This is a "condition" that both shortens the growth phase of the hair cycle and produces progressively shorter, finer hairs. Eventually these hairs totally disappear.

If your grandfathers and father showed evidence of a receding hairline and balding, and you are experiencing hair loss, you too are very likely to pass this genetic trait on to your sons and grandsons. By the way, we do inherit MPHL from either side of our family, so take a look at photos of both your mother's and your father's male relatives to see who had the most hair loss in your family lines. Biological aging is also an important, secondary determinant of both thinning hair and baldness. As we get older, less testosterone and more DHT are produced; when there is an excess of DHT, this contributes to our hair getting thinner and eventually to hair loss.

The Hamilton-Norwood Scale, initially created by James Hamilton in the 1950s and revised by O'Tar Norwood in the 1970s, details the way male pattern baldness (MPB) occurs. There are two variations: "anterior" and "vertex." Anterior MPB means that the receding starts from the front of your scalp; vertex MPB begins from the crown (top). Both anterior and vertex patterns of balding end the same (stages VI and VII)—the crown of your head is bald.

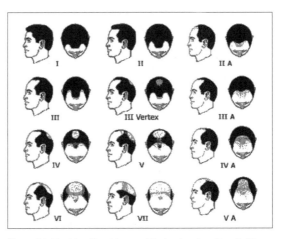

Figure 8.1. The Hamilton-Norwood Scale of male pattern baldness

Knowing that hair loss is caused mostly by genetics and aging ought to dispel most myths about men's baldness. Have you heard that wearing hats, helmets, or baseball caps makes you bald? If this were true, the hat (or helmet) would have to literally choke each hair follicle for weeks on end. Think about it: how many baseball players in the Baseball Hall of Fame still have a full head of hair, and many are old men when inducted. Was their cap loose fitting, whereas the guys with MBHL wore tight-fitting caps? Another set of wild tales market "cures" for hair loss and baldness caused by poor circulation. Blaming receding hairline on the amount of blood flow to hair follicles opens the door to all sorts of "doctor-recommended" products that purport to improve blood flow and/or nutrients to the blood and vitamins to the scalp. Ever heard the one about getting a cow to lick your head? Men faced with a receding hairline may try nearly anything, and research tells us that the typical man who seeks medical treatment for his MPHL has already engaged in considerable efforts to self-treat.[10] No matter what advertisements may claim about a treatment, receding hairlines and MPB are almost always genetic.

You might also have heard that stress will cause you to go bald. Stress does not cause baldness, but like chemotherapy, it can cause temporary hair loss. The chemotherapy involved in cancer treatment is designed to attack fast-growing (cancer) cells, and because hair roots are fast-growing cells, they too are attacked. Chemotherapy causes temporary hair loss all over the body, not just the scalp. Stress can stop hair growth. If you have overwhelming stress, the buildup of stress hormones causes the hair shaft to stop growing and forces a large number of hairs into a resting phase. In effect, your hair growth goes dormant. Within a few months, the affected hairs may fall out suddenly when washing or brushing your hair; they typically grow back 6–9 months later.

Under normal circumstances, the hair follicles on the scalp do not continuously produce hair. After 2 or more years, they revert to a resting stage for several weeks, up to 2 months, before beginning to grow new hair. At any time on a healthy human scalp, about 80–90 percent of the hair follicles are growing hair, which leaves up to 10–20 percent of scalp hair follicles in a resting state. The average life span of a single hair is 4½ years; the hair then falls out and is replaced within 6 months by a new hair. The average guy will lose 50–100 hairs from his head each day (about 0.1%). If you are among the small group of men in their sixties and seventies with a full head of hair, this process of shedding and growing new hairs remains unaffected.

Alopecia areata is an autoimmune condition where white blood cells attack the hair follicles and produce small, patchy areas of hair loss. It usually starts as a small circle of perfectly smooth baldness, and the hairs in the (bald) patches will usually regrow within 3–6 months without treatment. The hair that grows back may be white, leaving a small patch of white hair. Alopecia can affect hair on other parts of the body, too, such as the beard.

A recent study treated mice that had been genetically altered to overproduce the stress hormone called corticotropin-releasing factor (CRF). The study was designed to assess if a stress hormone inhibitor called astressin-B would diminish the effects of stress on the colon, yet what the researchers accidently found was that the stress hormone receptors in the skin and near or within the hair follicle were affected. If this hormone inhibitor proves to be reliable, there may someday soon be a treatment to prevent alopecia areata and the hair loss caused by stress.

No conditioner, shampoo, vitamin, or other product reverses baldness. Yet there are some medications that slow down hair loss and may stimulate hair growth when hair follicles still exist. When the hair follicles are gone, the hair is gone for good. Traditional methods of stimulating hair growth include minoxidil and finasteride, and surgical transplantation is also available to treat baldness.

The two basic U.S. Food and Drug Administration (FDA) approved options to slow down the rate of hair loss are minoxidil (Rogaine) and either finasteride (Propecia; not Proscar) or dutasteride (Avodart). The topical minoxidil can be purchased at any drugstore without a prescription, and if the product works, it works slowly, requiring 2–4 months before any noticeable results. Studies have confirmed that a twice-daily application of this topical cream can stimulate the growth phase of hair for some men. It seems to be most effective on the crown, rather than the frontal region, and if it works, it encourages live hair follicles to regrow a hair. Even so, applying Rogaine is basically a treatment for preserving what hair is already there. The drawback is the requirement to rub the topical onto the scalp twice daily, for as long as you want the result. It is necessary to continue to use the product for as long as you wish to keep the regrown hair.

The use of finasteride and dutasteride for hair loss involves a much lower dose of the same drugs that shrink an enlarged prostate. Both require a prescription. Taken once daily, the drugs are only effective for "fertilizing" and thickening *existing* scalp hair. Both have the same drawbacks: they are more costly, and they may lower sexual drive and (temporarily) cause erectile dysfunction. These side effects are reversible shortly after the drug is stopped.

Contemporary surgical treatment involves hair transplantation— surgically taking hair (several hundred plugs) from the side or back of the scalp and implanting it in the front. For reasons not fully understood, the hair on the side of the head seems to be "naturally resistant" to the hair-damaging hormones. Transplant procedures have improved greatly and produce much more natural-looking results than older surgical plug methods, which often left a checkerboard of hair stalks and bald spots. Many transplant patients also take Propecia (finasteride) to keep what they've transplanted. If you are considering a hair transplant, it is critical to triple-check the surgeon's credentials and experience treating other men.

Currently, there are countless new, controversial and experimental treatments marketed to address men's hair loss. One treatment recently approved by the FDA is low-level light therapy (LLLT). Advertised as a nonchemical, noninvasive treatment for hair loss, it seems that men who have more hair (perhaps in early stages of hair loss) tend to have better results. Low-energy laser light travels several layers into the scalp tissue without harming the skin and scalp, and the therapeutic light energy is absorbed by the cells, beginning the process of cell repair. One theory is that the laser light stimulates the cellular production of energy. There is minimal clinical evidence of the efficacy of LLLT, although most experts agree that it is safe.

Another "treatment" is to purchase a pair of hairpieces. A good hairpiece is custom made for you (taking into consideration the shape of your skull, your skin and hair color, the amount of your remaining hair). If properly cared for, a custom hairpiece can provide you with years of a self-presentation that reflects some receding hairline but no evidence of balding on the crown. By contrast, a bad hairpiece is a red flag that points to *your* concerns with balding. Good hairpieces are not inexpensive, and you will need two identical ones so that you can alternate their use while you clean one of the pair.

Maybe the best "treatment" is to let nature take its course. Nearly every man's hair thins with time; it's part of our bodies' aging. Our receding hairline can be a celebrated sign of our earned status as older men. As much as the vast majority of men with hair loss do not seek treatment for their hair loss, studies consistently reveal that men are upset by their hair loss.[11]

GRAYING HAIR

Whether wanted or not, graying hair slowly takes over. Gray hair once was considered the ideal in politics and business, and white or gray powdered wigs were all the rage in the eighteenth century among U.S. colonists, who gravitated to gray because they equated older age with respect, power, and prosperity.

The onset of graying hair is relatively predictable. Scientists are not completely sure *why* it happens. Nor is there certainty *how* our hair grays. The consensus opinion is that getting gray hair is a natural part of growing older. It results from a progressive loss of pigment (melanin) cells, whether it is our scalp, face, armpit, chest, or pubic hair.

The rate of our hair's graying is related to both aging and heredity. Each shaft of hair is basically colorless, and melanin (or the pigment) is produced by melanocyte cells inside the follicle. Each hair is made up of two parts—a shaft, which is the colored part we see growing out of our heads, and a root. The root of every hair is surrounded by tissue called the follicle, and it is the hair follicle that contains the pigment cells. These pigment cells continuously produce the melanin to give each hair its color. Once a hair follicle stops producing pigment and the hair shaft turns gray, there is nothing that can make it start producing pigment again.

For a long time medical researchers assumed that with age the melanocyte cells simply became less efficient at making pigment—they got old and tired, and we got gray. However, recent studies have shown that growing older brings about a steady decline in the number of new pigment-producing cells, and the stem cells within hair follicles responsible for color are the most impacted by irreparable DNA weathering that comes from our exposure to ultraviolet light, chemicals, and ionizing radiation. Our genetic makeup and heredity also play some role, since premature graying tends to run in families. There are racial differences, too. Among white men, hair starts turning gray often in their midthirties, but among Asians it begins in the late thirties and for African Americans in the midforties. About half of 50-year-olds are at least 50 percent gray.

Legend has it that some men's hair turns white virtually overnight as a result of a traumatic event. Although extremely unlikely, stress *may* accelerate the pace of our natural graying process. Stress hormones may impact the survival and the number of new pigment-producing melanocytes; however, no clear link has been found between stress and gray hair. Gray hair is simply a sign of biological aging, and once the graying starts, the proportion of (remaining) hair turning gray increases by 10–20 percent each decade.

Becoming Gray

Leo M. Cooney, professor and chief of geriatrics at the Yale University School of Medicine, argues that "people with premature graying of the hair don't die any sooner than anybody else . . . gray hair has something to do with your genetics and very little to do with premature aging."

Source: Parker-Hope, T. (2009, Mar. 10). Unlocking the secrets of gray hair. *New York Times*, Section D, p. 5.

Graying hair contributes to people's notions about our health and well-being. They presume we are less physically active, tire easily, and are less sexual.[12] The messages conveyed through television and magazines are rarely pro-gray. Americans are ambivalent about gray hair in the workplace or among middle-aged men, and even Presidents Ronald Reagan and George H. W. Bush preferred coloring their hair.

There are probably hundreds of other folk remedies (e.g., in Chinese medicine, fo-ti is a longevity tonic that is used to treat graying hair); people believe that a deficiency in folic acid (vitamin B9) causes graying, which can be prevented by eating foods high in folate, such as leafy greens, beans, and grain products that have added folic acid, but the sure way is to hide the gray by using hair coloring. Some men use a temporary dye, which coats your hair with distinct color molecules and is quick and easy to apply. Temporary dyes contain no ammonia and may result in less damage to the hair. Most of these commercial self-applied dyes characteristically begin to wash away after a half dozen morning shampoos, which means that you have to reapply the dye several times a month. An alternative is called progressive coloring. This is the "Grecian Formula" strategy that colors the hair gradually, and the change is not as noticeable as overnight regular dyes. Progressive hair colorants (and there are many, such as Gray-Ban, Grecian Formula, and Youthair) use lead acetate and sulfur as the active ingredients and cause the treated hair to darken when exposed to air. Several applications are needed to gradually color your hair, and you can decide how dark of an effect you want. The colorant both coats and penetrates the hair shaft.

A third option is a tone-on-tone semipermanent color. This method of coloring uses peroxide to permit the color molecules to penetrate the hair shaft and creates a more permanent color. This strategy to "remove the gray" usually takes 10–15 minutes to apply and will last nearly twice as long as direct dyes. But expect to invest time and money.

UNEXPECTED HAIR

As we age, the texture of hair changes—it becomes coarser. At the same time you are dealing with the graying, thinning, and slow loss of scalp hair, the hair that remains has become bristly. You recognize that your hair doesn't lie down as well as it used to when brushed. You also notice that you have some coarse, fast-growing bristly new hairs in all sorts of places—your eyebrows, ears, nostrils, and tops of the toes. You are dealing with the biology of aging. You are not suffering from "hypertrichosis," which is a medical condition that involves excessive growth of hair in areas where hair does not normally grow (e.g., palm of your hand), and for a very few cases excessive enough to be informally called werewolf syndrome.

If your eyebrows become bushy, and if your nose, toes, and ears sprout these bristly, coarse hairs, you are dealing with genetics and hormone changes, not a medical condition. The nose and the ears contain thousands and thousands of hairs. Most are so small you can't see them. For about three-quarters of men, the tiny little hairs inside the nose and ear canal and on the outside of the ear will eventually become thicker and coarser as they age. Similar to how science doesn't fully understand *why* our hair grays, we understand too little about why hair follicles in and around men's ears and nose begin growing coarser.

You can manage most of this new hair growth quite easily. Plucking the distinct, extra hairs on the tip of the nose or above the bridge of the nose with tweezers is an easy way to remove unwanted individual hairs on the face. But using tweezers isn't recommended for most other places—such as your ears and nose. There are electric trimmers that you or someone else can use (consider asking your wife, partner, or barber) to trim the length of the hair on your eyebrows and the outside of your ear. There also are inexpensive, battery-powered trimmers that safely cut down nose and ear hair and have external combs to protect the skin from being pinched or nicked.

FACIAL CHANGES

Years of the pull of gravity, adding a bit more facial body fat,[13] and loss of skin's elasticity—put these three together, and you have the basic ingredients to why wrinkles begin to appear, why men's ears and noses get bigger, why the cheeks look more sunken, and why "double chins" slowly emerge as we age.[14] The actual pace of the changes is affected by sun exposure, smoking, diets, and when men "turtle up" and have less active lifestyles.[15]

Facial anatomy is composed of three things: the skin; the underlying soft tissue, muscle, and fascia; and the bony, cartilaginous skeletal structure. With aging, the elasticity of skin declines, there is a weakening of the underlying soft muscular tissue over the cheek and jaw bones, and there is bone resorption. The more noticeable result is the sagging appearance of skin in the midface and nose and the likely formation of jowls. As the skin thins, becomes dryer, and loses elasticity, eyelids may begin to droop and the lower eyelids may begin to appear "baggy." Wrinkles develop on the brow, around the eyes, in cheeks, and next to the mouth. With age, the height/length ratio of the nose and ear progressively decreases, which means a lengthening of the ears and the prolongation of the nose and "drooping" of its tip. At the same time, the hairline moves upward, further making the upper part of the face look elongated, and the skin under the jaw sags down, making the skin fold and the man appear to have a second (or double) chin. Our once smooth, fuller face has slowly morphed to become more leathery, weathered, wrinkled, thinner, and longer, with occasional "age spots" to boot (discussed below).

Similar to graying hair, these facial changes may well make some men not appreciate getting older, nor feel good about their changing appearance. There are two basic kinds of strategies to manage the expected age-related changes in facial appearance. Upstream strategies prevent; begin by reducing your exposure to the factors that hasten facial aging—avoid cigarette smoking, reduce exposure to ultraviolet sunlight, and hydrate to reduce water loss that stiffens skin and weakens the facial musculature. Upstream strategies involve other forms of prevention, including engaging in jaw and neck exercises, eating well, and maintaining fitness. Men who are more sedentary slowly add weight by not burning enough calories through exercise, and this increases the risk of the double chin. The downstream strategies are treatment-oriented, ranging from noninvasive techniques such as skin care products that may tighten and firm skin to the more invasive cosmetic surgery that might remove wrinkles, tighten facial skin, remove the double chin, or restructure the nose. Do recognize that cosmetic moisturizers merely cover the skin with a water

Know the Nose

Like other organs, the nose changes as the body ages, and we become increasingly vulnerable to nasal problems and complain of nasal obstruction, nasal drainage and sneezing, coughing, nosebleeds, snoring, olfactory loss, and nasal-sinus pain. An especially notable age-related nasal change is the reduced efficiency of the nose for breathing.

Source: Edelstein, D. R. (1996). Aging of the normal nose in adults. *Laryngoscope, 106* (9), suppl. 81, 1-25.

barrier to slow the loss of moisture from the skin and give the skin a temporary appearance of plumpness and fullness.

SKIN

Skin is our body's largest organ. It is our principle organ of touch, sensuality, pleasure, and appearance. It varies in thickness, ranging from the soles of the feet (the thickest) to the thinnest areas under the eyes and on the eyelids. One square *inch* of skin on a healthy middle-aged man contains nearly 3 million cells, 75 feet of nerves, 600 sweat glands, at least 100 oil glands, and many hair follicles. Imagine what 1 square *foot* contains, and then consider that a male body is covered by 15–20 square feet.

The structure and function of skin change as we age. It loses some of its elastic quality and becomes looser. It loses its ability to retain water, resulting in drier skin. It becomes thinner. It heals more slowly. It is less able to resist being damaged. These changes bring about normal things like wrinkles and, for about two-thirds of adult men, skin problems.

Skin "thins"[16] with aging—more accurately, the epidermis (or outermost layers of cells) comes to involve fewer layers. The epidermis is composed of two basic levels that collectively measure little more than 1 millimeter in a healthy middle-aged man. The living cells of the epidermis aren't the very top layer; rather, they are just below several layers of near-dead or dead cells. Skin cells routinely move upward, replacing the 50–100 million dead, top-layer cells we "shed" daily. Dermatologists refer to the time it takes cells to move upward as "transit time," and the process is called *desquamation*. You are more apt to notice the "shedding" during the winter as you remove your socks and see white specks clinging to them. As we get older, the transit time slows down; the entire process of replacing skin cells takes as much as 40 days rather than 14–20 days, and without the faster rate of replacement we once experienced as young men, the skin thins.

Just beneath the surface skin is the thicker "dermis." This middle layer of skin is loaded with glands, nerves, blood vessels, hair follicles, fibrous proteins (called *collagen* and *elastin*) that determine the skin's elasticity and structure, and proteins that hold water in the skin and serve as skin moisturizers. The dermis also becomes thinner with age because of slower cell reproduction. Fibrous protein cells diminish in number at an annual rate of about 1 percent, causing the skin to become (and appear) looser and sag.[17] With less fibrous protein cells, the thinner and more flaccid dermal tissue also produces fine wrinkles all over the body surface.

Wrinkles. The best advice is to put on sunscreen and wear a hat. Compare the skin on your face and hands with the skin on your butt. Your hands and face haven't been hidden from the sun. Because it is the sun's radiation that largely determines the pace of developing wrinkles, most wrinkles appear on the parts of the body where sun exposure is greatest. There are two types of wrinkles: fine surface lines and deep furrows. Squinting your eyes when too vain to wear your glasses or when not wearing sunglasses, scowling all the time, or puckering your lips thousands of times a day while smoking cigarettes—all of these habits accelerate the pace of facial wrinkle formation. The skin has memory (called *mnemodermia*), and its memory is like an elephant's. When it is repeatedly pushed into the same folds with each frown, smile, or facial contraction, fine wrinkles become deep furrows.

For men who are troubled by their emerging facial wrinkles, there is some evidence that fine wrinkles can be delayed and reduced by using wrinkle creams that include retinoids, which are derived from vitamin A. There are lotions and creams that are able to reduce skin roughness. You are also encouraged to use "detergents" such as Dove soap, rather than (Ivory) "soaps" that contribute to dry skin because they are alkaline soaps. To manage deep furrow wrinkles, there are a variety of treatments, such as chemical peels, laser treatment, and dermabrasion, which involves an intense scrubbing and leaves the treated area sensitive and red for about a week.

Have you noticed "age spots," or what some people call "liver spots"? The spots (or *lentigines*) are brownish and appear over time on your face and body, similar to freckles. The spots are no more than distinct clusters of epidermis cells and the uneven pigmentation most prominent in sun-exposed areas of skin. All epidermis cells make the melanin (or pigment) responsible for freckles, skin color, birthmarks, and moles. As our skin ages, the melanin-producing cells will at times mass together to cause dark(er) patches; aging skin also has lesser ability to fend off UV rays from the sun, and this UV exposure is largely responsible for the dermal changes that lead to the development of so-called age spots.

Fungal skin infections (called *tinea*) such as athlete's foot and "jock itch" in the groin are noticed by others if you are constantly scratching the itch. Most of these infections are superficial, whether it is skin cracking between the toes, a scaliness over the sole of the foot, or red, raised scaly patches in the skin folds in the groin area. Beyond the itching and the unpleasant odor, the infections can be controlled with a daily application of an antifungal cream or powder for 4–6 weeks. Risk factors include sweating heavily, walking barefoot on damp public floors, weak immune systems, and smoking.

By contrast, a *fungal nail infection* is more difficult to treat and will continue indefinitely if left untreated. Nails are essentially hardened skin cells and made mostly of keratin, which is the same protein found in hair. The living cells begin in the hidden (half moon) area under the cuticle, and as new skin cells grow, the older cells are pushed forward, harden, and form a visible nail. As we age, nails thicken and become more susceptible to infection. The infection frequently begins as a white spot just under the tip of the toenail or fingernail, and as the fungi spread deeper into your nail, the nail discolors, thickens, becomes dull, develops crumbling edges, and has dark, smelly debris. It can be unsightly and is sometimes painful. Oral antifungal medication (e.g., griseofulin, terbinafine) works about 50–75 percent of the time. Unlike most antibiotics, it often takes 6–12 months to see if the treatment worked or not, because it takes that long for a nail to grow out.

Cellulitis is a bacterial infection involving a sudden, red skin rash. Microorganisms are always living on skin and can enter the body when there is a small crack or cut. Though cellulitis can occur anywhere on the body, it is more likely found on the legs and arms, starting on a crack in the skin, especially between the toes. The inflamed, infected area becomes red, hot, and irritated, and because you have an infection, other symptoms can include muscle aches, chills, fatigue, fever, and sweating. Men with compromised immune systems are at greater risk of a cellulitis infection, and those with a fungal infection are also at increased risk of cellulitis coming back multiple times. Typically, treatment involves a 7–10 day regime of oral antibiotic medication.[18]

Eczema is a common problem in the skin that involves itching, redness, and scaling. Less often, you might also have to deal with edema, or the accumulation of fluid beneath the skin. The actual cause of eczema is unknown. The most common form of eczema is *dry skin* (or xerosis), which is likely caused by dehydration and vitamin A deficiency. Sometimes called "winter itch," dry skin is more common in northern winter climates with low humidity and cold temperatures. It usually manifests as itchy, scaly, cracked, red plaques on the arms and, more commonly, the lower legs and shins. Dry skin can be prevented by reducing the effects of (harsh) soaps that remove too much of the skin's natural oils and keeping the skin hydrated via liberal and frequent use of skin care emollients and moisturizers.[19]

Psoriasis is an autoimmune, chronic inflammatory disorder of the skin (and, at times, joints) which occurs in many forms and is more common as we get older. It affects millions of men, has no known cure, and is not contagious. The most widespread form (plaque psoriasis) produces reddish, scaly lesions or thick lesions covered with thick silvery white scales that can erupt anywhere on the body. It commonly appears on the elbows, scalp, knees, ankles, groin, or torso, and the lesions may be itchy. Although the cause of psoriasis is unknown, it can break out as a result of psychological stress, an infection, a skin abrasion, or the side effects of prescription drugs, especially among men using multiple prescription and over-the-counter medications (called *polypharmacy*).[20] The prescription drugs most often associated with psoriasis are the nonsteroidal anti-inflammatory drugs (NSAIDs) we use to treat headaches, arthritis, and sports injuries; antibiotics such as penicillin; and diuretics.

Treatment aims at managing the symptoms. Corticosteroid creams and other topical products are usually the first line of treatment. Your doctor might recommend one of several forms of photo or light therapy in combination with a topical cream that might include synthetic forms of vitamin D or anti-inflammatories like corticosteroids. For severe psoriasis, there are biological therapies that have been approved by the FDA within the past 5 years. Unlike medicines, which are a combination of chemicals, biologics are primarily made up of proteins that are made from or taken from living cells and tissues, and they act as inhibitors to specific molecules thought to be essential in causing psoriasis inflammation.[21] The treatments can be taken orally or by injection (e.g., Enbrel, Stelara, and Humira). Because these biologics attack T-cells within your immune system responsible for causing skin problems, these new treatments do carry the risk of reducing the ability of your immune system to fight potentially serious and even life-threatening infections.

Shingles is a type of painful, blistering skin rash caused by the herpes zoster virus, which is the same virus that causes chickenpox. It is more likely to develop after age 60, especially if you had chickenpox when you were very young. Once you have had chickenpox, the virus remains dormant in certain nerve cells. Exactly what triggers the onset of the rash isn't known. The initial signs are little grouped blisters that cause pain, tingling, or a burning sensation; the tingling, burning discomfort usually begins before the blisters are noticeable. For most people, the blisters are clustered together and sit on a line of reddened skin that may begin on the back and will run around the ribs to the front of the belly. The line of blisters can be thin or as wide as your fist. Sometimes shingles are located on the neck, hands, and cheek. On rarer occasions, the rash may involve the eyes and mouth. Should an itching, *painful* rash develop in your eyes, see a physician *immediately*; blindness is one of the complications. Wherever shingles is located on your body, it can cause considerable pain because it involves an inflammation of spinal nerves, and there might be lingering pain after the flare-up.

Ironically, shingles usually gets better on its own; however, your physician can prescribe antiviral medication (e.g., acyclovir, famciclovir, valacyclovir) to fight the virus, and the medication typically shortens the course of the inflammation and helps reduce the discomfort. You can also soak the inflamed areas with a wet cloth to ease the discomfort or soak yourself in a colloidal oatmeal bath. The goal is to keep the blisters dampened until crusting occurs. Finally, a herpes vaccine is available (Zostavax, approved in 2006) and has been shown to reduce the risk of getting shingles by half, as well as reduce the pain associated with this condition if you still get it. The vaccine is recommended for adults 60 years and older.[22]

THE BELLY

Have you noticed that your once-chiseled chest seems to have sunk into your belly? That your waistline has expanded? Chances are you weigh more now than you did when you were younger, and even if you weigh the same as you did 25 years ago, your muscle/fat ratio has likely changed. Physiological aging causes muscle to diminish and fat to increase. In addition, as we get older, our bodies simply need fewer calories to maintain our weight and good health, so if you are still eating like a teenager and do not regularly exercise, you've probably put on pounds. If these added pounds are belly fat and you are now "pear" shaped, you are living with more than just a change in your appearance—there is a serious health risk.

> For my sixtieth birthday, I asked my wife to surprise me. She said, "Ahhh, give me some hints." So, I gave her two hints. I'd like something sleek and polished, and something that goes from zero to 200 in seconds. She gave me a scale!
>
> —Source unknown

The surgeon general argues that there is an "obesity epidemic" among middle-aged and older men in the United States.[23] Whether or not this claim is true, three-quarters of men age 40 and older have already added enough abdomen weight that they can be officially classified as overweight. Clinical studies have found that the size of a man's belly (waist circumference) is actually a better predictor of heart disease and mortality than general obesity.[24] The Mayo Clinic proposed a good way to measure your waist. Use a flexible tape measure—not one of the metal tape measures from your workbench. Pull the tape around your bare abdomen just above the hipbone until it fits snugly. Relax, exhale normally, and measure your waist without sucking in your belly. What's your waist size? Generally speaking, if your waist size is greater than 40 inches, you need to pay attention to things you do (and do not do) that will increase your risk of type 2 diabetes and heart disease.[25]

Even though the most common weight-related change for men is the accumulated fat around the abdomen, which makes men in their sixties and seventies look a tiny bit pregnant, too frequently men do not fret much about their weight. Nearly two-thirds of men age 50 and older in a Gallup poll reported that they rarely worry about their weight, and in a later Gallup poll nearly two-thirds of the men also described their weight as "about right."[26] As a result, men who are overweight (but not obese) are not likely to perceive themselves as overweight or think that their eating and exercise habits are unhealthy.[27]

Middle age is when your age begins to appear around your middle.

—Bob Hope

On occasion you will see a guy at the mall, workplace, or beach who sports a bulging beer belly. Unlike women's experiences, his largeness has long been accepted and has even been considered evidence of being powerful and "manly." Americans have normalized large breakfasts of steak and eggs, the "man-sized" frozen dinners in Hungry-Man advertisements (with 1,700 calories), and 300-pound, very fit professional footballers.

Being large is accepted, so long as you are fit. This could be why men whose weight is roughly 10–20 pounds more than their ideal weight are rarely judged by other people as "heavy" (though women are), and this lack of judgment could be why there is such a disconnect between the large percentage of men who are overweight and the small percentage who recognize themselves as such.

Even should we concede that our weight is higher than the ideal, barely more than half of adult men in the United States have ever tried to lose weight in their lifetime.[28] Men prefer to use exercise and going to the gym as a way of "correcting" an overweight body, rather than dieting.[29] As one 54-year-old man observed about men and dieting,

> It's not normally vanity. The men don't seem to worry that they are overweight, whereas the women are more inclined towards the sort of vanity of being overweight, y'know. Most of the men that I know up here were doing it for some sort of medical reason. Cause, y'know, something pushed them into it; otherwise they wouldn't have come [to the slimming club].[30]

Men who work out 30–45 minutes and burn off 200 calories are unaware that the athletic drink they downed right after working out added 130–300 calories right back.

All in all, by the time we are 60, most of us tend to be heavier than we were at 40. We might pat our flabby-looking stomach after a morning shower, think a moment about it, and then do nothing. That is the problem.

LEGS

As our bodies age, there are two appearance changes in men's legs. One is the slow loss of muscle mass in the thighs and calves, or what is thought of as the onset of age-related "skinny legs." The other is the arrival of varicose veins.

Have you discovered a ropy, blue, gnarled, and sometimes painful vein winding down your leg or ankle? If so, you are among the 20–50 percent of men who are likely to live with varicose veins or the milder spidery veins.[31] Varicose veins are most common in the surface veins of the skin. They tend to be inherited from either side of your family, and aging increases the risk. In normal veins, one-way valves keep blood moving toward the heart, but the wear and tear of aging causes weakened valves to no longer open and close properly, allowing blood to remain in or flow back into the vein. This pooling causes the vein to enlarge. As you get older, your veins also can lose elasticity, causing them to stretch, which can affect valve functioning.

Risk is increased by being overweight, being physically inactive, smoking, and having a poor diet, which are the same poor health habits that are linked to heart disease. Additionally, leg veins are subject to the effects of high pressure when standing, and men who run outdoors on hard surfaces can hasten the onset of varicose veins. Though varicose veins may be perceived as unattractive, they usually are not a sign of a serious problem. They are mostly a cosmetic concern. However, for some men varicose veins can be achingly painful.

Treatment begins by self-care—such as wearing compression stockings, elevating your legs at night, exercising, losing weight, and avoiding long periods of standing. Do you have a recliner with an extending footrest (or "easy chair") to elevate your legs? Compression socks (or stockings) ought to be your first effort to deal with varicose veins before you begin other treatments. They can be worn from morning to night, and as they steadily squeeze your legs, they help veins and leg muscles move blood more efficiently. Medical therapies include sclerotherapy, which entails injecting the small- and medium-sized varicose veins with a solution that causes the vein to absorb the solution and close. No local anesthesia is needed, nor is there a recovery time. You can immediately return to your planned activities for the day. After a few weeks, the treated varicose veins should fade. The same vein may need to be injected more than once. Other effective treatments are laser surgery, vein stripping, and catheter-assisted procedures where a physician inserts a catheter into an enlarged vein, heats the tip of the catheter, and pulls the catheter, leaving the heat to destroy the vein and causing it to collapse and seal shut.

By contrast, the onset of age-related skinnier legs (smaller calf and thigh circumference) is often preventable but isn't really treatable. Because the primary cause of smaller calf and thigh circumference is the loss of muscle mass, men who are not physically active—who prefer to ride the elevator rather than take the stairs, or motor around the golf course in a cart rather than walk or pull the clubs—do not counteract the effects of physiological aging. Their less active behavior teams up with nature's slow decline in muscle-producing testosterone to yield "skinny" legs.

Smaller calf circumference can also be the consequence of poor nutrition. As noted in chapter 3, basic nutrition is essential to maintaining our body's muscle mass. Calf and thigh muscles are less likely to shrink in size in your seventies and eighties if you maintain a healthy diet and are active. You ought to be aware that low leg strength and smaller calf circumference are linked to frailty and the risk of falling upon standing up. Our best defense against loss of muscle mass is an offense—to remain physically active and to eat well.

FEET CONCERNS

Rarely are your feet going to affect others' judgment of your appearance, or even grab your own attention. But they surely affect your mobility, quality of life, and self-presentation, which you and others notice. All day long your feet take abuse supporting your weight, yet most of us do not think about our feet or grasp how important they are until they don't work and we're incapacitated. Anyone who has broken a toe or faced the symptoms of Achilles tendonitis—pain and tenderness on the back of the foot or heel—after a weekend of activity knows how little it takes to feel hobbled. An injured foot—whether caused by a painful ingrown toenail, a nagging stress fracture, or even a blister—will keep you from enjoying life. Don't let this happen. And don't wait for a foot problem to restrict your activities. What follows is a list of common foot problems that can be easily treated and often prevented.

Flat feet (and fallen arches). As we get older, our feet enlarge. More specifically, they flatten. With age, the feet's tendons and ligaments lose some of their elasticity, become looser, and don't hold the bones and joints together as compactly. These changes are the effects of decades of weight-bearing use and ordinary aging, where the muscle mass declines and tissue weakens. The constant pressure of bearing weight causes two changes: the "fat" pads on the bottoms of your feet thin, and the tendon forming the arch in the foot stretches, which lowers the arch. As the arch lowers, the front of the foot widens and the foot becomes longer and flatter. Foot flattening causes two additional changes. With tendons and ligaments becoming more flexible, this lets the ankle roll inward and increases the chance for sprains. Foot flattening also pulls the big toe up, which often causes cramp-like pain in its own right.

You might not want to admit it, but as your feet flatten, you might need to change the way you engage in physical activity. There's no need to retire from an athletic life because of flat feet; rather, you just need to compensate for years of wear and tear. Purchasing customized insoles for your shoes is a smart decision, and being fitted for good athletic shoes is equally smart. Particularly for men who want to continue working out or whose jobs require long periods of standing and walking, insoles will very often reduce the sense of tiredness in the feet and noticeably reduce foot discomfort while working.[32] Shoes should have cushioning in the heel and sole to make up for the loss of natural padding.

For most men, after age 40 our shoe size gets bigger by a half size every decade. So, if you are 50 and wearing size 10 shoes, by age 60 you need to have your shoe size measured, because the odds are that you will be buying size 10½. Your new shoe also needs to fit the widest part of the foot, usually the front, which means you might be buying a 10½ wide rather than your former medium width. But most men resist and keep wearing the wrong-sized shoes. An interesting study of veterans visiting a clinic found that only 25 percent were wearing the right-sized shoe.[33] As noted next, three foot problems are related to improperly fitting shoes: calluses and corns, bunions, and ingrown toenails.

Calluses and corns. When narrow, too-tight shoes are worn, the skin of the foot will endure friction as the shoe rubs against parts of your foot. Where there is persistent rubbing against the skin, this friction causes hard bumps of skin, called *calluses* and *corns*, to form. Calluses are, in a sense, permanent blisters. They are thick, hardened layers of skin that usually develop under and around the heel area, under the ball of the foot, and under the big toe. A corn is a form of callus with a hard central core and typically develops on top and between the toes. They can be painful. Properly fitted shoes, with good support and cushioning, are an effective method of prevention. You might also consider podiatrist-developed insoles that realign your foot and reduce unnecessary pressure and friction. Both corns and calluses can be treated using over-the-counter pharmacy products that contain salicylic acid, which dissolves the protein in the thickened skin and cuts back the callus or corn. Don't attempt to cut away a callus or corn at home, for you risk an infection.

Bunions. Not as common among men as women, bunions can develop when you compress the toes of your foot with narrow, poor-fitting shoes. A bunion is when your big toe is bent inward toward the second toe and a boney bump forms on the outside edge of the large toe. The bump begins as red (inflamed) calloused skin and over time becomes larger, boney, and more painful. Stiffness may develop, and researchers find that our quality of life suffers.[34] If a bunion begins to develop, you need to wear wide-toed shoes. This alone might resolve the problem, but if it continues to get worse and causes severe pain, you are looking at surgery to remove the bunion and realign the toe.

Big toe stiffness and pain. As cartilage in the big toe joint wears away, stiffness and pain develop slowly. The big toe is one of the most common sites of arthritis, particularly among men, and has troubling consequences.[35] The big toe joint (called *metatarsophalangeal,* or MTP) is essential for normal foot functioning, for it allows the toe to bend upward with every step you take. Limitation of motion of the big toe is only one of the symptoms arising from mild to severe degenerative arthritis. When the joint starts to stiffen, walking becomes painful and more difficult. Stiffness interferes with maintaining balance on uneven surfaces and a normal gait. Big toe stiffness is an arthritic condition where the articular cartilage between the joints begins to wear out, causing the raw end of the two connecting bones to rub one another. Untreated, a bone spur may develop on top of one of the toe bones, and this overgrowth also reduces the toe's ability to bend. Pain relievers and anti-inflammatory medications such as ibuprofen usually reduce the swelling and ease the pain. Wearing a shoe with a wide toe will reduce the pressure on the toe. If the joint remains stiff and painful, seeking an opinion from a podiatric practice wouldn't hurt.

Ingrown toenail. When the sharp edge of the nail grows down and into the skin of a toe, the result is pain and discomfort, redness, and swelling around the nail. You're dealing with an ingrown toenail, and if it gets infected, you *will* be dealing with more pain, redness, swelling, and a very visible uneven gait as you try to walk. An ingrown toenail is usually the result of poorly fitting shoes and toenails that are not trimmed properly. As we get older and our feet get bigger, too often we keep using our older, too-small shoes. When a big toe is lifted up as a result of the arch flattening, it can rub against the top of a too-tight shoe. The skin along the edge of a toenail may become red and infected. The rubbing can also thicken the toenail and force it to grow down into the skin. The big toe is usually affected, but any toenail can become ingrown.

Heel pain and heel spurs. Heel pain is experienced with your first steps in the morning and is a common foot complaint. It is often a by-product of "fallen arches" and involves an inflammation. Usually, there is a sharp acute pain felt at the bottom of the heel area, and sometimes the pain extends to the back of the heel as you take those first steps. The pain diminishes as you walk around, because you are forcing the nerves to adapt to the discomfort. What is happening is that the band of ligaments under the foot (called *plantar fascia*) tightens when you are sleeping or driving and sitting inactive for a long period, and when you stand and put your body weight on your foot, the ligaments are forced to immediately stretch and lengthen. This (again) causes micro-tearing of the ligament, which causes the stabbing pain. Gently stretching your foot by standing on the ball of the foot and your toes will help. If the heel pain is ignored and left untreated, a pointed bony growth can form at the back of the heel bone or under the bone. This is a heel spur.

Since heel pain is usually caused by an inflammation, the first line of treatment is anti-inflammation medication such as ibuprofen. Equally important is to rest the injury—take a few days off from physical activity—and get shoe inserts that support your arch. Even though heel pain is most often caused by tissue inflammation, it can result from a broken bone, a tight Achilles tendon, a pinched nerve, or other problems.

Achilles tendonitis. Tendonitis involves an inflammation of the Achilles tendon, which is the large tendon at the back of the ankle that connects the calf muscle to the heel bone. Aside from an injury and inflammation, tendonitis is also related to a chronic degeneration of tissue and thus our aging-related, wear-and-tear loss of the normal fiber structure of the tendon. Fundamentally, it is an overuse injury. Whether acute or chronic, men with tendonitis will most often experience stiffness and a shooting, burning pain at the back of the ankle, just above the heel bone. This regularly occurs during the first few steps out of bed in the morning or when first walking after a long period of sitting. It is very noticeable when climbing stairs or walking up a hill. It usually develops from a sudden increase in physical activity, such as when men play weekend sports. You won't be limping around, but you will feel the pain. It is the stress on the Achilles tendon that causes the irritation, inflammation, and pain. Treatment is much the same as managing heel pain—anti-inflammatory medication such as ibuprofen,[36] icing and massaging the tendon, and adding an insole pad to raise the heel to reduce some of the strain on the tendon. If the pain is persistent, consult your physician or sports injury therapist.

Fungal nail infection (onychomycosis). Mentioned briefly as a skin infection, this topic is worth more attention. Infections caused by fungi in the toenails (and, much less often, the fingernails) become common with age. More than an embarrassing cosmetic issue involving ugly discoloration and nail disfigurement,[37] fungal nail infections can cause other health problems. Like all infections, they are contagious. It is a progressive, recurring infection that begins in the skin underneath the nail (or "nail bed") and migrates to the nail itself (or "nail plate"). Over time it causes the nail to become brittle, thicken, discolor, change in shape, and split. The outside edges of the nail crumble, and the debris of dead tissue is trapped under the nail. The fungi feed on nail tissue, leaving behind their messy debris. Untreated, the toenail can become so thick that when you are wearing shoes, the shoe presses against the nail and causes noticeable pressure, if not pain. Untreated, the collection of fungal microorganisms can spread from the toenail to other areas of the body. Wash your hands after touching an infected area.

What puts you at risk for fungal nail infection is both environmental and family history. You might be more susceptible genetically. But the fungi spores grow best in warm, moist areas. If you are living in a warm climate, wear socks made out of synthetic material that don't breathe and don't allow air to circulate around your foot (e.g., nylon, acrylic), regularly participate in fitness activities and end up with sweaty feet, and bathe in a communal gym shower, you are putting your toenails at risk. Prevention is the best defense: keep your feet dry, your nails short, wear socks made out of 100 percent natural material (e.g., cotton, silk, wool), select breathable footwear, and don't plod around barefoot in the gym, in the locker room, or on the pool deck. Most importantly, don't share toenail clippers with someone who has a fungal nail infection.

Historically, the medicines used to treat nail fungi were not very effective. But recent advances in oral antifungal medicines have made treatment much more effective, because they go through the body to penetrate the nail and nail bed within days of starting therapy. Although treatment is expensive and recurrence is very possible, the newer oral antifungal drugs require shorter treatment periods and yield higher cure rates. Usually taken once a day for at least 6 weeks and up to 3 months, terbinafine (Lamisil tablets) and itraconazole (Sporanox capsules) are the most widely used. The alternative fluconazole (Diflucan) is gaining acceptance, partly because it treats the yeast-based infections that can also cause the nail infection.[38] These oral medications are quite safe, yet they are never recommended for men with liver disease or congestive heart failure. They are also more effective than the available topical agents, which seem best used if only less than half the nail is involved. Topical treatments are less effective because they cannot penetrate the nail deeply enough, so they are rarely able to kill off the fungi spores and cure the infection. But they may be useful as supplemental therapy and are not very expensive.

Foot odor. Ever dread removing your shoes for fear of grossing out anyone close by with a nasty, unpleasant, and embarrassing stench? Smelly feet result from sweat confined in a sock and/or shoe, and men who wear socks made of synthetic materials are adding risk. Actually, the odor is the result of bacteria that flourish in warm, moist areas and release isovaleric acid.[39] The bottom of your foot is a perfect breeding ground for the bacteria when your foot is wrapped in an inorganic sock and embedded in a shoe or boot. It's a condition that's very easy to treat. Rotate your shoes, make sure you wear socks made of natural material that absorb perspiration, and don't bother spending your hard-earned money on costly shoe powders and sprays.

CHAPTER 9

Getting in Touch with Your Spiritual Self

with David C. Wihry

In this chapter we consider something that seems, at first glance, to be beyond the boundaries of a discussion of men's physical, mental and emotional, sexual, and social health. Yet understanding the importance of spiritual health and getting in touch with your spiritual self have the potential to positively impact all dimensions of your health and quality of life.[1] Repeatedly, narrative studies and surveys of middle-aged and older men tell us that spirituality is a positive influence as men face the challenges of aging and illness and confront the existential distress of dealing with questions about life's meaning or the uncertainty of an illness's trajectory.[2]

Although attendance at church, synagogue, or mosque tends to fall off in later life (largely due to health and mobility limitations), private prayer is more frequent, faith is strengthened, and spirituality is deeper.[3] The deepening sense of spirituality in later life, whether based in a religious tradition or not, is very likely because we become more contemplative or thoughtful.[4] This has been described as *gerotranscendence*,[5] and it reflects how men rely less on external definitions of themselves while their appreciation for connections across generations deepens. In the well-known Nun Study, researchers found that adults who aged well acquired deeper spirituality, a strong sense of community, and a high level of gratitude.[6] They suffered less—even when faced with the death of friends or their own life-threatening illnesses. Hundreds of studies have documented the links between spirituality and lower rates of cancer, heart disease and heart attacks, alcoholism, and mental illness; high levels of healthy practices; and even lower mortality or death rates.[7]

The topic of spirituality can be difficult to discuss, even taboo in some people's minds. Even so, it is important to consider spirituality in the context of men's health and aging, without moralizing about what is good or bad and right or wrong. It has been suggested that growing older has the potential to energize your spiritual self.[8] The opportunity to consider ourselves in relation to eternity, or thinking beyond the material and the present, presumably lends meaning and purpose to our existence and places us in the context of something larger and perhaps more lasting than our own mortality. This quest for meaning may or may not be associated with a particular religion or expressed in religious terms. Becoming in touch with our "inner soul" as we grow older may help reduce the fear and trepidation we often feel about dying and death, at the same time that it can reduce feelings of stress and improve our attitude when dealing with challenges associated with aging-related health problems and the experience of bereaving the loss of some aspects of our health.[9] Some men may see their spiritual quest as a journey, with an existential quality to it. For them, a great deal of value is placed on direct experiences of a sacred nature, however personally defined. Experiences of this type can change how we view ourselves and the world in which we live.

> The deeper we look into nature, the more we recognize that it is full of life, and the more profoundly we know that all life is a secret and that we are united with all life that is in nature. Man can no longer live his life for himself alone. We realize that all life is valuable and that we are united to all this life. From this knowledge comes our spiritual relationship with the universe.
>
> —Albert Schweitzer

In its simplest terms, spirituality can be seen as the search for the "meaning and purpose of life."[10] Few of us would presume that having meaning and purpose in life isn't a good thing. However, the concept inevitably grows more "fuzzy" as the relationship between spirituality and religion is considered. Spirituality means many things to any one man. Very similar to other "fuzzy" concepts—such as quality of life or love—spirituality is intrinsically personal. It is the very personal sense of "being"—being in the moment, being involved with more than your corporal self, being connected with an intangible other, being part of something much bigger. Spirituality can be rooted in (1) *God-oriented* spiritual experiences that are based in monotheistic Abrahamic theologies of the Christian, Jewish, and Muslim traditions; (2) *world-oriented* spiritual experiences that call attention to our interconnectedness with nature; or (3) *people-oriented* spiritual experiences that stress the human capacity to be intimately one with others.[11] Spiritual experiences are those moments when we are struck by wonder, awe, blinding moments of clarity, deep-rooted compassion, and/or a near-primal sense of our insignificance. These moments can occur standing on a beach and watching the majestic power of the ocean, hiking across a hill loaded with spring wildflowers, being "touched" by a television news story about a man and his family's suffering with unemployment, while praying, and being awed by a meteor shower or a waterfall. Many religions have institutionalized practices that are designed to try to promote spiritual experiences, from Catholics' communion or the greeting of others in neighboring pews, to the Shinto tradition of talking with dead elders, to the Navajo's community-witnessed purification rituals.

Because ideas about spirituality and religion are so diverse, it is useful to take a quick look at some statistical trends to get a general sense of how midlife and older men think of these matters. The Gallup Organization has done several nationally representative polls on the topic of religion and spirituality in America.[12] They reported that half of Americans identified themselves as being religious, and a third stated they were spiritual without reference to God or a higher authority. Similar findings—where spirituality is expressed in nonreligious terms—were reported in a study of hundreds of older adults' life reviews, despite the fact that it is the older generation that tends to equate spirituality with a religious culture.[13]

Men who call themselves spiritual may subscribe to various beliefs, philosophies, religions, and outlooks on life. Some men who perceive themselves as spiritual may have deep ties to an organized religion, while others may not. More of the men born after World War II tend to separate religion and spirituality and view spirituality as an "inner province," whereas they see religion in terms of a denomination.[14] The ideas and tenets of spirituality, such as beliefs about the interconnectedness of all things and the importance of overcoming the corporal self, have spanned centuries, even though the term *spiritual* might not have been attached to the experiences. To someone looking to further explore their spirituality, we provide a brief look at some of the perspectives on the following topics: the meaning of spirituality, how individuals start on the spiritual path, how some have established a spiritual practice, the challenges many face on that path to understanding their own spirituality, and how men struggle with spirituality.

WHAT IS SPIRITUALITY?

Understanding Meaning

A quest to understand meaning in life is one element of spirituality.[15] Being on a spiritual quest is a way to (re)discover significance and purpose in our lives. As we go to work, find love, raise families, and live our lives, continuing to search for meaning can help add purpose to what we do and tie our experiences together into a meaningful and coherent whole. Author Ian

Harris notes that spirituality lets us know that there may be significance to our lives that goes beyond our daily activities and challenges we face.[16]

One of the major aspects of spiritual experience involves a deep feeling of interconnectedness between all things. Robert Atchley, a scholar on aging and spirituality, commented, "As fully awakened spiritual beings, we feel our interconnectedness."[17] A spiritual understanding of interconnectedness can involve seeing our lives and the actions we take as being intimately caught up with the welfare of others. A realization of interconnectedness can also be an understanding of what our relationship is to the natural world.[18] This consciousness of our connectedness to human society and/or the natural world can direct our actions and sense of how things happen and why.

Transcending the Self

The word *transcendence* is something that is often mentioned in conjunction with spirituality. It, too, is a fuzzy concept, one that involves the idea of moving beyond ourselves to something greater. Transcendence is closely related to interconnectedness. For example, when we realize an interconnectedness with the lives of others, the universe, or Mother Nature, we have, at least for a moment, reached a new level of consciousness—one in which we have gone beyond our own narrow concerns and sensed that we are part of something terrifically bigger.

An Experience beyond Words

Spiritual experiences are not easy to grasp through just thoughts alone. One way to better understand spiritual experience is in the context of the emotions and feelings that such experiences evoke. Atchley states, "Experiences labeled spiritual are usually described by respondents in terms of qualities like wonder, compassion, clarity, stillness, silence, or expansiveness."[19] Watching a birth or observing a lightning strike is an experience that really cannot be retold.

Experiencing the Sacred

The concept of sacredness is another element of spirituality. There is no one definition of what is sacred, and that which is sacred can range from gods in various religions to sacredness in the natural world and beyond. Certainly, the word *sacred* often has a religious connotation in the sense that something might be sacred as opposed to being profane. However, what is sacred can be attached to places and things that we respect, revere, or embody with particular meaning. In this sense, things such as a vow, a picture of a lost loved one, or a friendship can also be sacred.

Turning Outward

There is often a tendency to perceive spirituality as a practice that is completely focused on the self—our awe, journey, or clarity of perception. Although spirituality focuses on the inner world of the individual, it is not necessarily a selfish activity. Spiritual experiences, practices, and understanding can be transformative, helping a man become more compassionate and concerned about the welfare of his fellow human beings. This is one way in which the contemplative nature and inner peace of spirituality can help a man turn outward to help make the world a more just place.[20]

In the Spirit of Things

Spirituality has been argued to provide us with

- meaning to life;
- guideposts for individual values;
- an internal sense of wellness and identity;
- a sense of commonality with people, community, and the environment;
- and a defined relationship with someone/ something beyond ourselves.

Facing Ourselves

Spirituality is not always a comfortable practice. To be spiritual can mean confronting the ugly and deficient aspects of ourselves. Death and pain in all its forms, whether mental or physical, reside within us all. Looking at these deficiencies in ourselves, however, can sensitize us to the struggles of others and, in so doing, can help us to become more compassionate individuals.[21]

Movement toward Spirituality

Like many things related to spirituality, the reasons why we may set out on a spiritual journey are diverse. As we age, men may have more time to look deeply at themselves, once the time-consuming demands of jobs and raising children become less pressing. Some men may also look to engage in searches for personal meaning as they work through the uncertainties in life.[22] A major impetus for a spiritual journey—whether within the Ananda spiritual community traditions, a mainstream faith tradition, or a nonreligious quest—could be the acknowledgment of suffering or our mortality, or a decision to take a mini-retreat (or vacation) to refresh.

Forgiveness

For some men, forgiveness may be at the heart of spirituality. Being able to forgive can benefit a man emotionally and physically, and in fact, as we grow older, forgiving frequently becomes easier. Working through the anger or distance that exists between you and a relative, a former friend, or a coworker can be a spiritual experience and can make you feel more whole and healthy. For men, in particular, forgiving someone often means giving up the desire to seek revenge. This appears to happen when we are able to give up long-standing views of what occurred between us and someone else and "imagine new and more hopeful endings" that allow us to focus on something greater than the original pain and hurt we felt.[23]

SPIRITUAL EXPERIENCES: WHAT DO THEY FEEL LIKE?

Spiritual experiences can be felt in different ways—through our bodies, through our minds, through our emotions, as well as beyond these means of perceiving the world. We might feel calm or peace. We may also have a spiritual experience when viewing a beautiful piece of art or hearing a piece of music that (temporarily) overwhelms us. Just being completely present in the activities in which we engage may also be spiritual. These experiences can come to us at any time. They can be found in many different contexts, even at work, in a conversation with others, or when engaged in community service. More than a few of us may well have discovered some aspect of our spiritual self while on a fishing trip, hunting in the forest, hiking up a mountain, or even exercising in the gym.

There have been some efforts to understand what happens in the bodies of individuals when they have a spiritual experience. Andrew Newberg, from the University of Pennsylvania, has been studying the relationship between brain activity and spiritual experiences using an imaging technique—single photon emission computed tomography (SPECT). He and his colleagues commented that the elusive nature of spiritual experience can be observed in the cardiovascular changes among Zen practitioners of meditation.[24] Studying Tibetan Buddhists in deep meditation, Franciscan nuns immersed in prayer, and Pentecostal Christians speaking in tongues, they found markedly similar changes in brain activity during their most intensely religious moments. The researchers argue that "spiritual experience, at its very root, is intimately interwoven with human biology."[25]

The SPECT scans showed the neurological effects of spiritual behavior. In an interview for Salon.com, Newberg stated, "We've hypothesized that when people meditate or pray—if they block the sensory information that gets into [the attention center of the brain]—they no longer get a sense of who they are in relation to the world. They may lose their sense of self, and they feel they become one with something greater—ultimate reality or God."[26] Of course, Newberg's research does not prove whether spiritual or religious experiences are authentic or god-given, but (and this seems important) it does shed light on the impact of spiritual experiences on the body.

Establishing a Spiritual Practice

If you are drawn to a particular religion or are intrigued by the mysteries of the universe, consider exploring the mystical traditions and philosophies of the world.

Even if you are not part of a religion, meditation and contemplation can be a valuable way to cultivate your spirituality.

Engage in the activities that evoke awe and wonder in you, whether this is just being with loved ones, being outdoors, or learning about the world you live in.

Tell your story. Examining your life can help you in your search for meaning and significance.

Spirituality and service go hand and hand. Serving others is one way to cultivate your spirituality.

SKEPTICISM

One recent review article on spirituality and mental health concluded that spirituality (as well as religiousness) was often a coping resource for individuals who were facing illness or other traumatic experiences.[27] The review also reported that, with some exceptions, conditions such as anxiety, depression, or substance abuse were uncommon among those who were found to be more spiritual. Yet, questions remain about how generalizable these findings are to other Christian and non-Christian traditions.

But can we simply say that men facing chronic illness should rely on their spiritual self to cope, and that men with a spiritual self are less likely to have mental health troubles? Healthy skepticism is invaluable when evaluating studies of religion, spirituality, and health. First is the chicken-and-egg analogy: does spirituality (or religiousness) protect midlife and older men from mental health troubles, or were depressed or alcohol-dependent men less engaged in their spiritual self to begin with? As also discussed earlier, there may be a close relationship between spirituality and religion in some men's lives, but spirituality and religion are not the same. Scientific studies may use religious affiliation or how often a person prays as evidence of spirituality. But neither affiliation with a religious culture nor prayer clarifies what it means to be spiritual, nor are they necessarily accurate measures of spirituality.

One article from a 1999 issue of the *Lancet* urged physicians to even rethink the religious affiliation–health connection.[28] The problematic aspect of interpreting the effect of religious involvement on health is that activities such as attending religious services or participating in prayer may not be spiritual. Rather, social contact may be the key factor in the maintenance of good health, and this is something that can be had by anyone, regardless of whether they are spiritual or not. The issues mentioned above may keep us from knowing exactly what aspects of a spiritual self have a positive influence on health. Despite the robust research literature that assures us that a spiritual self is associated with better health, this relationship is still not fully understood.

OTHER BENEFITS?

Aside from the persuasive evidence that spirituality (or religiousness) is positively associated with better physical health and quality of life, there are other benefits of being engaged in either spiritual practices or a faith community. For example, one study that looked at the life reviews of older adults discovered that when people compared themselves to their younger years, they had a greater store of confidence in themselves and had come to terms with the twists and turns along the way.[29] The study also found that an important element of spirituality was a willingness to view life and its challenges with humor. The strengths that these elders gained throughout their lives also allowed them to feel freer in the actions they were taking and the directions they were choosing for their lives.

SPIRITUALITY IN MEN

Spirituality is often discussed without reference to gender. However, there have been attempts to examine the spiritual concerns of men in terms of why we may, in particular, be reluctant to be open about our spirituality. Why have men shied away from showing their spiritual self? Various explanations have been suggested. One group of analysts has argued that men's "natural" yearning for spirituality is often pushed away while growing up and becomes hidden. They believe that men conceal the emotions that spiritual experiences evoke because men have been taught that people are not receptive to such displays from men. It almost seems as if being inexpressive is going to be accepted more readily than any display of behavior that appears to portray a man as passive, gentle, or "wimpish." It is true that, in our culture, men are still expected to mask their emotions, whether positive or negative.[30] To intervene, distinctive men's groups and philosophies have emerged to assist men whose quest is to get in touch with their "inner essence."[31]

ESTABLISHING SPIRITUAL PRACTICE

Establishing a spiritual practice is a deeply personal undertaking. The form of this spiritual practice will be largely based on the beliefs you hold and what feels most comfortable for you to engage in. If you are not religious, you may be more interested in practices such as meditation or yoga. Neither practice has an explicit spiritual context, yet engaging in these activities may help you see your connectedness with others and bring a sense of awe and wonder.

For those who identify with a particular religious tradition or spiritual philosophy, the contemplative practices associated with these faiths provide one avenue for starting a spiritual practice. Prayer, meditation, the reading of scripture, and similar practices have a long history within many of the world's religions. Mystical traditions are also elements of many of the world's religions and indigenous belief systems, although the exact nature of mysticism differs among them. Mysticism is the personal experience of spiritual or religious truths or understanding of reality that goes beyond our common perceptions. Mystical events are temporary, and because they must be experienced, they are difficult to convey to others.[32] Many of the world's religions and philosophies have writers who claimed to have mystical experiences, and to the extent possible, these writers have tried to convey in words what these experiences were like. These writers are a great resource for those who are interested in different spiritual practices. Mysticism is something that nonreligious individuals might want to explore as well, as there have been attempts to describe mysticism in naturalistic terms without any reference to the supernatural.

Telling a Life Story

Contemplating the course of a person's life is one spiritual practice. Simply finding a quiet place where a person can write or think about their life is an activity that can be used to engage in the search for meaning that is a key part of spirituality. Looking at the milestones in your own life, as well as the insights you have gained from those experiences, is one way to help yourself understand your own spirituality.

People who do not associate with a particular religion or philosophy can also benefit from spiritual practices. One practice, in particular, involves looking at our lives, whether through telling our story on paper or simply reflecting. This is, in essence, a search for meaning—a fundamental aspect of spirituality.[33] Meditation is a similar spiritual practice that is available to men who describe themselves as nonreligious. People meditate for various reasons: to promote feelings of peace or calm, to discipline the mind, and even to gain perceived health benefits. Many employer-based health coverage plans include wellness centers that teach meditation, to get you started. Meditation can take various forms, but there are some commonalities between meditation practices. They involve focusing on various aspects of the body and mind. Some meditation practices involve following one's breath as it enters or leaves the body, or focusing on the sensations that the body experiences. Often, the goal is not to hold on to sensations and thoughts that arise in meditation, but rather to let go of them as they arise and to bring the mind back to the original object of meditation. Meditation is most often done in a place that is quiet, which will aid in focusing on the object of meditation.[34]

The National Institutes of Health's National Center for Complementary and Alternative Medicine (NCCAM) has researched the role of meditation for the maintenance of good health. According to the NCCAM, it is theorized that meditation can impact portions of the autonomic nervous system to cause a decrease in your heartbeat and breaths per minute. In terms of safety, the NCCAM suggests that overall "meditation is considered to be safe for healthy people."[35] However, the NCCAM notes that meditation should not be used in place of conventional medicine.

Meditation

Meditation is one way to cultivate spirituality. It is useful for those looking to develop peace and calm, as well as for those looking to discipline the mind. Look for meditation groups in your area. Meditation is becoming increasingly common, and meditating with a group can help to provide a supportive, like-minded community to help sustain your own spiritual practice.

If you are drawn to a particular spiritual tradition, you might want to look at the meditative and contemplative aspects of that tradition.

It can be useful to look toward experienced meditators for guidance. Many books from various religious traditions, as well as with no connection to religion, provide techniques and instructions for meditation.

LEAVING A LEGACY

The idea of leaving a legacy for future generations has spiritual relevance and is a concrete way in which to share your philosophy of life and your view of the relationship you have with the world with family members and other significant persons in your life. It is a way to identify what you see as important and, in turn, to share it with those around you, without moralizing that your values are best. It can be an important part of a man's life planning and help you decide how you want to spend your time, energy, and money as you grow older. For example, have you geographically moved from where your parents and grandparents grew up and wanted to reconnect? Would you be interested in visiting their local newspaper's archives for photos of the way things used to be? Doing "legacy work"— whether looking backward in time or preparing a life narrative for your grandchildren—can be a powerful way for you to create meaning throughout the second half of your life and feel vital and healthy as you are aging. It can be a very effective way to heal or deepen relationships with those you love or care deeply about.

Meg Newhouse, founder of the Life Planning Network in New England, reminds us that a legacy can be as public as an architectural monument and as private as a letter written to your children or grandchildren.[36] It can also be a seemingly casual word of advice. Writing in *Social Work Today*, she argued that legacies intentionally left to the next generation are a way to reflect what you feel in your heart or soul. These "legacies of the heart" will probably be a testament to your spiritual view of life. The developmental "push" after midlife to find meaning or purpose can fuel the desire to leave a legacy, which may intensify with age or proximity to death.

Ways to Shape Your Own Legacy

- Think about what your passions, values, and dreams are as a way of helping to point to your purpose or calling in life.

- Try to visualize the legacies you would like to leave the world and who you might want to leave them with.

- Write your own obituary or epitaph.

- Share more fully in conversations with those you love in order to identify a legacy that defines who you really are.

- Write an ethical will (sometimes called a legacy letter), as a way to bequeath your inner wealth, which can include your important values, philosophies of life or life lessons, experiences, and specific messages to loved ones.

- Write, tape, illustrate, or assemble photographs in a scrapbook to document your personal reflections about life experiences, themes, lessons, and family history.

- List the tangible treasures that you wish to pass on with the story of their histories and the personal importance attached to them.

- Take on a public legacy project, individually or collectively, such as community volunteer activities, coaching, or mentoring, which allows you to share your ideas and resources with others.

Legacies can be private or collective, tangible or intangible. Examples of private, tangible legacies include family heirlooms and other family treasures, such as recipes and letters, arts and crafts creations, written or audio-visual recordings, family histories, memoirs, ethical wills, money, and real property. Private, intangible legacies include individual actions on your part such as mentoring, teaching, coaching, counseling, informal conversations, and caregiving. Collective or group legacies include volunteering, community engagement, political action, social entrepreneurship, and specifically formed groups for making charitable contributions.

SAGE-ING, TIMESLIPS, AND SERVANT LEADERSHIP

In many cases, thinking spiritually requires that we change our mind-set from "doing" to "being." This can be really difficult because, as men, we live in a world that emphasizes being active and involved. Successful physical aging tends to focus on the overriding importance of "using it or losing it" and remaining active. How then can you live a contemplative life as you grow older? For Anne Basting, the creator of the TimeSlips Program, it means getting involved in creative storytelling, which emphasizes the value of using your imagination when it comes to constructing your own life stories rather than fixating on remembering all the specific details of past experiences.[37] For Rabbi Zalman Schacter-Shalomi, who developed the term "sage-ing" to replace aging, it means a belief that older adults hold a special, even sacred, place in society as mentors and bearers of culture, and that getting older can be a time of great discovery.[38] Sage-ing is a non-denominational process of spiritual development that aims to deepen self-awareness, enhance interpersonal relationships, hone communication skills, and cultivate a valuation of elders as mentors and wise counsel in our community. For Robert Greenleaf and more recently Richard Leider and Larry Spears, it is the idea of "elder servant leadership," whereby elders teach by story, by example, and by caring about those who follow in their footsteps.[39] Elder servant leaders find deep satisfaction in giving all that they have to offer in ways that serve others rather than just themselves, and they embrace this as a critical responsibility of their elderhood. For them, the new elder spirit is one of "giving it away" because, they argue, elders know that people are strong not in proportion to what they can hold on to, but rather according to what they can give away.

For each man, the process of spiritual awakening is a gradual descent to find buried feelings, to discover his inner world, where he can pick up the threads of his personal story. It is necessary for men to find their myth and live it.

Source: Bolen, J. S. (1989). *Gods in every man.* New York: Harper & Row.

CONCLUSION

This chapter may have raised more questions than answers, and that is all right. Spirituality is a deeply personal issue, and the ways it can be approached are varied, which means that your understanding of spirituality and spiritual practice may be very different than those of someone else, or even the presentation in this chapter. To one person, being spiritual may mean seeing the truth in a particular religion or philosophy and immersing themselves in this truth. To another, spirituality may mean experiencing the awe of Mother Nature and living in our universe, even if that does not include believing in a higher power. Yet another may disagree with the concept of spirituality or find the practice of spirituality unhelpful in their own lives. And that is all right as well.

If you are interested, there are practices that you can use to develop spiritual insight. For those who are drawn to a particular religion, many of the world's faiths have strong mystical traditions, which can be a source of guidance for spirituality and spiritual practice. Reading scripture, prayer, contemplation, and other activities associated with a religion may be beneficial as well.

For those who do not or choose not to identify with a particular religion, there are other ways to establish a spiritual practice, such as reflecting on your life through writing, or just enjoying activities that give you a sense of wonder and interconnectedness. Meditation, taking a quiet walk, and other relaxation techniques can be used to further develop a spiritual practice. There are also conceptions of mysticism that don't involve supernatural elements which can be examined.

However you choose to think about the practice of spirituality, it is important that it not just be an inward, selfish activity. The sense of wonder, awe, and interconnectedness will help you to move beyond yourself. We can be transformed by these spiritual experiences and the peace that they bring us, and we can emerge with a more compassionate outlook on life, an outlook that allows us to better see the interconnections between all people and act on this insight.

CHAPTER 10

Alcohol and Drugs

with Kristianna Hall

Alcohol—just a particular combination of carbon, hydrogen, and oxygen molecules—can have complicated effects on our bodies as we age. Many of the traditions and customs men adopt and pass along to the next generation, including the continuing emphasis on our invulnerability, have been closely associated with alcohol. Bar hopping, beer festivals, bachelor parties, retirement celebrations, and numerous other well-established traditions surrounding the consumption of alcohol remain widespread. The consumption of alcohol is almost always an expected activity at major sporting events, and the 5 o'clock whistle continues to produce almost a knee-jerk reaction for both blue- and white-collar men alike to meet the boys at a local watering hole and hoist a few.

It is likely that many people reading this chapter may catch sight of its title and think "Well, that doesn't apply to me," or "Yeah, I have a few drinks, but I know I'm not a 'substance abuser.'" For most of you, you're exactly right. Although this chapter does address some of the signs, symptoms, and possible consequences of substance abuse, it is not intended to demonize the use of alcohol; nor is the intention to convince everyone who has a drink or two that they have a pending problem. Instead, it is important for middle-aged and older men to know *how* the process of aging changes the way our bodies respond to different substances and adds new risks associated with alcohol and medication use. On a more general level, this chapter will speak to the challenges and changing needs associated with becoming older while being on medications and/or using alcohol. Of course, many men can maintain a normal and healthy lifestyle that includes the consumption of reasonable amounts of alcohol as we age. Some men, however, might want to consider reducing their level of consumption in order to improve their physical and mental health and maximize their overall quality of life.

ALCOHOL: WHAT'S NORMAL AND WHAT ISN'T?

It is estimated that fewer than 10 percent of men age 60 and older are "at-risk" drinkers.[1] Low-risk drinking for men has been defined by the National Institutes of Health as no more than 14 drinks per week and no more than four drinks on any day within the week.[2] Drinking is not always physically or medically harmful, even among older men. There has been medical evidence to tell us that light alcohol consumption (e.g., an average of one or two drinks per day) among healthy older adults may have health benefits, especially in terms of men's heart health and longevity. There also has been criticism of this heartening finding, since most existing alcohol-use studies are based on averages and include many men who had previously decreased their alcohol consumption because of their older age and medication use.[3] While social drinking in light to moderate amounts can be relaxing and heart healthy, drinking that third drink daily is associated with numerous negative health effects—it can cause serious illness, worsen other medical conditions, interfere with needed medications, and greatly decrease overall quality of life.

Terms like *moderate* and *heavy* (or *excessive*) drinking can mean different things to different people. For men age 60 and older, the recommended ("moderate") amount of alcohol is one drink per day, with the allowance of two drinks on occasions. Clinicians and researchers agree that a "standard drink" is best viewed as a 12-ounce can of beer, a 5-ounce glass of wine, or a 1.5-ounce shot of liquor (see figure 10.1). You should compare this "standard" with what you actually pour as a serving. Heavy drinking has been defined by the Centers for Disease Control and Prevention as more than two drinks a day, on average.

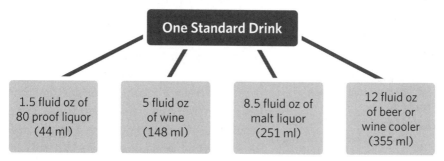

Figure 10.1. Standard sizes of alcoholic drinks

Given that half of men over age 50 drink "socially," which means occasionally and no more than moderately,[4] the safe use of alcohol versus its unsafe use needs to be addressed, along with the potential health benefits and risks of drinking in various amounts. Medical studies regularly show that consuming a safe amount of alcohol may be protective of our health.[5] Moderate alcohol consumption can improve appetite. As you've probably heard, alcohol can be beneficial for cardiovascular health, and research indicates that moderate consumption by older adults has also been shown to be protective against type 2 diabetes[6] and is associated with better cognition and well-being when compared with older adults who abstain from alcohol use.[7]

However, one key risk associated with alcohol use is our aging. As we get older, we are more sensitive to and less tolerant of even lower amounts of alcohol than we were able to consume in our forties and fifties. Frederic Blow, an expert on the topic of the use and misuse of alcohol in older adults, warns us that we may be at risk for severe consequences even from what we've always considered moderate drinking.

But why is this? As a man ages, his total volume of body water decreases. Alcohol is distributed in a person's body water, and older adults have less room to work with, so to speak. Older men also have less of an enzyme responsible for metabolizing alcohol in the stomach, which leads to more work for the liver and results in slower alcohol processing. These effects of normal aging cause the alcohol consumed to have a heightened impact as we get older; we will likely have a greater blood alcohol concentration (BAC), even when we drink the same amount of alcohol as a younger man. BAC refers to the amount of alcohol in a man's blood measured in terms of weight and volume and is routinely expressed as a percentage. Because alcohol in the blood travels directly to the brain, and because middle-aged and older men routinely experience greater sensitivity to the same amount of alcohol a younger man consumes, their higher BAC more severely affects reaction time, vision, hand-eye coordination, and brain function.

There are many other factors that affect your BAC when you drink. Some of these include your size and physical condition, what you have had to eat, how much sleep you have had, what

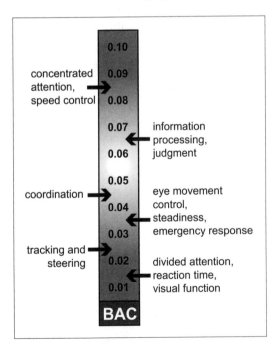

Figure 10.2. Blood Alcohol Content (BAC) scale. Courtesy of Campus Alcohol Abuse Prevention Center, Virginia Tech.

medications you are taking, and, importantly, the actual alcohol content of the chosen "drink." The effects of body weight on BAC are reflected in the BAC Chart for Men. The chart is intended as a guide for men, but it does not recognize how getting older increases the blood alcohol percentage.

BAC CHART FOR MEN

Drinks per hour	Approximate blood alcohol percentage								Driving Risks
	Body weight in pounds								
	100	120	140	160	180	200	220	240	
0	.00	.00	.00	.00	.00	.00	.00	.00	Only safe driving limit
1	.04	.03	.03	.02	.02	.02	.02	.02	Driving skills significantly affected
2	.08	.06	.05	.05	.04	.04	.03	.03	
3	.11	.09	.08.	.07	.06	.06	.05	.05	
4	.15	.12	.11	.09	.08	.08	.07	.06	
5	.19	.16	.13	.12	.11	.09	.09	.08	
6	.23	.19	.16	.14	.13	.11	.10	.09	Legally intoxicated
7	.26	.22	.19	.16	.15	.13	.12	.11	
8	.30	.25	.21	.19	.17	.15	.14	.13	Criminal penalties
9	.34	.28	.24	.21	.19	.17	.15	.14	
10	.38	.31	.27	.23	.21	.19	.17	.16	Death possible

Source: B.R.A.D. Be Responsible About Drinking. Retrieved from www.brad21.org/bac_charts.html.

ALCOHOL RISKS

The dictum "Warning: Alcohol can be dangerous to your health" isn't to be taken lightly. Consuming too much alcohol has severe adverse effects on our mental and physical health. Unlike the protective effect of moderate alcohol use against the development of many cardiovascular disorders, heavy alcohol consumption is associated with an increased risk of erectile dysfunction, dementia, hypertension, and nonischemic cardiomyopathy.[8] For example, it is thought that between 5 and 10 percent of all cases of dementia are causally related to alcohol abuse, while still other men diagnosed with conditions such as Alzheimer's disease may in fact be suffering from alcohol-related symptoms.

As already mentioned, a single drink can produce higher blood alcohol levels in older men than middle-aged men because of the increase in body fat relative to muscle as we get older. The percentage of total body weight consisting of fat for a typical male generally doubles from age 25 to age 60. Because alcohol does not dissolve in fat, the same alcohol dose results in higher blood alcohol levels in the older man.[9] In addition, as we get older, sensitivity to alcohol may increase because we do not metabolize or break it down as quickly. Also, because the amount of water in our body declines as we get older, the same amount of alcohol will result in a higher percentage in an older man's blood compared to a younger man. For all these reasons, older men cannot drink the same amount as they did when younger without noticeable effects.

We know the stereotype: men are more likely than women to take risks associated with drinking, such as driving after drinking. Say you and your wife go out for a nice dinner and share a bottle of wine. Quite likely, you drank more of it than she did; because of gender traditions, you will nevertheless be the one driving home. You think you are okay, but, as detailed above, our bodies do not "process" that wine as rapidly as when we were younger. Our driving capabilities are diminished as a result of the BAC.

Perhaps one of the greatest risks involved with social drinking is the potential to drink while taking over-the-counter drugs, prescription medications, or both. In one study of people using five or more medications, *nearly half* unwittingly misused medications and alcohol over a 6-month period.[10] Even some herbal remedies are harmful when mixed with alcohol, and alcohol can cancel out the effects of many different medications or cause them to be toxic to the body (see the section in chapter 11 on herbal remedies).[11] For example, alcohol in conjunction with acetaminophen (a common, over-the-counter headache medication) may lead to liver damage, and when alcohol is used with depressant-type medications such as sleeping or pain pills, it can have fatal repercussions. It is very easy to unknowingly misuse substances and encounter serious troubles.

Beyond the range of cardiovascular maladies related to consuming too much alcohol, heavy drinking causes many existing physical conditions to worsen, directly contributes to mental health concerns, and is the toxic substance related to more than 60 different disorders.[12]

WHAT IS "SUBSTANCE ABUSE," ANYWAY?

Probably most of us understand on some level what substance abuse *looks* like—perhaps we know someone who identifies himself as an alcoholic, or maybe we've seen someone take a few too many pain medications a few too

Alcohol and Its Effects

Physical Complications of Excessive Alcohol Use

- Liver disease (cirrhosis)
- Chronic obstructive lung disease
- Peptic ulcer
- Psoriasis
- Increased risk of falling
- Malnutrition
- Osteoporosis
- Anemia
- Coma
- Deterioration of brain and spinal cord
- Sleeping problems
- Worsening of high blood pressure
- Brain atrophy
- Potential for harmful medication interactions
- Potential for seizures; delirium tremens during withdrawal

- Esophagitis
- Alcoholic cardiomyopathy
- Increased risk of pneumonia, tuberculosis
- Enlarged liver; enlarged spleen
- Gastritis
- Atrophy of testes
- Peripheral neuropathy
- Decreased platelets
- Clumsiness
- Muscle problems
- Changes in the heart and blood vessels
- Worsened diabetes
- Potential for additional side effects if cigarettes are used with alcohol
- Potential risk of death from withdrawal

Mental Health Issues Related to Alcohol Consumption

- Depression
- Impulsivity
- Confusion
- Potential of hallucinations during withdrawal
- Delirium

- Anxiety
- Irritability
- Mood disorders
- Suicidality
- Forgetfulness

Source: Centers for Disease Control and Prevention (n.d.). *Frequently asked questions.*

many times. But when does it go from "a few too many" to a worrisome problem, and how does that happen?

The phrases *substance abuse* and *substance dependence* are frequently used interchangeably, but they refer to two separate (yet often interrelated) conditions. Substance dependence, in its simplest form, refers to the pervasive *need* to use a drug or alcohol and frequently involves a physiological component of tolerance and/or withdrawal. Substance abuse, however, refers to a *pattern* of excessive or harmful use of alcohol or drugs. The harm and negative life consequences involved in the abuse of alcohol or drugs include neglecting responsibilities, jeopardizing the health and well-being of others, legal problems due to drunk driving, and the inability to stop engaging in unlawful and/or dangerous behavior despite the consequences.[13] Psychiatric texts make it clear that abuse and dependence are two different conditions, yet the people we commonly think of and refer to as "substance abusers" have become habitually dependent on a drug or on alcohol. So then, how does dependence develop? Let's look at Ron's story for clarification:

> Ron, a man in his midforties, was recently laid off from the job he'd had for the past 20 years. Ron had always enjoyed a nip or two of Southern Comfort after getting home from work, but he never overdid it because he knew he would need to pick up his wife from her job later in the evening. After being laid off, Ron let his wife take the car to work every day while he stayed at home. Upset about losing his job, and having no need to drive, Ron started drinking a little more SoCo in the evenings before his wife got home. Eventually, Ron noticed that he did not feel much after three drinks, and still not much different after four. He needed to have almost five drinks to feel the alcohol's effects, and when he woke up in the morning his hands often shook. After a few mornings of this, Ron started to have a glass of whiskey in the mornings to steady himself. Ron's wife noticed his increased drinking and became concerned for her husband's health.

Ron's story illustrates the concept of substance dependence. When Ron upped his alcohol intake to three drinks per night, he felt a certain level of intoxication. However, after having three drinks per night for a while, Ron's body started to develop a *tolerance* to the alcohol, meaning that he needed to have more and more drinks to feel the original effects that he once felt after one or two nips of whiskey. This type of physiological tolerance often goes hand in hand with withdrawal—in Ron's case, his shaky hands in the morning indicated that his body was "suffering" from *not* having alcohol. For those who are dependent on a substance, physical withdrawal symptoms are unpleasant and often compel the user to seek more alcohol or drugs, simply to stave off withdrawal.

Figure 10.3 shows the beginning and end, respectively, of tolerance and dependence. The top shows a typical drinking experience: The user starts out feeling normal (baseline). After drinking, the user feels the "high" and then eventually sobers up and feels normal again. For people with alcohol dependence, however, like Ron, the bottom image is more applicable.

If Ron does not drink, his hands shake and he experiences uncomfortable withdrawal symptoms. Thus, Ron starts at below baseline (he feels bad) and then must drink simply to get himself to feeling okay.

The story of Ron's experience with alcohol dependence may not always hold true for the vast majority of adult men. Diagnostic criteria have generally been developed and tested on younger people, and while middle-aged and older adults may experience the same end results as their younger counterparts, the process of addiction can look quite different.[14]

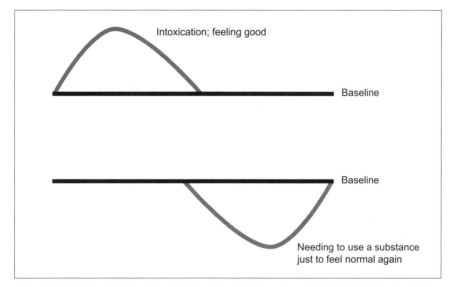

Figure 10.3. Drinking experience baseline

Differences in the Addiction Process as We Age

It is important to realize that men over 50 may become physiologically dependent on substances without meeting the standard criteria for dependence. Granted, this sounds nonsensical, but clinical guidelines for tolerance and dependence generally fail to account for adults' aging-related physical changes.[15] Going back to Ron, even if he had not developed a problematic pattern of alcohol use, his two drinks a night would have, most likely, eventually become too much had he continued to drink in the same manner when he reached his midsixties.

Research in the area of older adult addiction has identified two distinct types of problematic users. As you might guess, some older men are alcoholics or drug addicts who survived into older age. They are referred to as "early-onset" users or "survivors." Men who fall under this category are at high risk for continued substance use later in life and have a much greater risk of health complications as a result of their years of drinking or drug use.[16]

However, men sometimes develop a problem with alcohol or other substances for the first time later in life. They are known as "late-onset" users or "reactors."[17] Among these late-onset users are men who develop substance use problems after the onset of other health problems or a very troubling later-life event.[18] Experiences such as the death of a spouse or the postretirement loss of daily vocational rhythms can lead to severe distress and an increased use of a substance to cope. Older men who use substances to cope or "medicate" may have earlier used a drink to wind down, and now some of them turn to alcohol to try to cope with troubles and their depressive mood.[19] Early-onset alcoholics account for approximately two-thirds of all problem drinkers among older men, late-onset problem drinkers the other third.[20]

SUBSTANCE ABUSE IN OLDER MEN

According to the National Survey on Drug Use and Health, the evidence is that the use of illicit drugs and misuse of alcohol are increasing among older men.[21] More older men now disclose "heavy" than "moderate" alcohol use, and more also report occasional binge drinking (which is defined as five or more drinks in a sitting). Most experts concur that the problem of misuse and abuse of legal and illegal drugs in older adults is grossly underreported and likely to become more of an issue as baby boomers reach retirement age, because they have had a higher substance use level than previous generations of older adults.[22]

Why does substance abuse in older adults go so unnoticed? For one thing, because diagnostic criteria and clinical screening tests tend to be geared toward a younger population, a problem among older men can get overlooked by health professionals. Moreover, many medical practitioners are not able to differentiate symptoms that may be associated with aging, such as tremors or confusion, from drug- or alcohol-related side effects, especially given the fact that a small amount of alcohol may seem inconsequential to a health professional but could have deleterious effects on an older man's health.[23] Furthermore, the substance abuse that tends to be associated with life events such as losing a job or going through a divorce may not readily apply to older men, whose "late-onset" drinking practices are less likely to be publically viewed. For example, while the excess drinking by a man in his twenties or thirties may cause him to lose his job or be slapped with a DUI, a retired man in his seventies who depends on a daughter for rides may still have an alcohol abuse problem, but one that will never manifest itself and affect his daily life.

Criteria for Substance Abuse

A maladaptive pattern of substance use leading to clinically significant impairment or distress, as manifested by one or more of the following in a 12-month period:

- recurrent substance use resulting in a failure to fulfill major role obligations at work, school, or home;
- recurrent substance use in situations in which it is physically hazardous;
- recurrent substance-related legal problems;
- continued substance use despite having persistent or recurrent social or interpersonal problems caused or exacerbated by the effect of the substance.

Source: Diagnostic and Statistical Manual of Mental Disorders, 5th ed.

Misuse of Prescription Drugs

Men are not immune to the possibility of prescription drug misuse and abuse; in fact, it is much more common for middle-aged and older men to make unintentional mistakes with regard to their consumption of prescriptions than younger men. As we get older, we are commonly prescribed several different medications, often from more than one health care provider, and we are at an increased risk of experiencing medication interactions and other side effects that result from "polypharmacy," which is the concurrent use of four or more different prescription drugs.

Older men sometimes do not understand that their physical symptoms may in fact be related to the misuse of medications and/or abuse of alcohol. Just like their doctors at times, older men may mistake physical and mental symptoms such as hand tremors, dizziness and instability, sadness, and confusion for normal aging—they assume that they are "just getting old," when the real cause might be as simple as mixing alcohol with an over-the-counter medication, or mixing an over-the-counter medication with a prescription medication. As we get older, we need to be aware of our increased risk of "substance misuse," even when it is absolutely unintentional. Not only are our older bodies less able to process the alco-

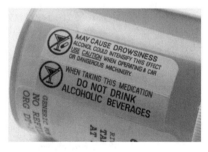

Figure 10.4. Prescription Rx warning

hol in a drink, but a single glass of wine along with our evening dose of a medication can cause instability, confusion, and many other physical and psychological symptoms. We can and should be our own best resource for monitoring substance use.

RISK FACTORS FOR SUBSTANCE ABUSE

Certain conditions put older men at greater risk for experiencing a substance use problem later in life. These include psychological conditions such as depression or anxiety, age-related health problems, and a previous history of substance abuse problems.[24]

Comorbid Psychiatric Conditions

A significant risk factor for substance abuse across all ages is a psychological problem. In fact, older adults with alcohol abuse or dependence are nearly three times more likely to have an underlying psychological disorder. Here we will briefly focus on depression, as it, much like substance abuse, is an underrecognized problem in older men.

Men's depression too often goes unnoticed. Most of the time, the complaints we voice that are associated with depression tend to be physical—fatigue, sleep disturbances, unexplained aches and pains, loss of appetite (see chapter 4 for more details). For older men these symptoms are too readily thought to be evidence of normal aging—slower movement, forgetting (to take medications), worrying about being a burden. The depression we *feel* is not sadness, but rather a lack of energy or a worsening of existing physical issues such as arthritis or headaches.

It may be tempting to try to manage our losses, grief, physical pain, and boredom by using alcohol and prescription drugs, but research shows that this can actually complicate our symptoms of depression. With alcohol especially, short-term rewards are not worth the long-term ramifications. Alcohol is a depressant drug and actually worsens conditions such as anxiety and irritability, and it also has a negative impact on the quality of your sleep. Moreover, it can interact in harmful ways with antidepressants.

Nonprescriptive Drug Use

Statistically, adults are less likely to use illicit (illegal) drugs as they grow older. It is middle-aged adults, age 50–54, who are the most likely to use marijuana, to purposely misuse prescription drugs, and to use other types of illegal substances, but according to the National Survey on Drug Use and Health, these numbers "declined dramatically" as respondents' ages increased. For men over 65, about 1 percent reported using prescription drugs for nonmedical purposes, and approximately 1 percent reported using marijuana.

Legal in an increasing number of states, medicinal marijuana is used by older adults who suffer from glaucoma or advanced macular degeneration and by cancer patients undergoing chemotherapy. It has also proven to be an effective therapy for a variety of other conditions, including inflammatory bowel disease, migraines, fibromyalgia, alcohol abuse, depression, hepatitis, digestive disease, bipolar disorder, and Parkinson's disease. Medical marijuana has also proven helpful in stimulating appetite in AIDS and cancer patients. It is available for sale in an authorized dispensary in those states permitting its distribution if you have medical authorization. For those older men suffering from chronic pain that has not been treated effectively by other means, the use of medical marijuana may be a treatment to consider in consultation with your physician.

Common Examples of Drug Misuse

Although there is potential for the abuse of many prescription drugs, most men genuinely try to take their medications the "right" way and are often unaware that some side effects they experience may be as a result of mistakenly misusing their prescriptions. One scenario in which prescriptions can be misused is medication sharing. You might start to develop a new ache or find that falling asleep is becoming increasingly problematic, and a well-intentioned friend might offer one of his or her unused prescriptions—"Oh, well that happened to me, and this cleared it right up. I've got half a bottle left, and it'll save you a trip to the doctor." In these times of increasing medical costs, it might seem very tempting to save time and money by accepting a "donated" prescription. However, this practice can be highly dangerous—you will not be able to know if the new medication will interact with your other prescriptions, what side effects it may cause in you (versus in your friend), or whether it really is the best treatment for your condition.

Despite the fact that it is expensive to seek medical help and fill a prescription, it is really important that the medications you take come from a health care professional who is informed of your personal history and knows about all of your current prescriptions.

Perhaps the most common example of drug misuse involves the interactions of different prescriptions with themselves, or with over-the-counter medications or alcohol. At this point we have not done our job if you do not realize that alcohol and prescription medications are a harmful cocktail, so we will focus on the former two scenarios. Naturally, the number of different prescriptions and/or over-the-counter medications a man takes will increase his risk of misuse. This is especially pertinent to psychoactive drug consumers, as they are generally on more medications than are nonpsychoactive drug users. Also, the use of several prescriptions from one class of drugs, such as combining two types of bronchodilators, is a common example of misuse in older adults. Over-the-counter medications are also commonly misused when combined erroneously with prescriptions. For example, using aspirin in conjunction with anticoagulant drugs increases your risk of bleeding, and combining aspirin with Clinoril, an anti-inflammatory drug used to treat arthritis pain, puts you at increased risk of gastrointestinal upset.

Studies have identified that accidental misuse is sometimes just that—an accident. Older adults may take either too much or too little of their prescriptions, which is often due to improper (or nonexistent) instructions that they receive from their pharmacists or health care providers. You may not know or remember the use for particular medications, or you may have trouble in appropriately following directions concerning proper dosage. Not only are older adults less likely than younger people to receive physician- or pharmacist-initiated counseling on proper usage of their medication, but older adults are unlikely to ask their health care providers questions about how to take their prescriptions. In one study it was found that older adults were more uninformed than younger adults about the potential risks of medications they were taking (in this case the drugs were potentially driver impairing).[25] *Do not hesitate to ask questions, and never be afraid to request clarification.* Your health care provider and pharmacist will be able to tell you what you need to know about your prescriptions. Don't let your physician assume that you already know everything you need to know about a new prescription; this is your health, and you have every right to stay as informed as possible.

COLLATERAL DAMAGE—MAKING SURE UNUSED MEDICATIONS DO NOT CAUSE HARM

Most of us probably have several old orange containers lurking in our medicine cabinets. For whatever reason, we seem reluctant to get rid of old prescription medications. Maybe we're worried they will fall into the wrong hands if we simply put them out with the garbage, or maybe we're environmentally conscious and prefer not to contaminate our water by flushing pills down the toilet, or maybe we just forget that we even have medicine left over from that annoying sinus infection that plagued us two years ago.

According to the U.S. Environmental Protection Agency, older adults are especially prone to the accumulation of expired or unused prescription medications; this is no great surprise, given that older people make up the largest prescription-using population. Medications pile up when health care providers switch patients' prescriptions or encourage them to discontinue using certain drugs, or when family members pass away and

Asking Questions about Your Medications: What You Need to Know

- Make sure you know the name and spelling of the drug you are being prescribed, as well as why your doctor wants you to take it.

- Ask your doctor to write down how often and for how long you should take it.

- Ask if you will need a refill, and if so, how to get one.

- Ask what changes you need to make when taking the medication: "Are there foods, drinks, other medications, or activities that I should avoid while taking this medication?"

- Ask what time of day you should take the medication.

- If a medicine says "take with food," ask whether that means before, with, or after food. If it does not specify, ask, "Should I take my medicine at meals or between meals?" or "Do I need to take the medicine on an empty stomach or with food or a whole glass of water?"

- Ask what you should do if you forget and miss a dose.

- Ask when the medicine will begin to work, and ask about any possible side effects that it has, especially for older people.

- And *always* bring a list of all prescription and over-the-counter medications you are currently taking, as well as when you take them, and show it to your doctor.

Source: NIH News (2007, July 26). *NIHSeniorHealth offers tips on how to talk with your doctor.* Washington, DC: U.S. Department of Health and Human Services.

leave unfinished medications, or when people stop using medications due to unpleasant reactions or just plain feeling better.[26]

These excess medications, left unused in your home, can cause a host of problems. You may have grandchildren who could gain access to potentially lethal amounts of medications. At the very least, having too many prescription bottles can lead to mistakenly taking the wrong medicine or confusing expired pills with newer ones. But we hang on to them because the problem of disposal seems sometimes to be just as risky and/or problematic.

There are, however, many resources available for medication disposal. The U.S. Drug Enforcement Agency, recognizing that people often have unused or unwanted prescription medications in their homes, has organized "Drug Take-Back" days. These national events involve participating collection sites where people can drop off their old medications for proper, environmentally friendly disposal. Your community may also have other local collection programs for safe drug disposal, such as those operated by senior centers, law enforcement, or pharmacies.

THREE COMMONLY PRESCRIBED DRUGS

Psychotropic Medications

The term *psychotropic medications* refers to drugs that are prescribed for a mental health condition. Also referred to as *psychoactive medications*, these types of drugs have the highest risk for abuse. They include benzodiaze-pines and opiates, which are arguably the most abused by older adults and merit their own discussion (see below).

Older men should take some comfort in the fact that, as a group, we are less likely than older women to abuse psychotropic (or other) prescription medications. Older men tend to be more likely, as mentioned earlier, to abuse alcohol and cannabis than they are to misuse or abuse prescription medications. However, risk factors for psychotropic medication misuse and abuse include having a large number of different prescriptions and other substance abuse problems (either previously or at the same time). Men are certainly not immune to unknowingly or purposively misusing medications.

Benzodiazepines

One type of psychoactive drug, benzodiazepines, or "benzos," as they are commonly called, is repeatedly mentioned in the medical literature as being a risk for both abuse and misuse by older men. Often prescribed to older adults for the treatment of anxiety and sleeping problems, benzodiaze-pine use can often result in physiological dependence after as little as 2 months. Benzos have largely replaced barbiturate-type drugs and other sedatives of the past as they are considered to be safer. But as a class of drugs they represent a significant threat. While this is *not* intended to scare anyone off their meds, it is important to realize that if you have been prescribed a benzodiazepine-type drug, you may experience withdrawal symptoms if you discontinue its use.

Benzodiazepines and Their Common Brand Names

Oxazepam:	Serax, Murelaz, Alepam
Lorazepam:	Ativan
Diazepam:	Valium
Temazepam:	Restoril
Triazolam:	Halcion
Alprazolam:	Xanax
Clonazepa:	Klonopin, Rivotril
Flurazepam:	Dalmane

Withdrawal from benzodiazepines is somewhat similar to withdrawal from alcohol in its symptoms and potential severity. This is because each of these substances has the same depressant effect on the body. Although withdrawal from any substance is uncomfortable and sometimes a painful process, those who are dependent on either alcohol or benzos (as opposed to most other substances) may actually run the risk of death when withdrawal is abrupt and not medically managed. Symptoms of withdrawal from benzos include increased pulse, hand tremors, insomnia, nausea, vomiting, and rebound anxiety. Grand mal seizures can occur. It is extremely important to seek medical advice before making the decision to stop a prescription; your doctor may only advise you to gradually step down your dose. Under no circumstances should you ever begin or discontinue taking a medication without first talking to your health care provider.

It cannot be stressed enough that the combination of benzodiazepines and alcohol can be deadly, with the possible result of a shutdown of the central nervous system. In one study conducted specifically on the misuse of prescription drugs by older adults, almost 15 percent of all misuse events involved alcohol, which suggests that many older men may unwittingly put themselves at risk by drinking in conjunction with their prescriptions.[27]

Opiates

Many older men are also prescribed opiate-type medications, often for the management of chronic pain. However, when used inappropriately, they can produce a euphoric "high" that may open the door for some men to become dependent on their pain medications for more than just physical relief. While most authorities agree that older adults are far less likely to abuse their opiate-type prescriptions than their younger counterparts, taking these medications puts us at increased risk for harmful side effects. Drugs such as codeine, for example, can lead to poor motor coordination, whereas stronger medications such as oxycodone can impair your vision, diminish your ability to pay attention, and be even more detrimental to your coordination.[28] While withdrawal should be medically monitored, the risks involved with ceasing the use of opiates are generally not as serious as they are with benzos and are confined to more uncomfortable side effects such as nausea, aches, insomnia, and diarrhea.

DO I HAVE A PROBLEM?

If you are concerned that you may have a problem, you are not alone. As many as one in five men over the age of 60 may face a serious health risk because of their alcohol abuse, and more older men may unknowingly misuse their prescription medications to the point where professional help is required. Fortunately, there is evidence that older adults respond to alcohol and/or drug abuse treatment as well as, if not better than, their younger counterparts. In addition, although withdrawal can be a longer process for older people than for younger individuals, older adults tend to experience less severe symptoms. On the other hand, treatment services may take somewhat longer to gain access to because you are older, and temporary hospitalization may be recommended if detoxification is necessary.

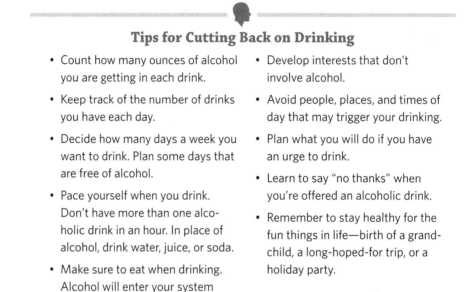

Tips for Cutting Back on Drinking

- Count how many ounces of alcohol you are getting in each drink.

- Keep track of the number of drinks you have each day.

- Decide how many days a week you want to drink. Plan some days that are free of alcohol.

- Pace yourself when you drink. Don't have more than one alcoholic drink in an hour. In place of alcohol, drink water, juice, or soda.

- Make sure to eat when drinking. Alcohol will enter your system more slowly if you eat food.

- Develop interests that don't involve alcohol.

- Avoid people, places, and times of day that may trigger your drinking.

- Plan what you will do if you have an urge to drink.

- Learn to say "no thanks" when you're offered an alcoholic drink.

- Remember to stay healthy for the fun things in life—birth of a grandchild, a long-hoped-for trip, or a holiday party.

Source: National Institute on Aging (2012, Mar.). *Alcohol use in older people.* Washington, DC: U.S. Department of Health and Human Services.

Older men who suffer from alcoholism can benefit from being prescribed naltrexone, which decreases alcohol cravings. Naltrexone also blocks the effects of opiate drugs, making it useful for people addicted to pain medications. When used in conjunction with substance abuse treatment, naltrexone can also give those in recovery an extra layer of protection from relapse. Furthermore, 12-step meetings, such as those offered by Alcoholics Anonymous (AA), can be helpful in recovery; about a third of all members are over the age of 50. Men who are in recovery from drug (rather than alcohol) abuse may actually find themselves more comfortable in AA than its counterpart, Narcotics Anonymous (NA), as NA generally tends to have younger members.

Types of Substance Abuse Treatment for Older Adults

Brief interventions: One or more counseling sessions involving direct feedback on screening questions, patient education, approaches to motivational and behavioral changes, and use of written manuals and materials to reinforce message

Interventions: Counseling sessions with patient in the presence of family or friends to confront drug-use problems

Motivational counseling: Intensive meetings with counselor to understand patient's perspective on the situation, assess readiness to change behaviors, help patient shift perspective, and consider alternative solutions

Specialized treatment: Inpatient/outpatient detoxification, inpatient/outpatient rehabilitation, outpatient services

Maintenance treatment: Psychotherapy, individual and/or group counseling, and self-help and 12-step programs

Source: Simoni-Wastila, L., & Yang, H. (2006). Psychoactive drug abuse in older adults. *American Journal of Geriatric Pharmacotherapy, 4,* 380–394.

EXAMPLES OF ALCOHOL SCREENING TESTS

If you are questioning your alcohol use or that of a loved one, consider the following two examples of evidence-based screening tests used by physicians and mental health professionals to assess for alcohol abuse. An "evidence-based screening test" is one that has proven to be valid (i.e., effective) based on the results of rigorous scientific evaluation.

CAGE Test

The word *CAGE* is an acronym for the first letters of the key words in the following four questions. A response of "yes" to any two questions may indicate a risk of alcohol abuse:

1. Have you ever felt you should *Cut* down on your drinking?
2. Have you ever felt *Annoyed* by criticism about your drinking?
3. Have you ever felt *Guilty* or bad about drinking?
4. Have you ever felt the need for an "*Eye-opener*" in the morning to steady your nerves?

Source: Ewing, J. A. (1984). Detecting alcoholism: The CAGE questionnaire. *Journal of the American Medical Association, 252,* 1905–1907.

Short Michigan Alcoholism Screening Test (S-MAST)—Geriatric Version

Two or more "yes" responses may be indicative of an alcohol problem.

	Yes (1)	No (0)
1. When talking with others, do you ever underestimate how much you actually drink?	○	○
2. After a few drinks, have you sometimes not eaten or been able to skip a meal because you didn't feel hungry?	○	○
3. Does having a few drinks help decrease your shakiness or tremors?	○	○
4. Does alcohol sometimes make it hard for you to remember parts of the day or night?	○	○
5. Do you usually take a drink to relax or calm your nerves?	○	○
6. Do you drink to take your mind off your problems?	○	○
7. Have you ever increased your drinking after experiencing a loss in your life?	○	○
8. Has a doctor or nurse ever said they were worried or concerned about your drinking?	○	○
9. Have you ever made rules to manage your drinking?	○	○
10. When you feel lonely, does having a drink help?	○	○

Total S-MAST-G Score (0–10)   ____   ____

Source: Blow, F. C., Brower, K. J., Schulenber, J. E., et al. (1992). The Michigan Alcoholism Screening Test—Geriatric Version (MAST-G): A new elderly-specific screen instrument. *Alcoholism: Clinical and Experimental Research, 16,* 372.

CHAPTER 11

Holistic Medicine

with Kristianna Hall

In today's world of rapid technological and medical advancements, it seems that there is a new breakthrough treatment or revolutionary prescription every day. With every doctor's visit, many older men may find that they return home with yet another pill to include in their daily schedule of medications. And while pharmaceutical breakthroughs undoubtedly do save lives and are necessary, there also exists the option to supplement our health care regimen with a variety of nontraditional approaches to the treatment of our bodies—sometimes called *holistic* health and medicine.

> The competent physician, before he attempts to give medicine to the patient, makes himself acquainted not only with the disease, but also with the habits and constitution of the sick man.
>
> —Cicero

So what is holistic medicine, and can it make a difference in the quality of our lives? The term refers not to a single approach or procedure but to an overarching mentality regarding human health and healing processes, which focuses on the idea that *all* aspects of our health, from the body to the psyche, should be considered in treatments. The defining approaches for holistic health professionals integrate humanizing health care and therapies from a whole-person perspective to address the biological roots of health problems and our lifestyle determinants of suffering. A more straightforward way to think of holistic medicine would be to envision a doctor who not only cares that you've physically had a heart attack but also needs to know how you felt about it emotionally and how it affected your relationships or other areas of your life. With that information, holistic medicine could be used in a variety of ways along with conventional heart health management: to speed recovery, to ease stress, and to aid in the prevention of further cardiac trouble.

Many health organizations, such as the National Institutes of Health, use the term *complementary and alternative medicine* (CAM) to encompass different aspects of holistic treatments.[1] *Complementary* medicine, as you might suspect, refers to the integration of holistic treatments with standard Western pharmaceutical care, whereas *alternative* medicine indicates that standard medical care is replaced by a different treatment. It is important to note that these areas overlap—for example, acupuncture can be considered as a complementary therapy by some, while others choose to make it their sole form of treatment for a given condition. In this chapter we will focus on types of holistic medicine that can be complementary and not limit the discussion to purely alternative treatments designed to replace conventional health care.

CAM includes an extensive group of healing methods and products such as herbal medicines, prayer, crystal healing, Reiki massage, homeopathy, acupuncture, and chiropractic care, and most CAM therapies are incompatible with each other. Some CAM practices come from Western traditions and others from "whole medical systems," which refer to the comprehensive systems of care found in different cultures and parts of the world, such as traditional Indian and Chinese medicines. While these systems came about as complete treatment plans in their respective locations, today we can find aspects of different traditions of medicine integrated into a care plan based on standard Western medicine (such as herbal medicines or massage therapy) or simply used as a supplement to a healthy lifestyle. According to the National Center for Complementary and Alternative Medicine (NCCAM), "CAM practices are often grouped into broad categories, such as natural products, mind and body medicine, manipulative and body-based practices."[2]

We realize, of course, that not all men will readily embrace the idea of using "alternative" or even complementary forms of medicine. Some will point to the traditions of Western medicine as having served them well, and they may unequivocally believe that Western medicine represents treatments that are endorsed by the professional community, familiar to the general public, and, not unimportantly, accepted by health insurance carriers. Even so, there is considerable value in appreciating the exceedingly wide range of CAM treatments, many of which boast a longer history than Western medicine and represent the standard of care for hundreds of millions of people outside the United States (not to mention tens of millions in the country). It is for that reason that we take a more in-depth look at

> A man may esteem himself happy when that which is his food is also his medicine.
>
> —Henry David Thoreau

holistic practices, focusing on some of the more pertinent applications for middle-aged and older men.

BIOLOGICALLY BASED THERAPIES

Biologically based complementary medicine is couched in the idea that better health can be achieved through use of natural products and dietary modification, particularly "functional foods," which refer to "processed foods containing ingredients that aid specific bodily functions in addition to being nutritious."[3] Foods that promote health and have medicinal properties include common berries, fruits, soy, vegetables, green tea, and herbs, as well as the "nutraceuticals" that are derived from many natural sources. In the United Kingdom, most nutraceuticals are regulated as drugs, and in the United States, while most natural health products are sold over-the-counter, the Food and Drug Administration (FDA) now maintains that any product that claims to impact disease must be categorized as a drug.

Functional Foods

One class of functional foods includes the *probiotics*, because they contain the same types of beneficial bacteria already found in your own body. The bacterial strains *Lactobacilli* and *Bifidobacteria* are found in many foods and supplements. Below are a number of examples:[4]

> *Yogurt*. Yogurt is the most popular and commonly used probiotic food, and depending on the brand, it can contain several strains of "good" bacteria, such as *Streptococcus thermo-philus*, *Lactobacilli (L.) acidophilus*, *L. casei*, *L. reuteri*, and *bifidus*. Make sure that you buy yogurt that has live and active cultures—some manufacturers pasteurize their product, which kills the bacteria and negates a probiotic effect.

> *Kefir*. Kefir (pronounced "keh-fear") is a fermented milk product derived from animal or plant milks. It is a beverage comparable in taste and consistency to drinkable yogurt products and is available in health food stores.

> *Dairy products*. Many "typical" dairy products are also available with probiotics. Some companies produce sour cream, cottage cheese, and the like with added live and active bacterial cultures. Cultured buttermilk and acidophilus milk are two other examples.

> *Cabbage*. Sauerkraut, kimchi, or any fermented cabbage product contains high concentrations of *Lactobacilli*. Make sure that you buy a

product that is unpasteurized. It should also need to be refrigerated, as the preservative ingredient sodium benzoate kills live bacteria.

> *Brine-cured olives, salted gherkins (cucumbers).* These foods also contain *Lactobacilli*, but again, beware of pasteurized products and/or those containing sodium benzoate.

> *Brand-name probiotic foods.* As probiotics become more widely recognized, companies are marketing products containing live and active cultures. From chocolate bars to cereal to juice, more options become available as consumer demand increases. Many of these companies tout the inclusion of probiotics as a major selling point, making their products more user-friendly for the shopper.

The European Food Safety Authority and the FDA sparked new debate when they recently questioned the science behind many companies' claim that supplementing your diet with probiotics has proven health benefits.[5] While more research is needed to confirm their effectiveness, evidence exists that the use of probiotics can have health benefits, especially for certain conditions. Most commonly recognized is their use in promoting healthy digestive function, as microorganisms in the gut help to regulate food absorption and nutrient processing. Research supports the NCCAM recommendation for the use of probiotics for treating diarrhea, preventing and treating urinary tract infections, treating irritable bowel syndrome, and reducing the recurrence of bladder cancer.[6]

Antioxidant-rich foods belong to another class of functional foods that promote health by removing cell-damaging particles called *free radicals*. Free radicals are produced during natural body processes, such as breaking down food for use; they are also created when people are exposed to cigarette smoke, pollutants, and radiation. When free radicals overwhelm our body's ability to regulate them, they adversely modify blood lipids, proteins, and DNA. These potentially harmful molecules are thought to be involved in the development of various diseases, such as cancer, Parkinson's disease, and rheumatoid arthritis. Your body produces its own antioxidants to counter free radicals, and antioxidants are absorbed from food. While antioxidant supplements are very popular among today's consumers, there is no conclusive evidence to show that they have any positive influence on our health. By comparison, consuming antioxidant-rich foods has been correlated with a reduced risk of disease.[7] The exception to this rule is that antioxidant supplements, when combined with zinc, appear to be effective in reducing the risk of developing advanced stages of age-related macular degeneration (AMD).[8]

Besides functional foods, dietary supplements are another example of biologically based complementary medicine. In general, they include vitamins, minerals, herbs, amino acids, or enzymes. While a healthy, balanced diet is the starting point, the addition of certain supplements can serve to enhance your physical and mental functioning. For older men, it is important to make sure to include several different supplements.

Foods That Pack a Punch

The USDA's top 20 antioxidant-rich foods are as follows:

1. Small red beans (dried)
2. Blueberries (wild)
3. Red kidney beans
4. Pinto beans
5. Blueberries (cultivated)
6. Cranberries
7. Artichokes (cooked)
8. Blackberries
9. Prunes
10. Raspberries
11. Strawberries
12. Red Delicious apples
13. Granny Smith apples
14. Pecans
15. Sweet cherries
16. Black plums
17. Russet potatoes (cooked)
18. Black beans (dried)
19. Plums
20. Gala apples

Source: Wu, X., Beecher, G. R., Holden, J. M., et al. (2004). Lipophilic and hydrophilic antioxidant capacities of common foods in the United States. *Journal of Agricultural and Food Chemistry, 52,* 4026–4037.

Vitamins

Vitamins for men to especially consider are vitamin B12, which we do not absorb efficiently from our food as we get older, and vitamin D, which we have greater trouble absorbing from foods or creating it during exposure to sunlight. Dietary guidelines suggest that if you are over 50 you should take a vitamin B12 supplement of 2.4 micrograms per day; similarly, because vitamin D is essential to prevent aging-related bone loss, men over 60 are recommended to get at least 1,000 IU per day.[9] Vitamin C is also especially important once you pass age 60 for the prevention of gout, an inflammatory arthritis condition that is most common in men. In a 20-year study, it was found that for every 500-milligram increase in vitamin C intake, men's risk for gout went down by about 17 percent.[10] Finally, if you do not drink milk daily, calcium supplements can strengthen bones and help to prevent the consequences of falls or other injuries. After age 50, it is recommended that men get 1,200 milligrams per day.[11]

However, a caveat about taking vitamins is to remember that more is not necessarily better—taking more than the recommended amount of any vitamin can be dangerous. For example, too much vitamin A can have an adverse effect on your bone health.[12] Also, there are limits to how much your body can absorb in the way of vitamin supplements. By the way, absorption is probably maximized by taking your vitamins with juice (the acid helps) or, better yet, during a meal (the fats and protein help promote absorption).

Supplements and Herbs

The claims of dietary supplements and the range of supplements available can create considerable confusion. You know this if you have wandered into a natural food store with its rows of medicinal products. It seems that each bottle claims to prevent or enhance certain aspects of health, yet in reality it is extremely difficult to prove any one substance's efficacy.

Many of us relate to the dilemma of hearing a product hailed as a breakthrough in health, only to read about that same product's woeful ineffectiveness or even threat to our health some time later. By and large, this is the case with supplements—while some research shows their effectiveness, other studies cannot find significant benefit.

Certain supplements, however, have shown great promise in promoting health, such as fish oil. Not surprisingly, fish oil and omega-3 supplements are the most commonly used natural products among adults in the United States who take dietary supplements. Omega-3s, which are polyunsaturated fatty acids, are necessary for human health. They are found in foods like walnuts, vegetable oils, and (most famously) fish. The Mediterranean diet, which is high in healthy fats (olive and canola oil), fish and poultry (not red meat), fruits, vegetables, and flavoring derived from spices and herbs rather than salt, reinforces a belief in the value of fish oil. Although more research is needed to determine omega-3's specific effects on the human body, the substance has been shown to be effective in helping to reduce the risk of heart attack, especially for those who have suffered one already.[13] Omega-3s also seem to improve brain health, as well as reduce the risk of Alzheimer's disease.[14]

Should middle-aged and older men take fish oils daily? Many physicians are skeptical, but many scientists recommend use of fish oil in a number of circumstances. There are a certain number of oils our body can't make, and two are the omega-3s and the omega-6s. Omega-3s seem to decrease inflammation and can assist men who are having joint pain or any sort of autoimmune issue. Men with rheumatoid arthritis often benefit. There's also some evidence that fish oil can be helpful for mood-related issues, especially once we move toward middle age. As far as dosing, there isn't a standard. Some people say somewhere in the range of 1–4 grams per day, and it seems wise to start with a low dose.

Perhaps the most alluring facet of biologically based CAM is the use of herbal supplements and remedies. Widely touted by consumers, the use of herbs for a healthy lifestyle dates back to ancient times and remains widely practiced throughout the world. Herbal products largely fall into the same gray area as do other supplements—the scientific evidence is inconclusive when it comes to their effectiveness. Some herbal supplements may interact with your medications, so do ask your physician or pharmacist about what you decide to take. Many herbs have long histories of use for specific conditions; some medicinal supplements commonly used by older men are as follows:[15]

> *Saw palmetto*: used by men to help treat urinary conditions caused by an enlarged prostate. This herb can influence the results of a prostate cancer screening test (be sure to tell your doctor you are taking it).

> *Glucosamine and chondroitin*: used in combination to treat arthritis pain.

> *Ginkgo:* used to prevent and treat memory problems; also used for depression and anxiety.

> *St. John's wort*: used to treat a depressed mood; can influence the effects of prescription medications.

> *Kava*: used to ease anxiety; relaxes muscles, prevents seizures, and decreases emotional distress.

> *Ginseng*: used to increase energy; may help with erectile dysfunction (ED).

> *Valerian*: used to improve both ability to fall asleep and quality of sleep.

> *Chili pepper (capsicum)*: used in cream form for topical arthritis pain treatment; also used for diabetic nerve pain and improvement of pain associated with fibromyalgia.

> *Echinacea*: used to boost the immune system.

> *Garlic*: used to help the cardiovascular system; lowers cholesterol.

Some other herbs might also be effective in treating ED; however, some may be dangerous. Herbs and other natural remedies to treat ED have been used outside the United States for a long time, including in Africa and China. It is still very difficult, however, to speak with certainty about their effectiveness and safety. Unlike FDA-approved medications, natural remedies haven't undergone the rigorous testing and long-term monitoring required by federal regulatory agencies to endorse herbal medications as safe and effective. As reported by the Mayo Clinic, some herbal ED therapies can cause side effects or interact negatively with other medications.[16]

Be Smart

For those of you using vitamins or supplements of any kind, it is important to inform your primary care physician and pharmacist. If you are considering a new natural herb or supplement, consult your physician first. A 2007 study conducted by the American Association of Retired Persons (AARP) found that even though large numbers of men and women choose to use herbs and other natural remedies to treat their health problems, 7 in 10 people over age 50 (69%) who make use of CAM treatments did *not* talk about it when they last saw their physicians, leaving themselves open to potentially dangerous interactions with prescription drugs and other side effects.[17] A number of reasons appear to explain why such poor communication exists between patients and physicians about this, including the fact that some men think that their doctors are not going to be receptive to the news and are not adequately informed about nontraditional treatments. Another reason is that their doctors don't take the time to ask them, and men might be embarrassed to ask because they may have their own doubts about whether the treatments are effective or not.

While many products may be natural, they could still be potentially unsafe, because they could interact in potentially dangerous ways with other over-the-counter medications, prescriptions, or medical procedures. Supplements like garlic, green tea, celery, arnica, fenugreek, ginkgo, chamomile, dong quai, and ginger can increase the chances of bleeding and experiencing difficulties clotting when taken in combination with blood thinners and anticoagulants (especially during surgery). If you are taking a low-dose (81 mg) aspirin and drink green tea, you increase this risk. Ginseng can also increase your risk of developing a blood clot when taken in combination with blood thinners and anticoagulants. If you combine diabetes medications with sage, fenugreek, garlic, ginseng, or chromium nettle, it may cause your blood sugar level to drop more than you want. If you combine digoxin (for treating congestive heart failure) with ginseng or kyushin, the result could be inaccurate readings of your digoxin levels. Combining digoxin with licorice root can lower your potassium levels and increase your sensitivity to digoxin, and combining digoxin with St. John's wort can also decrease digoxin's effectiveness.[18]

CONSIDERING SUPPLEMENTS

Herb/natural supplement	Does it work?	Is it dangerous?
Dehydroepiandrosterone (DHEA)	Supports the production of sex hormones. May increase levels of testosterone.	May alter the natural balance of sex hormones, causes acne, and may lower high-density lipoprotein (HDL) cholesterol.
Epimedium (horny goat weed)	May help with erectile dysfunction.	May cause thinning of the blood and lower blood pressure.
Folic acid and vitamin E	May help with erectile dysfunction.	Minor risk unless taken in high doses.
Ginkgo	May help with erectile dysfunction and reduce the sexual side effects when taking antidepressants.	May increase your risk of bleeding.
Ginseng	Used for a number of conditions and may help with erectile dysfunction.	Considered safe although it may lower blood sugar levels and may promote abnormally elevated mood and irritability when taken in combination with certain antidepressants.
Yohimbe (African tree bark)	May help with erectile dysfunction.	Has been linked to anxiety, elevated blood pressure, and fast/irregular heartbeat.
Zinc	May help with erectile dysfunction.	High doses can damage your immune system.

Taking herbal supplements alone may also pose a risk to your health. Herbs affect individuals differently as a result of factors such as age, weight, sex, and individual biochemistry, and you should never assume that adding any type of supplement to your diet will be safe, despite the fact that the products may be labeled as "natural." It is important to make sure that any diagnosis of a disease or condition you are trying to manage has been made by a health care professional who has substantial conventional medical training and experience with providing therapies for that disease or condition. Proven conventional treatments should not be replaced with an unproven CAM treatment.

If you plan to start using a new natural product, here are some important tips recommended by the NCCAM:[19]

> Don't wait for your health care providers to ask about your use of herbs, supplements, and other natural remedies; start the conversation yourself.

> Keep a current list of all of your therapies and treatments, including over-the-counter and prescription medicines, as well as any CAM products such as dietary and herbal supplements. Note any medical specialists or CAM practitioners you see. Take the list with you whenever you visit health care providers. Be sure to tell them about all of your therapies and treatments. They want to know, even if you think their response is dismissive. They are listening for problems. List all therapies and treatments on any patient history form you are asked to fill out.

> Gather information on the CAM therapy you're interested in and take the information with you to your doctor, so you and your doctor can refer to them as you talk, and your doctor can help you evaluate the information.

> Make a list of the things you want to talk about. For example, you might include the following:
  • Why I want to take the supplement.
  • How I found out about it.
  • Is it safe for me to take? Will it interact with any of my medications?
  • Is it likely to help me?
  • What else should I know about it? Where can I find more information?
  • Should I try this? If not, why not? Might something else be better?

> Take a notepad or tape recorder with you. Listen carefully and keep a record of what you find out. You may want to ask a family member or friend to accompany you, so you can compare notes after your visit.

> If something is unclear to you, or if you want more information, don't be afraid to ask. Your health care providers may not be able to answer every question, but they can help you find the answers.

MANIPULATIVE AND BODY-BASED PRACTICES

As defined by the National Institutes of Health, the second category of CAM is manipulative and body-based practices. As you might assume, these holistic approaches focus on the body itself, specifically its structures and systems. Bones, joints, soft tissues, and the circulatory system are chief targets of this mode of treatment. Some examples of manipulative and body-based methods include reflexology, massage therapy, and chiropractic therapy.

Reflexology

Reflexology, which is rooted in traditional Chinese medicine, supports the notion that we have reflex points in our hands and feet which can be used to aid in the healing of other body parts.[20] Reflex points (also called "pressure points") can be bundles of nerves or sensitive areas of veins, muscles, or ligaments and may be manipulated in such a way as to cause pain or pleasure. The philosophy behind these points revolves around their function as warnings to the body. For example, should applied pressure continue, injury will occur. Moreover, when the brain sends out pain signals, their purpose is to try to provoke a corrective reaction, like removing the pressure so that the body can return to its natural functioning. Reflexology promotes the stimulation of these pressure points, temporarily disrupting the body's normal routine so as to almost trick it into restoring its proper flow and balance of energy.[21]

By examining your hands and feet, a reflexology practitioner can then make decisions about what your overall health condition may be. A key belief of this type of medicine holds that the nerves within the hands and feet are specifically related to certain parts of your body's larger systems and are affected in ways that are identical to the way in which a larger organ system is affected. In other words, if you are experiencing pain in your kidneys, a reflexologist would find that a specific area of your hand or foot was also tender. By manipulating the areas of the hands and feet that correspond to pain or swelling in the body, reflexology improves blood flow and helps the body to regain its energy balance, which is self-corrective and can lead to improvements in symptom management and overall health.

Massage Therapy

The number of older adults making use of massage therapy has grown within the past few years.[22] There are over 80 variations of massage therapy. The goal of massage is generally to decrease tension and pain, to increase the flow of blood and oxygen to soft tissues, and to promote both circulation and relaxation. Physically, massage helps to maintain natural joint lubrication, which alleviates some of the pain surrounding conditions such as arthritis or just the normal aches and pains associated with the aging process.

Acupressure, also called "shiatsu," combines the ideas of pressure points and healing massage by concentrating the massage to the pressure point locations. Unlike reflexology and more like acupuncture, acupressure is concerned with pressure points throughout the body and not just those on your hands and feet. Pressure point massages can help to improve your circulation, release muscle tension, and ease joint stiffness. These improvements have a positive effect on your strength, coordination, and stability, minimizing the risk of balance-related injuries.

For middle-aged and older men, massage therapy has a variety of different benefits, both physical and psychological. Massage has also been shown to be effective in treating insomnia and other sleep disruptions that many of us experience as we age, and with better and more restful sleep, our health and mood improve. Emotionally, many aging men can find themselves troubled by feelings of isolation. Therapeutic touch has been shown time and time again to have incredibly beneficial effects on our mood, and the importance of the human contact aspect of manipulative and body-based practices such as massage cannot be overstated.

Chiropractic Therapy

Use of chiropractic care ranges from around 6 to 12 percent of the population, and most men who seek chiropractic care do so because of low back and/or neck pain and not for organic disease.[23] Chiropractic services remain among the top three most frequently used CAM therapies in the United States.[24] Most practitioners are certified DCs (or Doctors of Chiropractic) and use some form of spinal manipulative therapy; more than 90 percent also provide nutritional advice and recommend nutritional supplements, therapeutic exercises, and physical activity or exercise.[25] They are not the "bone crunchers" so commonly stereotyped in the media. Chiropractic care recognizes the importance of the nervous system to our body's function and capabilities. The underlying holistic philosophy of chiropractic therapy is based on the belief that the structure and condition of our body influence how the body functions, and our mind-body relationship is crucial to maintaining health and healing.

MIND-BODY MEDICINE

The third subcategory of CAM, mind-body medicine, supports the philosophy that not only do your mind and body influence each other, but your mental state has the potential to positively influence your physical being. Mind-body medicine can take the form of meditation, guided movements such as yoga or Tai Chi, or the use of creative outlets such as art or dance. All seek to enhance your ability to find a harmonious balance between mind and body. Mind-body medicine practices share some commonalities with practices based on natural energy fields—Reiki massage, qigong, and acupuncture are examples of healing modalities that incorporate both principles. We include energy medicine as a subcategory.

Energy Medicine

The holistic practice of energy medicine is based on the principle that people are surrounded by energy fields, and that a positive change in your energy field can foster a positive change in your health. One example of scientifically measured energy is a magnetic field, which is the basis for magnet therapy in CAM and is taken for granted in magnetic resonance imaging (MRI) within traditional medicine. In magnet therapy, magnetic devices are used to alleviate pain and other troubling symptoms associated with various conditions.

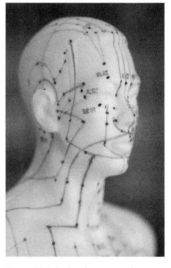

Figure 11.1. Paths of energy in the body known as meridians. Courtesy of Scotshot/Shutterstock.com.

Energy medicine also includes practices based on biofields, which support the principle that people have a subtle form of energy and that any disturbances in this energy field can lead to illnesses. Practitioners who implement healing touch therapies, a practice of gently touching their clients' bodies, try to detect these energy field disturbances and alleviate them. You might be familiar with the word *qi* (pronounced "chee"), which refers to the Eastern concept of life energy—a natural force flowing through your body. According to traditional Chinese and Japanese medicine, qi flows throughout the body by way of paths known as "meridians," and health discomforts are caused by deficiencies, excesses, or obstructions in an individual's qi that prevent its natural movement in the meridians. Therapies such as Reiki and acupuncture seek to promote health by balancing your qi flow.

Reiki

Practitioners of Reiki ("ray-key") support the belief that a universal source of healing energy exists which enhances and supports your natural well-being. Like healing touch, it involves the use of touching or holding the hands lightly over the body in order to help you access this fundamental source of healing energy.[26] Reiki, which is concerned with achieving balance and harmony, ascribes to the philosophy that the practitioner can act as a conduit for this universal energy, channeling it to the person through his or her hands. People who have been treated with Reiki often describe sensing heat or coolness, total body relaxation, and a sort of internal vibration in a part of their body regardless of whether the Reiki practitioner actually placed his or her hands on or around that spot. While the ways in which Reiki works are as yet unproven by science, it has been incorporated into clinical care as a complementary therapy and may have positive effects on immune function and endorphin production.

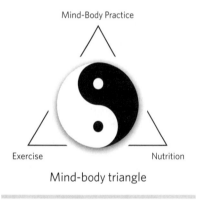

Mind and Body

Eastern medicine believes that optimal health cannot be achieved by exercise and diet alone, but must include mind-body practices.

Mind-Body Practice

Exercise   Nutrition

Mind-body triangle

Non-contact Therapeutic Touch

When the energy therapy only involves light or near-body touch, it is called either *healing touch* or *non-contact therapeutic touch* (NCTT). The practitioner's "touch" influences the energy field that surrounds and penetrates the body. A study conducted at the University of Missouri showed that 73 percent of patients who were receiving NCTT after surgery experienced more significant reductions in pain, slept more comfortably, and requested fewer pain medications than the control group. Guy McCormack, the lead researcher, reported that "there seems to be some subliminal aspects we are not aware of that may have to do with the connectivity between people. . . . If people believe that NCTT is going to be beneficial and are knowledgeable of it, it will be beneficial."[27]

Qigong

Qigong ("chee-gung") is another holistic medicinal approach that is part of traditional Chinese medicine. According to the Qigong Research and Practice Center, "It is the art and science of using breathing techniques, gentle movement, and meditation to cleanse, strengthen, and circulate the life energy (qi). Qigong practice leads to better health and vitality and a tranquil state of mind."[28] As an interesting side note, it is estimated that over 60 million Chinese people have a daily qigong regimen. While traditional Chinese medicine divides qigong into several action-based categories, whether it be movement oriented, meditation oriented, or breathing oriented, for our purposes we will consider the three to be integrated in the same form, as the health benefits of any one style do not outweigh the others. Moreover, our experience seems to suggest that qigong resources readily available to the average person already use a combination of movement and breathing techniques.

Qigong has many health benefits particularly pertinent to older men's issues. One 30-year study conducted on high blood pressure found that patients who took traditional hypertension medication combined with a 30-minute session of qigong two times per day experienced stabilization in their blood pressures. Moreover, the doses of blood pressure medication required for the qigong group over the 30 years decreased, and for 30 percent of the hypertensive patients it was altogether eliminated.[29] Qigong has also been shown to have positive effects on aging men's bone density and heart function, while decreasing the decline in the production of sex hormones inherent to older age. Use of the practice also contributes to the health of your immune system, and it has been found valuable in the prevention of a second stroke for people who have already suffered one.[30]

In addition to its physical benefits, qigong is also believed to contribute to positive emotional health. Qigong incorporates meditation, which helps to focus the mind and calm the nerves. It also makes use of breathing techniques, which are proven relaxation methods. Use of qigong by older men can help to increase spirituality, enhance a personal sense of well-being, and restore energy to both body and mind.

ACUPUNCTURE

The principle of acupuncture is that it stimulates the natural healing processes of the body and can be used to treat stress, nausea, pain, and other conditions. It is perhaps one of the most well-known forms of CAM—and arguably also one of the most daunting. Acupuncturists place small needles just below the surface of the client's skin. Although more visually impressive, acupuncture functions in much the same way as acupressure and reflexology, with an intent to restore the balance of a person's qi in order to promote healing. A form of traditional Chinese medicine, acupuncture clears blockages in qi by inserting small needles at pressure points throughout the body. They are then left in for a period of 20–40 minutes, with most recipients reporting greater relaxation and a deeper sense of well-being. Benefits for health conditions, such as the alleviation of pain, usually require more than one treatment, although people who suffer from a sprain, for example, may only require one session for relief.[31]

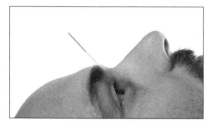

Figure 11.2. Man receiving acupuncture. Courtesy of Merlin/Shutterstock.com.

Acupuncture has been used to treat a variety of medical conditions for thousands of years. Middle-aged and older men may find acupuncture helpful not only for its promotion of well-being but also for its ability to ease symptoms associated with aging. One study of older adults who suffered from arthritis in their knees found that a 6-month course of acupuncture resulted in less pain and increased agility.[32] Acupuncture has also been found to be useful for relieving chronic pain, headaches, and pain after surgery. It is used by many to help maintain heart health, as acupuncture can be used as a weight-loss aid and may lower cholesterol and blood pressure.[33]

The World Health Organization also classifies certain diseases and symptoms as showing potential for treatment with acupuncture, but which are as yet unproven by clinical studies. The rather long list includes conditions such as cancer pain, asthma, insomnia, ED, Ménière's disease, osteoarthritis, substance abuse, chronic prostatitis, acute spine pain, and non-insulin-dependent diabetes. While the future of acupuncture in Western health care looks promising, many Americans are already turning to the practice as a supplement to their existing health care plans as a way of avoiding further prescriptions and medical costs. With an extremely low

Conditions for which Acupuncture Has Been Proven Effective through Clinical Trials

- Adverse reactions to chemotherapy
- Depression (including depression following stroke)
- Headache
- Facial / neck / knee / low back pain
- Hypertension (essential)
- Hypotension (primary)
- Nausea/vomiting

- Pain in dentistry
- Rheumatoid arthritis
- Stroke
- Postoperative pain
- Sprain
- Leukopenia
- Sciatica

Source: World Health Organization (2003). *Acupuncture: Review and analysis of reports on controlled clinical trials.* Geneva, Switzerland: World Health Organization.

occurrence of serious side effects (only 10 incidents of internal injury in the U.S. from 1965 to 1997) and a positive effect on one's mental well-being, older adults are becoming more active users of acupuncture.

OTHER SYSTEMS OF COMPLEMENTARY AND ALTERNATIVE MEDICINE

While this chapter has primarily focused on the use of different modalities of CAM, it is worthwhile to touch on a few other systems of alternative medicine before closing. We briefly explore homeopathy and Ayurveda.

Homeopathy

Homeopathy is a system of treatment developed in the late 1700s by Samuel Hahnemann, a German physician. The practice of homeopathy flourished in the United States in the 1800s, and by the early 1900s there were over 100 homeopathic hospitals in the country. Although it fell out of favor in the 1920s, following the Flexner Report that established MDs as "proper" medical providers and allopathic medicine as the curriculum in medical schools, homeopathy is regaining popularity in the United States. It has remained a mainstay of medicinal practices in many other countries. Homeopathic remedies are regulated by the FDA, including the manufacture, labeling, and dispensing of remedies.[34]

Homeopathy is based on the principle that "like cures like." Hahnemann, while developing medicines, found that rather than using a larger dose of a substance, diluted doses of the same substance could work as a curative, because the small dose stimulates our body to produce an antidote to fight the ailment or disease. This is the exact principle for immunizations: our body is injected, for example, with a small dose of polio when we get the polio vaccine, and that triggers the immune system to develop antibodies. In homeopathic medicine, the "like cures like" principle is best illustrated in the following:

> No substance is poisonous when taken in its correct dose.
>
> —Samuel Hahnemann, creator of homeopathy

Can you remember the last time you were stung by a bee? The stinging, burning pain, swelling, heat, and redness are probably etched in your memory. These are the symptoms that you experience when an angry bee injects its venom into your healthy body. How can a poisonous substance like bee venom (*Apis mellifica*) be used as a medicine? It is precisely the fact that it *causes* symptoms that makes it useful as a medicine. Bee venom, when used as a homeopathic medicine, can relieve the pain and discomfort of bee stings as well as other illnesses that have similar symptoms. People suffering from conjunctivitis (pink eye), who complain of stinging or burning pain, redness and swelling of the eyelids, often benefit from *Apis*. The type of arthritis that is hot, red, and swollen with stinging pains may also be cured or helped by a dose of homeopathic bee venom.[35]

Homeopathic remedies are available in different potencies, and the medicinal system contains over 200 remedies for various conditions. Because homeopathy focuses on the whole person, diagnostically, homeopathic practitioners are concerned not only with physical symptoms but also with the client's personal characteristics—the person's food preferences, sleep patterns, and general outlook on life are taken into account when deciding what remedy is appropriate.

Below are just a few examples of homeopathic remedies for a problem many middle-aged and older men live with—an enlarged prostate (benign prostatic hyperplasia, or BPH):

> *Pulsatilla*. Derived from a perennial flower, pulsatilla may be recommended if you have prostate problems characterized by pain or discomfort after urination (including yellow discharge from the penis) and accompanied by pain traveling to either the pelvis or into the bladder. You are a strong candidate for this treatment if you are emotional, enjoy receiving affection, and prefer to be in open-air surroundings.

> *Lycopodium*. This, too, is derived from a natural plant, a small distinct fern called a ground pine. Lycopodium may be recommended if the prostate is enlarged, urine discharges slowly, and you feel pressure in your prostate during and after urination. You are a particularly strong candidate for this treatment if you have digestive problems such as gas and bloating and lack energy late in the day.

> *Staphysagria*. Part of this colorful plant may be recommended if you report a burning pain whether you are urinating or not, have difficulty retaining urine, and experience impotence. Strong candidates for this treatment consider themselves to be romantically inclined, shy, and sentimental.

As these three examples suggest, homeopathic remedies are designed to incorporate facets of the entire individual—personality, likes and dislikes, and immediate symptoms. Once you have selected the appropriate remedy and potency, the dose is then dissolved under the tongue. Given that the actual substances are so diluted, the remedy itself is generally tasteless or slightly sweet. Side effects are generally mild and can include a rash or, at times, a dramatic but temporary worsening of symptoms. Homeopathic practitioners regard both of these occurrences as indications that the disease is being pushed out of the body.

Ayurveda

Ayurvedic medicine originated in India and is one of the world's oldest health care systems. Like other holistic approaches, it focuses on integrating body, mind, and spirit and will use a combination of treatments both to cleanse the body of impurities and to promote healthy balance. Cleansing the body of harmful substances is believed to be one of the key goals in achieving wellness.[36] In Ayurvedic medicine, the practitioner assesses which of your *doshas* (life forces) are imbalanced by a number of diagnostic methods, including touch, observation, and questioning the person about digestion and personal habits, among others.

Basic to Ayurvedic medicine is its philosophical premise about our "interconnectedness." Not only are both living and nonliving things in the universe linked together, but the body's constitution and life forces contain elements found in the universe. To have good health, your body and mind (*prakriti*) must be in harmony and every cell in the body must contain a balance of the life forces (*doshas*); disease and psychological ill health emerge when your *prakriti* is not in harmony with the universe and, in turn, your life forces are imbalanced. *Prakriti* refers to our body's constitution and its three life forces (*doshas*) that control the activities of our body. Each *dosha* is a combination of two of the five basic elements in the universe—air, fire, water, earth, and ether (distant space)—and each *dosha* uniquely affects bodily functions. For example, the *pitta dosha* (which represents water and fire) controls metabolism, whereas the *kapha dosha* (earth and water) controls structure—muscle, bone, and cell organization—and helps maintain immunity and strength. Each of us represents one of the 10 unique ways the *dosha* can combine to yield a different body and behavioral type.

Ayurvedic treatment practices[37] focus on eliminating impurities through cleansing and managing symptoms through meditation, breathing, physical exercises, and changes in diet. Cleansing (*panchakarma*) detoxifies the body, strengthens your immune system, and restores balance. The underlying logic of *panchakarma* is that we can't completely digest our emotions, food, and experiences; as a result, toxins accumulate in our bodily tissues, creating imbalance and, eventually, disease. The toxic is known as *ama*, and *panchakarma* is a cleansing process that is recommended annually and earlier when needed to restore the body to its own balance and healing ability. Pent-up anger, for example, needs to be cleansed. A daily dose of *bastis*, a medicated oil and herbal preparation, to aid digestion and reduce the accumulation of *ama* from foods, as well as less frequent cleansing of the upper respiratory tract and sinuses, helps to keep the body balanced. Yoga, exercise, lying in the sun, and meditation help manage physically and psychologically troubling symptoms and promote spiritual healing.

Ayurvedic medicine is widely used in India, and to be an Ayurvedia practitioner you now need to be credentialed. However, it is important to note that in the United States there is not yet a standard for licensing Ayurvedic practitioners. Because Ayurvedic medication also uses hundreds of herbs, plants, and minerals in its pharmacopeia, there may be a danger for toxicity and harmful medicinal interactions. Make sure you seek a licensed practitioner. If you are interested in using Ayurvedic medicine, remember these tips from the NCCAM:[38]

> "It is important to make sure that any diagnosis of a disease or condition has been made by a provider who has substantial conventional medical training and experience with managing that disease or condition.

> Proven conventional treatments should not be replaced with an unproven CAM treatment.

> It is better to use Ayurvedic remedies under the supervision of an Ayurvedic medicine practitioner than to try to treat yourself.

> Before using Ayurvedic treatment, ask about the practitioner's training and experience.

> Find out whether any rigorous scientific studies have been done on the therapies in which you are interested."

In conclusion, CAMs and holistic medicine can be a great addition to your health. While Western medicine is undeniably capable of treating most ailments, it is important not to ignore healing approaches from other traditions or schools of thought. Supplementing your diet, freeing your energy, getting a massage, and practicing qigong or yoga are all excellent ways to ensure your continued health or to recover from an illness.

PART III
BODILY HEALTH

CHAPTER 12

Heart Health

with Katherine Guardino and Stefanie Tedesco

Heart health boils down to lifestyle choices. It is becoming aware of our own risk for heart disease and what we can to do to keep the heart muscle strong and pumping and our arteries unclogged. Much of the danger of heart disease lies in the fact that it can go undetected, and there is no period at which prevention is not useful, even after an infarct. Someone may have smoked for 40 years, but it's still very useful to quit. So why do men take their heart for granted until they encounter debilitating chest pain or are told by a physician that they must make major lifestyle changes just to survive? Is it because each of us thinks we are not a "coronary candidate"?

Heart disease doesn't discriminate very much. Other than among some Asian Americans (e.g., Vietnamese, Chinese), it holds the position as the leading cause of death among men in the United States in all racial/ethnic groups (see table).[1] And even recent Asian immigrants (Vietnamese, Indians, Pakistanis) are increasingly at very high risk. For more than three decades, heart disease has been responsible for 25 percent of deaths in men annually. It used to be the cause of death for an even greater proportion of men, before American diets replaced animal fats with vegetable oils in home and restaurant

Heart Health

- Become—and stay—physically active
- Eat well—balance calorie intake with the calories burned
- Choose foods low in saturated and trans fat, sugar, and salt
- Choose more fruits, vegetables, and whole grains
- Control your weight, or lose some if you're overweight
- Don't smoke—or stop if you do
- Manage your blood pressure and cholesterol level

cooking,[2] before the dramatic reduction in men who smoke, and before blood pressure (BP) and cholesterol medications became an option.[3]

These factors—changing cooking oil, the decision not to smoke, and added medications—signal just how much health habits can delay dying from heart disease and improve the quality of men's lives. Whether you fully appreciate it, it is not being selfish to prioritize your (heart) health. Taking 30 minutes a day for getting the heart pumping in physical activity or asking family members to join you in eating a heart-healthy diet isn't selfish; it's smart. So is an annual physical exam that can identify problems earlier and start you on heart medication. Heart health involves becoming aware of what puts each of us at risk and then changing the habits that weren't problems when we were younger. For example, drinking cup after cup of coffee isn't necessarily a challenge to heart health; rather, it is the cream and sugar you add to the coffee.[4] Learn to enjoy the coffee without the sweet, creamy taste. It is never too late to start to amend existing health habits. Adopting a healthier lifestyle quickly lowers the odds of dying from heart disease by 50 percent or more,[5] even for men already age 70–80.[6]

LEADING CAUSES OF DEATH BY RACE/ETHNICITY

Rank	White	Black	American Indian or Alaska Native	Asian or Pacific Islander	Hispanic
1	Heart disease	Heart disease	Heart disease	Heart disease	Heart disease
2	Cancer	Cancer	Cancer	Cancer	Cancer
3	Chronic lower respiratory disease	Stroke	Diabetes	Stroke	Stroke
4	Stroke	Diabetes	Chronic lower respiratory disease	Chronic lower respiratory disease	Diabetes
5	Diabetes	Chronic lower respiratory disease	Stroke	Influenza and pneumonia	Chronic lower respiratory disease

Sources: CDC/NCHS.

Are You at Risk?

Cardiovascular diseases have many causes, not one. Here are a number of factors that accumulate and increase your likelihood of developing some type of heart disease (discussed more thoroughly in the chapter text):

- Being a man age 45 or older
- Living by the manhood code
- Having a blood relative with heart disease
- Getting little or no exercise
- Having an abdominal bulge (or beer gut)
- Being seriously overweight
- Living with a lot of stress
- Eating a fatty diet and/or one high in salt
- Having high cholesterol
- Having high blood pressure
- Having diabetes or high blood glucose
- Being a smoker
- Drinking cup after cup of coffee with cream and sugar; it's not the coffee, but the cream and sugar
- Using medication that elevates blood pressure
- Drinking more than two drinks every day

A man's lifetime risk, *on average*, of developing heart disease will be 50 percent after reaching age 50,[7] and as we age we accumulate more significant challenges to our heart health. Most of the challenges are things we can control. To illustrate, a condition called *metabolic syndrome* refers to a combination of biological risk factors that coexist in men, such as abdominal obesity, poor cholesterol levels, insulin resistance, and hypertension, which, along with the normal decline in testosterone levels, boost the risk for both cardiovascular disease and diabetes. Our lifestyle habits serve as the escalator for each of these clinical problems, raising some men's chance of being affected by heart disease much faster than other men. Research confirms that heart health is seriously challenged by inactive lifestyles, diets that involve foods high in fat and cholesterol, obesity, cigarette smoking, drinking more than moderate amounts of alcohol, and chronic stress. These lifestyle-determined risks work alongside genetics, normal aging, and socioeconomic status to accelerate the deterioration of our cardiovascular system. This chapter calls attention to the nature of the heart, to the heart diseases that men commonly experience, to the gendered character of our experiences, and to living with heart disease.

THE HEART

About the size of a man's clenched fist, the heart is a muscular, four-chambered pump supplying oxygen-rich blood to the rest of the body. It is located under the ribcage in the center of your chest between your right and left lungs (and not under your left breast or pec). The heart is divided by a partition ("septum") into two halves, and each half is divided into two chambers. The upper pair of chambers are the atria, and the lower two are the ventricles. The ventricles pump blood out of the heart, and the atria receive blood returning to the heart. In healthy men, the heart beats (or contracts) in a regular rhythm that makes up the two sounds "lub-dub." It does this somewhere between 60 and 90 times (an average of 72 times) per minute for a 60-year-old.

Visualize the process: the right atrium receives the blood that is returning from the body and is oxygen and nutrient depleted and high in carbon dioxide. A valve (the *tricuspid*) opens, and the blood floods down into the larger right ventricle, which passes the blood through the pulmonary artery to the lungs, where the carbon dioxide is released (and exhaled) and fresh oxygen is added. The oxygen-replenished blood flows back from the lungs into the left atrium, held momentarily until another valve (the *mitral*) opens, and then flows into the larger left ventricle. From there it is pumped through the aorta, the largest artery in the body, into smaller and smaller arteries and then into the capillaries, where the cells of the body are fed.

Those capillaries are tiny—so small that blood cells line up in single file—and they link the arteries (outflow from heart) to the veins (return vessels). While the blood is in the capillaries, the oxygen and nutrients are off-loaded from the blood cell and the carbon dioxide and other waste products are loaded. On their way back to the heart through the veins, 10 percent of the blood travels through the kidneys, where wastes are filtered out; some cells head to the intestines, where good nutrients are loaded from food. It takes about a half

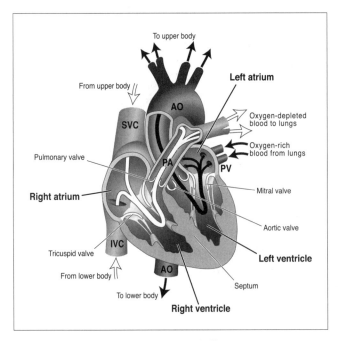

Figure 12.1. Heart. Illustration by Jacqueline Schaffer.

ed full circle,
through the

ract, or beat,
ıg 6 quarts of
l,800 gallons
ɔly a "pump";
ı and volume
d what your
g, your heart
ch it pumps
ɪte" of 15–20

normal for standing in the kitchen and
h is somewhere in the range of 60–80
ɛen exercising or climbing stairs, your
requently per minute) to pump more
uscles and affected cells. The maximum
ɪt 160 beats a minute for a 60-year-old

tbeat with the noticeable "lub-dub," and
hen your hand is over your chest or you
ɪalf is when the heart is contracting (the
ɛartbeat is when the heart is at rest (the
ion. When you take your pulse, you feel

ɛs your heart
ᵀhenever you
mbers repre-
-contraction/
P reading of
ɪastolic pres-
ɪoner reports
ing action (or
of nerve cells
ɪm, called the
sinoatrial node (SA node), and a second bundle
located in the center of the heart, called the
atrioventricular node (AV node). Cardiologists
refer to these bundles of nerve cells as "natural pacemakers," because they
regulate sleeping, standing, and working heart rhythms and the flow/volume of blood the heart pumps.

Blood Pressure: Behind the Numbers

>160/>100:	High blood pressure
140/90:	Borderline high
130/85:	High normal
120/80:	NORMAL
110/75:	Low normal
90/60:	Borderline low

Check Your Pulse

A normal resting pulse rate for a middle-aged or older man is somewhere near 60–80 beats per minute.

50 or less:	Amazing; likely an athlete
55-65:	Good
66-80:	Ordinary
≥80:	Trouble

HEART DISEASE

To this point, *heart disease* has been referred to as if it was a specific disease, but it isn't. Heart disease is synonymous with the medical umbrella *cardiovascular disease* (CVD), which includes all of the problematic conditions associated with the heart (*cardio*) and blood vessels (*vascular*), particularly the arteries that supply oxygen to the organs and tissues throughout our body. Two common forms of CVD are high BP, or hypertension, and problems with heart rhythm, called *arrhythmias*, where the expected "lub-dub" rhythm becomes irregular. Another type of CVD isn't as common but has the terrifying name *chronic heart failure*, and its technical name, *congestive heart failure* (CHF), isn't much friendlier to the ear. The most common CVD is *atherosclerosis*, which results from the progressive buildup of fats on the inner walls of the arteries, chokes blood flow, causes hypertension, and may result in a stroke (cerebral infarction) or heart attack (myocardial infarction [MI]). Atherosclerosis is also referred to as *coronary heart disease* (CHD), *coronary artery disease* (CAD), or its medical term, *ischemic heart disease* (IHD).

Men's CVD Risks

Each of these distinct types of heart disease is reviewed later in the chapter. But first, because particular heart diseases are more common among some men than others, it is useful to begin by identifying who is at greater risk for what heart disease.

Cardiologists, clinical researchers, and the American Heart Association have systematically identified a number of social factors and biological conditions that differentially increase men's chances of CVD.[8] It is ultimately in a man's best interest to know what puts him at risk for heart trouble in later life. This removes many of the uncertainties and gives us greater control to do what we can to live a healthier, longer life.

Periodontal Disease and Cardiovascular Disease

There appears to be a connection between gum disease and people's greater risk of cardiovascular events—heart attacks and strokes. Periodontal (gum) disease also has a hereditary basis. Because signs of periodontal disease may be warning signs of CVD, men should be especially vigilant for red, swollen, tender, or bleeding gums; persistent bad breath; or loose teeth.

Source: Humphrey, L., Fu, R., Buckley, D., et al. (2008). Periodontal disease and coronary heart disease incidence: A systematic review and meta-analysis. *Journal of General Internal Medicine, 23,* 2079–2086.

Family History

Early on when seeing a health care professional, you are going to be asked about the health status of your parents or, if they've died, their cause of death. High BP, high blood cholesterol, and diabetes are common hereditary diseases, and you also may have a genetic predisposition to some types of CVD.[9] If your father, his brothers, or your brother had a heart attack or stroke by age 55, or your mother, her sisters, or your sister had angina (chest pain usually felt under the breastbone) or a heart attack before age 65, you're also vulnerable. Because men develop heart disease about 10 years earlier than women, our attention may be initially drawn to the men in our families, but don't ignore health histories of the (older) women. If any of your immediate family members have had "heart troubles," it's particularly important for you to pay attention to your heart health. You very likely learned many unhealthy habits while growing up, and it is your (family's) lifestyle habits more than genetics that increase CVD risk. For the men predisposed to a CVD, many medications are available to help manage the risks we inherit.

Masculinity and Our Gendered Lifestyle

For reasons not fully understood, men develop CVD about 10–15 years earlier than women. This gender gap in onset cannot be explained by our biological differences (e.g., men's vs. women's hormones). The consensus of expert opinion is that our gendered lifestyles increase or reduce our risk of CVD. Researchers began questioning whether there is a link between being a man and CVD in the 1950s. Their thinking was that the social pressure men faced to be and act "masculine" results in greater CVD risk. Men raised in the 1950s and 1960s were expected to live up to an idealized standard of masculinity that projected an image of strength, bold risk taking, and utter independence. Repeatedly bombarded with messages and images of how "real men" ought to act and think, most men didn't recognize how often these gender messages were counterproductive to healthy living.

One researcher interviewed patients in a coronary care unit shortly after their heart attack to assess their gender characteristics. Men, and even women, who scored high on negative "masculinity" (i.e., describing themselves as dictatorial when necessary, at times as impatient) experienced a more severe heart attack.[10] Other researchers equally made the case that hostility, anger, and irritability increased the risk of CVD in men.[11] This research called attention to the Type A behavior pattern (or Type A personality) and its hostility component that represented the ideal of masculinity in the United States, especially during the 1950s and 1970s.[12]

Recent studies also found that men with lower femininity scores (i.e., reporting that they did not necessarily see themselves as warm, sensitive, or understanding) were at a greater risk of CVD death. The researchers concluded that men who pushed themselves to be the powerful alpha male and turned away from so-called feminine characteristics are at an elevated risk of having an MI and dying of heart disease.[13]

More than how our personalities reflect the gender script, the social pressure to be "masculine" puts us at greater risk of CVD in many under-handed ways. When men are expected to be (naturally) more competitive, intense, and impetuous, experiencing these charged emotions not only ele-vates BP but also results in hurried eating, greater use of alcohol, and other health habits that increase our risk of heart disease. Men who keep up the tough-guy persona are almost 50 percent less likely to use preventive health care services[14] and do not believe they are at risk of a cardiac event. When we are encouraged to "tough it out," we develop a wariness to admit a need for help, even from a physician.[15] We ignore heart disease symptoms by renaming them tiredness, getting older, or heartburn, not because we cannot feel the pain but because we have learned to "read" our bodies as other men do—the masculine way. But there are costs. Complying with the dictates of job- and relationship-related masculinities has knotted men's lives into many stressful lifestyle practices that accelerate our likelihood of experiencing heart disease.[16]

Why should it still be considered "unmasculine" to want to engage in healthy, preventative care; to stop kidding ourselves that a recurring symp-tom like shortness of breath will go away; or to think that our identities as men are at risk if we want to consult a physician? Whoever came up with these ideas? The men of past generations, who routinely died early. As ma-ture men, we've been taught to think for ourselves. Unhealthy "manhood rules" have ruled too long, and it is time to abandon them.

Socioeconomic Status

Socioeconomic status (SES) refers to an individual's social and economic po-sition in society relative to other men. It reflects men's education, occu-pation, and housing status more than our income. For example, a skilled electrician or plumber who chose not to complete high school could earn much more than a high school math teacher. But in American society the teacher's SES would be defined as stable middle class, as opposed to the electrician's undervalued work[17] and working-class status.

SES is another umbrella construct, bringing together a host of distinc-tive CVD risks.[18] Our parents' SES, for example, contributes to our CVD risk through dietary habits as much as a lifetime of stress.[19] The lower a man's SES at birth, the greater his likelihood of also living within (chron-ically) stressful surroundings, and chronic stress is a significant risk factor for CVD. As adults, men with lower SES are more often time bound, find fewer opportunities for engaging in regular exercise, and end up with less exercise capacity; have less access to healthy foods; more often work in a high-demand/low-control job that adds stress and without employment-supported health insurance; and have less access to routine diagnostic and preventive care.[20] As the nation moves toward a national health plan, some of the SES disparities in getting to and receiving medical care will diminish. But this is a "downstream" solution, well after the "upstream" effects of SES intrude on men's heart health and, by creating a vicious spiral, have a pronounced negative effect on men's stress level and overall physical health.[21]

Race

CVD differs markedly by race/ethnicity, and much of the difference is attributed to histories of discrimination and SES. As a group, African American and Native American men have some of the highest premature CVD mortality rates in the United States, whether caused by stroke, high BP, or heart failure, particularly if they live in impoverished communities. Remarkably, when not living in impoverished communities, the race difference in CVD nearly disappears. This strongly suggests that it is being from a poorer SES that escalates the risk of CVD among African American and Native American men.[22] Researchers have recently discovered that some African Americans carry a gene mutation that also puts them at greater risk for having a rare kind of abnormal heart rhythm.[23] Heart disease risk is also higher among Mexican Americans, native Hawaiians, and some Asian Americans. This is principally due to a predisposition to insulin resistance, obesity, and diabetes, which are also related to SES. For example, Native Americans historically had the lowest rates of heart disease, until their segregation and impoverished lifestyles led to high-fat diets.[24]

Older Age

Myocardial aging, or the age-related changes in our cardiovascular functioning, is expected. Aging affects the heart muscle by thickening it—it "beefs up" a bit as it endlessly works—yet this thickening seems determined more by hypertension or other CVD than intrinsic aging. The vessel pathways also normally develop fibrous tissue and fat deposits, which narrow the vessel walls of arteries and make the heart muscle work harder to pump the oxygenated blood into the body. As the arteries and arterioles become less elastic as we age, they cannot relax as quickly during the rhythmic pumping of the heart. As a result, BP increases. Together, these changes cause wear and tear on the heart itself, and one result is a slight increase in the size of the heart.

Men age 50 and over ought to have regular BP and blood cholesterol testing to chart their heart health. Elevated BP and blood cholesterol and arrhythmias can be clinically managed to add many years of healthy living. Similar to some men's genetic predisposition, myocardial aging is something none of us can directly control, but its effects can be managed when we partner with a physician.

Hypertension (High Blood Pressure)

BP is the force of blood against the walls of arteries and veins, and hypertension is high BP in the arteries. It is a type of CVD. An advantageous BP is 120/80, or preferably 110/70. The lower the better, so long as you are not dizzy. When a man's ordinary systolic pressure is greater than 130 and the diastolic is greater than 80, his BP is considered "borderline high" (and prehypertensive). High BP for middle-aged men is defined as a systolic pressure at rest that averages 140 or more, a diastolic pressure at rest that averages 90 or more, or both. Clinicians previously thought that any systolic BP over 140 is abnormal and worrisome, but clinicians now take into account the effects of myocardial aging and define hypertension by your age and CVD history; an 80-year-old man who earlier had a stroke, for example, may have a higher "normal." But you ought to continue to strive for a lower BP when you are 80. Not everyone's arteries stiffen with age, and despite your age, a BP greater than 140/85 is evidence of hypertension. This is because as we age (as mentioned above), our arteries gradually stiffen and small arteries (the arterioles) can become partially blocked, thus increasing resistance to the flow of blood.[25]

More than half of men by age 50 in the United States have high BP (>140/90). Hypertension is much more common among African American men. It is also common among smokers, as well as men who are overweight, have a high salt (or sodium) diet, or are sedentary. You can have your BP checked at no cost in most places of work and even some grocery stores, gyms, and pharmacies. When the systolic BP is greater than 140 and the diastolic is greater than 90, consult a health care provider and find out how you can lower it. Drug therapy is available; lifestyle changes also will be recommended that emphasize eating well, staying active, and stress management.

Blood Cholesterol Levels (Lipids)

Cholesterol is a waxy, fat-like substance (a lipid) in the body's cells and is used to build cells and some hormones. Cholesterol itself is not a disease. It is both produced in the body and consumed through our diet. About 75–85 percent of cholesterol is made by the liver and other cells and transported in the blood by carrier molecules called *lipoproteins*. The other 15–25 percent comes from the animal products we eat, such as meat, poultry, fish, eggs, butter, cheese, and whole milk. Food from plants (e.g., fruit, vegetables, cereals) has no cholesterol.

Cholesterol is only needed in small amounts—the optimal level is less than 200 mg/dL (milligrams per deciliter). Men's cholesterol level is "borderline high" when it ranges between 200 and 239, and a level over 240 is classified as "high" and worrisome. Cholesterol levels move up (or down) as a result of what and how much we eat, whether we stay active, and the age-related accumulative effect of diet and exercise habits.

There are two major types of lipoproteins (or cholesterol molecules). Each cholesterol molecule is wrapped in a protein "jacket," and the more protein a lipoprotein has, the denser it is. High-density lipoproteins (HDLs), dubbed the "good" cholesterol, are the molecules returning from tissues and organs to be treated by the liver, where the cholesterol is recycled and passed from the body. HDL molecules make up about one-fourth to one-third of the total blood cholesterol. Their partners are the low-density lipoproteins (LDLs), or "bad" cholesterol, that supply cholesterol to tissues in the body. When the proportion of LDL molecules is great, cholesterol synthesis in the liver is not well regulated and cholesterol-saturated LDL molecules are not recycled; rather, they return to the blood stream and stick to blood vessel walls, slowly narrowing (or "clogging") the vessels and restricting circulation flow. The HDL/LDL ratio is an indicator of men's risk of atherosclerosis. This cardiac risk is calculated by a simple formula—total cholesterol ÷ HDL—and the optimal number is less than 4.9 (e.g., 220 ÷ 45 = 4.89).

Another blood fat is triglyceride. Calories eaten in a meal and not converted immediately to energy are converted into triglycerides and transported to fat cells to be stored. They are released between "meals" when you need energy. Overeating, however, produces too many triglycerides, and excess triglycerides are linked to heart disease. Whenever you have your lipid profile assessed in a blood draw for the "cholesterol test," the optimal triglyceride level is less than 120. Triglycerides are amazingly sensitive to your intake of sugar, saturated fat, and alcohol.

Beneficial Berries

The antioxidant effects of blueberries, blackberries, raspberries, and strawberries increase HDL cholesterol, lower systolic blood pressure, and reduce the risk of blood clots that may result in a myocardial infarction.

Glucose (Blood Sugar)

Researchers are confident that mild to moderate hyperglycemia ("high blood sugar") is a significant cardiovascular risk,[26] and men who later develop type 2 diabetes are at two to four times greater risk of CVD than people without diabetes.[27] Glucose regulation becomes problematic and is more common among older men due to the age-related metabolic changes that result in insulin secretion and insulin action; however, it is important to understand that hyperglycemia and diabetes are not a necessary part of aging. Recent estimates suggest that more than 20 percent of men age 60 and above have issues with high blood sugar because of their weight gain. If you have been told that your glucose level is high, you also have heard the expectation to change your lifestyle habits well before your health care provider will propose the option of drug therapy to help control your blood sugar.

MINIMIZING RISKS

Most risks, as you already know, are unhealthy habits, which are more easily preventable. Continually putting off getting physically active or changing your diet can become toxic. Most men are aware that when we choose to do nothing to change unhealthy habits, we are choosing to add more risk. There are several decisions that men should make to maintain (or regain) a healthy heart.

Quit Smoking

People who smoke are six times more likely to experience a heart attack and more likely to face the disabling effects of heart disease 10 years earlier than nonsmokers. An exceptional British study investigated the 50-year cumulative risk of illness and death among *physicians* who smoke.[28] About half of the persistent cigarette smokers were killed by their habit, and a quarter were killed in middle age. Those who continued to smoke cigarettes lost, on average, about 10 years of life compared with nonsmokers; stopping at age 60, 50, 40, or 30 gained, respectively, about 3, 6, 9, or 10 years of life expectancy compared with the physicians who continued to smoke. Why? Breathing smoke into the lungs damages the lining of the arteries and contributes to the buildup of plaque. The nicotine in cigarettes is a stimulant, causing the heart muscle to work harder and hastening the thickening of the heart muscle. If you give up smoking this week, you immediately begin to lower the risk of heart disease, and after only a few years your risk returns to the baseline of a nonsmoker.

Maintain Physical Activity

Being physically active burns calories—even standing burns more calories than sitting. Put the printer down the hall, use the door you have to push open instead of the one that opens automatically, and walk the flight of stairs rather than ride the elevator. Being physically active and engaging in exercise are among the best things you can do for your heart. If you exercise for at least 30 minutes of moderate-intensity physical activity on most days, you are increasing "good" cholesterol levels and, in turn, decreasing your risk of CVD. The link between physical activity and CVD is complex; physical activity is what is needed for survival, and it is when we are not active that we increase our risk of being overweight, having high blood sugar and cholesterol, and atherosclerosis, which can cause a stroke or heart attack.

Lose Weight

If you are 15 pounds or more overweight—and more than half of men age 50 and older are overweight and on the edge of being obese—you are playing Russian roulette with developing both diabetes and CVD. Diabetes jacks up the odds of an early stroke or heart attack among men. Overweight men have a 20 percent increased risk of CVD, and abdominal obesity (the pregnant gut look) can make men age 50–64 have a 440 percent greater risk of stroke.[29] Shedding those extra pounds around your abdomen is a way to raise HDL cholesterol and reduce the heart's workload. Review your options with your health care professional, as well as the information on staying physically active and eating well in chapters 2 and 3.

Adjust Your Diet

Trans fats are unhealthy man-made fats that raise bad (LDL) cholesterol and have no nutritional benefit. They are manufactured by adding hydrogen to vegetable oil, which makes the oil less likely to spoil—and utterly unhealthy. Trans fat is found mostly in commercial baked goods, such as crackers, cookies, and cakes, but also in many fried foods, such as french fries and doughnuts. A heart-healthy diet consists of limiting your saturated fat; eating fruits, vegetables, and whole-grain high-fiber foods (aim for five servings of vegetables and two servings of whole fruit daily); eating red meats no more than twice a week; eating fish (especially oily fishes such as salmon) at least twice a week; limiting alcohol intake to no more than two drinks per day; limiting sodium (salt) intake; and avoiding all trans fats that are regularly listed as "hydrogenated oil" in the ingredients section. See chapter 2 for more details.

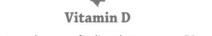

Vitamin D

Researchers are finding that men age 50 and older with low (15–30 ng/mL) or very low (<15 ng/mL) levels of vitamin D are 45 percent more likely to develop coronary artery disease and 75 percent more likely to have a stroke than men with normal levels of vitamin D (>30 ng/mL). Men with low vitamin D levels should talk with their doctors.

Source: Anderson, J. L., May, H. T., et al. (2010). Relation of vitamin D deficiency to cardiovascular risk factors, disease status, and incident events in a general healthcare population. *American Journal of Cardiology, 106,* 963–968.

Eliminate Heavy Drinking

Protect your heart by reducing your amount of alcohol intake to one drink (at most two) per day. Some argue that light drinking, especially red wine, can actually lower the risk of CVD, because it may have a beneficial effect on LDL cholesterol.[30] But the therapeutic/toxic ratio is very narrow. One drink is okay; two drinks—marginal. Drinking more than two often raises the level of the triglyceride fats, results in a greater intake of empty calories that can settle in the gut, and leads to high BP. Be careful.

Manage Stress

Researchers first recognized in the 1950s that stress is a CVD threat and that trying to live in line with masculinity expectations quietly ratchets up stress levels.[31] By the 1980s, chronic stress was distinguished from acute stress and recognized as the insidious, deadly aspect of men's everyday lives, especially among men with lower SES (see chapter 5).[32] Because the experience of stress is a normal part of life, the health objective is to manage stress with exercise and other strategies that can lower emotional distress and cardiac risk.[33]

DIAGNOSIS OF CARDIOVASCULAR DISEASE

There are a variety of ways to assess whether you have heart-related problems, and many of the "tests" are integrated into a routine medical exam. A *blood test* is used to measure the amount of cholesterol in your blood. Determining your BP identifies whether you are hypertensive. Even though having someone in a doctor's office use a BP "cuff" might provoke a little anxiety and increase your BP (known as the "white coat syndrome"), if your BP is high, it is usually rechecked within a few minutes to eliminate the likelihood of a "false positive."

Another common painless, noninvasive test is having an *electrocardiogram* (EKG or ECG) to identify abnormal heart rhythms. Routine EKGs are no longer recommended; they are a waste of money unless there is a clear clinical need. During a standard EKG, electrical leads are placed on your chest, arms, and legs while you are lying down. The leads detect small electrical signals that are charted on graph paper. Sometimes, an *exercise EKG* (a "stress test") is done while you are exercising on a treadmill or bike, and it might uncover problems with either heart rhythm or blood supply to the heart which cannot be found when an EKG is taken at rest. At times, if the standard stress test does not provide sufficient information, a nuclear stress test, where an isotope is injected that shows when blood flow in the heart is limited, can be useful. (Radionuclide imaging is discussed more thoroughly below.) Another variant is wearing a portable EKG (called a *Holter monitor*) for 24 hours to provide your physician a longer record of your heart's functioning.

An *echocardiogram* uses ultrasound waves that come from a small hand device placed on your chest. The sound waves bounce to the heart and back to a detector to produce a picture of the heart beating. A physician can see the structure of your heart and whether it is functioning properly. This method is also noninvasive—nothing other than the sound waves penetrates the skin—and it isn't expected to cause discomfort or pain. Similarly, *magnetic resonance imaging* (MRI) can be used to produce very detailed pictures of your heart.[34] For the MRI scan, you lie inside a "donut- or tunnel-like" scanner that has a magnet around the outside. The scanner uses a magnetic field and radio waves to produce detailed images. Because this procedure is expensive, it is typically used only for men with a CVD history and when prior testing requires better imaging.

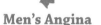

Men's Angina

Angina is a symptom of a problem, not the disease itself. As plaques of cholesterol build up on the walls of the coronary arteries, the arteries narrow, restricting the flow of oxygen-rich blood to the heart. When any area of the heart muscle fails to receive enough oxygen, it can result in intense pain or discomfort in the chest. This is angina.

Angina can be best described as pressure or tightening in the chest area, a feeling that is akin to significant indigestion or heartburn. The pain isn't localized; it's more widespread. When untreated, the pain can spread to the man's neck, arms, and other parts of the body.

During times when the heart has a greater demand for oxygen, there is an increased likelihood of angina to occur. This includes periods of activity involving physical exertion, situations of emotional stress, and whenever there are extremely hot or cold temperatures. While angina is not a heart attack, it strongly reflects the risk of having a heart attack.

The presence of angina is often tolerated (or ignored) by old men, but it is important to investigate any chest pain as a means of preventing further risk to your heart health. Angina cannot be cured once it develops, but it can be treated. The most common drug used for angina is nitroglycerin, which functions to relax both veins and arteries, easing the demand on the heart and increasing its blood supply. Other drugs that lower blood pressure and slow the heart rate, such as beta blockers, are useful in easing the heart's demand for oxygen.

For men with CAD, *angiography* is a study using a cardiac catheterization procedure to view blocked vessels. It is the gold standard for diagnosing CAD. With a local anesthetic, a catheter is inserted into an artery in the groin (upper thigh) or wrist and guided into the heart. A "contrast agent" is injected through the catheter into the coronary arteries, and motion X-rays detail blood flow and the condition of these arteries. A "cath" is a very useful procedure to determine whether your primary arteries are blocked and whether you need either bypass surgery or stents.

Radionuclide imaging uses a "gamma camera" following injection of a small amount of a short-lived radioactive material, usually thallium (^{201}Tl), to create a computerized image of the heart. It is part of the stress test, and it may be the test of choice when a cardiologist is called in for a consult by an ER physician assessing a man arriving with "chest pain."[35] By comparison, it would absolutely not be used to assess the status of a current heart attack. Basically, the test is used to evaluate the severity of CAD. The radioactive material is injected into a vein, circulates with the blood, and ends up in the heart, where the gamma rays can be used to image the heart's structure. Radionuclide imaging exposes patients to very little radiation, yet because the radioactive material is retained in the heart briefly, sophisticated radiation alarms may be triggered for several days following such testing.

CARDIOVASCULAR DISEASE(S)

Without intending to be disparaging, to say that someone has CVD is about as helpful as saying that someone has cancer. All we know is that his heart and circulatory system are no longer entirely healthy, but there are no specifics on the type of heart disease and its severity. CVD is a construct that lumps together a number of different chronic illnesses, and by the time we are in our seventies, many men have more than one type of CVD. Reviewed next are the most common CVDs men experience.

Arteriosclerosis and Atherosclerosis

The thickening and hardening of the arteries is called *arteriosclerosis*, and a specific type of arteriosclerosis called *atherosclerosis* refers to the narrowing (or "clogging") of the arteries. Long-term demand on the arteries to deliver oxygen and nutrients to organs can cause them to become stiffer and thicker, which impedes blood flow. Over time, the normal elasticity of the arteries stiffens (or hardens) a bit, much as the elasticity of a flexible garden hose becomes stiffer after a number of years. It is possible to grow

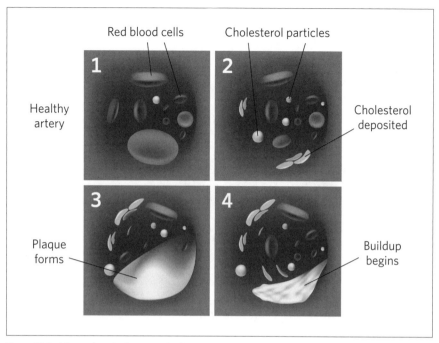

Figure 12.2. Atherosclerosis. Courtesy of Alila Sao Mai / Shutterstock.com.

old without any atherosclerosis, as it is almost exclusively a function of an unhealthy lifestyle.

The progressive buildup of fatty deposits in and on the walls of the arteries, smaller arterioles, and vascular microvessels causes the vessels to "clog." This clogging actually involves plaque formation. As white blood cells try but are unable to digest all the LDL cholesterol, the accumulating mix of protein and calcium becomes plaque on the wall of the blood vessel (see figure 12.2). The smooth vessel surface transforms into microscopic mountain ranges of plaque. Imagine a clean straw pushed into a milk shake, the straw withdrawn and dried, and then reinserted and withdrawn again several times. When you look through the straw, the passageway is no longer clean and smooth, but "blocked" by some of the dried milk shake. When people speak of older men with "clogged" arteries, atherosclerosis is the condition that is being referred to.

This condition increases the risk for angina and MI. If untreated, atherosclerosis can ultimately cut off blood flow to the heart or brain, resulting in a major heart attack or stroke. Routine screening tests for your levels of individual lipids (HDL, LDL, and triglycerides) are a necessary, early step toward managing atherosclerosis. If warranted, various statin drugs are available and quite effective in helping to reduce LDL cholesterol and postpone atherosclerosis.[36] What is most important to know is that atherosclerosis can be prevented and treated, but it is lethal if ignored.

Erectile Dysfunction and CAD

Erectile difficulties affect over 50 percent of men age 50–70, and ED's common cause is vascular disease. ED might be another early warning sign of heart disease, which too often remains "silent."

Source: Jackson, G. (2006). Erectile dysfunction: A marker of silent coronary artery disease. *European Heart Journal, 27,* 2613–2614.

Many more men with ED develop coronary artery disease symptoms within several years than men without ED. ED can predict a cardiac event such as a heart attack or stroke within 3–5 years.

Source: Jackson, G., Boon, N., Eardley, I., et al. (2010). Erectile dysfunction and coronary artery disease prediction: Evidence-based guidance and consensus. *International Journal of Clinical Practice, 64,* 848–857.

This is not a rare disease, and the greatest danger of "athero" is its status as a "silent disease." Atherosclerosis is responsible for 25 percent of all men's deaths in the United States annually. The combination of a silent disease with a "silent" man is even deadlier. Too often his disease goes undetected because he does not have routine (annual) lipid levels assessed and because he is stoic and ignores the early warning signs—angina (chest or arm tightness) during exertion, a weakness on one side of the body that comes and goes, or recurring pain in the calf muscle when walking.

As with many CVD conditions, lifestyle changes are the best bet to the prevention of atherosclerosis. Taking up a healthy diet, instituting regular exercise to maintain a lower resting heartbeat, and stress management training will ultimately decrease the demand on the heart and lessen cardiovascular risk more than medical care alone.[37] Management of LDL cholesterol and hypertension with medications is also almost always recommended.

Coronary Artery Disease (Ischemic Heart Disease)

CAD is atherosclerosis of the coronary arteries—the exact condition just discussed, but the focus shifts to the large branches of the main arteries that encircle the heart and supply it with oxygenated blood. The process in which fatty plaques gradually and irregularly accumulate in and on the wall of the coronary arteries results in ischemia (inability to provide adequate oxygen to the heart muscle), which eventually causes damage to the heart. Complete blockage of an artery leads to a heart attack—in medical terms, a coronary thrombosis or MI. Preventing a heart attack is the goal of all treatment strategies, such as taking low-dose aspirin; aggressively managing BP, cholesterol, and blood sugar levels; and tackling "lifestyle" risk factors (smoking, excess weight, inactivity).

The "silent" character of CAD is best illustrated in the case of a 62-year-old physician who is a regular on a morning British television news program. Dr. Chris Steele decided to undergo a heart scan using a new 3-D scanner just to show viewers how much science and technology could reveal about our bodies. He did not anticipate that the heart scan would reveal that half of his main coronary artery was blocked. He wrote,

> Minutes later when the radiologist . . . told me the result, I went numb. It was such an immense shock that I could hardly take it in. The film crew were completely taken aback and asked if I wanted them to stop recording. I vaguely remember mumbling "no, carry on" while Dr. Jenkins told me: "I'm sorry but it's serious and you need to be seen urgently by a heart specialist." I was reeling. . . .
>
> So as far as I was concerned there was no reason to suspect that anything was wrong. But in fact—possibly in common with millions of other people—I was walking around with a ticking time bomb inside me. That's why I'm sharing my story . . . my condition which is thankfully only a 50% narrowing of one of my coronary arteries can be controlled with medication and regular daily exercise (I now walk for 30 mins everyday nonstop).[38]

Essential Hypertension

Hypertension is a very prevalent CVD, as well as a major risk factor for many other CVDs. Approximately 50 percent of mid- to late-life men are hypertensive, with BP bordering 140/90. Similar to atherosclerosis, hypertension can be a silent killer. It remains hidden because the symptoms of hypertension—increase of warmth in the body, heavy perspiration, nose bleeds, and tiredness—are so ordinary that most of the time they are ignored.

Because it is such a common type of CVD and isn't immediately disabling, you might not realize the silent damage years of high BP does to the circulatory system. It makes us prone to earlier heart attacks, heart failure, and strokes, as well as a progressively poorer quality of life. Early diagnosis depends on having your BP checked regularly, minimally twice a year by age 50. Think of the pressure put on the inside of a garden hose when the water pressure is cranked up but the nozzle isn't spraying full volume; this is similar to the pressure an increased heart rate has on vessel walls. Now add to the image the fact that the hose is old, sun-dried, and hardened, and you can better imagine your aging blood vessels being strained even more and the walls nicked and scratched by the high-pressure blood rapidly passing through. The "erosion" of the vessel walls isn't much different than the way water systematically erodes the walls of a streambed. But rather than widening the vessel, the nicked walls become primed for plaque buildup and tiny blood clots. It is the premature wear and tear on vessel walls that make us more susceptible to atherosclerosis, blood clotting, and consequently early heart attacks and strokes.

Mild hypertension can best be managed without medication and with a heart-healthy lifestyle that involves reduced salt intake, weight loss, exercise, and stress management. When your health care professional advises you that you're prehypertensive, consider that your wake-up call. Think of a heart-healthy lifestyle as food/exercise *therapy* (see chapters 2 and 3). Second, as discussed more thoroughly in chapter 5, stress cranks up the heart rate, taxing not just the heart muscle but the vessel walls.

When your hypertension becomes severe, there are many different medicines/drugs that are used to treat high BP, including alpha blockers, angiotensin-converting enzyme (ACE) inhibitors, angiotensin II receptor blockers (ARBs), beta blockers, calcium channel blockers, diuretics, and vasodilators. The first drug health care professionals prefer to try is usually a thiazide diuretic (such as Diuril, Esidrix, or Zaroxolyn), or "water pill," which causes for a short time more frequent urinating. This reduces the volume of fluid in the body and helps void unneeded sodium. With less fluid and salt, BP is lowered and there is less work for the heart. Diuretics are powerful drugs, and you are advised to only use them after a health care professional's recommendation. Don't self-diagnose and seek your own medication from a pharmacy. At times, though rarely, a diuretic can bring about an arrhythmia (discussed below). Much more often this family of drugs reduces potassium and magnesium levels in the blood and increases the odds of muscle cramps and weakness, headaches, and symptoms of dehydration. The American Heart Association recommends that men taking diuretics monitor themselves for dehydration (signaled by greater thirst, dizziness, and decreased urine output).[39]

If diuretics alone aren't enough to lower your BP, your health care professional may also recommend adding a medication such as calcium channel or beta blockers or ACE inhibitors. These classes of medications/drugs are prescribed to block different metabolic functions that affect BP. For example, ACE inhibitors block some of the production of a hormonal compound in the blood (angiotensin II) which causes a narrowing of blood vessels. ACE inhibitors allow blood vessels to widen, which lowers BP and improves heart output. But this class of drugs can cause a persistent, dry hacking cough and, less often, light-headedness, dizziness with standing, rash, and muscle pain. A very similar group of inhibitors are the ARBs;

they too widen blood vessels to lower BP, and they rarely cause the hacking cough, yet some people experience dizziness, tiredness, and abdominal pain.

Calcium channel blockers are a class of medications designed to reduce the amount of calcium available to the muscle cells in vessel walls and the heart. Because calcium is necessary for muscle cells to contract, blocking (or inhibiting) the flow of calcium within the blood relaxes the muscle cells, so that the vessels can dilate. Once dilated, both BP is lowered and the spasms of the coronary arteries (which cause the angina pain) are diminished. Side effects such as dizziness, constipation, and headaches vary considerably by the medication used; most are quite benign and well tolerated.

Beta blockers are a family of drugs that effectively block adrenaline and some functions within the sympathetic nervous system which naturally increase heart rate and BP when we experience stress and/or engage in moderate or intense physical activity. But since hypertension already involves an increased BP equivalent to "working out," the beta blockers "trick" the electrical system to lower BP by decreasing the rate and force at which the heart pumps blood. Beta blockers have a relaxing effect on muscle function; they slow heart rate. They also decrease the minor tremor that everyone has, which can improve target shooting and is why they are banned in the Olympics.

Alpha blockers are an even earlier class of medications that relax the vascular muscle in the walls of blood vessels. They are now hardly ever used except in cases of severe hypertension. Because these drugs seem to increase the risk of developing heart failure, they are no longer regularly prescribed. Vasodilators are another family of medications that used to be used to manage severe hypertension. They relax the smooth muscle of the blood vessel wall, dilate the vessel, and increase blood flow. When blood vessels dilate, their capacity to hold blood is increased, allowing less blood to return to the heart. As a result, BP decreases, and angina patients are often benefitted.

Experience has taught cardiologists that a combination of various hypertensive drugs is usually more effective than a single medication. As men get older, using low-dose combinations seems to better counteract (and chemically manage) the different causes of hypertension. In addition, there are now many different drugs within the same families of medication, and if you are being treated for hypertension you might find that a particular drug within a family of drugs has a better result—that is, fewer side effects—for you. Never hesitate to discuss the side effects of your meds with your health care provider, and if you are having troubles, do ask if alternative meds can replace yours. There are also many less expensive "generic" substitutes that are chemically nearly exact copies.

Arrhythmias

Arrhythmias involve irregular electrical activity in the heart and lead to a peculiar heartbeat, whether the heart rhythm is too fast (*tachycardia*), too slow (*bradycardia*), or simply irregular. For an arrhythmia to exist there is a hitch somewhere within the heart's natural pacemaker—the nerve bundle regulating the atrioventricular (AV) node or the sinoartial (SA) node. Some arrhythmias are evidence of heart disease and can be life threatening. Yet two of the more common arrhythmias are not due to heart disease and are harmless. The first, an extra heartbeat arrhythmia, can originate in either the atrial (upper) or ventricular (lower) pumping chambers and will cause a "premature" (or extra) contraction. Occasional premature contractions are a normal variation and not reason for concern. The second, a sinus arrhythmia, is a transient slowing of the heart rate when breathing in; since our heart and lungs are close together, if you take a deep breath while taking your pulse, you might find that your heart rate slows for a moment. This is a normal phenomenon, more common in young people and in athletes and others in good physical condition. It is generally a sign of health.

An EKG is used to diagnose the worrisome arrhythmias. Rather than finding a steady, coordinated heart contraction and muscle relaxation of 60–80 beats per minute (BPM), a bradycardia-type arrhythmia involves fewer than 60 BPM. As a caveat, men in excellent athletic condition often have BPMs below 60, but for the average man over age 50, a low BPM more often reflects a problem with the SA node or an interruption in the electrical pathways, and it causes a gap in the timing between the systolic "lub" (heart contraction) and the diastolic "dub" (relaxation). If the rhythm is quite irregular, fainting can occur because the heart does not pump the normal supply of oxygen to the brain. More common as we get older are the bradyarrhythmia symptoms, which include fatigue, dizziness, and light-headedness. Although this condition can contribute to high BP, angina, and/or heart failure, the first line of management is watchful waiting. A set of EKGs is needed for your physician to determine if the same arrhythmia regularly shows up. The set of EKGs can also provide evidence of a challenged heart muscle that would benefit from surgically implanting a pacemaker to manage the bradycardia.

By comparison, a tachycardia-type arrhythmia involves a resting heart rate of 100 or more BPM. It typically indicates a problem that starts within the atria (upper chambers) or AV node, where aberrant electric signals originating in the atria override the natural pacemaker. These abnormal electrical signals spread throughout the atria in a fast, sometimes disorganized manner, causing the heart to contract rapidly. It can be experienced as a racing, uncomfortable heartbeat. Other symptoms include palpitations,

Keeping the Pace

The bundle of nerves in the upper aorta that make up the heart's "natural pacemaker" can be supplemented with an artificial pacemaker. It is a small device surgically implanted in the chest or abdomen to help control abnormal heart rhythms.

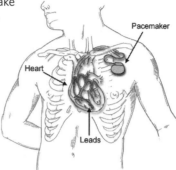

The procedure takes at least an hour, and it will be a few days before you can go back to your normal activities. You have to visit your physician several times the first year to check the pacemaker's signals.

The battery lasts 5–10 years, and when its life is near ending, a new pacemaker has to be implanted. The battery is encased in the device and cannot be changed.

Pacemaker. © Boston Scientific Corporation or its affiliates. All rights reserved. Used with permission of Boston Scientific Corporation.

sweating, chest pain, dizziness, and fatigue during light exercise. Treatment ranges from a large family of medications that slow the heart rate to electrical cardioversion, which shocks the heart back into normal rhythm.

The most common tachycardia is called an *atrial fibrillation* (AF), and men who have AF have a "fluttering" type of rapid heartbeat. There is no organized atrial activity, which means that the heartbeat does not consistently allow time for the atria to fill and fully empty before the chamber contracts again, depriving blood flow into the ventricular chambers and to the rest of the body. By not emptying, blood "pools" in the atria and clots can form, ultimately causing dangerous embolism. Clotting does not occur in many other atrial tachycardias. There is a large family of medications to prevent blood clotting, and surgically implanting a pacemaker and/or surgically altering the electrical pathways that cause AF are common treatments.

Tachycardia also can originate with a problem in the lower heart chambers, which is called *ventricular tachycardia*. These arrhythmias can be very dangerous and need immediate medical attention. They usually follow other heart problems—CVD, a prior heart attack, or a weakened heart muscle. The problem is that errant electrical signals within a lower chamber override the natural pacemaker, causing the ventricular chambers to pump at a rapid rate for a few seconds or longer and to not fully empty. Arrhythmia episodes lasting for more than a few seconds are threatening, often becoming ventricular fibrillation (or V-fib). When the heart rate goes into V-fib, it is always a medical emergency. In V-fib, the heartbeat is so fast that blood pumping basically ceases, and without blood flow to the brain the person goes unconscious within seconds and into cardiac arrest. Untreated, death occurs within several minutes. Dramatic television programming involving surgery or ER situations often depicts a V-fib scenario, where "paddles" are used to shock the heart out of V-fib and back into a more stable rhythm. Cardiologists believe that most of the sudden cardiac deaths in the United States result from V-fib. Outside the hospital, immediate treatment begins by calling 911 and starting and continuing cardiopulmonary resuscitation (CPR) until medical help arrives.

Heart Attack (Myocardial Infarction)

Heart attacks, the leading cause of death in most countries, usually occur after age 60 but can happen much earlier. Even when we maintain a healthy diet and regularly exercise, in the presence of risk factors, lipid-laden cells accumulate in the vessel walls, contributing to CAD. A heart attack occurs when the blood vessels leading to the heart are first "narrowed" and then become obstructed, starving the heart of needed oxygen-rich blood and killing part of the heart muscle. Sometimes, a heart attack follows a plaque deposit cracking away from a vessel wall, and then as a healing mechanism blood platelets attack the plaque deposit to produce a clot. When one of these clots (a thrombus) blocks the passage of blood in a coronary artery, it deprives the heart of oxygen and nutrients and part of the heart muscle dies. Very rarely, except when there is already underlying disease, severe stress can push your heart rate so high that it deprives the heart of enough oxygenated blood to cause a heart attack. The medical community calls all of these *acute myocardial infarction*, because they involve the death of an area of the heart muscle.

Middle-aged men frequently abstain from an annual doctor's visit when they are not feeling specific pains or symptoms. But to be blunt, this decision to forgo annual preventive checkups after age 50 often proves fatal. Men need to renounce the downstream "fix it when broken" mind-set and, instead, preserve their options for survival with upstream prevention. We need to focus our attention on preventing heart attacks before they happen—not adapting to a less functional lifestyle after the fact. Though the survival rate for men hospitalized with MI is approximately 90–95 percent, nearly a third of men experiencing an MI never make it to the hospital. It is important to understand that older men sometimes experience very little or no chest pain or other heart attack symptoms. As we get older, we have "silent" heart attacks. To prevent a heart attack from sneaking up, men need to have routine heart screenings in which BP, blood chemistry, and heart rhythm are charted and discussed.

Heart Attack Symptoms

- *Palpitations.* Actually feeling your heart beating fast, and it is, probably more than 120–150 beats per minute.

- *Angina.* Intense pain that feels like a tight band squeezing around your chest, or a pressure and heaviness in the chest. But do not count on pain to warn you. Some heart attacks are painless.

- *Upper torso discomfort.* A low-grade discomfort radiating from your breastbone to your back, jaw, and/or arm.

- *Sweating, shortness of breath, feeling very weak.* Your heart is working "overtime" and starving for oxygen-rich blood, so you feel as if you just ran a 5K and you actually might have been sitting. You have shortness of breath not relieved by rest.

- *Lightheadedness or dizziness.* Similar to the feeling we sometimes get right after rapidly standing up; your brain is not getting enough oxygen-rich blood.

Few men experience all of the symptoms. Should you experience any, don't wait to seek help—better safe than sorry.

It is vital that healthy men know the symptoms of a heart attack. Men's average age of the first heart attack is 66, and our risk of a heart attack starts to climb after age 45. Getting medical help right away increases the chance of survival.[40] A man's delay in recognizing the meaning of symptoms or asking for medical attention prompts complications and a greater risk of death. Aspirin can have a protective and therapeutic effect but carries a risk of intestinal bleeding. In consultation with your physician, if you have a history of angina, taking low-dose (81-mg or "baby") aspirin daily is probably smart.[41] And if you even *think* you are experiencing a heart attack, immediately chewing (not just swallowing) an adult aspirin (325 mg) as emergency therapy is not just smart but lifesaving.[42] But call 911 first.

Treatment for an MI begins with the immediate administration of aspirin, whether by you, an EMT, or the ER physician. The goal of all MI treatment is to restore normal blood flow and thus salvage the maximum amount of heart muscle. While being transported by EMTs and on arrival at the hospital, oxygen is administered to flood the lungs and assure what blood flow is occurring is enriched. Nitroglycerin is also immediately administered, usually through an IV. The added nitrates relax vascular smooth muscle and dilate vessels, thus increasing blood flow. Next is pain medication (usually morphine), since an MI causes intense pain, and most often beta blocker therapy is initiated to manage the body's natural response to stress.

Once stable, attention immediately shifts to identifying the obstruction that caused the MI and then restoring coronary blood flow. During the past decade, heart attack survival has improved greatly as a result of clot-busting medication (thrombolytics such as tissue plasminogen activator [tPA] and streptokinase). This typically involves cardiac catheterization, when available. A skilled catheterization team inserts the long, thin, flexible catheter into a blood vessel in your arm, groin (upper thigh), or neck and threads the tube to the blockage. Through the catheter, the team does a diagnostic angiography (live X-ray images, called *fluoroscopy*, taken from inside the blood vessel) and then angioplasty (inserting a guide wire with an attached, collapsed balloon to the obstruction, inflating the balloon with water to crush much of the obstruction and widen the vessel) and stenting, which leaves a wire mesh tube, known as a stent, in place after the balloon is deflated to keep the artery open (see figure 12.3). Other than catheterization, some men's blockage is severe enough to require a thoracic surgeon to perform coronary artery bypass grafting (CABG) to restore blood flow. CABG involves traditional chest surgery; if it is a vein graft, the surgeon takes a healthy vein from the body (usually your leg) and then splices (grafts) one end to the aorta and the other end to the coronary artery bypassing the blockage. If the left mammary artery is used as a bypass, which is exceedingly common, the beginning of the artery is left as it is and as it travels down the chest wall it is disconnected and used to bypass the blockage in the coronary artery.

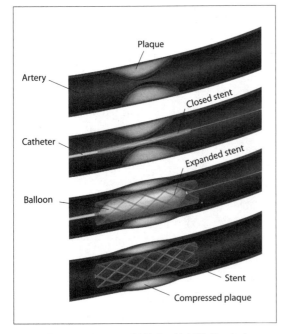

Figure 12.3. Stent. Courtesy of Alila Sao Mai / Shutterstock.com.

Finally, treatment turns to getting the man on a long-term post-MI treatment plan that includes different medications and lifestyle changes such as dietary modification, smoking cessation, stress management, and regular exercise. After hospitalization, some men worry about overexerting themselves and triggering another MI; they avoid physically stressing activity and become "cardiac invalids."[43] Or, a man's wife worries, tries to do everything for him, and prevents him from "straining" his heart.[44] Fifty years ago, medical advice urged men to take it easy following their heart attack. Now, however, health care professionals involved in cardiac rehabilitation recognize that exercise is heart building.

Sex after a Heart Attack

A noted cardiologist argues that sex is just another form of exercise as far as the heart is concerned. He writes, "As you become aroused, your heart rate begins to increase and you breathe a little faster; as excitement increases, both the heart rate and blood pressure increase, reaching their peak at orgasm. . . . The average duration of sex is 15 minutes and the heart is really only stressed for three minutes" (p. 212). He continues, "You can die at any time, and this includes during sex! The risk during sex is very low indeed" (p. 213).

If you experience angina during other types of exercise, you might also experience angina during sex.

Casual sex with a new partner can be more stressful to your heart, and problems may occur because of the newness of the encounter. Sex within a long-standing relationship is less stressful, because people are comfortable with one another.

Source: Jackson, G. (2000). *Heart health.* London: Class.

Experiencing uncertainty about the future is quite ordinary. You might be encouraged, for example, to take a post-MI "stress-EKG" to decide how much exercise is safe for you and for planning a rehab program. Cardiac rehab emphasizes exercise, (re)education, and nutritional and emotional counseling. Following the advice you've been given is essential to preventing recurrence. Men are urged to adopt a healthy lifestyle and to try to "lead a normal life," including returning to work. But what was "normal" is what got most of the men into trouble in the first place. After the heart attack, you are also urged to "put the MI behind you" but pay attention to your heart health. This "go-ahead-but-be-careful" message can be confusing. Don't be afraid to ask a health care professional for further explaination.

Stroke (Cerebral Infarction)

Stroke is the leading cause of disability and the third leading cause of death in the United States, and it is more common among African American and Hispanic men.[45] As with several other CVDs, the modifiable risks are high BP, too high blood cholesterol, physical inactivity, abdominal size, and smoking; strokes are also associated with AF and diabetes.[46]

A stroke occurs when a blood vessel in the brain either bursts or is blocked by a clot. A hemorrhagic stroke is the type where the blood vessel carrying oxygen and nutrients bursts and spills blood into the brain, causing that portion of the brain to be deprived of oxygen and die. This type of stroke usually is the result of chronic hypertension, and the first symptoms are a sudden vicious headache; sudden numbness or weakness of the face, arm, and/or leg on one side of the body; and, less often, loss of consciousness. When there is an "intracerebral hemorrhage," it is more often disabling, if not fatal.

Ischemic strokes are much more common. They occur when a blood vessel becomes blocked, impeding blood flow to that portion of the brain. One type of ischemic stroke is less worrisome because the blood clot breaks up on its own within an hour and the stroke effects disappear shortly afterward. When this happens, it is called a *transient ischemic stroke* (or *ministroke*). However, most ischemic strokes involve a clot that lodges in a cerebral artery or a branch of one of the carotid arteries supplying the brain. The blockage chokes off the blood and oxygen supply, resulting in the death of an area of brain tissue. Much like an MI, a cerebral infarction begins suddenly, and moments afterward we experience the blinding, disorienting symptoms—dizziness and vertigo, difficulty speaking, feelings of weakness, perhaps loss of vision in one eye, confusion, and sometimes unconsciousness.

Symptoms get worse a few minutes after they start, because this type of stroke can continue to cause the death of brain tissue over a few hours. After this, most ischemic strokes cause little or no further damage; when the stroke remains unchanged for several days, it is clinically referred to as "completed." There are, however, "evolving" ischemic strokes that do not fully stabilize right away and affect an increasingly larger area of brain tissue. They result from clots in a narrowed artery (*arterial thrombosis*) and progressively starve brain cells. For instance, a piece of a blood clot formed when blood "pools" in the fibrillating atria can break off from the left atrium and travel directly toward the brain, causing a stroke. This is why blood-thinning medication (e.g., Heparin, Warfarin) is regularly prescribed for men who have a history of AF or abnormal blood clotting.

Knowing the symptoms for ischemic strokes is essential to getting treatment fast and lessening subsequent disability. The FAST acronym in the boxed insert summarizes key symptoms. Identical to the advice following a heart attack, getting to medical care as rapidly as possible is critically important. Physicians identify which artery in the brain is blocked based on the side of the face and the arm most affected. Immediate (ER) treatment stabilizes the man's heart rate and breathing, and if the stroke is very severe, the man will be treated with drugs to reduce further swelling and pressure in the brain. Other treatment involves powerful medications to dissolve clots and reopen the artery (thrombolytic agents such as tPA) and to prevent the formation of further blood clots (antiplatelet agents such as aspirin and clopidogrel).

Once the ischemic stroke is completed, imaging tests are commonly used to determine if the internal carotid arteries and other accessible arteries are blocked or narrowed. Imaging can involve the noninvasive Doppler ultrasonography, magnetic resonance (MR) angiography, and CT angiography, or the slightly more invasive cerebral angiography. Sometimes surgery is needed to remove the clot or fatty deposits ("atheroma") that continue to block an artery, and when needed a carotid endarterectomy is performed. Usually a vascular surgeon, sometimes a neurosurgeon, opens a very small space in the side of the neck and then the artery to remove the blockage while you are awake with a local anesthetic. There is no more discomfort than visiting a dental hygienist for a cleaning. Different types of post-stroke rehabilitation are frequently needed, ranging from retraining the brain to move muscles needed to walk to learning new ways of performing tasks to circumvent or compensate for any residual disabilities. About two-thirds of men with an ischemic stroke survive and will need some type of rehabilitative therapy. The National Institute of Neurologic Disorders and Stroke identified five types of disabilities: movement problems or paralysis, problems speaking or understanding written and spoken language, cognitive problems involving thinking and memory, loss of ability to feel touch or pain, and emotional disturbances following the trauma of the stroke and resulting physical and mental losses.

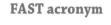

FAST acronym

F = *Face:* Is one side of the face drooping?

A = *Arm:* Can the person raise both arms, or is one arm weak?

S = *Speech:* Is speech slurred or confusing?

T = *Time:* Time is critical. Call 911 immediately.

Aneurysm

An aneurysm is an abnormal balloon-like bulge in an artery due to a weakness in the vessel wall (see figure 12.4). Between 2 and 8 percent of men age 65 and older have an aneurysm, and, not surprisingly, the likelihood of having an aneurysm increases with age because of the diminished elasticity of vessels.[47] High BP, atherosclerosis, and smoking are key risks,[48] yet clinical researchers are not certain exactly what causes an aneurysm. They suspect that the weakness in a vessel wall could be present at birth, a genetic predisposition, or the result of inflammation or a traumatic head injury.[49] Aneurysms can occur within any part of the body and rarely cause symptoms; however, a large cerebral aneurysm can press on nerves to cause vision problems and/or numbness in the face. By far the most common aneurysms occur in the aorta, the main artery carrying blood from the heart, and can be abdominal (near where the aorta divides to the legs) or thoracic (up higher). But aneurysms occur in smaller arteries, including arteries in the brain. Similar to aortic aneurysms, most cerebral (brain) aneurysms develop at the forks or branches in arteries because the walls in these sections are weaker.

If the aneurysm is identified before it ruptures, it often can be successfully treated with surgery or drug therapy. Typically, various drugs may be administered to lower the risk of rupture by lowering BP and relaxing blood vessels. Surgery is the gold standard. Depending on the size of the aortic aneurysm, vascular surgeons may propose traditional surgery where your belly is opened and a graft replaces the damaged portion of the aorta; the alternative is called *endovascular repair*, which involves inserting a stent graft through the artery to where it is above and below the aneurysm.

Should an aortic aneurysm rupture, life-threatening bleeding begins inside the body and the situation is most often fatal. The person typically loses consciousness immediately, since blood flow to the brain has been markedly interrupted. The rupture of an existing cerebral aneurysm causes a hemorrhagic stroke.

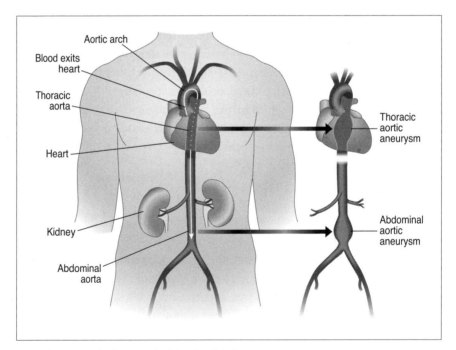

Figure 12.4. Aneurysm. Illustration by Jacqueline Schaffer.

Heart Valve Diseases

Under normal conditions, the heart valves let blood flow in one direction through the four chambers. The four heart valves open and close in sequences that keep blood circulating, much as the intake and exhaust valves in a car engine open and close in sequence. The narrowing (stenosis) of an aortic valve is mostly due to years of wear and tear and is more common among older men with another CAD. Aortic stenosis restricts blood flow, causes the heart to work harder to pump blood across the valve, and results in chest pain, shortness of breath, and fainting—symptoms similar to a heart attack. If untreated, the risk of death is significant—30–50 percent within a year. Left-sided narrowing is the more prevalent problem and reflects a gradually developing structural defect, usually caused by scarring and plaque buildup that keeps the valve from closing or opening as expected.

Narrowing of the mitral valve is most frequently related to prior rheumatic fever or an infection in the heart and is much less common than it used to be. When the mitral valve does not close properly (called *mitral valve prolapse*), blood flows backward through the mitral valve when the heart contracts. This reduces the amount of blood that is pumped out to the body and is harmless for most men; in a small number of cases, however, the problem can progress to serious mitral regurgitation (also known as mitral insufficiency), and surgery is necessary to restore valve function.

Valve "repair" is a surgical procedure that involves replacement of the damaged valve with a "tissue" valve from a pig heart or a mechanical prosthesis. The mortality rate associated with this surgical procedure has decreased significantly since the 1990s—less than 5 percent for men under age 75 and about 10 percent for men over 80.[50] While the odds of survival with surgical intervention do not seem so rosy themselves, they are *much* better than doing nothing. The quality-of-life outlook is very good after a successful valve replacement, even for 80-year-olds.[51]

(Congestive) Heart Failure

Heart failure is often the final consequence of injury to the heart muscle or long-standing hypertension. This is when the heart can't pump enough blood to meet the body's needs. Heart failure is a progressive disorder involving a weakening of the entire cardiovascular system. It results from the sum of different causes. Aging wears on the heart, causing it to stiffen. Then add the cumulative effects of unhealthy dietary habits[52] and other lifestyle habits that prematurely damage the heart's function. A history of untreated hypertension or AF will contribute to heart failure. A prior heart attack that damaged heart muscle also contributes to the heart's diminished pumping ability.

Whenever the heart is unable to pump the necessary amount of blood to the rest of the body's organs, CHF develops. Because many medical advancements and life-prolonging therapies are successful and enable men to survive minor heart attacks and other health assaults (e.g., diabetes, hypertension), heart failure is predicted to become more prevalent as men continue to live longer.

The prognosis associated with heart failure is fairly poor. The process of heart failure impairs the kidneys' function to extract sodium (salt) and water, and this increases the likelihood of leg swelling, fatigue (tiredness), and shortness of breath. Heart failure therapies aim to enhance quality of life while maintaining independence and reducing hospitalization for as long as possible. Multiple drug treatments are available, including the use of beta blockers and loop or potassium-sparing diuretics to alleviate symptoms (discussed above as hypertension treatments). Innovative exercise training and relaxation therapy in older men with heart failure, which work to lower anxiety levels, also add to quality of life.

HEART HEALTH REVISITED

Stopping heart disease before it debilitates is a reasonable goal. To this end, beyond the useful publications that the American Heart Association has available about heart-healthy living and beyond the "diets" that are as tasty as beneficial, it is vital for *men* to step back and assess how much trying to be "the big wheel" comes at the expense of time for yourself, for physical activity, and for enjoying family and friends. Rarely discussed in news reports about heart health is how debilitating the social pressure to be "masculine" is to *our* heart health. Be a rebel: eat better, get active, lose the gut and get to a healthy weight, control cholesterol, reduce blood sugars, manage BP, and by all means stop smoking.

CHAPTER 13

Cognitive Health

MEMORY AND MEMORY LOSS

with Elizabeth Conner and Alexandra Leichthammer

We have all bumped up against the experience of momentarily not remembering an acquaintance's name or simply "brain freezing"—when you know what you were about to say (or write down), but because of a momentary lapse in brain function you do not recall what it was, and you stand there in the fogginess of no thought. Maddening, sometimes embarrassing, but in fact no big deal. Did you know that forgetting some information is as indispensable as remembering? Otherwise, our short-term and recent memory would be overwhelmed. Memory lapses are more likely to occur when you are tired, distracted, under stress, and have to draw on long-term memory.

Think of your brain as a filing cabinet, where images, smells, conversations, and other information and memories are stored. We cannot possibly file everything; the brain is a finite storage system, so things have to "go" as one ages. Researchers have found that healthy middle-aged and older men experience predictable changes in brain health[1]—we improve our ability to reason things out better than when we were young (complex reasoning), and we have a better understanding of what others are going through (empathy). Both changes are signs of becoming wiser. Because there is less available "free" space in our brain, we do one thing at a time better and lose our edge at multitasking.[2] A hallmark of normal cognitive aging is that it takes more time (measured in nanoseconds) to recollect something stored and more time to encode new information, which neuroscientists attribute to changes in brain chemicals (or neurotransmitters).[3]

Despite occasional memory glitches, our ability to continue to develop memories based on new experiences and information, to consolidate new information into long-term memory, and to recall these and even older memories at a future time is not sacrificed as our brain ages. Our wisdom, our complex reasoning ability to think through alternatives, and our performance of habitual actions are all unaffected by normal brain aging. All in all, our short-term (or recent) memory and ability to recall detailed events from our past hold up well as we age. Our memory for factual and conceptual information remains intact. Moreover, if there is no health challenge (such as diabetes or cardiovascular disease) nibbling away at brain function, the skills we learned earlier in life and practiced over the years—acquired chess and poker strategies, or understanding the mechanics of throwing a curve ball—may remain flawless.

Healthy men do experience a slight decline with age in some areas of cognitive function. These changes can occur in visual and verbal memory, immediate memory, or the ability to name objects. Beginning in middle age, it takes longer to think of a word, recall a name, or retrieve a date from our memory (discussed later), and the clumsy moments where we do not recall something can be expected to occur a bit more at age 65 than at 50. When these moments occur, they may be alarming because they *suggest* a loss of personal control and may be socially awkward.

Without enough knowledge about brain aging and brain health, too many men accept myths about aging as truth and view memory lapses as a sign of old age, even senility. When several memory lapses occur in close proximity, you might quietly wonder, "Am I losing my marbles?" "Do I have Alzheimer's disease?" Your diagnosis, however, is very doubtful—forgetfulness is a common experience at all ages, as well as part of normal aging. But we understandably question whether our memory lapses represent symptoms of Alzheimer's disease (AD), much as we question whether sudden chest pain is predicting a myocardial infarction. For healthy men, the fear of becoming cognitively inept is rooted in the extensive and pejorative media coverage of AD[4] as much as the expectation for us to always be self-sufficient.[5]

Other than being bothersome, instances of forgetfulness and absent-mindedness should not evoke apprehension. They are characteristic of the normal forgetfulness that increases in later life and is clinically known as *benign* senescent forgetfulness. Men who worry whether their forgetfulness is dementia are unlikely to actually suffer from a serious memory disorder; instead, it is more common for people with memory impairment to be unaware of their lapses. To cease feeling uneasy, it is useful to recognize that the memory changes of normal aging differ markedly from memory disorders. There are three types of memory loss that are associated with illness, not normal aging:

1. A number of illnesses (and their medications) are linked to mental loss, such as the mental confusion caused by the posttraumatic distress of a heart attack or stroke or any underlying vascular disorder. Vascular disorders can starve the brain of needed oxygenated blood and particularly affect memory, as opposed to general cognitive functioning.[6]

2. Problems with memory may arise as a result of what is called *mild cognitive impairment* (MCI). MCI is a condition characterized by mild to moderate memory problems, and sometimes by some loss in a man's thinking (or cognitive) abilities; it is often described as a stage midway on a continuum between normal forgetfulness due to aging and dementia. People with MCI are aware of their forgetfulness, and most only have minor problems with thinking; thus, they experience little interference with going about most everyday activities. Even the majority of people with MCI do not develop dementia. If you are forgetful, this adage should reassure you: you need not worry if you momentarily forget your ATM pin number; you only need to worry if you forget what the ATM is used for.

3. Late-life dementia is a progressive decline of memory and other cognitive function, such as thinking, learning, remembering, organizational skills, and complex visual processing. It is a disease, not a normal part of aging. *Dementia* refers to a group of diseases of the brain that are irreversible and progressive, eventually thwarting a person from distinguishing a nickel from a dime or engaging in conversation.

BRAIN HEALTH

Neuropsychologists contend that brain health is analogous to body health. Similar to muscular strength, our ability to remember and analyze improves when we keep the brain active and look after it with a good diet and other healthy habits.[7] We have the ability to maintain brain health; we can increase our brain's functioning, whether at age 80 or 50. Taking on intellectually challenging or just new activities builds new connections in the brain. Have you recently cited the alphabet backward, eaten a bowl of soup with the spoon in the "other" hand, or challenged your brain to decipher what's on television without your glasses on? The brain has the ability to produce new cells and store new information at any age. Just as we can modify our behavior to improve our heart health, we can also make changes in our environment and lifestyle to significantly slow if not prevent cognitive decline and to improve cognitive ability.[8]

Good for the Brain

Physical exercise, which we know is good for the body, also turns out to be good for your brain.[9] Though any exercise can help, daily aerobic exercise is best, and research shows that regular aerobic exercise improves memory.[10] Regular exercise increases oxygen flow to the brain and reduces risk of diseases that contribute to cognitive decline such as diabetes and cardiovascular disease. Engaging in physical activity has several other beneficial effects: it reduces stress, positively affects mood, and increases the production of "feel good" brain chemicals, which protect brain structures and result in better memory. Most (but not all) longitudinal studies also find a decreased risk of dementia in individuals who exercise regularly.[11]

Cognitive exercise such as working on a jigsaw puzzle and reading (not skimming) the newspaper are "thinking" challenges, and whenever the brain is challenged, it bolsters memory functioning and builds reserve.[12] There also is some reliable research that suggests that frequent participation in cognitively stimulating activities may reduce the risk of AD.[13] Take up anything that challenges your mind— from mulling over the best aperture setting on a camera to capture the light coloring a leaf, to volunteering to work with children who are poor readers, to learning a new game of strategy such as Mahjong Titans or cribbage. Take a hands-on course in a field you don't know much about, such as furniture refinishing or Oriental brush painting, or cook some recipes in an unfamiliar cuisine. These are effective ways to keep your brain dynamic.

> I think that the main thing is staying active. To me, exercise the brain whenever you get the opportunity because I think that the brain goes idle real quick if you don't use it.[14]

Healthy eating, particularly food with antioxidants (berries of any type, cherries, raisins, oranges, red grapes, spinach) and fishes with omega-3 fatty acids (salmon, tuna), reduces your risk of cognitive decline and may also lower your risk of AD. Omega-3 fatty acids are also good for the heart. Most research

Common Causes of Memory Change

Health Related

- High blood pressure
- Prescription drugs
- Bad nutrition
- Low blood sugar
- Depression and/or anxiety
- Taking several prescriptions

Lifestyle Related

- Lack of sleep
- Too much sleep
- Lack of activity
- Stress

What You Can Control

- Anxiety
- Tiredness
- Diet
- Cholesterol
- Stress/depression
- Inactivity of mind/body
- Overuse of alcohol/drugs
- Smoking
- Stress

showing a possible benefit for cognitive health uses fish consumption as a yardstick for the amount of omega-3 fatty acids eaten. Studies suggest that a so-called Mediterranean diet, representing the usual dietary habits of the populations bordering the Mediterranean Sea, with lots of fruits, vegetables, fish, whole grain bread, and olive oil, can improve brain health.[15] If you want good brain food, blueberries—one of the richest sources of healthful antioxidants—protect memory,[16] and eating fish improves cognitive abilities.

Sleep is necessary for memory consolidation, being attentive, and efficiently thinking through problems.[17] Make sure you're getting a good night's sleep to ensure brain health. Sleep-related problems such as insomnia and sleep apnea leave you tired and unable to concentrate. Sleep loss also impairs memory consolidation; one theory is that while we sleep, we are processing experiences while dreaming, and memories are being consolidated.

Bad for the Brain

Heavy drinking. Having a drink a day isn't a problem for either the heart or the brain, but heavy drinking, which is typically defined as consuming an average of more than two drinks per day, has a significant negative effect on the brain's ability to make, retain, and recall memories. Put simply, drinking results in many types of memory problems. Well-known lapses are the "brownouts" where people do not remember the details of experiences such as who won the game they were watching on television.

Overeating. New research suggests that consuming between 2,100 and 6,000 calories per day may double the risk of memory loss. In their study of people between the ages of 70 and 89 and free of dementia, researchers found that high-calorie eaters experienced MCI twice as frequently as people with low-calorie diets.[18] Perhaps, given the diets of men, this partly explains why memory loss may be more common in men than women.[19]

Smoking. Research shows that smoking causes white blood cells to attack and kill off healthy brain cells, increasing the risk for dementia.[20] In addition, nicotine causes deterioration of the brain which affects sexual arousal, emotional control, and sleep.

Stress. The chronic stress of juggling work demands or even ongoing low-level noise from neighborhoods creates an overproduction of the "stress hormones" cortisol and glucocorticoids (see chapter 5). Too much stress is like constantly driving a car with the pedal to the metal, flooding the body and brain with stress hormones and somehow increasing the permeability of the blood-brain barrier (BBB), which is a network of literally hundreds of miles of blood vessels and capillaries within the brain.

Elevated levels of cortisol are thought to damage brain cells in the memory encoding center (the hippocampus), as well as damage the shield of the BBB to allow toxins in the blood to cross into the brain, causing you headaches or worse.[21] Harnessing chronic stress, even by prescription medication to stop the brain from speeding, is protective. Managing stress without chemicals is preferable. Hence, start saying "yes" to pleasurable opportunities in your life, like stepping away from work and its stresses by going to lunch with friends or holing up somewhere to read a chapter of a mystery novel as a work break. Building into your day both 30 minutes of exercise and quiet "breaks" that provide some form of relaxation will increase your productivity and protect your brain's health.

Ignoring your health. If a health condition is undermining your learning ability, you won't have much luck with memory improvement unless you take care of the problem. Medical problems that become increasingly common as we age can interfere with cognitive functioning and cause memory loss. For example, the surges in blood sugar associated with type 2 diabetes reduce blood supply to the brain; medication and exercise improve blood sugar levels and, thus, memory and thinking. Memory lapses and confusion also result from reduced flow of oxygenated blood to the brain, which is characteristic of men with untreated high blood pressure and high LDL cholesterol; again, diet, exercise, and medication improve blood flow and HDL cholesterol levels.

BRAIN MYTHS AND MEMORY MISCONCEPTIONS

Not long ago we were told that we inevitably lose "gray matter" as we age, and that once brain cells are lost, they are not replaced. That information is not even half correct. There is no massive die-off of brain cells with age. Brain researchers have learned that if we do not have a disease that causes brain cells (neurons) to die, then nearly all of the neurons remain healthy until death.[22] There also is the misconception that *some* brain cells are lost as we age, just as we lose skin cells. But in reality, few neurons die over our lifetime. We start with more than 100 billion neurons, and if there is any "loss," it isn't the same as thinning hair. The remaining nerve cells compensate for lost neighbors, similar to the neighboring trees in a forest sprouting new branches to restore the canopy.[23] You should also know that several areas in the brain—including the hippocampus, where new memories are stored—regularly generate new brain cells.

What does happen with brain aging is that the neurons (brain cells) shrink in size. Typically, information moves as an electrical signal from one nerve cell to another. The gap between the sender neuron and its neighboring neuron is the synaptic connection (or synapse) and is only thousandths of a millimeter wide. When neurons shrink as the brain ages, this causes the gap to increase in size. With neurons no longer almost "touching" and the synapses wider, the chemical messengers (neurotransmitters) transporting information and memories across neurons are not able to retrieve information or deposit new memories as fast. In addition, starting in middle age, the brain produces smaller quantities of the neurotransmitters that relay information between nerve cells. Altogether, these bring about changes in processing speed, similar to having slower Internet service or the minor dimming of an incandescent lightbulb in a flashlight with aging batteries. This may be annoying at times, but our brains continue to function and function well. Age-related brain changes should not affect our ability to think, analyze, or recall odd words while playing Scrabble.

When elders say, "My memory just isn't what it used to be," typical brain aging is *not* likely the cause. In the absence of disease, researchers advise that any noticeable reduction in memory most probably results from boredom and inactivity. It is likely that our eyesight and hearing also reduce the efficiency of memory. When the brain isn't regularly challenged, brain aging is accelerated. The cliché "use it or lose it" is operative. The more you work out your brain, the better you'll be able to process and remember information.

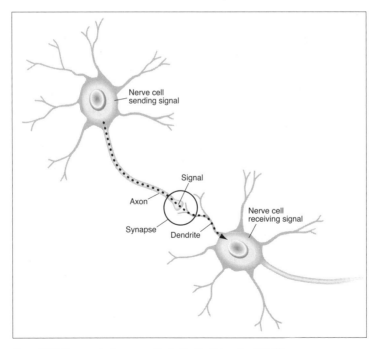

Figure 13.1. Neurons and synapse. Illustration by Jacqueline Schaffer.

The brain is full of chemicals, and memory studies make it clear that age-related changes in memory are the result of different chemical reactions in the brain that occur over time, not brain cell loss. Too little biochemical activity significantly affects the regions of the brain related to memory; by contrast, eating well and physical activity affect brain chemistry and lessen the odds of sensing that our memory is "not what it used to be." Among the brain chemicals are endorphins and dopamine, which are the "feel good" chemicals associated with happiness and pleasure. An extended reduction in using your brain (or becoming physically inactive) reduces levels of endorphins and dopamine. New studies tell us that the pace of brain aging is slowed when endorphins and dopamine are enhanced by a healthy diet, engaging in both physical and mental exercise, and lessening stress. The message is clear: although the brain volume becomes less, brain function in healthy men does not change much and normal memory loss doesn't get much worse over time.

THE MEMORY SYSTEM

Our brain collects and stores memories in different parts of the brain. Memory is grouped into three categories: working, recent/short-term, and long-term. The area of the brain involved in *working memory*[24] has a very limited capacity and can only hold a handful of information (about five to nine thoughts) at the forefront of the mind. Working memory allows for the manipulation of information for comprehension, learning, and reasoning. We can only "recall" information in our working memory for a few seconds, up to a minute, unless we are exposed to the information again. If you are consciously aware of a noise, for instance, then that noise is in working memory and the information is processed to conclude a "noise." Have you ever forgotten someone's name almost immediately after they introduced themselves; made a mental list of five to six things to do before leaving the house and, once you got to the car, had to go back to retrieve something forgotten; or forgot part of a phone number you just looked at? If so, you have your working memory to blame. When a new thought, noise, or observation enters working memory, another must be released—either transferred to another part of the brain or forgotten.

When information is transferred from one part of the brain to another along pathways involving billions of neuron-and-synapse connections, it is stored either in recent or in long-term memory. Keep in mind that the neuron-and-synapse connections are not linked in simple lengthy chains, like cars on the highway during rush hour. Each neuron has a web of synapse connections, similar to the roots and branches of a tree. When information is stored in either recent or long-term memory, a message from one nerve cell may diverge to multiple neighboring cells and cascade into a forest of thousands of other neurons.

Recent (or *short-term*) memory stores things such as your schedule for the week, what you ate for dinner last night, and about half of what your wife or partner was talking about at dinner. In contrast, *long-term memory* can hold much more information and for a longer amount of time (potentially forever). It seems to be less affected by aging. Frequent exposure to a certain stimulus (e.g., the voice of someone) or repeating a particular action (e.g., the keypad of a calculator)—that is, learning something and encoding it in the brain—greatly increases the chance that the information will be stored in long-term memory.

MEMORY CHANGES THAT ACCOMPANY AGING: BENIGN SENESCENCE

Benign senescent memory lapses occur as the result of age-related changes in different parts of the brain. In recent decades, the medical community has changed its point of view about these memory changes. Viewed in the past as inevitable, they were referred to in the popular press as "senior moments" or "middle-age pauses." Researchers have accumulated enough information about brain functioning among middle-aged and older men to recognize that brain aging does not result in much progressive memory loss. From about age 50, normal brain aging begins to show more evidence of twisted fibers inside nerve cells (called *neurofibrillary tangles*) and neuritic plaques (also called *amyloid plaques*), which consist of deteriorating neuronal material surrounding deposits of a sticky protein called *beta-amyloid*. The neurofibrillary tangles populate the medial temporal lobe regions associated with memory function and seem to be present among all men, including those without cognitive deficits.[25]

These findings strongly suggest that neurofibrillary tangles may contribute to memory lapses in normal aging as much as MCI and AD; their presence is part of brain aging. They are also associated in greater number with some dementias. It is the large number of neurofibrillary tangles and neuritic (amyloid) plaques and the location within the brain that distinguish late-life dementia.[26] This new way of thinking about the memory changes that accompany brain aging is similar to the way we now know that atherosclerosis is evidence of both normal aging and cardiovascular disease. It also seems that older men use different brain regions for working memory than used by younger men when performing the same tasks,[27]

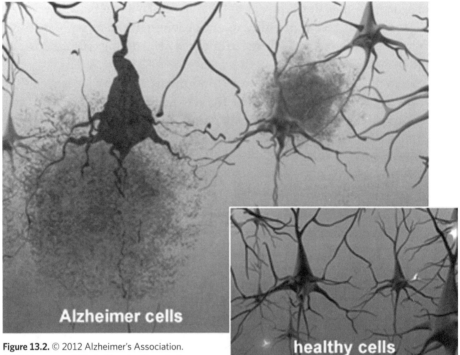

Alzheimer cells

healthy cells

Figure 13.2. © 2012 Alzheimer's Association.
All rights reserved. Illustrations by Stacy Janis.

and when the medical community used to compare younger and older men on only one brain region, the false assumption was that "senior moments" and cognitive decline were normal.

While the inability to recall the six to eight items on a grocery list is a familiar experience for almost everyone, if memory lapses occur more often, they should not be written off as "normal" aging. Rather, they are "suspect" of a problem such as chronic stress and persistently high levels of the "stress hormone" cortisol, or a medication side effect, or an underlying cardiovascular disease that affects the brain, or a neurological disorder that leads to memory loss such as Parkinson's disease (PD).

Even "ordinary" memory loss does not occur in the same way for all men. The hippocampus, which is the part of the brain largely responsible for forming new memories and moving short-term information into long-term memory, is susceptible to age-related wear and tear. This is more severe among men who smoke or drink more than moderate amounts of alcohol, who work(ed) in noxious environments exposing them to unhealthy chemicals, who have cardiovascular problems related to high cholesterol, who are on medications that affect cognitive functioning, and who live with high levels of stress.

Even though age-related neurological changes should be no more worrisome than the minor weakening of bones and lessening of muscle mass that accompany the aging process, brain aging may cause worries when we compare ourselves to our past. Forgetting a phone number that you have dialed many times before, getting too little accomplished when multitasking, and not being able to remember just *why* you walked into the living room are examples of a typical 40-year-old man's forgetfulness as much as signs of brain aging among healthy middle-aged and older men. Men need to stop feeling uneasy about absentmindedness. Just in case the takeaway message didn't get stored in long-term memory, "senior moments" are the result of a *slowing* of the memory process described above, not memory *loss*; if there is memory loss, there is some underlying medical pathology affecting brain function.

Managing Memory Changes

When memory lapses (or loss) disrupt our everyday life, we notice and others may too. Men coping with memory loss confront fears of dependence and lack of control. Although there is no "one size fits all" technique, there are strategies that can be employed to make living with memory lapses easier to manage and less fearsome. These slight changes are simple modifications and can be extremely effective in reducing the distress.[28] Keeping one's day organized is strategic:

> Minimize potential problems/obstacles by putting things such as your keys and other important items in central locations so you don't have to search for them every time you need them.

> Be sure that memory problems don't interfere with taking medicines as prescribed. If you take some medication several times a day, setting reminder alarms can be helpful.

> Memory aids—a personal digital assistant, wall calendars, and posted reminders—will help ensure that you remember appointments and important dates (especially your wedding anniversary).

> Because procedural memory involves visualizing, make some important reminders unconventional, such as putting a shoe on the kitchen table, to increase recall that you need to make an important call.

Normal Memory Loss

Forgetting the following is part of normal aging (if occurring on an *occasional basis*):

- Where you placed something
- Names of acquaintances
- An appointment
- Something you had just read
- Why you walked into a room
- Details of conversations
- Information that seems to be "on the tip of your tongue"

> ❭ Develop a habit of carrying a memo book and writing things down—including a "to do list." Start the day reviewing what's on the agenda to help retain personal control and to avoid the frustration of forgetting.

> > I suddenly realize that she asked me to do something, and I haven't remembered to do either of the two things. That frustrates her a bit, of course.[29]

> ❭ Forgetting the location of one's car in a parking lot is inconvenient and potentially dangerous if you wander the parking lot in a rainstorm or late at night. Write down the row, or park your car near a landmark (light pole, tree), even if it is farther away.

> ❭ Simplify your physical environment. Remove some of the "noise." Getting rid of some of the distractions encourages a greater focus on tasks at hand. Our multitasking skills just aren't as awesome as they used to be, so why swim upstream?

MEMORY LOSS: ILLNESS AND MEDICATION

Sleep disorders, chronic stress, vitamin B12 deficiency, physical illnesses (e.g., cardiovascular disease), psychiatric disorders (e.g., depression), and the medications prescribed to treat various conditions inhibit memory function and can cause memory loss by disrupting brain chemicals. With care these memory problems are reversible.

Medications

Many medications to treat one condition, or the interaction between various medications, can result in memory loss. Certain medications can impair memory directly; however, memory loss and cognitive functioning also may develop as a side effect of specific medications. Zolpidem (Ambien), for example, is a commonly prescribed sleep medication for short-term insomnia. Though uncommon, amnesia and short-term memory loss are side effects associated with the sedative.

More common is "polypharmacy," where a few prescription medications individually are not a problem but together result in additive or interactive adverse side effects that cause mental confusion, mental sluggishness, and memory loss. Be cautious when taking four or more prescription drugs and over-the-counter medications at the same time (this is the common threshold after which increased adverse drug reactions and drug-drug

Looking Out for a Friend

One unusual case of someone with cognitive troubles involved a 69-year-old man who began to have a difficult time remembering things, forgot to eat regularly or enough, and soon lost interest in seeing his retired buddies at their breakfast café. Knowing that the man was a widower, one of his breakfast buddies called the man's brother, and together they took him to his physician. The man was having an adverse reaction to one of his newer heart medications. After discontinuing the high-dose statin drug (which had been prescribed to reduce his elevated cholesterol), his neuropsychiatric reaction slowly but surely ended. He agreed to try a different statin drug, and as nearly all other men using statin drugs, he fares well.

Not all cases of neurological changes are as quickly noted or easily re-solved. The same man's cognitive problems and social withdrawal could have been caused by the onset of later-life depression and its biochemical effects. In addition, men who are feeling sad, lonely, worried, or bored will too often "self-medicate" with alcohol, causing even more serious cognitive problems.

interactions can be expected). For example, using prednisone (to manage either symptoms of cancer or allergic reactions) in combination with aspirin or some blood thinners can significantly increase the risk of mental confusion, delirium, and dizziness. If the medication has a long half-life, it may take weeks of near disability before the drug is fully out of your system. If you have started a new medication and find yourself more forgetful and mentally sluggish, consult your physician or pharmacist. The

Memory Loss and Medication

Many over-the-counter and prescription medications can greatly impair memory and cognitive functioning. Most high blood pressure medications (e.g., Aldomet and Aldoril—methyldopa; Inderal—propranolol), antidepressants (e.g., Elavil—amitriptyline; Prozac—fluoxetine), pain medications (e.g., Motrin—ibuprofen; Duract—bromfenac), diabetes medications (e.g., Dymelor—acetohexamide), and antibiotics (e.g., Chibroxin—norfloxacin) warn that the side effects may include impaired cognitive function.

Even the over-the-counter sleep and allergy medications and cold remedies such as Tylenol PM, Advil PM, and Benadryl have a sedating side effect that impairs memory. It is vital that you closely examine your prescription and non-prescription medications and ask the pharmacist if their additive and interactive effects can contribute such unwanted experiences as slower thinking, memory loss, and confusion.

effect of certain prescription drugs also can join the effects of common over-the-counter pain medication (e.g., Advil) to exacerbate your mental sluggishness.

Many prescription and over-the-counter anticholinergic drugs (including medical marijuana) interfere with or block the production of the neurotransmitter acetylcholine (a chemical in the brain), and without sufficient acetylcholine your attention and memory are impaired. As you get older, you are more likely to experience anticholinergic effects because your body produces less acetylcholine.

Alcohol

The current accepted standard is that one drink or glass of wine a day has a protective benefit, slowing the progression to dementia among men who already have MCI.[30] However, if you drink more, recognize that alcohol adversely affects the brain. Even a single drink can produce higher blood alcohol levels in older men than middle-aged men, as a result of the increase in body fat relative to muscle as we get older. The percent of total body weight consisting of fat generally doubles from age 25 to age 60. Because alcohol does not dissolve in fat, the same alcohol dose results in a higher blood alcohol level in the older man with more fatty tissue.[31] In addition, the brain becomes more sensitive to the effects of alcohol as we get older. Older men cannot drink the same amount as they did when younger without noticeable effects.

One common effect is memory loss—the "buzz" in fact dulls the brain's ability to process the stimuli seen and heard. For some men the issue isn't foggy memory, but rather the tremors and poor coordination that emerge as alcohol damages the cerebellum. The fact is that chronic alcohol abuse can lead to reductions in brain volume (mostly in the white matter). Researchers have observed serious alcohol-related deficits in cognitive functions among heavy drinkers. The most extreme are cases of alcohol-related dementia. A drink a day remains unproblematic; however, the "green light" to have a nightly drink becomes a "red light" if *you* recognize that you are among the class of men whose mental functioning is dulled with even one drink, or if you are depressed. Being depressed and drinking double the adverse effect on memory.

MILD COGNITIVE IMPAIRMENT

If cognitive decline were charted on a continuum, MCI would be an intermediate step between the expected memory loss of normal aging and the striking decline of cognitive function in dementia, particularly AD. People with MCI have more memory problems than normal for people their age, yet their symptoms are not grave and they are able to carry out their normal daily activities.

Because MCI isn't typically assessed in routine patient care, it may go undiagnosed. There are several subtypes of MCI. The most common is amnestic mild cognitive impairment (aMCI). It presents as memory

SYMPTOMS OF NORMAL FORGETFULNESS VERSUS COGNITIVE DISORDERS

Normal age-related forgetfulness	Mild cognitive impairment	AD
Sometimes misplaces keys, eyeglasses, or other items	Frequently misplaces items	Forgets what an item is used for or puts it in an inappropriate place
Momentarily forgets an acquaintance's name	Frequently forgets people's names and is slow to recall them	May not remember knowing a person
Occasionally has to "search" for a word	Has more difficulty using the right words	Begins to lose language skills; may withdraw from social interaction
Occasionally forgets to run an errand	Begins to forget important events and appointments	Loses sense of time; doesn't know what day it is
May forget an event from the distant past	May forget more recent events or newly learned information	Has serious impairment of short-term memory; has difficulty learning and remembering new information
When driving, may momentarily forget where to turn; quickly orients self	May temporarily become lost more often; may have trouble understanding and following a map	Becomes easily disoriented or lost in familiar places, sometimes for hours
Jokes about memory loss	Worries about memory loss; family and friends notice the lapses	May have little or no awareness of cognitive problems

Source: Editors of Johns Hopkins Health Alerts (2009). *Guide to understanding dementia.* New York: MediZine.

impairment more than cognitive problems with language, thinking, and judgment, and it can progress to AD.[32] A recent study suggests that approximately 19 percent of men age 70–89 who were free of dementia were affected by MCI. The prevalence of MCI increases with age and is higher in men than in women across all age ranges.[33]

Men diagnosed as having aMCI know they are having cognitive problems. They've experienced critical incidents and sense that something is no longer right. It could be getting confused or having memory lapses. As one man reported,

> Well, I've been playing [cards] with a foursome for a number of years. . . . So one day when I was playing a hand, all of a sudden I said to them, "I don't remember what trump is" and that's when I started thinking, "I wonder why would I forget that, that's basic?" So that's what happened . . . I became aware of it.[34]

Other than some confusion and memory lapses, men with aMCI essentially have normal cognitive function and are able to successfully complete activities of daily living.

Though aMCI increases the risk of later developing a dementia, a good proportion of men with aMCI never get worse. Symptoms include recognizing that you are forgetting things more often, including important events such as appointments, returning phone calls, and meeting up with friends. Men with aMCI also lose their train of thought and sometimes become confused with the plot in a book or movie. If the memory loss is somewhat more severe, a man may become exasperated by having to plan and make decisions—his working memory gets overwhelmed while trying to manipulate the different bits of information.

The exact causes of aMCI are still unknown. Because it is an accelerated pace of brain aging, the evidence shows that there are more neurofibrillary tangles and amyloid plaques and some shrinkage of the hippocampus, a brain region important for memory. Factors that seem to contribute to the etiology of MCI include too little participation in mentally and physically stimulating activity and the "silent" cardiovascular diseases of high cholesterol, hypertension, and coronary artery disease. At present, there is no approved treatment for MCI.

LATE-LIFE DEMENTIA

Dementia, in particular AD, is among the most common, debilitating, and feared age-related conditions, making it the subject of intense public

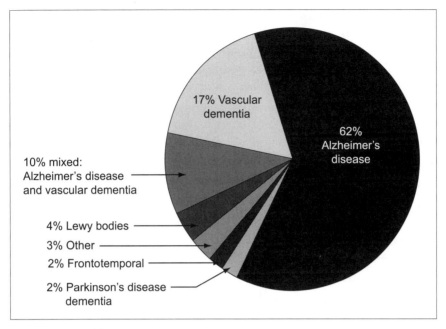

Figure 13.3. Types of dementia

interest. Dementia involves a group of brain disorders and is found in only 1 percent of men age 60–64. The risk of eventually living with dementia noticeably increases every 5 years, to yield up to nearly 40 percent of men who are older than 85. This truly is a late-life disease that was rarely found in the U.S. population when men's average life span ended before age 70. Aside from a few treatable causes (e.g., chronic drug use, brain tumors, subdural hematoma, metabolic disorders involving B12 deficiency), nearly all dementing disorders are progressive, degenerative diseases and may become particularly devastating. There are several types. There is the familiar AD, which accounts for close to two-thirds of dementia diagnoses. Vascular dementia is considered to be the second most common cause of dementia in both Europe and the United States. Rarer is dementia with Lewy body, Parkinson's disease dementia (PDD), and frontal lobe (frontotemporal) dementia; these three account for less than 10 percent of all dementias.[35]

Memory loss is the key sign of most types of dementia; also involved are deficits in reasoning and judgment, personality changes, and an inability to remain socially engaged. Dementia is distinguished by cognitive decline in multiple domains—memory and intellectual ability (thinking, planning, analyzing, and judgment). If it progresses far enough, it might cause an inability for men to involve themselves in the simplest everyday activities. It is not uncommon for people with dementia to have little or no awareness of some or all of their cognitive problems. Neuropsychiatric symptoms such as apathy, agitation, and depression are common. With increasing loss of function, a person with dementia may slowly (or suddenly, depending on the rate of progression) be robbed of his independence, and placement in a nursing home could eventually become necessary. Men with dementia usually survive 7–10 years after the onset of symptoms, yet some live as long as 20 years.

Vascular Dementia

High blood pressure (hypertension), coronary artery disease, high cholesterol, diabetes, smoking, and alcoholism increase a person's chances of having a serious vascular disease, especially a stroke or heart attack. As that risk increases, so too does the risk of vascular dementia, in which many small cerebral infarcts (strokes) and the subsequent alteration of the brain's blood supply destroy some brain tissue by depriving the area of oxygenated blood and nutrients. Most strokes involve a blood clot (thrombus) that lodges in a cerebral artery or a branch of one of the carotid arteries supplying the brain (see chapter 12). Symptoms of vascular dementia can vary, but they usually begin much more rapidly than AD. Depending on where in the brain the strokes occurred and how severe they were, the accumulated damage can seriously affect the person's memory and language skills (speech and ability to understand speech), judgment, vision and visual field (ability to see to the side), and coordination or motor function on one side of their body. Because some areas of the brain produce emotions, just as other parts produce movement or allow us to see, hear, or smell, vascular dementia commonly involves mood and personality changes. Men with vascular dementia may cry easily and have sudden mood changes (called *emotional lability*).

Unlike AD, vascular dementia is largely preventable, if the person engages in a heart-healthy lifestyle to prevent heart disease and strokes. In addition, the same heart-healthy lifestyle lowers the risk of type 2 diabetes, which is a known risk for cerebral infarcts. For no clear explanation other than the effect of diabetes, African Americans are more likely to develop vascular dementia.

There is no "life preserver" that can be thrown to remedy the ill effects of a high-risk lifestyle that involves smoking, overeating, and carrying too much weight. However, men with vascular dementia can take steps to prevent further strokes, such as controlling high blood pressure, getting treatment for high blood cholesterol and diabetes, not smoking, becoming more physically active, and regularly visiting a health care provider to monitor blood pressure.

Alzheimer's Disease

Unlike with MCI and vascular dementia, men are less often diagnosed with AD than women, yet men's risk of developing AD isn't much different than women's. Because the majority (95%) of AD cases are late-onset, men's relatively shorter life span explains why fewer men than women develop AD early enough to be diagnosed. Early-onset AD, striking people younger than age 60 and even as young as 30, often runs in families. However, it is rare, accounting for fewer than 5 percent of AD cases.

AD involves microscopic changes in the structure of the brain and abnormalities in brain chemistry that resemble but are qualitatively and quantitatively different from normal aging. Chemically, AD seems to reduce the presence of acetylcholine, which is the primary neurotransmitter enabling neurons to electrically communicate with one another. Structurally, the disease also involves a rapid, progressive reduction in healthy nerve cells. Evidence at autopsy can reveal the presence of many dying neurons and at their core the amyloid deposits (discussed earlier); there is also much greater evidence of neurofibrillary tangles within neurons. MRI scans can detect shrinkage in specific regions of the midbrain attacked by AD, yet postmortem studies suggest that there also is a lot of AD that goes undiagnosed.[36]

Rapid cell death occurs most in the hippocampus (the structure within the brain most closely associated with memory). After 7–10 or more years of the progressive destruction of nerve cells, the actual structure of the brain is noticeably different. Magnetic resonance imaging (MRI) brain scans, which either compare a healthy man to a man with AD or compare one man's images across time, dramatically depict the way this disease literally erodes brain matter. The degeneration of neurons results in spaces (or vacuoles) that become filled with fluid and metabolic waste. Researchers think that what distinguishes AD is the rapid rate of atrophy in healthy brain cells.

The left panel of figure 13.4 shows a normal brain, revealing no atrophy. Notice the structural changes and reduction in

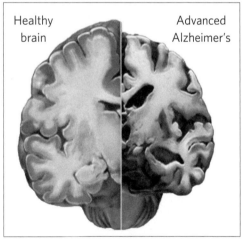

Figure 13.4. Alzheimer's brain. In the Alzheimer's brain, the cortex shrivels up, damaging areas involved in thinking, planning, and remembering. Shrinkage is especially severe in the hippocampus, an area of the cortex that plays a key role in formation of new memories. Ventricles (fluid-filled spaces within the brain) grow larger. © 2012 Alzheimer's Association. All rights reserved. Illustrations by Stacy Janis.

mass in the image on the right. The image shows severe atrophy in the hippocampus and entorhinal cortex, indicative of AD. As the disease progresses, the person's functioning typically deteriorates.

It remains impossible to predict the timing and exact sequence of cognitive decline and overall loss of functioning. Some men plateau and remain level for years, whereas other men may push right through the earlier levels and then remain for a long time in a moderately severe level of impairment.

For everyone involved—the man with the disease, his family, his health care providers—AD is a stressful, personally challenging experience. For a man with AD, the decline in cognitive functioning progresses from the problems with memory that characterize MCI toward more severe problems in judgment, thinking, and use of language. The AD pattern of decline starts with lost complex functioning (although we only see the confusion and memory troubles) and moves toward loss of simple functioning, such as losing the ability to appropriately name objects or distinguish monetary denominations.

In the early phases of the disease, the symptoms of confusion and memory loss emerge, partly because declarative memory is initially affected. For example, the secretary of the board of directors of a nonprofit organization may be unable to take detailed notes of a meeting, and later when preparing the minutes of the meeting, misinterpretations are made. Slowly, as the disease worsens, the same man misses deadlines and meetings, and even though he was once outgoing, he is now more withdrawn. Later in his illness trajectory, as brain integrity and cognitive function continue to deteriorate, there is evidence of his disorientation in time and space, declines in personal hygiene, and inappropriate social behavior. Eventually behaviors dependent on procedural memory become problematic, including how to use a fork and knife or what to do with a toothbrush. The pace of deterioration and specific functioning lost are determined by the sites of the brain most affected.

Typically, symptoms are worst in the late afternoon or evening; this is referred to as *sundowning* and is symptomatic of AD. A man with mild to moderate AD may become unusually demanding, abusive, or suspicious; exhibit mood swings; and perhaps see or hear things that are not there as the day wears on. Still others will remain quite passive and gentle throughout much of their decline. In general, because men have gendered histories of being more demanding and "negative" than women, some men's sundowning may be mistaken as personality rather than evidence of disease. Similarly, their histories of being quietly independent may mask their early wandering, another symptom of AD; he and others might perceive his agitation as boredom and/or his wandering as a purposeful decision to take up a frivolous walk about the neighborhood. People with AD increasingly communicate through behavior instead of speech.

Currently, the diagnosis of AD is more likely to follow an earlier diagnosis of MCI than it was just a few years ago. While some men with aMCI

Global Deterioration

Level 1: No cognitive decline

- No complaints of memory loss and no problems in daily living

Level 2: Very mild cognitive decline
"Forgetful"

- Some complaints of short-term memory loss; forgets names and location of things

Level 3: Mild cognitive decline
"Early confusion"

- Has difficulty managing money or traveling to new locations; makes mistakes driving (including minor fender benders); feels frustrated and may become depressed; rambling and repetitive in conversations

Level 4: Moderate cognitive decline
"Late confusion"

- Decreased sense of time; has difficulty with complex tasks (finances, adjusting thermostat); increased irritability; disoriented at home and becomes emotionally unstable; loss of sense of humor

Level 5: Moderately severe cognitive decline
"Early dementia phase"

- Needs help grooming and when to bathe; occasionally doesn't recognize family members; decreasing awareness and more withdrawal; repetitive behaviors and questions; pacing; may become agitated and assaultive

Level 6: Severe cognitive decline
"Dementia"

- Needs help dressing, bathing, and decreased use of toilet (maybe incontinent); eating with fingers; toddler-like affect

Level 7: Very severe cognitive decline
"Late dementia"

- Speech erodes; dependence on others for all activities of daily living (walking, toileting, bathing); weight loss; restricted to bed or a wheelchair

Source: Reisberg, B., Ferris, S. H., de Leon, M. J., et al. (1982). The Global Deterioration Scale for assessment of primary degenerative dementia. *American Journal of Psychiatry*, 139, 1136–1139.

progress on to dementia, the medical community now believes that AD is an appropriate diagnosis that only fits individuals who are no longer on a Level 3 plateau (see Global Deterioration insert). An AD diagnosis can be derived after a clinical workup rules out other explanations for the dementia symptoms. Often, this will include a mental status examination screening for cognitive deficits in orientation, naming, memory, and perceptual skills. Most commonly used is the Mini-Mental State Examination (MMSE, often just called the "mini-mental"), which screens for cognitive impairment. Recent advances in neuroimaging using MRI or positron emission tomography (PET) scans can also help make a diagnosis. Yet, AD can be conclusively diagnosed only after death by microscopic examination of brain tissue at autopsy.

Early diagnosis renders a chance to plan treatment and construct opportunities that will have a significant impact on the quality of life of the person with AD and his family. Planning ahead is crucial. Typically, the monetary costs all too often get greater and greater as the disease progresses. We must recognize that people with AD likely have years in front of them that provide excitement and enjoyment as much as challenges. The person with AD does not regularly see the same problems and worries that caregivers face (see chapter 22 for further discussion), and talking frankly is better for all than pretending that the disease doesn't challenge one's integrity or future.

Sometimes what appear to be personality changes as a result of dementia are caused by sheer boredom and frustration at a misunderstood situation. Sometimes the person with AD forgets that they have just had sex and may try to initiate more sex than their partner can cope with. Men may be obstinate about their personal freedom and view their AD as a threat to their masculinity. An old cliché is, "Threaten a man's masculinity and he's likely to get macho."

There is no cure for AD or pharmaceutical treatment that even halts the disease. There are, however, medications that may help slow the pace of brain cell deterioration for some men. The predominant medications treat the brain chemistry changes that affect memory, language, judgment, planning, and ability to pay attention. Cholinesterase inhibitors, such as donepezil (Aricept), rivastigmine (Exelon), or galantamine (Razadyne), aim to avert the breakdown of acetylcholine and are modestly helpful for a small number of people. Like many drugs, however, their side effects may not be well tolerated and include gastrointestinal problems and nightmares.

At different points in the disease process people may experience emotional distress, restlessness, irritability, and hallucinations. Some men may experience reduced sexual interest or, less often, sharply increased sexual interest known as hypersexuality.[37] There are a range of effective environmental adaptations and nondrug approaches, and some medications are successful in controlling agitation, sleeplessness, loss of appetite, night wandering, delusions, and other "behavioral symptoms." Anyone caring for someone with AD would benefit by reaching out and talking with the professionals at their local Agency on Aging (there is one in virtually every county in each state) and the closest AD association. They can put you in touch with a wide array of strategies to live with this disease, as well as with nurses, social workers, and occupational therapists to help modify the home and everyday environment.

PARKINSON'S DISEASE

PD is the second most common neurodegenerative disorder and the most common movement disorder that may or may not involve memory loss. It too is a late-life chronic disease affecting about 1 percent of older adults in the United States, and twice as often men.[38] Very often the diagnosis occurs early enough that men will be living with PD for 20 or more years. About 20 percent of men with PD go on to develop a dementia that includes loss of memory and impairment in other cognitive functions. Men living with PD who develop dementia may develop the AD dementia or what is called PDD.

Being told they have a neurodegenerative disease, but not too troubled by its initial mild symptoms, some men try to go about their lives as usual. They may keep the news to themselves, choosing not to let their family know and braving the burden "like a man should." However, researchers find that men who see themselves as highly masculine have a harder experience.[39] By emphasizing their independence, or by not depending on others, men forego treatments that can help manage symptoms, as well as the social and emotional support that others can provide.

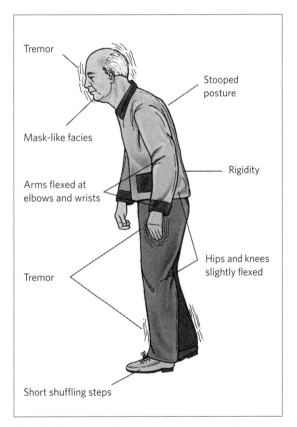

Figure 13.5. Parkinson's signs and symptoms. From F. D. Monahan & M. Neighbors. (1998). *Medical-surgical nursing: Foundations for clinical practice*, 2nd ed. Philadelphia: WB Saunders.

The side effects of PD can alter appearance and hinder a man's physical abilities. Research has shown that men's quality of life diminishes if they believe that their PD affects their public appearance and results in feeling like they are less than a whole man; the men in this study were most uncomfortable with whether others somehow saw their loss of strength, and they worried that their poor posture made them appear vulnerable or weak.[40]

PD is a neurological disease related to the degeneration of dopamine-producing neurons in the midbrain and thus dopamine deficiency. Dopamine is the brain chemical that controls muscle movement and makes it possible to reach for and drink a cup of coffee with smooth, coordinated muscle movement. The decrease of dopamine is what eventually disrupts motor functioning and causes the involuntary tremors, shuffling, speaking difficulties, and facial masking (or an expressionless, mask-like face). Slowed movement (called *bradykinesia*), resting tremors, stooped posture, and overall stiffness (or *rigidity*) are the common and frustrating symptoms. The causes of PD are ambiguous and varied, ranging from genetics, to exposure to the toxins in insecticides, to head trauma.

The majority of people diagnosed with PD have "idiopathic PD," which means that there is no specific cause. Nevertheless, research shows that a very small number of men may be genetically predisposed to PD. This does not mean that the disorder is passed down through generations, but that some gene groups are more predisposed to developing the disorder. Spurred by the discovery that PD is distributed in an uneven geographical pattern, some researchers argue that exposure to certain pesticides or mercury can increase one's chances of developing PD, though this hypothesis remains just an educated guess.

Currently, there is no cure for PD. Medication, physical therapy, and surgery (in extreme cases) are available forms of treatment for the PD symptoms that are most bothersome. The best treatment is based on individual needs, so there is no "gold standard" of therapy. Regular exercise and good nutrition do help with the physical symptoms of PD and improve men's quality of life. There are also medications to help manage the tremors and rigidity, even though these tend to lose their potency (or efficacy) after several years of use, and there are medications to stimulate the production of dopamine. As one man reported, "That small daily dose of Sinamet certainly did the trick," and he went on to enjoy his retirement.[41] Sinamet is a combination of carbidopa and levodopa for the treatment of PD symptoms. Treatment with the drug rivastigmine also seems to mitigate dementia symptoms such as word recall, ability to follow commands, and comprehension of spoken language.[42]

BRAIN HEALTH REVISITED

Dementia isn't inevitable, nor is substantial memory loss. Most clinical researchers and health care practitioners argue that we *can* maintain our brain health and prevent (or at least delay) the onset of dementia symptoms. We can now die in our eighties or nineties *with* cellular evidence of dementia (and prostate cancer), rather than *from* it, and stay smart, strong, and active. Researchers at the Mayo Clinic and the University of California, San Francisco, two locations where some of the newest research on MCI and AD occurs, all agree that the real risk to our brain health is us. If you smoke, are physically inactive, drink heavily to relieve stress, regularly overeat and shun healthy foods, or prefer watching sitcoms over reading a newspaper, you are giving up many years of independence.

CHAPTER 14

Men and Diabetes

with Kaitlyn Barnes

Has your brother always had a "big" appetite, hungry for large portions—
"like three Big Macs, a whole big old trail of French fries"[1]—and can't get
satisfied, craving foods high in starch and sugar, and drinking more than a
few sodas daily to try to satisfy that unquenchable thirst? Does he urinate
often—for example, once every 20 minutes for 2 hours after a bottle of
water? More recently, however, have you noticed that his cuts and bruises
are taking longer to heal? Maybe he has begun to notice some tingling or
coolness in his hands and feet, and despite how much he eats, there's a bit
of weight loss? No big deal, you think; he says he feels fine. And he probably
does feel okay. You probably think that all these little changes are symptoms
of normal aging, right?

Well, they are not. What is happening is that he is developing, or has
developed, diabetes—his blood sugar level (BSL) is too high. Diabetes, particularly the adult-onset (type 2) diabetes just described, has been increasing at a rapid rate in the United States, nearly doubling in the past 30 years,
and is more common in African Americans, Latinos, American Indians, and
Native Hawaiians. Rarely found among indigenous peoples, this disorder is
very prevalent in modern societies with our "Western diets." For example, a
century ago diabetes was unknown among the Pima and Tohono O'odham
Indians of southern Arizona, but once their agricultural economy was disrupted and their traditional foods were replaced by commodities like white
flour, lard, processed cheese, and canned foods, two generations later half
of the adults are now diabetic.[2] According to the Centers for Disease Control and Prevention (CDC), diabetes affects about 12 percent of men age 20

and older in the United States, altering the lives and lifestyles of nearly 13 million men.[3] This estimate is equivalent to the entire population of Illinois or Pennsylvania, which are the fifth and sixth largest states, respectively.

Even if you are not (yet) diabetic, why should statistics about the increasing prevalence of diabetes concern you? One reason is that type 2 diabetes is most likely to develop as we get older, and since men in recent generations are living longer, we are more vulnerable. More than one-quarter (26.9%) of men age 65 and older have diabetes, and this proportion will certainly increase. In 2010, over 1 million new cases of diabetes were reported for people ages 45–64, and the biggest jump occurred among Hispanic/Latino, African American, and Asian men.

As another reason for concern, it is estimated that millions of men living with diabetes have not been diagnosed. Perhaps as many as 35 percent of men age 40–60 and 50 percent of men age 65 and older have what is called *prediabetes*—the stage right before the development of full diabetes. Completely unaware that they already have diabetes, the odds that they are living a healthy diabetes-management lifestyle would be a long shot. Their health is seriously at risk, even though they may feel okay. Diabetes is the sixth-leading cause of death for men in the United States, and it is a leading cause of other health problems such as kidney failure, nerve damage (neuropathy), lower-limb amputations, blindness, hypertension, heart attacks, and strokes. Every man 40 and older will benefit by paying (very) close attention to his blood sugar and lifestyle. Although there is no cure for diabetes, the disorder can be effectively managed to fight off its complications.

WHAT IS DIABETES?

Diabetes is a metabolic disorder that interferes with the way our bodies turn food into energy. What defines the onset of diabetes is when the level of blood sugar in our bloodstream is too high (*hyperglycemia*). When food, especially carbohydrates, is digested, it is converted into the sugar energy source called *glucose* to feed muscles, tissues, and organs. Normally, glucose constantly travels through our bloodstream and will enter cells when the hormone insulin is present. Insulin is produced by the pancreas and released into our bloodstream throughout the day, and more is released when we eat. It acts as the "key" and "opens" up passageways on the surface of each cell to take the glucose molecules from the blood into the cells. When your body does not produce enough insulin, sugar levels rise in the bloodstream. Similarly, when we acquire type 2 diabetes, our body does not efficiently use the insulin it produces. Cells become resistant to insulin, leaving a greater amount of glucose to build up in our bloodstream. Other cells needing the glucose are not getting it for their essential energy and/or growth. Finally, the excess glucose eventually damages the small blood vessels throughout the body, especially affecting our eyes and kidneys, as well as skin, nerves, muscles, intestines, and the heart.

Diabetes can emerge in three ways. The pancreas—the spongy gland located behind the stomach that controls the digestive enzymes—involves three cell clusters: alpha cells, beta cells, and delta cells. The beta cells (β-cells) are the cells that produce insulin. One scenario is that there is no insulin being produced by our pancreas's β-cells. A second scenario is that some of the β-cells in the pancreas are destroyed for some reason and we are not producing sufficient insulin for the amount of glucose present in our bloodstream. The final scenario is that our pancreas is producing enough insulin, but our body for some reason or another has become

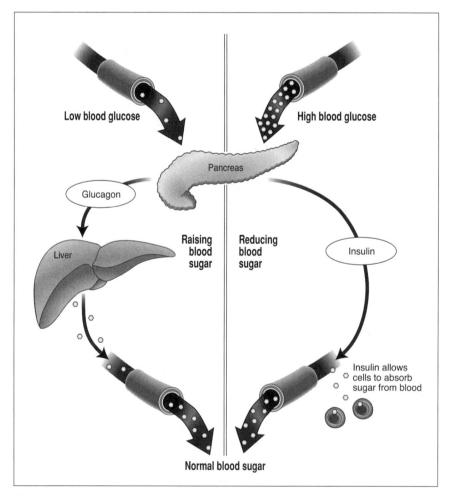

Figure 14.1. Regulating blood glucose levels. Illustration by Jacqueline Schaffer.

resistant to the insulin. In each scenario, the passageways on our cells stay closed, and glucose is not able to get in to be converted into life-sustaining fuel. Instead, the glucose is left to build up in our bloodstream. The elevated level of glucose is sometimes described as a poison.

The anguish all diabetic men face is that they are usually unaware of its presence until one of its *serious* complications shows itself. Diabetes develops so slowly that it is easy to normalize (or ignore) the signs and symptoms of craving sugary and starchy foods, always being thirsty, and going to the bathroom again and again. Health complications and men's complaints prior to a diagnosis also include disturbed sleep because of the frequent need to urinate, feeling full because of the slowed digestion of food in the stomach, erectile dysfunction (ED), unexplained feelings of fatigue, numbness in feet or hands, and blurry vision.

You may be saying to yourself at this point, "I'd rather not know I have diabetes." If so, you wouldn't be alone; like most other men, you probably do not want to admit you are sick. In some racial/ethnic communities, men feel that having diabetes is discrediting, because of the lingering stigma that having diabetes equals being *very* sick or because of the myth that diabetes is self-induced.[4]

Diabetes is a bear in every sense of the word. Deny its existence, pretend it isn't there, walk right through it, and you can wind up mauled and destroyed.

Source: Lodewick, P. A., Bierman, J., & Toohey, B. (1999). *The diabetic man.* Los Angeles, CA: Lowell House, p. 81.

Unlike other chronic diseases (such as tuberculosis or cancer), studies have shown that the crippling effects of type 2 diabetes can be avoided. If you (or people close to you) pay attention to the signs and symptoms and figure out early enough that you have an elevated BSL, you can adopt a new, reasonably easy lifestyle that holds in check most if not all of the negative effects of the metabolic disorder. It is not that simple, however. BSLs rise every time you have eaten more than you should have, have eaten foods that are not recommended, or have not exercised. Psychological stress can have the same effect as the foods we eat; when there is some sort of stress going on in our life (problems at work, a family member causing us to worry), our BSLs will rise. Diabetics often have to go against the grain of their community's and family's food traditions to eat healthily; men who routinely eat white rice are prime examples. Some diabetic men also do not have the financial means to adopt a healthy meal plan that includes fresh (or canned) non-starchy vegetables, whole grains, fruits, and a limited amount of saturated fat.

For all prediabetic and diabetic men, self-management of their diabetes isn't a simple "you can do it." Yet managing our BSL to give us a good quality of life (without the amputations and blindness) isn't insurmountable. For most men, becoming conscious of and altering our lifestyle is difficult at first. Changing from an eat-anything-you-want lifestyle to healthy meals doesn't happen at the snap of a finger, but it is achievable. More and more men, particularly in the African American community, have family and friends willing to change diets and help them.[5] Their wives, partners, and women kin are protective and willing to change family traditions and life-styles to help their man with his self-management.[6] Commenting on his wife's contribution to whether he checked his blood sugar, took medica-tions, engaged in physical activity, and ate properly, one Mexican American man noted,

> She's the one who's . . . you have to do this and you have to do that and she's always on me. And she's always, you know if it wasn't for her, I wouldn't be here now probably.[7]

WHY TWO TYPES OF DIABETES?

Diabetes comes in two principal forms: type 1 and type 2. The two differ in how and when they are typically developed and in their treatment plans. You may have heard the term *juvenile diabetes* or *insulin-dependent diabetes*, which begins earlier in life and has the tendency to affect young children or young adults, though it could start as late as someone's midthirties. It is an autoimmune disease that damages and destroys the body's β-cells. This causes the body to produce very little or no insulin at all. Without the production of insulin, people with type 1 quickly build up glucose in their bloodstream. They are inevitably "insulin dependent," and this means that they have to take insulin every day, usually in the form of an injection. They also must pay particular attention to their meal and exercise plans for the remainder of their lives.

Adult men are much more at risk for developing type 2 diabetes, which emerges when the body becomes resistant to insulin, or when the pancreas does not produce enough insulin to meet demand. Adult-onset diabetes (type 2) has been found to be inheritable in families. But nutritional con-siderations and a sedentary lifestyle seem to be the main determinants of its onset. When we eat more calories than we expend, whenever it is difficult to engage in enough physical activity to burn these calories, and when we eat simple sugars and fats that have many more calories than nat-ural "healthy" foods, it is up to our pancreas to produce a lot more insulin to try to counteract our choices. This increase in insulin production and the calories that cannot be stored (fats and sugars in the blood) are what probably lead to the insulin resistance at the cell membrane sites. Basically, this occurs when cells become compromised and less sensitive to the effects of insulin. In addition, the frequent or constant demand for a large production of insulin can cause the β-cells to essentially become "worn out," leading to slower production. When insulin is undersupplied or cannot be used by cells, our tissues and organs become fuel depleted at the same time that the glucose and fat levels in the bloodstream elevate.

Hyperglycemia means high blood sugar. You are "hyperglycemic" when your BSL goes too high, because either there is too little insulin in your body or your body is not properly using the insulin it has. Every diabetic has his own individual BSL range, though anything above 200 mg/dL is bad for anyone. A BSL above 400 is approaching a dangerous level. The best treatment for hyperglycemia is not to allow it to happen in the first place. If you follow a healthy meal plan and engage in moderate exercise, your BSL should not go too high. However, whenever it is above 300, because you couldn't pass up a fast-food fill-up of a burger and fries, it may be necessary for you to postpone exercising until your BSL returns to a safer range.

Your body will alert you to high BSLs. The more noticeable hyperglycemic alarm is that you feel very thirsty at a time when you should not be that thirsty (for example, you have not just exercised). Other symptoms are an unusually frequent urge to urinate, shortness of breath, soreness in your muscles that wasn't there before, and a very dry mouth.

Hypoglycemia means low blood sugar. Blood sugar dropping too low (below 70 mg/dL) happens from time to time to every diabetic, especially for men with type 1 diabetes during and after moderate exercise (e.g., shoveling light snow, taking a 30-minute walk). Symptoms of low blood sugar include shakiness, dizziness, sweating, hunger, headache, tingling around the mouth, unusual clumsiness or confusion, difficulty paying attention, or sudden mood swings with no cause. The common rule for hypoglycemia is, "When in doubt, treat." The quickest way to treat hypoglycemia is to raise your BSL, that is, to ingest some form of sugar. Low blood sugars are dangerous because you will pass out if the level goes too low. With good diabetes control hypoglycemia should not be too much of a problem. The key is to learn your body's early signs of low BSL so that you can treat it sooner (with just orange juice, for example).

RISK FACTORS FOR TYPE 2 DIABETES

There is not one main cause of diabetes; rather, many environmental (or lifestyle) factors put us at greater risk. It is important to understand that type 2 diabetes is preventable, mostly by not ingesting more calories than our bodies can use. It is equally important to note that it is rare to find any man who eats perfect proportions of carbohydrates, fats, proteins, and vegetables all the time and who maintains regular exercise and near perfect weight. We all eat differently depending on our family traditions, our busy schedules, stress, loneliness, anger, sadness, and other various reasons. Some of us will develop diabetes because of our lifestyle, and some will not. That being said, the "couch potato" syndrome is a significant risk for type 2 diabetes. The prevalence of diabetes is more than four times as high among men who are obese (having a body mass index >30), compared to men of normal weight. Diabetes is twice as prevalent among African American, Hispanic/Latino, and Native American men as Caucasian men, mostly because of diet and weight, and all Pacific Islanders are also at great risk of developing type 2 diabetes.

Diabetes Risk Factors for Men

- Family history of type 2 diabetes
- Being overweight or obese
- A diet heavy in carbohydrates and starches
- Being sedentary, or physically inactive
- Stress for men over 45
- High blood pressure (hypertension)
- Lipid abnormalities (high cholesterol)
- Use of certain medications (e.g., diuretics, cortisone, prednisone)
- Being of African American, Native American, Pacific Islander, or Latino (especially Mexican American) heritage

Chronic stress is indisputably related to the onset of diabetes, and stress management is crucial to controlling diabetes (and heart disease). When distress caused by work-family conflicts, getting older, or other stressors is not well managed or managed by eating more salty fats and sweet foods, this results in increases of cortisone.[8] The stress response (see chapter 5) involves stimulation of epinephrine and cortisol release. These hormones oppose insulin and are thought to lead to our body's insulin resistance.[9]

Yearly checkups with your physician can help monitor your BSL and make you aware of your status, saving you a lot of diabetes-related complications down the road. If you let diabetes' symptoms go unchecked, you increase your risk for developing one or more of the other medical conditions closely associated with this metabolic syndrome. Your risk for diabetes can be determined by a simple blood test.

YOU HAVE BEEN DIAGNOSED. NOW WHAT?

Being told we have diabetes can set off a range of emotions. Men will commonly be shaken and experience anger, guilt, or depression, or else deny it all together. It is expected that you will feel temporarily overwhelmed by the diagnosis, but it is important that you not "puddle" too long or shift into an "aw-heck-with-it" type of denial. It is also understandable that your frustration may escalate when you have trouble keeping your blood glucose level down, or when other people provide unwanted advice and ask meddling questions about your body and lifestyle choices.

As soon as you can, you need to initiate the actions necessary to live with diabetes, and this begins with talking to your family. It is understandable that you might first want to conceal your diabetes. You might be thinking of your family's pleasure in eating large meals or certain foods and how you do not want to negatively affect their lives.[10] However, the worst thing you can do is deny the fact that you have a serious, chronic illness that will definitely get worse if it's ignored. Balancing a desired quality of life with recommended care for this disease isn't something you can do alone. As one Chinese American man commented about his wife's effort to help him,

> A couple of times, I went out for social events, and ate a lot of foods I wasn't supposed to eat, my blood sugar level went up so high, to 300 something. So my wife is good to me, very concerned about me. Sometimes in the morning she will check my chart, the record. [She] checked it and was angry. She said, "Hey, this isn't going to work. If something happens, if you don't even care about yourself, then in the future I'm not going to care about it." When she said this, I . . . thought, hey, that's not nice. . . . Later after I calmed down a little, and thought about it, it really is true that you have to be persistent yourself.[11]

Asking for and accepting others' attention isn't selfish, nor is it an admission of personal failure, and there is no need to apologize for needing to make lifestyle changes.

Too few people realize that diabetes is a disease that can often be turned back once it has started. While you may not be able to turn back the hands of time, you can dramatically reverse your body's insulin resistance by changing lifestyle habits; you may also need oral hypoglycemic drugs to increase the responsiveness of the β-cells (such as one of the drugs from the sulfonylurea class). Once a man comes to accept his diagnosis, changing his meal plan and level of exercise also will trim down his waist. These lifestyle changes reduce the cells' insulin resistance, and often he can bring blood sugars back into normal ranges (e.g., "normal" for the hemoglobin A1c test is between 4% and 6%).

Many men come from communities where diabetes is prevalent and believe that the negative complications of diabetes are inevitably linked with getting older, because they have witnessed the terrible effects (such as renal failure, blindness, and loss of limbs) in the lives of older family members.[12] These complications are preventable. Too many men with diabetes also must deal with the dual challenges of diabetes management and maintaining a sense of themselves as nondependent and in control of their body and life. They oppose being "policed."[13] Don't resist being dependent, and recognize that diabetes management *is* taking control of your body and life.

SELF-CARE AND LIFESTYLE MANAGEMENT

You've likely heard the saying "knowledge is power." This is especially true when it comes to managing diabetes. Few men, especially those who come from at-risk backgrounds (such as a family history of diabetes, being African American or Latino), are knowledgeable about diabetes before their diagnosis. But you can quickly gain the knowledge necessary to take control and to feel the relief and confidence that it is possible to live a long life without diabetes complications.

The first step is to assess the level of your confidence with the physician who made the diagnosis. Was the explanation clear, and were you presented with an action plan? As men, we don't have the best track record of fully listening to the advice provided. But your doctor will be the main person helping you self-manage your diabetes. You're going to want someone who is direct and listens to your thoughts and answers your questions—for example, someone who asks you straight up about your experience of erectile difficulties[14] and appreciates the importance of men maintaining their erectile function. Without a plan of action clearly discussed, it is predictable that men newly diagnosed will experience more diabetes distress and poor self-management.[15]

If you do not feel like your current doctor can be *your* partner in treatment, you need to look for someone else or find a clinic. You want to make sure that your health care provider recommends an action plan that you can live with; hopefully, you can find a diabetes care team you can count on to help you—dieticians, diabetes nurse educators, and exercise physiologists. Remember, you are the captain of your team. Put yourself first, but don't ignore the advice.

Although you will (or should) have a health care provider as your treatment partner, a lot of the care will be your own responsibility. Here are four questions you should be asking your physician or others on the team at each visit:

1. What is your A1c level? The hemoglobin A1c (HbA1c) test determines how well you are managing your blood glucose over a period of time; your HbA1c level ought to be tested every 2–3 months. Your goal is to get your A1c level under 7 percent.

2. Should you be checking your BSL? Your doctor will let you know how often you should monitor your blood glucose, based on your

recommended treatment plan. Diabetics who are on insulin treatment must monitor their blood glucose more often than diabetics who are only on lifestyle or medication interventions.

3. What is your blood pressure (BP)? High BP is very common among diabetic men, because coronary heart disease and diabetes are often co-occurring. Your goal is to keep your BP at least at 130/80. High BP along with high blood sugar can damage the blood vessels in your eyes and cause blindness.

4. What is your cholesterol level? High cholesterol and other blood fats are very common in men with type 2 diabetes. You should have a simple blood test called a *complete lipid panel* or *lipid profile* done to evaluate the four types of fats in your blood. These four are low-density lipoprotein (LDL) cholesterol, high-density lipoprotein (HDL) cholesterol, triglycerides, and total cholesterol. LDL cholesterol is the "bad" cholesterol. You should aim to keep your LDL level below 100. HDL is the cholesterol that protects us from heart disease and ought to be at least 50 mg/dL, preferably 60 mg/dL. Triglycerides are what your body converts calories into if they aren't used right away, and your goal should be to keep them at 150. Total cholesterol is just the sum of all our blood cholesterol content and should be below 200.

Holding yourself accountable for your day-to-day care is the most effective diabetes treatment. You may be in charge of monitoring your BSL at home; you certainly will be in charge of watching what you eat, increasing your activity level, and following the prescribed plan of action to reduce blood glucose, blood cholesterol, and BP. Eating less and eating healthy are very important to everyone, but even more important once someone has diabetes. Our body will not set off "alarms" to warn us right away, should we stray from the recommended amount of calories in a "healthy diet" and go back to calorie-packed sugars and fried foods. But you will be silently doing damage to your body. A healthy person's body keeps blood glucose levels in a normal range when the pancreas is able to release insulin to lower glucose levels and glucagon, which raises glucose levels for men who are hypoglycemic.

The best meal plan reduces calories and omits the calorie-packed sugars found in fruit juice and white sugar, which are quickly converted and digested into the bloodstream as glucose. While cutting back on simple carbohydrates and sugar may be mentioned in brochures as a common approach to managing diabetes, it's not the essential one. The American Diabetes Association says that cutting back on sugar helps only if it's part of an overall effort to manage total carbohydrate intake. The most important aspect of living with diabetes is becoming carbohydrate savvy; for this, reading food labels is empowering. *Carbs* is the general name for starches and sugars. While they have different names, starches and sugars have the same effect on your body. Starches are the things made out of grain, flour, and corn—like breads, cookies, cakes, and beer. Sugars are pretty self-explanatory—anything with natural or artificial sugar counts as a sugar, whether it is in a donut or a glass of sweetened tea. So, while you might think eating a bagel is okay because it is not filled with as much sugar as a donut, it may actually be worse because of its starch. It's best not to eat either. You also might think that eating an orange a day is healthy, but all the sugar in that orange is having the same effect on a diabetic man's body as other "sugary" food would.

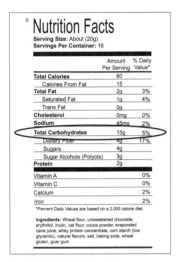

Figure 14.2. Nutrition Facts label for low-carb chocolate brownie mix

If weight loss is part of the recommended action plan, the good news is that the amount of weight reduction does not have to be extreme. Many studies have found that losing just 10–12 pounds can reduce insulin resistance. Here are a few easy suggestions made by Harvard medical experts[16] that can help us get started on our transition to a healthier lifestyle:

> Losing weight can be the best treatment for diabetes, and it is essential for lowering BSLs. Try to lose 5–10 pounds. Here's one strategy: reduce or completely eliminate sweetened or naturally sweetened drinks. These drinks include bottled tea, sodas, sports drinks, and fruit juices. These drinks cause our blood sugar to rise quickly and are full of many empty calories.

> Attempt to eat several very small meals at regular time intervals each day. Spacing out meals (and snacks) relieves the stress on our pancreas to produce insulin. With smaller meals, our pancreas only has to produce small amounts of insulin to deal with the glucose in our bloodstream.

> Gradually increase your daily activity level. Many men think that when they are diagnosed with diabetes they have to immediately join a gym and exercise, exercise, exercise. But you are busy and just do not have time to devote an hour or two at a gym; thankfully, it is recommended that you only increase your activity level to 30 minutes a day, five to six times a week. This does not mean weight lifting or hard aerobic exercise. You can divide the recommended 30 minutes a day

into three 10-minute "workouts," which might involve parking the car farther away from the store and later walking up the stairs instead of using an elevator. Going for a 15-minute walk counts as increased activity. We can count the number of steps we take by wearing a pedometer. The average healthy person walks 10,000 steps per day. If you wear a pedometer, work to increase your number of steps each day. Whether it is taking three 10-minute walks a day or just getting up to change the television channel instead of using the remote, no alteration in physical activity is too small to make a difference in reversing our diabetes diagnosis.

DIABETES MEDICATIONS AND INSULIN TREATMENT

If lifestyle changes do not decrease your BSL, you may be prescribed diabetes medications. There are currently six classes of oral drugs that work in different ways to lower our blood glucose levels. According to *Consumer Reports*,[17] taking effectiveness, safety, adverse effects, dosing, and cost into consideration, the most recommended (and most commonly prescribed[18]) is Metformin, which is a generic and is in the biguanides class. This type of medication helps lower blood glucose level by inhibiting the amount of glucose produced by our liver and making our muscles more sensitive to the

MEDICATIONS USED TO TREAT DIABETES

Type of drug	Individual drugs
Sulfonylureas	*Brands:* Amaryl, Diabeta, Glynase, Glucotrol, Glucotrol XL *Generics:* Glimepiride, Glipizide, Glyburide
Biguanides	*Brands:* Glucophage, Glucophage XR *Generics:* Metformin
Thiazolidinediones	Actos, Avandia
Alpha-glucosidase inhibitors	*Brands:* Precose, Glyset *Generics:* Acarbose
Meglitinides	*Brands:* Prandin, Starlix *Generics:* Nateglinide
Dipeptidyl peptidase 4 inhibitors	Januvia, Onglyza

Source: American Diabetes Association.

insulin we do produce. Metformin is typically prescribed by itself, but if its effect on blood glucose starts to dwindle, another oral medication may be added. It is very likely that you will need another type of medication after several years to keep your blood sugar controlled.

Another drug class strictly for type 2 diabetes is the thiazolidinediones (TZDs). These drugs help reduce insulin resistance, increase HDL lipids, and lower glucose production by the liver. Some TZDs, however, may have a link to increased cardiovascular events.

A drug from the sulfonylurea group, from which the first oral diabetes medication was available, is a common second choice. These drugs, along with drugs from the meglitinide class, stimulate the β-cells in our pancreas to produce and release more insulin. Drugs from the sulfonylurea and meglitinide groups have a higher incidence of low blood sugar (hypoglycemia), so they are usually taken in small dosages throughout the day.

Alpha-glucosidase inhibitors work to block our body from breaking down starches such as those found in bread, potatoes, and pasta. They also slow the breakdown of some sugars. This helps delay the rise in blood glucose right after eating a meal. The final class of drugs is DPP-4 inhibitors. They are designed to prevent the breakdown of GLP-1, which is a natural compound in our body that contributes to reducing blood glucose. By protecting GLP-1, the drugs allow for a "natural" lowering of blood sugars. This new group of drugs does not seem to cause the hypoglycemic effect of some of the other drugs.

Sometimes people with type 2 diabetes are treated with insulin because they have become "insulin deficient." Oral medications along with exercise and eating healthy may not be enough to keep your blood glucose within a healthy range. This isn't unusual, and one theory is that our β-cells become depleted from having to produce extra insulin for a long period of time. When this happens, you will need to take up using insulin, which can be injected or delivered by an insulin pump.

Historically, insulin was thought to be a "last resort" option, but it is becoming valued because it lowers the risk of the long-term complications of diabetes, keeps the BSLs controlled, and doesn't seem to negatively affect people's quality of life.[19] Nevertheless, some people resist moving from oral drugs to insulin because they have negative beliefs about insulin, needles, and/or blood glucose monitoring.[20] You might be one of the men who worries that his need of insulin injections will be embarrassing. Researchers find that some men think they need insulin because they have "failed" other therapies or failed to control their disease by not properly caring for themselves, and they feel that they need to hide their injections to avoid broadcasting their illness.[21] This is unsolicited and uninformed advice—don't apologize for needing to use insulin. It is a life saver.

COMPLICATIONS OF DIABETES

Hyperglycemia is the cause for nearly all diabetes-related complications. The diabetes-related complications that can be prevented or delayed include cardiovascular disease (atherosclerosis, heart attack, and stroke), nerve damage, renal disease, retinopathy, ED, and depression. In the section that follows, the key complications are summarized (and elsewhere in this sourcebook, many are discussed in more detail).

Cardiovascular Disease

Impaired glucose metabolism causes blood vessel damage, which then puts many diabetics at greater risk of hypertension, heart attack, stroke, amputations, and vision loss. Diabetics are two to four times more likely to develop heart disease or suffer a stroke as nondiabetics. This added risk is because diabetes weakens and damages any organ or tissue that blood flows through and progressively injures the cells that line blood vessel walls. Recently, researchers at Washington University identified two enzymes that diabetic men have less of, and it is their relative absence that *likely* causes the deterioration at the microvascular level.[22] However, what causes the deterioration still isn't fully understood.

What is known is that diabetic men are at much greater risk to develop atherosclerosis (the clogging and "hardening of the arteries"), which is a key determinant of heart attacks and strokes (see chapter 12). The damage to the blood vessels is due to fatty substances, or plaque, building up on artery walls; among diabetics, it noticeably affects the skin on your legs, the arteries beneath, and the vessels in your eyes. While many older people develop atherosclerosis, diabetics are affected much earlier and more severely. Even a tiny scrape on your leg can take weeks to heal and possibly even grow into a large open wound. This is because not enough blood can travel through your arteries to get to the cut to heal it. If wounds like these go untreated, they often become infected, which only causes more problems. In the most extreme cases, atherosclerosis can result in amputation of toes, feet, and partial or whole legs.

Neuropathy

About two-thirds of diabetic men suffer from at least a mild case of nerve damage. High BSLs eventually damage your nerve cells, which makes it harder if not impossible for the brain to control the functions of the body that it is supposed to, contributing to urinary dysfunction (resulting in incontinence) and bowel dysfunction (resulting in diarrhea). Severe forms of nerve damage do not occur often, and sometimes symptoms go away just as fast as they arose. But for some diabetics nerve damage can become painful and disabling. You can have a tingling feeling in parts of your body, or lose the ability to feel cold, hot, pain, or tactile sensation in general. This can result in not feeling the pain of an infection and thus not realizing that you have one. Nerve damage can also cause your feet and toes to become deformed, curling up and twisting in odd ways.

Feet and Lower Extremity Amputations

When diabetic men need to be hospitalized, about 20 percent are seeking help for foot problems—chiefly, infections and ulcers.[23] Diabetes can cause the sweat glands in your feet to stop working, which may sound good at first, if you are thinking about your history of "smelly" feet. But when sweat glands begin to fail, this causes the feet to dry out and the skin to crack, especially in between the toes, allowing bacteria and fungus to flourish. Untreated, these "minor" infections become major problems. Poor circulation is the key problem, leaving your feet with reduced blood flow to combat the infection.

In addition, the diabetes-caused nerve damage leaves little or no feeling in the feet, which eliminates any cue to the diabetic that he has a problem, until it has grown out of control. Toe and foot infections that rage out of control and are not noticed will too often end up needing amputation. Diabetes is the reason for more than half of the nontraumatic "lower extremity" amputations performed annually in the United States, especially among ethnic minority men. One study reported that diabetic men who undergo an amputation are, on average, older, being treated for other health problems, and more likely to belong to an ethnic/racial minority; American Indians had the highest risk of amputation, followed by African Americans and Hispanics/Latinos.[24]

Retinopathy—Eyes

Many diabetics have problems with their eyes due to "diabetic retinopathy," or damage to the small blood vessels in the eyes. This is the term used for all disorders of the retina caused by diabetes. Anyone can develop disorders of the retina (cataracts, glaucoma), though diabetics have a higher risk than nondiabetics (see chapter 18). The key to saving your sight is to catch and solve high blood sugar problems early. For anyone over the age of 30, a yearly eye exam is important, but for diabetics it is vital. Almost every diabetic will develop some form of an eye problem, reducing vision and threatening blindness. Risk of eye problems increases with the number of years you've been a diabetic; the deterioration of eye blood vessels is caused by years of a high glucose level. If you feel that your vision is deteriorating more than normal, or your vision becomes spotty or blurry, contact your doctor as soon as possible.

Mouth/Gums

Gum disease, also called *gingivitis*, is a very common diabetes-related complication. Gum disease and teeth with cavities can happen to any person (see chapter 17), but diabetics' high glucose level makes the gums and teeth more likely to be attacked by cavity-causing bacteria or become infected. Again, it is related to how excess blood sugar compromises cells. The advanced stages of gum disease are called *periodontitis*, which basically involves your gums deteriorating and pulling away from your teeth. This causes pockets to develop between the gum and tooth, allowing germs and bacteria easy access to the bone holding your teeth in place. Eventually this leads to bone loss and losing your teeth. Men with diabetes have a greater number of missing teeth than nondiabetics. Other complications of diabetes affecting your mouth can be dry mouth and poor healing if you cut the inside of your mouth.

Kidney Disease

Diabetes is the leading cause of kidney failure, or end-stage renal disease. Diabetic nephropathy (kidney disease) has caused over 40 percent of cases of kidney failure; however, the odds of developing nephropathy are getting smaller because of better treatment. Using historical patterns, between 10 and 20 percent of diabetics may develop kidney disease at some point in their lives. Diabetic nephropathy isn't an equal-opportunity disease. African Americans, American Indians, and Hispanics/Latinos develop diabetes, kidney disease, and kidney failure at rates much higher than Caucasian men. In the United Kingdom, people from an Asian or Afro-Caribbean origin with type 2 diabetes are twice as likely to develop diabetic kidney disease.

Our kidneys are the body's filters. Inside your kidneys are millions of little blood vessels that filter out all of the waste products from the blood. High levels of glucose in a diabetic's blood make the kidneys work extra hard, and after many years they become tired and worn out. The better that a diabetic is able to control his BSLs, the less likely he is to develop kidney damage. If someone has been diabetic for 40 years and has no signs of kidney damage, he most likely never will.

The symptoms of kidney disease are almost none; the kidneys work at full force until almost all function gives out and they just cannot work that hard any longer. If kidney disease is caught early, its deterioration can be limited with strict BSL and BP control. BP has a striking effect on the rate at which the disease progresses. Rising BP can quickly make kidney disease worsen, and BP can be lowered by managing (or treating) your stress level (even with quiet 5-minute breaks), eating less salt, avoiding tobacco, exercising regularly, and, of course, controlling your weight.[25] You might also need oral hypertensive medication. The lower your BP and BSL, the longer your kidneys will last.

Once the kidneys fail, dialysis is more common than a transplant. There are 10 times as many people on waiting lists for a kidney transplant than annually receiving a kidney donation and successful transplant. Dialysis itself is not easy or inexpensive. There are two different kinds of dialysis, and both aim to clean the blood through other organs. One way, hemodialysis, consists of hooking the patient up to a machine for a few hours, during which an artificial kidney cycles the blood out of the patient, cleans it, and then cycles it back into the body. The second method, peritoneal dialysis, has the same goals, but instead of using a machine, another bodily organ is used—the peritoneum, which is a thin membrane that lines the stomach. In this method a catheter is placed in the patient and stays there indefinitely, unless there is an infection.

Erectile Dysfunction

ED affects at least 50 percent of men with diabetes,[26] nearly three times greater than men without diabetes. To get and maintain an erection, men need healthy blood vessels and unimpaired nerves. The erectile difficulties among diabetic men are caused by their diabetes-related vascular disease and damage to the cavernosal nerves. Simply put, diabetes prematurely impairs the blood vessels and nerves that control an erection, introducing erectile failure 10–20 years earlier than for men without diabetes. Even many younger diabetic men who do not yet have the age-related reduction in testosterone level are not able to achieve and sustain a firm erection.

As addressed in chapter 20, ED negatively affects men's quality of life and psychological well-being, and diabetic men are no exception. Diabetic men often have more severe ED than other men, and their earlier ED seems to have a greater impact on their quality of life.[27] Men with diabetes can consult their physician or diabetes clinic and obtain an oral ED medication like Viagra, Cialis, and Levitra to help achieve an erection. Don't be embarrassed. Men are asking, and diabetic men rated ED the third most important complication of their condition, only behind kidney disease and blindness.[28]

Diabetes and ED

Erectile problems are common for men who have undiagnosed diabetes. Often, it is the erectile difficulties that become the first symptom men may notice that leads them to their physician. Only after they seek medical help for the ED do they discover their diagnosis of diabetes.

ED is also a symptom of underlying cardiovascular disease (CVD). Should you experience erectile problems, have a physician or clinic assess your blood chemistry for evidence of both diabetes and CVD.

Source: Ma, R. C.-W., So, W.-Y., Yang, X., et al. (2008). Erectile dysfunction predicts coronary heart disease in type 2 diabetes. *Journal of the American College of Cardiology, 51,* 2045–2050.

Depression

Men with diabetes are at risk of living with chronic depression. Studies show that people with diabetes report more depressive symptoms than reported by people without diabetes, and far more men who are members of ethnic minority groups experience higher levels of depressive symptoms than found in diabetic men of white European ancestry.[29] These ethnic/racial differences in rates of diabetes distress seem to be by-products of income and education differences, not ethnicity itself. Importantly, diabetic men from all ethnic/racial backgrounds are equally at risk of both diabetes distress and depressive affect.[30]

There's a bit of a chicken-and-egg issue, however, when it comes to depression and diabetes. Researchers find that men experiencing depression are more at risk of the onset of type 2 diabetes, yet type 2 diabetes is associated with only modest increased risk of depression.[31] Whatever comes first, the fact is that for diabetic men there is a considerable risk of living with and needing to treat both diabetes and depressive feelings.

Ketoacidosis

Ketoacidosis (diabetic coma for type 1 diabetics) is a serious complication of type 1 diabetes that needs immediate treatment. When you are without enough insulin to convert food into energy, your body is energy starved and begins to break down fats to use as energy. When this happens, waste products called *ketones* are made and disposed within urine. However, should your kidneys not reduce the ketones fast enough, they build up in the bloodstream, and high levels can result in ketoacidosis. Warning signs are dry skin and mouth, flushed face, deep and rapid breathing, muscle stiffness, abdominal pain, and mental stupor.

Hyperosmolar Hyperglycemic Nonketotic Coma (HHNC)

This is ketoacidosis in type 2 diabetics. It happens to about one in eight type 2 diabetics who become "insulin dependent," and it is more common than ketoacidosis is for type 1 diabetics. Basically, this condition is severe hyperglycemia; it does not involve the ketones. Called HHNC, it is most common among older diabetics (70 years of age or older), partly because of the lack of physical activity and partly because of dehydration. A man suffering from HHNC may appear confused and tired and have pasty, clammy skin. Hydrating and administering insulin are effective treatments for most cases of HHNC, but if the problem is severe, you might be hospitalized so that an IV can be administered to rehydrate.

COMMON VOCABULARY OF DIABETES

Your doctor will most likely go over all the information you need to know about diabetes, but in case you don't absorb all the information at your doctor's visit, here are some important terms and numbers that you should know:

> *A1c*: This is a test that measures our average BSL over the past 2–3 months. Your A1c level should be less than 7 percent.

> *β-cell*: These are the cells in our pancreas responsible for insulin.

> *Blood glucose*: This is also known as blood sugar. It is the main source of energy for our body.

> *Blood glucose level*: The amount of glucose present in our blood.

> *Body mass index (BMI)*: This is a measure that evaluates our weight relative to our height. It can determine if we are underweight, normal, or overweight.

> *Calorie*: A unit that represents the amount of energy provided by food.

> *Carbohydrate counting*: A meal-planning method that diabetics use to count the number of grams of carbohydrates in food.

> *Certified diabetes educator (CDE)*: A health care professional who has met the requirements to teach diabetes education.

> *Cholesterol*: A type of fat that is produced by our liver and found in the blood.

> *Combination therapy*: The usage of different medications together by type 2 diabetics to manage their BSLs.

> *Comorbidity*: The presence of one or more diseases in addition to a primary disease; often occurs with diabetes.

> *Endocrinologist*: A type of doctor who treats people with endocrine gland problems such as diabetes.

> *Euglycemia*: The term for the normal level of glucose in the body.

> *Fasting blood glucose test*: A check of our BSL after we have not eaten for 8–12 hours. It can be used to diagnose prediabetes or diabetes.

> *Glycemic index*: A ranking of foods based on their effects on blood glucose.

> *HDL cholesterol*: This is your good cholesterol. Men should aim for values over 40.

> *Hyperglycemia*: This refers to an excessive amount of blood sugar.

> *Hypertension*: Also known as high BP, it is a condition in which the blood flows through the vessels with a force greater than normal. A normal level of BP for diabetics is 130/80.

> *Hypoglycemia*: This is when one's blood glucose level is too low.

> *Neuropathy*: A disease of the nervous system; the most common form of neuropathy among diabetics is peripheral neuropathy, which affects the legs and feet.

> *Nutritionist*: A person with training in nutrition.

> *Obesity*: A condition where you have above the normal amount of fat in your body—a BMI greater than 30.

> *Pancreas*: The organ that makes insulin and enzymes used in digestion.

> *Polydipsia*: This means excessive thirst.

> *Prediabetes*: When blood sugar is at a higher than normal level but not high enough for the diagnosis of diabetes.

> *Retinopathy*: An eye disease that is caused by damage to the small blood vessels in the retina.

> *Sucralose*: A sweetener made from sugar but with no calories and no nutritional value.

> *Team management*: This means managing medical care with a team of health care professionals including a doctor, a dietician, a nurse, a diabetes educator, and others.

CHAPTER 15

Genitourinary Matters and Sexual Health

with Kaitlyn Barnes

Genitourinary (GU) simply refers to our genital and urinary organs—prostate gland, penis, testicles, urethra, the bladder, and the kidneys. These are grouped together because of their physical proximity in the body and because our reproductive organs and urinary system both use the urethra. The health problems that arise and compel men most frequently to seek medical care will involve disorders of the GU system, which can encompass prostate infections, erectile problems associated with aging and/or illness, and sexual diseases. Reviewed in this chapter are the GU and sexual health issues that become the concerns of middle-aged and older men more than younger men: prostatitis, benign prostatic hyperplasia, kidney stones, erectile problems, and sexually transmitted diseases (STDs) in later life. The two urogenital cancers—prostate cancer and bladder cancer—are addressed in chapter 19.

PROSTATE HEALTH

Physicians and medical researchers actually do not know all that the prostate gland does, but what is known is that the prostate contributes to both sexual and urinary function. So, take note: a healthy prostate is another reason to exercise, avoid obesity, eat your vegetables, keep fat intake low, quit smoking, and drink alcohol only in moderation. Each lifestyle decision directly affects your prostate and, in turn, your sexual health and risk of earlier death.

Contrary to popular belief, the prostate doesn't just start getting larger as we become older. In fact, it never stops growing after puberty, and it is the eventual enlargement of the prostate that causes most GU problems. It is natural for the prostate gland to enlarge as we age, but if it grows more rapidly than is ordinary, it is likely that you may encounter some type of prostate problem earlier in your lifetime than other men do. Nearly half of men after the age of 60 show evidence of at least one type of prostate trouble. Here's one common example:

> David mentioned that he's feeling frustrated. Because he has to get up sev-
> eral times each night to urinate, he isn't sleeping well. Sometimes he can't
> go back to sleep, which leaves him groggy, tired, irritable, and unable to
> concentrate for most of the day. What's especially driving him nuts is that
> David also has an urge to urinate while commuting, during his after work
> walks, and often while sitting in short meetings. He's stressed. (Reported
> by Brendan, a nurse practitioner)

To begin, it is important to know where your prostate is and what it does, as well as what distinguishes a healthy prostate from three different prostate problems: prostatitis (an inflammation), benign prostatic hyperplasia (BPH), and prostate cancer. If you are like most men, you probably are not exactly sure where the prostate is located, or what it does. The prostate is a gland found only in men and most other male mammals. About the size of a walnut in a healthy adult man, it was the size of a pea when you were born. It is somewhat firm; 30 percent of it is made up of muscular tissue, and the rest consists of glandular tissue. It is located between the

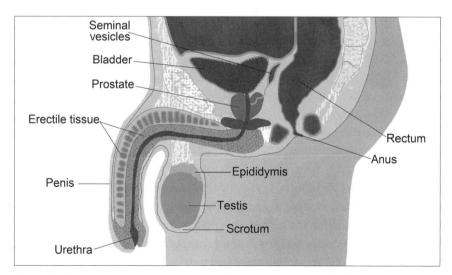

Figure 15.1. The male reproductive tract. Courtesy of ducu59us/Shutterstock.com.

bottom of the bladder and the base of the penis, and it backs onto the front wall of the rectum. The urethra (the tube that empties urine from the bladder through the penis) runs through the center of the prostate. The outer surface of the prostate gland is a layer of muscle called the *prostatic capsule*.

The prostate is a key part of men's reproductive system and has several purposes. The glands in the prostate produce nearly three-quarters of the milky white seminal fluid that is ejaculated during an orgasm. The urethra carries the seminal fluid through the penis, and as the prostate gland begins to empty during orgasm, it tightly squeezes the upper part of the urethra to prevent urination during ejaculation. During our climax, the muscular glands of the prostate pulse and propel forward the seminal fluid (and the sperm that was produced in the testicles). Men who have had a vasectomy ejaculate only the seminal fluid that is produced and stored in the prostate and none of the sperm cells made by the testicles. The prostate-specific antigen is the enzyme produced primarily by cells lining the ducts of the prostate gland to help keep the seminal fluid in its liquid form.

Problems with the prostate will not affect your ability to have an erection or ejaculate; however, prostate problems interfere with urination. In short, the prostate makes some of the fluid for semen, keeps urine out of the semen, and enhances pleasurable sensations of arousal and orgasm.

Prostate Exam

Since the prostate sits right in front of the rectum, the back portion of the prostate can be felt during a digital (or finger) rectal examination by your physician.

> No one likes the idea of [a rectal exam], and you certainly don't go around talking about it. (A man in his seventies)

> The [digital exam] might worry some guys, but it didn't worry me at all. It's all over quickly, and that's that. (A man in his sixties)[1]

The examination takes only a minute and should be entirely painless. If the exam is your first, you can expect that your physician will tell you that he needs to insert a single, gloved finger into your rectum in order to examine your prostate gland. Usually you will lie down and roll to one side, away from the physician, or you may be asked to simply bend over and rest the upper half of your body on the examination bed. The physician will cover a finger with a lubricant and insert his finger an inch into your rectum. Most men report that they feel a little pressure without any pain or physical discomfort. The discomfort you might experience is the odd sensation of having someone touch your anus and knowing that someone is doing this. A few seconds may elapse as the doctor waits for the sphincter muscle to relax, then he touches the rectal wall to determine the size of the prostate gland and moves his finger in a tight circular motion to feel the lobes and groove of the prostate gland. Most physicians continue to talk with you during the exam, and they let you know when they are removing the finger and using a premoistened wipe to remove excess lubricant. The exam is done.

Your physician would expect to have felt a firm and hard rubbery prostate gland. An enlarged, spongy gland may indicate either nonbacterial prostatitis or BPH. By age 50, about 25 percent of men suffer from symptoms of an enlarged prostate, and by age 80 up to one-third experience symptoms severe enough to require treatment.

Prostatitis

Prostatitis is an inflammation of the prostate gland and does not increase your risk of prostate cancer. This disease can affect men of any age, yet it begins to become common before we reach age 50 and triggers nearly 2 million physician visits annually.[2] Anywhere between 9 and 16 percent of men experience prostatitis; it accounts for one-quarter of all physician visits involving men's GU system, and perhaps as many as 50 percent of men will suffer from nonbacterial prostatitis / pelvic pain during their lifetime. Symptoms of chronic prostatitis—primarily pelvic pain and urinary burning, urgency, frequency, and hesitation—cause havoc on the quality of men's lives.[3]

Prostatitis can involve one of several types of inflammation and has been divided into four clinical categories: acute bacterial prostatitis, chronic bacterial prostatitis, nonbacterial prostatitis, and prostatodynia. Only 5–10 percent of prostatitis cases are caused by bacteria. With acute bacterial prostatitis, you experience the symptoms of an infection—fever, chills, nausea, body aches, and feeling lousy. This usually results from a bacterial infection from another area of the body which has invaded the prostate. The infection can also be caused by some of the bacteria within our urine. As the urine is being voided and traveling through the urethra, the bacteria may cross over and affect the adjacent prostate gland. Sometimes, though rare, men experience chronic bacterial prostatitis, because trace amounts of the bacteria "hide" in the prostate and didn't die with initial antibiotic treatment. Whether acute or chronic, bacterial prostatitis symptoms most often involve problems with ejaculation and urination: burning sensation when urinating (dysuria); difficulty urinating, such as dribbling or hesitant urination; frequent urination, particularly at night; urgent need to urinate; and pain or discomfort in the area between the penis and rectum (perineum), which you particularly notice when you sit. The infection is treated with antibiotics, and on occasion some men with a severe infection may need to be briefly hospitalized to flood the body with antibiotics.

You can also experience prostatitis that doesn't involve bacterial infection, and this is eight times more common than having an infection. The least understood and most difficult type of prostatitis to treat is called *chronic prostatitis* (or chronic pelvic pain syndrome), and it accounts for 80–90 percent of prostatitis diagnoses. The prostate is "inflamed" (swollen, irritated, painful), yet the causes are not clearly known. Urologists think that stress, irregular sexual activity, or a history of allergies might be contributing factors. Antibiotics are of no use, because there is no infection. Weirdly, the urine and semen usually contain higher-than-expected counts of the white blood cells that are typically produced to fight an infection, yet no bacteria is found when the urine specimen is examined. The other main type is *prostatodynia*, in which the pain and other symptoms tend to be localized to the prostate, with no obvious inflammation of the gland and no white blood cells in prostatic secretions.

The symptoms of nonbacterial prostatitis include frequent urination and urinary burning, genital pain, intermittent discomfort/pain in the lower abdomen and back for 3 months or longer, and an occasional discharge through the urethra during a morning bowel movement. For some men the symptoms persist, and for others the symptoms go away and return without warning, with the cycles varying in severity. Like other poorly understood conditions, nonbacterial prostatitis remains irksome. No single type of treatment is the gold standard. Some men use medication to reduce uric acid associated with gout, hot baths to provide symptom relief, anxiety/stress medication, biofeedback and relaxation training, and an added course of antibiotics just in case.

The exasperating symptoms of prostatitis will surely affect your quality of life. Whenever symptoms arise, it is best to immediately consult a physician. Episodes of prostatitis can have serious consequences if left untreated, even if treatment is not very effective. Pain is never a good sign, and it can be treated. Whenever you experience pelvic pain, painful urination or ejaculations, or difficulty urinating, see a doctor.

Benign Prostatic Hyperplasia

Of the hundreds of species of mammals, all of which have prostate glands, only men and man's best friend, dogs, are known to suffer from enlarged prostate.[4] Usually simply referred to as prostate enlargement, BPH is part of aging and can be maddening. As indicated by its name, BPH is

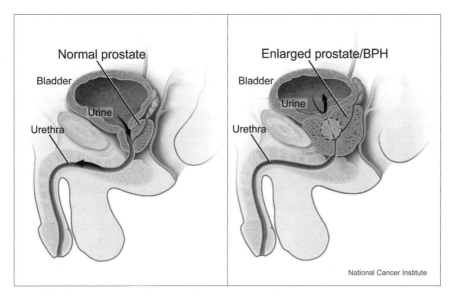

Figure 15.2. Normal and enlarged prostate. Courtesy of National Cancer Institute.

noncancerous. Perhaps half of men in their fifties and sixties begin to develop BPH. By age 80 it is likely that 90 percent of men will experience BPH, and only a third of these men will have symptoms that warrant treatment.

The prostate gland has two noticeable growth periods: one during early puberty and the other starting after age 40. Scientists are not certain why this second growth period starts and why the prostate enlarges as we age. One theory is that prostate gland cells are programmed to "reawaken" and trigger prostate growth. Other clinicians think that it is related to the gradual reduction in testosterone and the parallel increase in estrogen that occurs as we age. Whatever the actual cause(s), the gradual enlargement of the prostate to the size of a golf ball takes place as men age. As it enlarges, the prostate will often squeeze the urethra like a fist around a hose, making urination more troublesome. While benign, BPH is certainly bothersome.

The symptoms of BPH can vary greatly, but the most common ones involve changes or problems with urination—a need to strain or push to get the urine flowing; a hesitant, interrupted, weak stream while urinating; leaking or dribbling a bit after urinating; and more frequent urination, especially at night. Not welcomed are getting up to go to the bathroom two, three, four times a night; having difficulty urinating; and experiencing incomplete emptying of the bladder because of the difficulty in voiding when BPH squeezes the urethra. The American Urological Association has a symptom index (see p. 293) and raises the quality-of-life question: "How would you feel if you had to live with your urinary condition the way it is now, no better, no worse, for the rest of your life?" Rated on a scale from 0 to 6, would you say you would feel "delighted," "pleased," "mostly satisfied," "mixed feelings," "mostly not satisfied," "unhappy," or "terrible"?

Treatment options. Men who have BPH end up seeking treatment to relieve symptoms. Most physicians are wary of too early treatment when the gland is only mildly enlarged and the symptoms are not awfully troubling.[5] They recommend what is sometimes called "watchful waiting" as the first line of treatment. This is because the symptoms of BPH can completely disappear without treatment in a third or more of mild cases.

The Food and Drug Administration (FDA) has approved a handful of medications to relieve common symptoms. Most of the drugs are alpha blockers (technically, alpha-adrenergic blockers), which also are used to treat hypertension. In treating BPH, they relax the smooth muscle around the prostate to reduce the squeezing of the urethra and improve urine flow. The frequently used alpha blockers are doxazosin (Cardura), tamsulosin (Flomax), terazosin (Hytrin), and alfuzosin (Uroxatral). There are the standard precautions—tell your physician and pharmacist what prescription and nonprescription medications, vitamins, nutritional supplements, and herbal products you are taking or plan to take. There are serious complications when using some other medications, and feelings of drowsiness and dizziness are regularly experienced.

Another class of drugs known as *5-alpha inhibitors* is also regularly prescribed. Both finasteride (Proscar™) and dutasteride (Avodart™) treat BPH by blocking the body's production of a male hormone that causes the prostate to enlarge. Actually, they interfere with the enzyme that converts testosterone into an androgen, called *dihydrotestosterone* (DHT). Greater amounts of DHT are associated with prostate enlargement and male pattern baldness. These 5-alpha inhibitors appear to prevent further enlargement of the prostate and may actually shrink the prostate in some men. However, both drugs can also cause erectile difficulties and decreased libido and increase your risk of male breast cancer. This trade-off needs to be weighed carefully and discussed with your sexual partner.

A recent study[6] reported that men given a combination of dutasteride and tamsulosin had significantly improved symptoms of BPH compared to men who took either one alone; the combination significantly reduced the occurrence of the acute urinary retention problems. Consequently, the FDA approved Jalyn™ (dutasteride and tamsulosin), a single-capsule drug that combines the two popular BPH medications. This combination yields both sets of side effects: dizziness, drowsiness, sexual problems, and increased male breast size.

Many nonpharmaceutical therapies are also available and helpful. One of several types of microwave treatments and laser therapies is an option when the prostate becomes too large for good quality of life. Transurethral

AMERICAN UROLOGICAL ASSOCIATION SYMPTOM INDEX FOR BENIGN PROSTATIC HYPERPLASIA (BPH)

Symptom	Not at all	Less than 1 time in 5	Less than half the time	About half the time	More than half the time	Almost always
				Frequency		
1. Over the past month, how often have you had a sensation of not emptying your bladder completely after you finished urinating?	0	1	2	3	4	5
2. Over the past month, how often have you had to urinate again less than 2 hours after you finished urinating?	0	1	2	3	4	5
3. Over the past month, how often have you stopped and started again several times when you urinated?	0	1	2	3	4	5
4. Over the past month, how often have you found it difficult to postpone urination?	0	1	2	3	4	5
5. Over the past month, how often have you had a weak urinary stream?	0	1	2	3	4	5
6. Over the past month, how often have you had to push or strain to begin urination?	0	1	2	3	4	5
	None	1 time	2 times	3 times	4 times	5 or more
7. Over the past month, how many times did you most typically get up to urinate from the time you went to bed at night until the time you got up in the morning?	0	1	2	3	4	5

Total symptom score _____

Source: Barry, M. J., Fowler, F. J., O'Leary, M. P., et al. (1992). The American Urological Association symptom index for benign prostatic hyperplasia. The Measurement Committee of the American Urological Association. Journal of Urology, 148, 1549–1557.

Note: Your score will be between 0 and 35 points. Finding out whether your symptoms are mild (0 to 7), moderate (8 to 19), or severe (20 to 35) will help your doctor determine the best treatment for you.

microwave therapy (TUMT) uses microwave heat to burn away excess prostate tissue; it takes about an hour and can be completed as an outpatient. Similarly, photoselective vaporization of the prostate (PVP) is a minimally invasive procedure that uses a special high-energy laser. Both procedures reduce BPH symptoms and preserve sexual function. Treatment usually does not require general anesthesia and is performed in the urologist's

BPH Treatment for Moderate to Severe Symptoms

1. **Watchful Waiting**

2. **Medical Therapies**

   Alpha blockers

   - Alfuzosin
   - Doxazosin
   - Tamsulosin
   - Terazosin

   5-alpha reductase inhibitors

   - Dutasteride
   - Finasteride

   Combination therapy (alpha blocker and 5-alpha reductase inhibitor)

3. **Minimally Invasive Therapies**

   TUMT (transurethral microwave heat therapy)

   - TherMatrx™
   - CoreTherm™

   TUNA (transurethral needle ablation)

   HoLAP (holmium laser ablation)

4. **Surgical Therapies**

   TURP, laser, and similar surgeries

   - Transurethral electrovaporization
   - Transurethral incision of the prostate
   - Transurethral holmium laser resection
   - Transurethral laser vaporization
   - Transurethral laser visual laser ablation

   Prostatectomy

office or an outpatient setting. Your urologist will usually provide medication to reduce discomfort and help you relax during the procedure, and you might have the option to listen to your iPod or read during the procedure. Most men do not require a catheter after either procedure, and those who do typically are catheterized for less than 24 hours.

Another treatment strategy uses either high or low radiofrequency energy to burn away the excess prostate tissue. This noninvasive treatment applies precision-focused ultrasound waves to heat and destroy the targeted tissue. The procedure (called *transurethral needle ablation*, or TUNA) also involves inserting a scope into the urethra and then placing two small needles into the prostate. The needles permit electrodes to pinpoint and deliver radiofrequency energy directly to the obstructing prostate tissue.

As gruesome as any of these procedures might initially sound, they represent much more a psychological hurdle than having to deal with actual physical pain. Much like the oddity of your initial rectal exam, men are wary of the procedure until they've gone through it.

These less invasive strategies, however, may not fully relieve severe BPH complications. When this occurs, prostate surgery may be the last resort. The transurethral resection of the prostate (TURP) procedure is the most common of prostate surgeries. This surgical procedure involves no external incision. Instead, after general anesthesia, the surgeon reaches the prostate by inserting an instrument (a resectoscope) through the urethra and removes piece by piece the tissue squeezing the urethra. Most doctors and former patients swear by the TURP procedure—the disturbing symptoms of BPH are erased. Even though it takes several months after surgery to no longer pass blood in your urine and again achieve an erection without any difficulty, post-surgery most men are free of the maddening symptoms of their enlarged prostate.

Other surgical procedures (called *radical prostatectomy*) remove the prostate, are much more invasive, and have troublesome side effects such as incontinence and erectile dysfunction (ED). One study[7] reports that fewer than half of the men who had surgery (specifically, bilateral nerve sparing radical prostatectomy) felt that their sex lives had returned to normal within a year.

Although an enlarged prostate will eventually occur for nearly all men, there are some complications you don't have to accept and can treat. Most men who experience BPH can manage their mild to moderate symptoms with nonsurgical therapies and, often, nonpharmaceutical therapies. There are some herbal treatments. Even making some lifestyle changes can help control the symptoms and prevent your condition from worsening. For example, staying active rather than being a couch potato helps reduce symptoms, and it is commonly advised that you reduce your caffeine and alcohol intake, as well as not drinking anything for 2 hours before heading to bed.

KIDNEY STONES

Your kidneys are bean shaped and about the size of a man's fist. They really do look like kidney beans, just larger. They are located below the rib cage, one on each side of the spinal column. They regulate the body's fluid volume and electrolytes (which include sodium and calcium) by daily cleaning about 200 quarts of (dirty) blood, separating out roughly 2 quarts of extra water and waste products from the blood. The extra water and waste become urine, which is stored in your bladder until you urinate.

A kidney stone is a hard, crystal rock that forms in the kidney and is developed from calcium crystals and other salts that separate from the urine (see figure 15.3). The most common type of stone contains calcium in combination with either oxalate or phosphate. Kidney stones (sometimes called urinary stones) may be as small as a grain of sand or BB or, less often, even as large as a marble or golf ball.

Kidney Stone Symptoms That Warrant Seeing a Physician

- Extreme pain in your back or side that will not go away
- Cramping that causes vomiting
- Blood in your urine
- Burning feeling when you urinate
- Urine that looks cloudy and/or smells bad

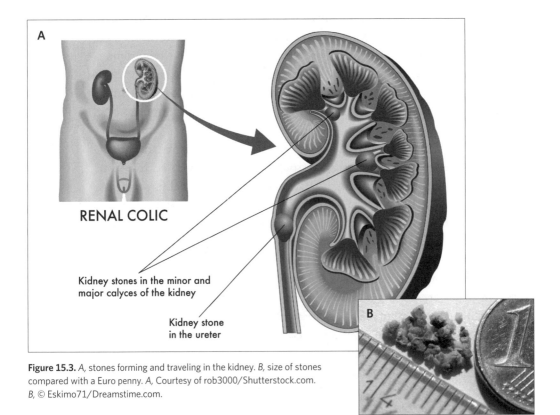

RENAL COLIC

Kidney stones in the minor and major calyces of the kidney

Kidney stone in the ureter

Figure 15.3. *A*, stones forming and traveling in the kidney. *B*, size of stones compared with a Euro penny. *A*, Courtesy of rob3000/Shutterstock.com. *B*, © Eskimo71/Dreamstime.com.

If you get one stone, you are at risk for another, and men's risk of kidney stones becomes more an issue as we get older. Kidney stones are common, affecting at least 12 percent of North American men by age 70.[8] For reasons that are not yet known, the percentage of people with kidney stones has been rising since 1980, and while the gender ratio is narrowing some, men are at three times greater risk than women.[9] Environmental and lifestyle factors play an important role in who is at risk. It is becoming apparent that kidney stones are associated with type 2 diabetes, hypertension, body size, and a diet that's high in sodium and sugar.[10] Some medications also raise men's risk of kidney stones, particularly some of the diuretics and calcium-containing antacids.

Normally, urine contains chemicals that prevent or inhibit calcium crystals from forming. These chemical inhibitors do not seem to work for everyone, causing some men to form the stones. Kidney stones may not produce symptoms until they begin to move down the tubes (ureters) through which urine empties into the bladder. When the crystals remain tiny (e.g., grains of sand), they will travel through the entire urinary tract and pass out of the body in the urine without being noticed. Bigger kidney stones, the size of a BB or so, also can be passed while urinating but not without discomfort. These "larger" stones may impede or block the flow of urine out of the kidneys. This causes swelling of the kidney and pain. The pain is usually severe.

Men who have never passed a kidney stone may not realize the severity of the symptoms. Some men report an abrupt piercing, cramping pain in the lower back or side near a kidney or groin. As a rule the pain increases and decreases in severity, somewhat like the rhythm of ocean waves. Compared to the discomfort of an enlarged prostate when voiding, a kidney stone is significantly more painful. As the (smaller) kidney stones work their way down into the bladder and through the urethra, they will normally cause some blood in the urine—the stones are most often jagged or knotty (resembling coral more than marbles), though some are smooth.

Quite obviously, stones as large as a marble will not pass through the urethra. This type of stone usually stays in the kidney, and if it becomes troublesome, your urologist will take steps to get rid of it. No longer is invasive surgery the first line of treatment. Urologists now use a range of more effective treatment alternatives. For example, when the stones are marble sized, extracorporeal shock-wave lithotripsy (ESWL) can be used to send shock waves directly to the kidney stone from outside your body. Lying on a table, a medical technician uses ultrasound or low-energy X-ray images to identify the exact location of the stone(s), followed by ultrasonic waves (or shock waves) to break up stones into tiny pieces. These pieces leave the body in the urine. Multiple ESWL treatments may be required, especially for multiple stones.

Larger and/or harder stones will necessitate more invasive intervention. The preferred method is percutaneous nephrostolithotomy, or "tunnel surgery." *Percutaneous* means that the procedure is done through the skin. The procedure involves a small skin puncture in your back and passing a tubular medical instrument (called a *nephroscope*) directly into the kidney. The scope creates the tunnel to the stone, which can be fragmented using ultrasonic waves, a laser, or electrohydraulic pressure (much like used in mining). The procedure necessitates general anesthesia and, often, a plastic tube (nephrostomy) temporarily left in the kidney and exiting from the back to assist in drainage of the urine for a few days.

The best prevention is to drink (more) water. Drinking lots of water helps to flush away the substances that form stones in the kidneys. Ironically, the good news is that regularly having a beer can help prevent kidney stones because beer provides an increase in magnesium intake, which helps prevent the calcium crystals from being formed in your kidneys; it is the stouts, porters, or other beers with lots of hops that are best.[11] Do not misinterpret this research, however. Beer is also a source of empty calories associated with men's belly fat (beer belly), and being overweight creates a greater risk for kidney stones and heart disease than the benefit of a beer is to preventing stones. If you are overweight, drink water.

SEXUAL HEALTH

In a society that is focused on and arguably obsessed with maintaining healthy lifestyles and now "healthy aging," it comes as no surprise that sexual health is also at the forefront of our attention. The cultural maxim suggests that so long as the man sexually performs, his manhood is unquestioned. But should he fail to get and sustain an erection, his sexual health is not in question; his masculinity is. For most men, our sexual well-being is equated with the expectation that sexual function should be reliable. As a 58-year-old man reported, "I suppose in the most simplistic terms, I associate getting an erection with being a man." Sexual performance proves masculinity, and impotence signals "failed" masculinity.

It is very likely that when men are partnered, healthy, and sexually active, sexual intercourse remains a routine dimension of a relationship. Researchers who study aging report that the salience of sexual activity slowly diminishes in its importance to relational intimacy as we age; however, "diminish" does not mean "end." Sexual desire and activity continue to play a vital part in most men's sense of self throughout their later years, whether gay or heterosexual.[12] Being partnered and remaining bodily unchallenged, men regard their sexuality as a dimension of a *relationship*, something managed by their own and their partners' sexual interest. Their sexuality is a taken-for-granted asset, like a heartbeat, until confronted by its failure.

Physiological aging and a decline in sexual function are not inevitably linked, even though much of the advertising for ED medication suggests as much. When, or if, sexual performance becomes a problem, the man first experiencing sexual difficulties may be turning 90, not 55. And, unlike his father's generation, he has options. Since the introduction of the oral drug sildenafil citrate (Viagra™) in March 1998, drug advertising airing during the evening news and baseball games has encouraged men to remain "forever functional."[13] At first, the advertisements targeted older men and presented ED drugs as a magic bullet to solve a man's impotence; however, the advertising now emphasizes a *couple's* sexual interests. Lifestyle sexual health medications such as Tadalafi and Cialis can be taken daily and remain active in the man's body for 24–36 hours.[14]

For more than a decade, the *AARP Magazine* has commissioned studies to better understand middle-aged and older men's (and women's) sexual lives and sexual attitudes. By all accounts, men's self-reported frequency of sex and the quality of their sexual relationship(s) have improved over the past 30 years. Indeed, though it's a pleasure that's falsely assumed to dwindle with aging, sex continues to play a very important part in many older men's and their partners' lives. Researchers regularly find that more middle-aged and older couples are having sex (and enjoyable, satisfying sex) than was found in earlier generations.[15]

Among men who maintain sexual interest—and most men do[16]—only one man in four is obliged to reformulate the meanings of sexual intimacy to bring it in line with his ED, which emerged as a result of an age-related health problem (such as diabetes) or a reaction to certain prescription drugs. Among older men who remain sexually active—and most men are[17]—their sexual activity may eventually shift to emphasize kissing, hugging, and sexual touching. The evolution of sexual activity from strictly coital sex to include other forms of sexual intimacy seems key to what sustains men's sexual satisfaction. As we get older, our sex becomes more interactive. There is more time allowed for foreplay and talking and laughing. Older lovers are more pleasure oriented, and we enjoy the process of warming up much more than when we were younger. We don't limit sex play to the genitals (see chapter 20).

Men's Birth Control: Vasectomy

Vasectomy is a safe and virtually foolproof birth control method. Men who have sought vasectomies are mostly white, married, and in their midthirties, and roughly a half million men seek a vasectomy every year in the United States. The surgical procedure takes about 30 minutes and involves blocking or cutting the tube (vas deferens) so that the man's ejaculate no longer contains sperm. "No scalpel" vasectomies are most common.

How an Erection Works

The penis comprises three long cylindrical chambers (see figure 15.4). The single, smaller chamber on the bottom (called *corpus spongisum*) encircles the urethra, which is the tube for urine and ejaculate. The two large chambers on top (called *corpora cavernosa*) comprise most of the erectile tissue. Erectile tissue is structured like a sponge, containing irregularly sized spaces. When you are aroused, the arteries running through the corpora cavernosa open up and the expandable erectile tissues in all three chambers fill with blood. This produces the erection. The erection begins when a man becomes sexually aroused from a touch, a thought, something seen, or even something heard. Nerves from the brain send messages to the penis, which allows blood to enter but not exit. The penis will grow in size and stiffen. It does not become erect by itself. Erection requires sensory or mental stimulation, or both—interaction between the brain and the body. Hormone messengers sent from the brain to the local nerves in the penis cause the smooth muscles of the corpora cavernosa to relax, allowing blood to flow in and fill the spaces—much like a dry sponge expanding as it soaks up liquid. Once the muscles in the penis contract and begin to stop the inflow of blood, they open outflow channels and the erection is reversed.

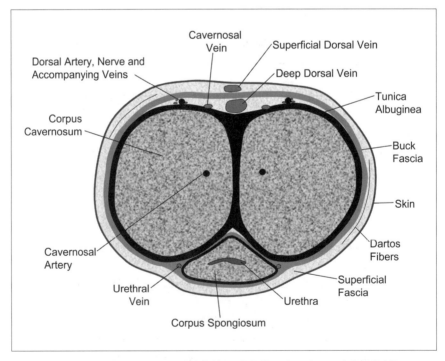

Figure 15.4. Anatomy of the penis. From A. P. S. Kirkham, R. O. Illing, S. Minhas, et al. (2008). MR imaging of nonmalignant penile lesions. *Radiographics, 28,* 837-853, figure 1.

Expert opinion in sexual medicine indicates that having erections—with or without sex—helps preserve our sexual function. The clinical evidence suggests that men age 55–75 who have long periods without sexual arousal more likely have erectile difficulties. In addition, should you stop engaging in sexual activity, including masturbation, you've added to the risk of not being able to get or sustain an erection. Sexual arousal causes oxygenated blood to flow into the penis, and when this occurs, the health of the smooth muscles, nerve fibers, and blood vessels responsible for erectile function is maintained. A European study of nearly 1,000 older Finnish men found that the men who had infrequent sexual intercourse (less than once a week) doubled the risk of developing erectile difficulties.[18]

Is the message that we need to "use it or lose it"? Maybe not. Most men have several spontaneous erections each night while sleeping. Just by having erections at night, even in the absence of sexual activity, we have built-in neurobiological protection against any erosion of our erectile capabilities.

It is the smooth muscle of the penis, a type of muscle that can only relax and contract around the blood vessels, that lets blood flow into the three chambers to cause the penis to become erect. The pharmaceutical revolution that occurred in the late 1990s targeted those smooth muscles. Viagra, Levitra, and Cialis are PDE-5 inhibitors designed to block phosphodisterase type 5 (PDE-5), the enzyme that breaks down the erection-producing chemical in our bodies. The ED drugs relax smooth muscle cells and widen blood vessels to enable the penis to fill with blood, enhance the hardness and duration of an erection, and increase the ability to achieve a new erection shortly after ejaculation.

ERECTILE DYSFUNCTION

Occasional erection problems happen to most men. If you can't maintain an erection long enough to have successful intercourse in over half of your attempts, you are experiencing ED. This varies in severity: it can be a total inability to achieve an erection, an inconsistent ability to do so, or an inability to maintain an erection for satisfactory sexual relations. ED severity has been assessed by the five-item International Index of Erectile Function, IIEF-5, which is also referred to as the Sexual Health Inventory for Men.[19] Summing the responses to the five items provides you an IIEF score, and, based on the sum, ED severity is classified into the following five categories: severe ED (5–7), moderate (8–11), mild to moderate (12–16), mild (17–21), and no ED (22–25). Very few men have ED severe enough that they have no erectile response at all. But many men, especially as we get older and our heart health has been compromised, may experience some problems with erections.

It is estimated that nearly one-quarter to one-half of men will report some erectile difficulties,[20] and roughly 5 percent of 40-year-old men versus 25–30 percent of 60-year-old men experience moderate to severe erectile problems.[21] The pervasiveness of the condition is a result of the greater number of older men in the nation's population. Erectile problems are associated with higher rates of chronic health problems—diabetes, obesity, hypertension, heart disease—and the medications and treatments used to manage these chronic conditions.[22] Many drugs, both prescription and nonprescription, also interfere with the erectile response, particularly medication for lowering cholesterol or blood pressure. If you are taking regular medication for any health issues, do check your drugs for their side effects.

The onset of ED usually occurs slowly as a result of our health, but ED can be an unexpected side effect of surgery, trauma, or a new medication. By whatever way ED emerges, being unable to either have or sustain an erection causes distress, challenging men's self-esteem and, at times, their sexual relationship(s). Commenting on how his self-esteem was rocked, one man disclosed,

Common Causes of Erectile Dysfunction

- Coronary artery disease
- Diabetes
- Hypertension
- Kidney disease
- Medications (e.g., antidepressants, antiarrhythmics, antihypertensives)
- Smoking
- Heavy alcohol use
- Prostate surgery
- Trauma to spine or pelvis
- Anxiety

> Oh it was knocking [me] terrible. . . . I work with other men and I think it [my ED] knocked my confidence in certain ways. Not outwardly. Outwardly, it always seemed that I was one of the lads and that I was okay . . . but inside . . . I didn't feel that I was matching up to them. I just felt I wasn't as good as them basically.[23]

As a result of direct marketing to consumers, researchers find that more middle-aged and older men now feel an unrelenting pressure to be as sexually fit as they were when younger.[24] Is it surprising that Pfizer sold approximately 1 billion pills in the first decade after Viagra™ was introduced?[25]

The first line of defense that will protect your sexual health and erectile functioning isn't taking ED drugs; rather, it is to take steps to improve your overall health, especially your heart health. If you smoke, this means quit smoking. The incidence of ED is nearly twice as great in men who are smokers compared to nonsmokers.[26] Study after study shows that cigarette smoking has an awfully negative effect on a man's ability to have or sustain an erection.[27] In one study, for example, men who smoke more than 20 cigarettes a day had a 60 percent higher risk of ED, compared to men

INTERNATIONAL INDEX OF ERECTILE FUNCTION (IIEF-5)

Over the past 6 months

	Very low 1	Low 2	Moderate 3	High 4	Very High 5
1. How do you rate your confidence that you could get and keep an erection?	Very low / 1	Low / 2	Moderate / 3	High / 4	Very High / 5
2. When you had erections with sexual stimulation, how often were your erections hard enough for penetration?	Almost never / 1	A few times (much less than half the time) / 2	Sometimes (about half the time) / 3	Most times (much more than half the time) / 4	Almost always / 5
3. During sexual intercourse, how often were you able to maintain your erection after you had penetrated your partner?	Almost never / 1	A few times (much less than half the time) / 2	Sometimes (about half the time) / 3	Most times (much more than half the time) / 4	Almost always / 5
4. During sexual intercourse, how difficult was it to maintain your erection to completion of intercourse?	Extremely difficult / 1	Very difficult / 2	Difficult / 3	Slightly difficult / 4	Not difficult / 5
5. When you attempted sexual intercourse, how often was it satisfactory for you?	Almost never / 1	A few times (much less than half the time) / 2	Sometimes (about half the time) / 3	Most times (much more than half the time) / 4	Almost always / 5

who never smoked.[28] To improve your erectile health also means taking up a healthy low-fat, low-sodium, and low-cholesterol diet; cutting back on the alcohol; and getting more exercise. Exercise alone improves blood flow, gets the (bad) cholesterol out of your blood, and improves libido and mood. Cutting back on the alcohol decreases the risk that you will experience a limp penis.

When health problems or one of your medications interfere and lifestyle changes are not enough to overcome your erectile difficulties, there are effective ED medications. Viagra, Levitra, and Cialis have revolutionized the treatment of erectile troubles and virtually replaced the complicated and painful options that existed before the mid-1990s. But these ED drugs are not miracle cures. The medications work via a very complicated series of biochemical reactions to help create an erection. The drugs do not produce desire, nor do they affect your libido. You have to be sexually aroused for the drugs to have any effect. When you are "turned on," the medication kicks in.

You also need a partner who accepts or supports your use of the erection-assisting medication; otherwise, the sexual experience will not result in a pleasant experience for either you or your partner.[29] When you and your partner are in sync about you using an ED drug, the research suggests that there are significant improvements in the quality of sexual relations, men's self-esteem and hardness confidence, and partners' reports of sexual satisfaction (see also chapter 20).[30]

Side effects, when reported, can include temporary vision changes (in the case of Viagra), back pain and muscle aches (in the case of Levitra), indigestion, headache, flushing of the skin, and a stuffy or runny nose. It is rare, but a few men have reported hearing and vision loss and an erection that will not go away.

Sex researchers caution that it can be difficult for heterosexual men's wives to fully understand what effects ED has on men. To bridge this gap, you should talk to your partner about your feelings, your erectile difficulties, and your sexual preferences going forward. Without the conversation, it is understandable that your sexual partner might use sexual myths to guide him or her and falsely presume that your erectile difficulties equal impotence, or he or she might mistakenly believe that avoiding sex altogether is helpful. Hence, have an in-depth conversation with your partner about your sexual health and your and your partner's sexual intimacy preferences.

SEXUALLY TRANSMITTED DISEASES AND INFECTIONS

Most sexually transmitted infections (STIs) and STDs are passed from one person to the next through contact with an infected sexual partner's bodily fluids such as semen, pre-ejaculate (the few drops of semen that are released before ejaculation), vaginal secretions, and blood. Yet some types of STIs (e.g., human papillomavirus, or HPV) and STDs (e.g., herpes, cytomegalovirus, syphilis) can be transmitted simply through intimate contact, including kissing and touching. STDs are caused by viruses, bacteria, or parasites that survive in moist, warm surroundings such as your mouth, urethra, anus, and a woman's vagina. Take note: there are more than 25 different infections or diseases that may be spread from one person to another when the contact is vaginal intercourse, oral sex, anal sex, or (sometimes) even kissing. The surest way to avoid transmission of STDs is to be in a long-term mutually monogamous relationship with a partner who is known to be uninfected.

STDs are more widespread among middle-aged and older adults than you might first think, and your risk of getting an STD does not decrease just because you are getting older. In fact, the risk of getting an STD has more than doubled in the past 10–15 years for men age 50 and older.[31] Experts attribute this marked rise of infection rates among boomer-age and older men to sociological trends, such as higher midlife divorce rates and the straightforwardness of online dating services to meet new sexual partners, as well as to a greater open-mindedness among Americans about having sex (or a sexual relationship) outside a marriage or monogamous partnership. Expert opinion also acknowledges that the principal reason for the escalation of STDs is a lack of sexual knowledge and failure to engage in safer sex.[32]

What increases a mature man's risk? The risk boils down to one basic lesson: you're at risk of contracting an STI if you take on a new sexual partner, and you are at great risk if you do not practice "safer sex." It isn't unusual for boomer-age and older men to have a new partner or multiple partners. Many divorced and widowed men begin dating again, and they are very likely to become involved with multiple new partners. Perhaps as a consequence of the "newness" of dating again and the availability of multiple partners, research shows that this group of men engages in sex more often than same-age married men. The use of ED drugs by some of these men also seems to further add to their risk of an STD, by making sex possible and by engaging in higher-risk sexual behavior, whether by the number or type of sexual encounters or not using a condom.[33] The lesson is that dating again fuels the risk of picking up an STD and passing it to a partner, often without knowing it.[34]

In addition, more middle-aged and older married men are having sex outside marriage compared to prior generations. A 2009 AARP study found that one-fifth of the men (age 45 and older) acknowledged already having had a sexual relationship outside their primary relationship. And a report from the Centers for Disease Control and Prevention (CDC) estimated that 6 percent of married men had sexual contact with more than one opposite-sex partner during the past year.[35] Because these estimates are based on what men report and there has been a stigma against having sex outside marriage, the AARP's and CDC's estimates are surely conservative. The likelihood of a married man becoming involved in what is sometimes still called an "extramarital" relation is highest during the early years of marriage, decreases to a low point until about the time of the eighteenth wedding anniversary, and thereafter increases continuously.[36] Knowing this, is it surprising that 40 percent of middle-aged men and one-third of older men say they did *not* feel it is "always wrong" to have sex with someone other than a partner, particularly when their partner either has dementia or is physically ill and cannot have sex?[37]

Experts say that we are more likely to find a new sexual partner when we are involved in a "sexless marriage"—one in which a couple make love no more than 10 times a year, whether the cause is someone's physical health or loss of interest. Among men age 50–65, roughly 20 percent of their marriages fall into this category.[38] In the same study, 85–90 percent of the men felt that a satisfying sexual relationship was important to their quality of life. The takeaway message here is that men who value the importance of sex are apt to pursue a new sexual liaison.[39]

The risk of an STI among middle-aged and older men is markedly increased because they are less likely to use condoms. One study reveals that roughly 90 percent of men over age 50 did not use a condom when they had sex with a date or casual acquaintance, and 70 percent didn't even do so when they had sex with someone they just met.[40] In another study, just 12 percent of the sexually active men age 50 and older who were unmarried and actively dating reported regularly using a condom.[41] Perhaps after years of being with one partner, men build up a false confidence that they're not at risk of an STD. This is, of course, magical thinking and puts you at great risk.

In addition, most boomer-age and older men who used condoms 30 years ago didn't enjoy the experience, and many aren't aware of the new generation of thin condoms that do not take away from erotic sensations. Condoms are now sold in various colors, tastes, shapes, and packaging to match personal preferences. All condoms must comply with FDA requirements—they must be constructed to be protective. Correct and consistent use of condoms will sharply reduce the risk of getting an STD.

Whatever the cause—midlife divorce, widowers dating again, a sexual liaison outside marriage, online dating, high-risk sex, or simple ignorance—imagine the following: You have just been to the doctor and received the devastating news that you have an STD. Do not be hesitant to find out what this means for your health and your future sexual activity. Can you control the symptoms, and are the effects of men's STDs more serious than just embarrassing?

Chlamydia is the most commonly reported bacterial-based STI men encounter and is spread through vaginal or anal intercourse. Chlamydia can be diagnosed using a sample of urine. The most common site of the infection is inside the urethra (the tube through which men urinate and pass sperm). During unprotected sex, the bacteria are transferred through genital fluids from one partner to the other. Symptoms include watery discharge from the penis or anus, burning pain during urination, and painful intercourse; a symptom *may* show up within 1–3 weeks after having sex, yet one-quarter of men with chlamydia remain symptomless and unknowingly affect their partners' sexual health. Because it is bacterial, it can be treated with antibiotics; if untreated, it can lead to pneumonia, serious urinary tract infection, and even eye infections.

There really are new, super thin, and not-so-tight condoms on the market these days. The thinner condoms balloon slightly over the penis, with a layer of lubricant, and then there's an outer thin skin that makes sure that sperm can't leak out. Men tell me they feel great and are very sexy and effective.

Source: Schwartz, P. (2010, May). Not your grandma's condoms. AARP.

HPV and *genital warts* are closely related. There are more than 40 different types of HPV, and most have no symptoms among men. As of this writing, there is no test to find HPV in men. Though most men who get any type of HPV are asymptomatic and never develop noticeable health problems, passing on this virus to a female partner can lead to serious and irreversible damage, such as causing her cervical cancer. HPV is transferred through genital contact, usually during vaginal and anal sex. It may also be passed on during oral sex. Practicing safer sex (using a condom) protects the health of all of your partners, present and future, as well as yourself.

Some types of HPV infect men's genital areas, including the skin on and around the penis or anus; other types can infect the mouth and throat. The more common HPV infections cause genital warts; some forms of HPV can cause penile, anal, or head and neck cancer. The types of HPV that cause genital warts are not the same as the types that can cause cancer. Genital warts are small, flat or raised, cauliflower shaped, and found on the penis, testicles, or anus. They can show up in just a few weeks but up to even 8 months after having sex with someone infected with HPV. The warts don't go away on their own, and left untreated, they can be painful, eventually growing to block the opening of the urethra. Because HPV cannot be cured, topical medication (involving trichloracetic acid) or laser surgery can remove the warts, yet the warts may recur since the virus stays in your body.

Hepatitis B (HBV) is a viral infection involving the liver; there is no cure for men already infected. You may have already contracted hepatitis B and do not know it, because most men who are infected are asymptomatic. This virus is spread during vaginal, oral, or anal sex, and it's "incubation" period lasts 6 weeks to 8 months. If you are having sex with an infected partner, your risk is greatest when exposed to blood and a bit less when exposed to other body fluids (e.g., semen, vaginal secretions). Men having sex with men are at greater risk than men exclusively having sex with women. The onset of symptoms causes flu-like feelings that don't go away, nagging tiredness, discolored or dark urine, and liver damage and consequently becoming jaundiced (or yellowing of the skin). Even though there is a possibility that this infection may clear up on its own, some men suffer through chronic infections for many years.

Gonorrhea ("the clap") remains a common STD. This, too, is bacterial and treatable with antibiotics. Gonorrhea is spread through contact with the vagina, anus, penis, or mouth; to reiterate, you can become infected without intercourse or ejaculation occurring, since transferring the bacteria from the infected person to you occurs simply by direct contact. The bacteria usually grow in your urinary track, but they can also be found in your anus, mouth, and throat. Roughly 10 percent of men with gonorrhea have no symptoms at all. Most men, however, begin to have symptoms within 2–5 days after infection, while some symptoms can take as long as 15–30 days to appear. The typical symptoms include a pus-like discharge from the penis, a burning or painful sensation when urinating caused by urethritis, or a rectal infection that includes discharge, soreness, and anal itching caused by proctitis. Many men will also experience epididymitis, a painful condition where bacteria has spread from the urethra into the ducts attached to the testicles. Untreated, gonorrhea is dangerous—it can cause heart problems, kidney problems, arthritis, and disorders of the central nervous system. Once diagnosed, the disease is easily treatable with an antibiotic, either in pill form or by injection; if it's an injection, a single dose is usually all that is required. Oral antibiotics require a longer course of treatment. Common antibiotics are ofloxacin, cefixime, and ceftriaxone.

The *herpes* simplex virus has two variations: type 1 (or HSV-1) isn't common and most likely affects the lips and mouth in the form of cold sores; the more common strain (HSV-2) emerges in the genital and anal area. HSV-2 is one of the most common STDs and will show up 2–7 days after having sex, though the symptoms can emerge as late as 30 days after having sex. A small proportion of men can have no symptoms, but most do. Common symptoms include small, painful blisters on the penis or mouth that will burst, leaving small, equally painful sores; itching or tingling sensations in the genital or anal area; and flu-like symptoms that involve swollen glands or fever. The blisters last 1–3 weeks and will go away untreated, but you still have herpes. Herpes cannot be cured. Once the first outbreak of blisters subsides, the herpes virus goes dormant and hides in the nerve fibers near the infection site. Symptoms may come back later, particularly during times of stress, in less severe and shorter episodes.

HIV/AIDS is a viral-based STD that is the most serious and potentially deadly of all STDs. The number of men age 50 and older living with the human immunodeficiency virus (HIV) has been increasing in recent years; this age cohort accounts for 15 percent of new HIV diagnoses and roughly 25 percent of all HIV/AIDS cases.[42] The increase has multiple causes; for example, many boomer-age and older men are having unprotected sex with new partners,[43] and the antiretroviral therapy (HAART) has made it possible for many HIV-infected men and women to live longer, even though their HIV can never be cured and can continue to be spread through unsafe sex.

HIV is primarily transmitted during vaginal, anal, or oral sex. One-third of all new cases of HIV/AIDS occur among men exposed through high-risk heterosexual relations; half of the new cases occur among men who have sex with men. The rates of HIV are 12 times greater among black men than white men, and five times higher among Hispanic men than white men.[44] HIV symptoms develop slowly, usually showing up over the course of several months, but maybe not until several years have passed after contact with the virus. Men and women living with HIV may not know that they have it, since they could remain asymptomatic and undiagnosed for several years; it is this group that is most likely to unknowingly spread the virus when engaging in unsafe sex.

It is difficult to first notice that you have HIV; the most common symptoms are weight loss and tiredness, flu-like symptoms that just don't go away, diarrhea, and, sometimes, white spots in the mouth. Because of the stigma of HIV/AIDS, middle-aged and older men may be reluctant to see a physician or seek HIV testing. If you have been recently dating, regular HIV testing is recommended. When you see your physician for a regular checkup, it's likely that he or she will underestimate your sexual activity or else not discuss it at all and, in turn, not offer HIV testing or discuss prevention. Take charge and talk to your physician. While treatment for this infection can significantly prolong an infected man's life, for far too many men (and women) this infection eventually progresses to AIDS and, in the end, death.

Syphilis ("the pox") is another bacterial infection that is usually transmitted through vaginal, oral, and anal intercourse, as well as kissing. It's very contagious when the infected person has sores, yet not as contagious when the infection is temporarily inactive. It is very easy to cure in its early stages. A single injection of penicillin will cure a person who has had syphilis for less than a year. For someone who has had it for longer than a year, additional doses of an antibiotic are necessary. Not many cases of syphilis occur among people aged 50 and older, and two-thirds of recent cases of syphilis were among men who have sex with men. The CDC recommends that men who have sex with men be tested for syphilis annually.[45]

When syphilis is undiagnosed and untreated, the infection can go through three phases, and its symptoms can be difficult to recognize. During the first phase, the symptoms include painless sores (or ulcers) on the mouth, lips, genitals, or anus; they show up sometime between 3 and 12 weeks after exposure and last roughly a month. These sores (called *chancres*) not only spread syphilis but also make it easier to transmit and acquire the HIV infection sexually. The sores fade away after a month, but you still have syphilis. Left untreated, the infection progresses to the second phase, and new symptoms appear, ranging from body rashes, even on the soles of the feet and palms of the hands, to flu-like feelings such as fever, fatigue, weight loss, muscle aches, and swollen glands in the groin. These symptoms may also come and go for 2 years. Finally, should the infection continue to be untreated, it becomes a tertiary infection that eventually damages the brain and heart. This occurred too often for men several generations back. Whatever damage was caused by the infection before it is treated cannot be undone. This STD can be diagnosed through a blood test and/or examination of the fluid that oozes from the sores.

SAFER SEX

Aside from sexual intimacy in a trustworthy monogamous relationship, there's only one foolproof way to avoid an STI or STD—to abstain from sex. But this isn't a realistic option for men who enjoy sexual intimacy. The best alternative is to practice "safer sex" (not safe sex). *Safer sex* means taking precautions during sexual activity to protect yourself from getting an STD and to help prevent STDs from being spread to your partner. It recognizes that the risk of STD transmission isn't assured, because there is no way of knowing with certainty that a new sexual partner is not already infected. Practicing safer sex doesn't mean eliminating sex from your life, nor does it mean eliminating erotic feelings. What it does mean is being smart and staying healthy. It requires prior planning and good communication between partners. It means showing love and respect for your partner(s) and for yourself. Safer sex means enjoying sex to the fullest without acquiring or transmitting sexually related infections.

One of the best methods to lower the per-act risk of STD transmission is for men to use condoms when engaging in vaginal, anal, or oral intercourse. Condom use isolates body fluids and thus helps us avoid contact with vaginal fluids, semen, or blood, should your partner be infected and absolutely unaware of being infected. Incorrect condom use, not just the bad decision to not use a condom, may also lead to STD transmission, since transmission can occur with a single act of intercourse with an infected partner (see insert on correct condom use).

All in all, condoms and communication make sex much safer. Typically, condoms are meant to fit any average-sized penis (approximately 4–7 inches). Early studies on heterosexual transmission of an STD established that male-to-female transmission to the vagina was significantly more likely than female-to-male transmission from the vagina, and the early evidence also showed that being the receptive partner in unprotected penile-anal intercourse is associated with a high risk of an STI.[46] These patterns urge us to recognize that protecting the health of our partner (and ourself) is best accomplished by discussing and using safer sex practices and being honest about our sexual history. Step up, be responsible, and have fun experiencing the sexual intimacy you want and deserve.

How to Use a Condom Correctly

- Use a new condom for every act of vaginal, anal, and oral sex throughout the *entire* sex act (from start to finish).

- Before any genital contact, put the condom on the tip of your erect penis with the rolled side out.

- Do not unroll the condom before placing it on the penis.

- If the condom does not have a reservoir tip, pinch the tip enough to leave a half-inch space for semen to collect.

- Holding the tip, unroll the condom all the way to the base of the erect penis.

- Make sure to always eliminate any air in the tip to help keep the condom from breaking.

- If you feel the condom break, stop immediately, withdraw from your partner, and put on a new condom.

- After ejaculation and before the penis gets soft, grip the rim of the condom and carefully withdraw from your partner.

- Remove the condom by gently pulling the condom off your penis, making sure that semen doesn't spill out.

- Wrap the condom in a tissue and throw it in the trash where others won't handle it.

- Ensure that adequate lubrication is used during vaginal and anal sex, which might require water-based lubricants. Oil-based lubricants (e.g., petroleum jelly, shortening, mineral oil, massage oils, body lotions, and cooking oil) should not be used because they can weaken latex, causing breakage.

Source: Department of Health and Human Services (2010). *Male latex condoms and sexually transmitted diseases: Condom fact sheet in brief.* Atlanta: Centers for Disease Control and Prevention.

CHAPTER 16

Bone, Joint, and Muscle Health

with Alison Ashley

There are few sure things in life, but one certainty you can rely on is that as long as we are living and breathing, our bodies will be changing. The very good news for all of us is that with medical advances, improved living conditions, and increased understanding of healthful practices, we are living longer and without as many health problems. However, our bodies are bound to experience wear and tear over time, and this certainty is compounded by the physiological changes that occur naturally as we age. Understanding the changes taking place in your musculoskeletal system will help you identify what part of your destiny you have control over and how best to take hold of that control. This feeling of control is particularly important when coming to terms with the strengths and vulnerabilities of your body's skeletal and muscle infrastructure.

"Oh my aching back!" Few if any mature men have escaped back pain. As we get older, it also seems that a common dinner conversation can turn to the new ache and pain that we experience. This is why we thought it so important to devote an entire chapter to topics such as basic back mechanics, bursitis, tendonitis, arthritis, sports injuries, osteoporosis, and fall prevention. Given that there are many factors that impact the health of men's bones, muscles, and joints, this chapter will also point to topics such as exercise physiology, nutrition, kinesiology, alternative medicine, and health practices such as acupuncture, biofeedback, yoga, Tai Chi, meditation, homeopathy, and massage. We outline steps that you can take to increase your chances of living successfully with various musculoskeletal conditions. Although musculoskeletal changes naturally occur over time as we age, many of the problems we experience are not always age related or inevitable as we grow older.

BONES, CARTILAGE, MUSCLES, AND TENDONS

The musculoskeletal system is made up of bones, cartilage, joint configurations, muscles, and tendons. Bones provide us with physical structure, as well as support and protection for soft tissue structures (like the heart and brain). Like all mammals, our skeleton first begins as cartilage tissue, which is slowly replaced by bone through a process known as *ossification*.[1] Think about that soft spot on a newborn's head and how it slowly "disappears." The cartilage surrounding joint surfaces, however, does not develop into bone, nor does it contain blood vessels or nerves. It remains a tough, elastic, flexible tissue that forms protective coverings at the ends of bones and is vital to healthy joint function.

The rigid elements of our skeleton meet at joints, or "articulations," and our joints differ by their structure and amount of movement. To make quick sense of this, think about the movement found in the ball-and-socket (or *synovial*) joints of our knee and shoulder versus a slightly moveable joint that may not contain a fluid-filled joint cavity, such as where two vertebrae meet in the spine. All healthy, moveable joints are composed of bones with smooth cartilage coverings (figure 16.1) and are lubricated with a thin layer of synovial fluid. There is actually a capsule covering the joint that contains the synovial membrane, and the capsule is reinforced with fibrous ligaments that link bone to bones to provide stability to the joints during their motion.[2] With normal aging, the cartilage in joints thins, the synovial fluid decreases in quantity and quality, and our ligaments become stiffer and lose flexibility, collectively preventing us from leaping out of a chair when sitting.

Muscles and tendons are the other key musculoskeletal structures. Muscles turn into tendons close to where they join the bone, and our tendons are more fibrous and thinner than our muscles. Together they provide stability to the joint when it is moving. If you touch the back of your heel, you will feel the biggest tendon in your body, the Achilles tendon, which connects the calf muscle to your heel bone. With normal aging, both muscle mass and the diameter of tendons decrease and the tissues become drier and stiffer, causing a natural decrease in strength and endurance.

A healthy musculoskeletal system is like a fine-tuned machine. However, injury, overuse, or just plain old wear and tear result in problems that are often first noticed when pain becomes a factor. Pain is like a check engine light coming on in your car. If you don't take care of the underlying issue, the problem will not go away and the vehicle (whether your body or car) may ultimately break down and become immobilized when you least want it to.

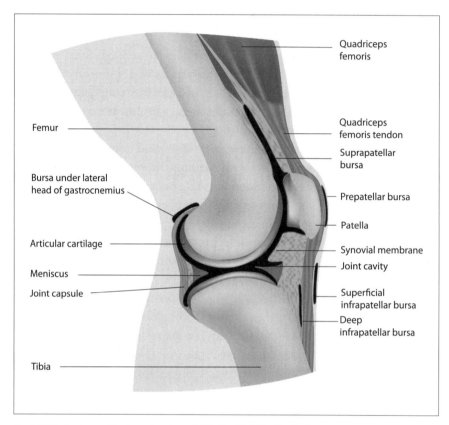

Figure 16.1. Anatomy of the knee. Courtesy of Alila Sao Mai / Shutterstock.com.

BACK PAIN

According to the National Institutes of Health, back pain is one of the most common reasons that Americans see their physician. Studies suggest that back pain bothers men and women equally, despite the fact that men are more often overweight, have an unhealthier lifestyle, and have more physically stressful types of work and job-related injuries.[3] Men do complain of exercise- and sports-related back pain more often than women. Fortunately, most back pain is temporary and will go away with time or when using over-the-counter pain relievers (acetaminophens such as Tylenol) or anti-inflammatory medication (ibuprofens such as Advil and Motrin). Not to be misconstrued, there are episodes when back pain can be caused by serious, lingering conditions such as compressed nerves and inflamed muscles.

Let's consider the mechanics of back pain. The spine is composed of bones, joints, nerves, and soft tissues, and it's the soft tissues that usually cause back pain. The discs—the structure that lies between the vertebrae (spinal bones)—definitely can be the source of pain, but more often it is the soft tissues (muscles and ligaments) in the back that become injured. Because the lower back supports most of the body's weight, a back ache may come from standing or sitting too long, lifting a heavy object, an athletic injury, or an accident. When standing or lifting, the soft tissues are constantly moving and can get pulled or strained. Strains may happen abruptly while lifting something heavy, but more commonly they come about slowly as a result of activities that involve repetitive movements such as prolonged bending when using a belt sander or weeding a garden.

It might initially seem unbelievable, but sitting can actually be worse for your back than standing or bending. Sitting is more complicated than standing. The soft muscles can get more tired when only the lower discs in the spine carry the weight of our torso and head. This is especially true if we are overweight or out of shape. Your center of gravity shifts to your "sitting bones" (or bones in your buttocks) and tailbone at the base of the spine, and in this position it takes considerable muscular force to sit upright. Riding in motor vehicles is notoriously hard on your back, because it involves prolonged periods of sitting and exposure to vibration. By contrast, when you stand, you are able to distribute your weight throughout your spine and back muscles, rather than the few discs and muscles in the lower back.

When is a chair not a chair?

When it becomes an instrument of torture.

Research also has shown that psychological factors such as stress, anxiety, and negative mood all increase the likelihood of developing acute or longer-lasting back pain.[4] Smokers are at greater risk, and being physically out of condition is an important reason why men have a recurrence of the "sprain and strain" type of back pain. Low doses of certain antidepressants, particularly tricyclic antidepressants, have been found to relieve chronic back pain, perhaps because chronic pain and depression depend on the neurotransmitters serotonin and norepinephrine to produce the sensation of pain. Importantly, people with lower back pain may get relief by regularly doing yoga, and many men rely on hands-on therapies such as chiropractic care and massage rather than pharmaceutical therapies.

MUSCLES AND MUSCLE INJURIES

Perhaps the most common problems with muscles throughout your life, regardless of age, are the aches and pains that result from their daily use.

We all have experienced the overuse of a muscle and how this causes soreness and discomfort, or a strain or tear resulting from extreme overuse of that same muscle. Muscle aches also can be the result of a fever or nervous tension.

Muscle cramps differ from aches. They are always sudden, painful, involuntary muscle contractions, and they are the most common problem in leg muscles. Have you ever been virtually frozen by the piercing pain of a Charlie horse? Cramps usually occur when a muscle is overworked from a long period of exercise or physical labor, and they especially occur if you are dehydrated. The best advice to prevent a muscle cramp is to stretch out the muscle and to be sure to hydrate prior to engaging in strenuous activity. Once you get a cramp, the best "medicine" is to stretch the cramped muscle and gently rub it to help it relax. Should you get a calf cramp, try to put your weight on your cramped leg while bending your knee slightly and rub your knotted calf muscle.

SPORTS INJURIES

Sports injuries happen to people of all ages while participating in a range of sports and activities that place exertion on different parts of the body. Sprains, strains, dislocations, and breaks cause varying degrees of disability when they happen and as they heal. Additionally, the ability to heal from injuries changes across our life span. As we get older, those old injuries that we thought we had left behind in our youth may decide that it is time to resurface.

A common feature of many injuries is, of course, pain, which is often accompanied by varying degrees of tenderness, swelling, and limitation in mobility. Injury-related symptoms often vary depending on the intensity of the injury. Injuries sustained through more intensive trauma often result in more significant pain and other physical symptoms. When you have experienced a significant injury, it is important to promptly consult with medical professionals to determine what course of treatment and rehabilitation will ensure that you avoid further damage to the affected part of your body while maximizing your healing potential. This is true when pain is brought on suddenly by a violent act such as a knee popping out of joint or an ankle twisting and extends to pain that increases over time due to repetitive motion injury (such as the bursitis of a golf or tennis elbow).

A sprain is the stretching or tearing of ligaments. Sprains occur when sudden force is placed on ligaments, such as when an ankle is twisted or your wrist is severely bent during a fall. By comparison, strains are the result of overstretched or torn muscles or tendons. When you strain a muscle or tendon, the injury may be acute, such as pulling your hamstring after trying to sprint to catch a fly ball (hamstring muscles run down the back of the leg from the pelvis to the bones of the lower leg). Injuries can also occur over a longer course of time, such as the tendonitis in a hand or wrist that golfers, tennis players, and men who work out on a rowing machine often encounter.

Common symptoms of both sprains and strains include localized swelling, tenderness, and sometimes severe pain at the site of injury or radiating from the injury, as well as the presence of a popping or tearing sound or feeling at the time of injury.[5] Bruising may or may not be present. Regardless of injury symptoms, there are some clear recommendations to follow that will help you prevent becoming injured in the first place.

Repetitive Motion Injuries

Tendonitis and bursitis are injuries that come from repetitive actions and are classified as overuse injuries. These injuries may result from playing certain sports or from activities such as swinging an axe repeatedly, working on an assembly line, keyboarding, or other tasks that require a repetitive motion that recurrently stresses the same body part. Tendonitis is the inflammation of a tendon located close to a joint. Familiar names for different types of tendonitis include tennis elbow, golfer's elbow, jumper's knee, and pitcher's shoulder. Bursitis is the inflammation of the fluid-filled bursae located near joints, and it occurs often in a hip, shoulder, or elbow.[6] The bursae are thin sacs located throughout the body that contain lubricating fluid and serve as cushions between bones and soft tissues, such as between the elbow and skin.

Overuse injuries often occur as a person adjusts the way they are carrying out an activity in order to avoid some initial pain that has become bothersome. Over time, pain develops as a result of the adjustment made to the motion that initially alleviated pain. When this issue is treated and resolved, the remnants of the initial injury return in the form of pain. Newly aggravated repetitive motion injuries often result from a sudden change in activity. Common culprits include developing new skills requiring repeated

Take Control of Sport Injuries

- Perform a proper warm-up and cooldown routine to prepare your body and help it recover.

- Engage in strengthening exercises, changing your activities to use different muscle groups. This is also known as *cross-training*.

- Wear equipment suitable for the sport, including proper footwear.

- Learn proper technique—and practice.

- Protect areas of past injuries—this may include wrapping or taping the injury site.

- If you experience pain, pay attention to it.

- Pain should be a signal that something is not right. Taking corrective action to stop pain can keep you in the game longer. Isn't that where you want to be?

practice; increasing the time, duration, or intensity of a workout; or even tweaking what had been an established training regimen.[7]

Symptoms of repetitive use injuries involve pain that increases over time. The pain can either be limited to a particular part of your body or radiate from the location where the injury took place to one or more other parts of your body. For example, if you have tennis or golf elbow, you may have difficulty gripping an object. Your elbow may be swollen, as well as tender and even warm to the touch. You may feel discomfort both when you are moving your elbow and when it is resting.

Diagnosing Sports and Overuse Injuries

In many cases it should be obvious what you need to do when you get injured. In those situations, following the general rule of resting, icing, compression, and elevating an injury will do the trick. However, there are times when this standard regimen will not be adequate and seeing a medical professional is advised. Some injuries clearly call for immediate medical attention, such as dislocations, spinal and head injuries, when there is considerable bleeding, or when someone loses consciousness or experiences severe, sudden pain.

Sometimes it can be tough to determine whether or not to consult with a doctor. However, it is important to remember that pain resulting from untreated or reoccurring injuries has the potential to further limit activity, and this, in turn, can erode your health and quality of life. Taking prompt action is more important to determine the extent of an injury than "watchful waiting"; it is an injury, and you need to know how to actively treat and rehabilitate the injury, as well as prevent reinjury.

Treating Sports and Overuse Injuries

"Aches and pains? Come on. They're normal for an athlete. You learn to deal with it. No one gets ahead running to the doctor whenever they feel a twinge of discomfort." Does that sound like you? Maybe running to the doctor for every ache and pain is a bit excessive. However, when an ache or pain comes on suddenly, exists over time, continues to happen every time you participate in a particular activity, or keeps you from engaging in activities that you have been able to do in the past, it is time to seek medical advice.

It is also essential to learn how to care for and manage injuries. Simply treating pain and not addressing the underlying issue leading to the pain will not benefit your long-term physical health. Do you love golf or gardening or jogging? Simply depending on an ibuprofen or pain reliever masks the injury and puts you at risk of further injury. Furthermore, if the pain exists for long enough, it is likely that "treating the pain" will mean a prolonged absence from activity. The real question becomes, what means more to you, the need to prove your vigor and independence and unconscious acceptance of the potential loss of control of the situation by avoiding care, or the knowledge of having the power to change your future by finding out what steps you can take to heal and resume control of your life once again?

The Truth about Healing

As we age, our musculoskeletal system goes through normal physiological changes that impact our body's ability to heal. Again, here are the facts—like them or not. Bone mass decreases, cartilage covering the ends of bones thins, synovial fluid in joints decreases in quantity and quality, joint spaces decrease, tendons decrease in diameter, and muscle mass decreases with increasing rapidity of deterioration after age 50. Other factors increasing the risk of musculoskeletal injury as you get older include decreased vision and hearing, a decreased sense of balance, and an increased likelihood of falling. Furthermore, because cell function slowly decreases, the ability to repair physiological damage sustained from an injury diminishes.[8] Additionally, having experienced an injury at some point in your lifetime increases the likelihood of the injury recurring later on.[9] As we get older, injuries that once healed within weeks can take much longer to heal and may recur with less provocation than was present with the initial injury. You can expect that it will be more difficult to return to the same level of functioning that had been achieved before an injury.

Taking Charge

Taking charge of your healing process initially may mean stopping participation in an activity that is causing pain. Initially, when you experience pain, rest the injured area. Seek medical advice if pain is recurrent, severe, or requires you to change activity choices. After seeking medical advice, do follow recommendations. If you do not like the recommendations or are not sure that the recommendations are correct, get a second opinion.

For Strains and Sprains, Remember *RICE*

Rest the injured area as soon as you are aware of the injury.

Ice the area for 30 minutes, warm for 15 minutes, and then repeat the cycle for up to 3 hours. Seek medical advice.

Compress. Wrap the injured area with an ace bandage or similar material to help decrease swelling. Remove immediately if circulation is being cut off to area.

Elevate the injury above the heart to decrease pain and swelling.

Source: Griffith, H. W. (2004). *Complete guide to sports injuries: How to treat fractures, bruises, sprains, strains, dislocations, head injuries* (3rd ed.). New York: Body Press / Perigee.

What to Take Away from This Information

If nothing else, recognize the need to address problems that result in pain. Consult your physician. Continue to be physically active, but remember to build up your strength and endurance over time and to warm up and then stretch both before and after exercising. Ignoring these simple rules can lead to undesirable consequences, including extended periods in which you are unable to be active and engaged to the degree you want to be in your life.

BONE AILMENTS AND DISEASES

Bones

Men's bones usually reach maximum strength, otherwise known as peak bone mass, around age 30.[10] From that point on bone mass begins to decrease, albeit *very* slowly. The slow and gradual reduction of bone mass is a normal part of the aging process, because new bone growth occurs at a slower pace than old bone death. There are things you can do to keep your bones healthy and strong. Eating foods rich in calcium and vitamin D and getting plenty of exercise contribute to your bone health.

Bone Facts

Your bones are constantly undergoing remodeling. Throughout life, bone-forming cells (osteoblasts) lay down new bone, and bone-removing cells (osteoclasts) resorb old bone. Bone modeling and remodeling preserve skeletal function.

Bone Density Tests

The effects of bone loss can be experienced when, all of a sudden, a stumble and fall leave you with a broken arm, leg, or hip that would not likely have broken when you were 40. In addition to engaging in healthy lifestyle practices, getting a bone density test is another way to be proactive with your bone health.

This test utilizes X-rays to measure the amount of calcium and other minerals in a section of bone, providing information directly related to your risk of fracture.[11] Bone density tests help identify a person's potential risk for fractures and monitor treatment. One type of bone density test that is used if you are 65 years or older or at risk of osteoporosis is the dual-energy X-ray absorptiometry scan. This test can report your risk for a bone fracture at the same time that it tells you whether you have normal bone density, low bone density, or osteoporosis. The National Osteoporosis Foundation recommends bone density tests for men ages 50–70 who have at least one risk factor related to osteoporosis, or for all men age 70 and over.[12]

Bone Spurs

Bone spurs are best understood as the bony projections that form on the edges of bones that meet in a joint. Common places for bone spurs involve the shoulders, spine, hips, knees, feet, and hands. While bone spurs themselves aren't painful, when they rub against nerves and ligaments, tendons, and other soft tissue, they cause considerable discomfort. Bone spurs themselves cause no symptoms, and until they irritate nearby nerves or tissue, they may go undetected for many years. There is no treatment for bone spurs; however, you can receive relief from local inflammation and the related pain. Should a bone spur grow significantly in size, surgery that files down or removes the spur is an option.

Bone Spurs Can Be Found in Many Places on Our Body

- *Fingers.* Here, they will feel like you have hard lumps under your skin and your fingers will actually look like they are disfigured.

- *Neck.* Spurs here can sometimes make it painful to swallow or take a breath, and if they are pushing up against veins, the result can be a restriction of blood flowing to your brain.

- *Shoulders.* Spurs on your shoulders can end up rubbing against your rotator cuff, which in turn can cause limitations in arm movement, tendonitis (swelling), and even tears in muscles and tendons.

- *Spine.* Spinal bone spurs can press against your spinal cord and nerves, resulting in pain and numbing elsewhere.

- *Knees.* Bone spurs on your knee commonly result in difficulty bending your leg and using your knee because they interfere with both bones and tendons.

Source: Mayo Clinic Staff (2010, Jan. 5). *Bone spurs.* Rochester, MN: Mayo Foundation for Medical Education and Research.

Because most bone spurs cause no signs or symptoms, you often don't even realize you have them until an X-ray for another condition reveals the growth. Should an undetected bone spur cause both pain and lost or restricted motion in your joints, the pain or swelling should compel you to make an appointment with your doctor. Early diagnosis and treatment can help prevent or slow further joint damage. Sometimes, bone spurs can be symptomatic of other diseases and conditions—commonly with osteoarthritis (discussed below). As osteoarthritis breaks down the cartilage in your joint, your body attempts to repair the loss. Often this means creating new areas of bone along the edges of your existing bones, and the new bone isn't an even, smooth addition.

The formation of bone spurs may accompany natural aging. They have been found in older people who don't have osteoarthritis or other diseases. Why this occurs is not fully understood. It appears that our body may create bone (spurs) to add stability to aging joints. The ever-increasing new bone growth may help redistribute our weight to protect areas of cartilage that was beginning to break down. If the new bone (spur) remains asymptomatic and does not harm neighboring soft tissue, it may actually provide a benefit, instead of only being painful.

Osteoporosis—Not Just a Woman's Issue

As a result of normal aging, bones become thinner, but with osteoporosis—a disease marked by the loss of calcium from bones and reduced bone strength—they become much thinner, porous, and brittle and are easily broken or fractured. Osteoporosis is the most common bone disease that involves the loss of bone density.

If you had an opportunity to take a close look at the inside of bone, it would look something like a honeycomb. When you have osteoporosis, the spaces in the honeycomb grow much wider, the bone also becomes smaller,

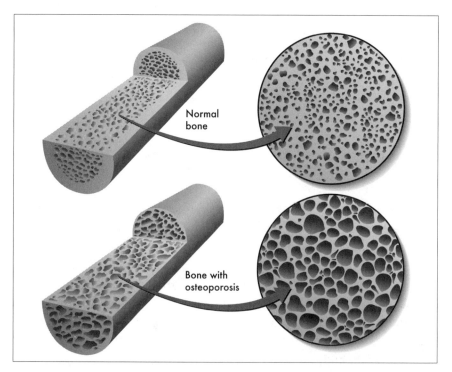

Figure 16.2. Bone cellular structure. Courtesy of rob3000/Shutterstock.com.

and the outer surface thins. While women far outnumber men diagnosed with the disease (because of their postmenopausal drop in estrogen and men's larger skeletons to begin with), you need to know that 6 million American men are living with osteoporosis and 20 million American men already have low bone mass (or osteopenia) and are anticipated to be living with the disease by 2020.[13] Osteoporosis is more common in Caucasians and Asians than in men of other ethnic or racial groups.

The American College of Physicians asserts that men's osteoporosis is substantially underdiagnosed, undertreated, and inadequately researched.[14] It is called a "silent disease" for two reasons. First, the way information on osteoporosis is presented on most posters and pamphlets shows only photos of women; nothing is mentioned about men.[15] Second, it advances without any visible symptoms; your first fractured vertebra is the initial symptom. Vertebral compression fractures (broken vertebrae) are the hallmark of osteoporosis; most commonly they are felt in the middle to lower part of the spine and cause a decrease in height. These fractures may occur suddenly and create piercing pain, or they can develop gradually and cause back pain to slowly build up. Anywhere from 3 to 6 percent of men have osteoporosis, and our risk increases as we age. Keep in mind that as many as one-seventh of all vertebral compression fractures and one-fourth of all hip fractures occur in men, and the older you are, the more serious and long-lasting the consequences of these breaks.[16]

Men's Osteoporosis Risk Factors

- Genetics—men whose parents have a history of fractures also seem to have reduced bone mass and are at risk for fractures
- Low levels of testosterone (hypogonadism)
- Heavy upper body weight
- Living with certain conditions (e.g., low body weight, rheumatoid arthritis, hyperthyroidism)

- Lifestyle choices
  - Staying sedentary and not exercising
  - Alcohol use
  - History of smoking
  - Eating choices that fail to incorporate enough calcium and vitamin D
  - Using medication for acid reflux
- History of cortisone treatment

What are some contributing factors that lead to men's osteoporosis? According to the National Institutes of Health, there are a variety of risk factors, and most are indirectly causal.[17] For example, acute fractures occur more readily among heavier white men—when the weight of a man's upper body exceeds the ability of the bone within the spine to support the load. Similarly, because exercise increases bone mass by reducing blood fats and increasing oxygen in the blood, a sedentary lifestyle adds risk to bone loss. Some commonly used medicines for asthma and arthritis also can cause loss of bone mass. Because cigarette smoking interferes with calcium being absorbed, when a smoker's body needs calcium, it will rob the bones. Other risk factors for men's osteoporotic fractures include frequent earlier bone fractures and declining quadriceps strength, falls, and moderate to high alcohol consumption.[18] Basically, older men who have a family history of osteoporosis, do not consume enough calcium or vitamin D, exercise very little, have low levels of testosterone, consume significant amounts of alcohol, take certain drugs, or smoke are at greatest risk.

CURRENT OSTEOPOROSIS TREATMENTS

Treating osteoporosis is aimed at slowing the pace of bone loss and rebuilding bone. Diet and exercise will surely help, but that may not be enough if you already have a great deal of bone density loss. The first line of treatment is to make sure that you are getting enough vitamin D and calcium. Our body needs the vitamin D to absorb the calcium, and without sufficient calcium in your diet, you body will draw from the calcium stored in bones to meet other needs. The daily recommendation for men under age 70 is 600 International Units (IU) of vitamin D and 1000 milligrams of calcium, and for men older than 70 the recommendation increases to 800 IU and 1200 milligrams, respectively. If you do not get enough of these two from what you are eating (see chapter 3), inexpensive supplements can be taken every morning.

Exercise and Weight Training Programs to Consider

Proper exercise stresses bones in a positive way, and when bones that are stimulated by exercise stress, there is an increase in density and overall strengthening. There are many exercise programs available that promote maintaining bone health. One such program called "Bone Builders" is an osteoporosis exercise program that relies on mild weight training to increase muscular strength and bone density. Balance training is also a key component of these classes. Originally developed from the Strong Living Program at Tufts University and based on research there, the Bone Builders program is designed to prevent and even reverse osteoporosis, improve balance to protect against falls and fractures, and enhance the participant's energy level and sense of well-being.[19] There is also an educational component to

Bone Builders training classes. Weekly discussions about an osteoporosis-related health topic are included, and leaders will share information you can use to improve your health. Bone Builders classes are located in many communities across the country, frequently affiliated with a Retired and Senior Volunteer Program, an Area Agency on Aging, or a local senior citizens center, hospital, or health care clinic.

Medication

The National Institute on Aging informs us that there are several medicines available to treat the disease which can be used by men. You are advised to talk with your doctor to see if any of them might work for you if you break bones easily or are at risk of the disease. These medications include the following:

> *Bisphosphonates.* This class of oral drugs (alendronate, or Fosamax; ibandronate, or Boniva; risedronate, or Actonel) aims to slow the rate of bone thinning in order to increase bone density, which makes it less likely that you will break a bone if you fall. There are some occasional side effects (nausea, heartburn, stomach pain), and the meds are usually taken in the morning.

> *Parathyroid hormone.* Given by injection daily to men with serious osteoporosis and at high risk for broken bones, the objective is to better regulate the level of calcium in your blood. The parathyroid glands are responsible for cueing how much calcium needs to be released from our bone, and should these glands become overactive, they call for too much calcium to be released. This is parathyroid disease, and its treatment is to take a synthetic parathyroid hormone called *teriparatide*, which stimulates bone growth and curbs the robbing of bones for unneeded calcium.

> *Hormonal therapy.* Men with osteoporosis and low levels of testosterone have been found to benefit from *testosterone replacement*. The level of this natural hormone is highest around age 40, tapering as we get older. Should your testosterone level be lower than normal for your age, its absence accelerates bone thinning and calcium loss. Using testosterone replacement—whether by rubbing a gel on your shoulders daily, wearing a patch at night, or monthly injection—can help curb bone thinning.[20]

For men who have osteoporosis and normal levels of testosterone, there is another natural hormone, calcitonin, that might be causing bone thinning. Calcitonin replacement (by either injection or a nasal spray) inhibits the bone resorption process, and this preserves or increases bone mineral density and lowers the risk of vertebral fractures.[21]

LIVING WITH ARTHRITIS

Arthritis is a chronic condition that involves inflammation of the joints and neighboring tissue, causing pain and stiffness.[22] Arthritis actually is an umbrella phrase that describes at least 100 different rheumatic conditions and diseases, including the most common for men: osteoarthritis, rheumatoid arthritis, and gout.[23] It is the main cause of disability in the United States, and it becomes more common as we get older. According to the Centers for Disease Control and Prevention (CDC), arthritis isn't as common in men as women; however, nearly 20 percent of men in every age group are coping with at least one type of arthritis. The chances of developing arthritis increase with the wear and tear of getting older, being overweight, smoking, and a family history.

While it is true that arthritis is found more frequently in people who are inactive and who are overweight or obese,[24] the pain, stiffness, and physical limitations brought on by arthritis can become problematic even for someone who is normal weight and has been active throughout his lifetime. Osteoarthritis (degenerative joint disease) involves the degeneration of the cartilage in a joint, which leads to increased friction and ultimately inflammation, pain, stiffness, crackling, and restricted motion in affected joints. Overuse of joints and injury are the primary causes for developing osteoarthritis.[25] It is diagnosed by pain that worsens with activity and lessens with rest. Medications can reduce the inflammation in order to relieve pain and prevent or slow joint damage. Over-the-counter nonsteroidal anti-inflammatory drugs (NSAIDs) are most often recommended, such as the ibuprofen medications Advil and Motrin.

By comparison, clinical researchers do not know what brings about rheumatoid arthritis, which results in its signature inflammation of many (not one) joints, where, as with other autoimmune diseases, immune cells attack healthy tissue and affect not only joints but internal organs. Rheumatoid arthritis primarily affects the synovium (lining of the joint), not the joint itself. For many years the theory was that an infection brought on by a virus, bacteria, or fungi was the cause; however, there is still no evidence to support this theory. At present, there is no cure for rheumatoid arthritis. A gentle massage is very effective in relieving the pain. In addition to ibuprofen medication, you eventually might need to consider corticosteroid medications, such as prednisone, to reduce the inflammation and pain.

What is certain with either type of arthritis is the associated pain, which is often severe enough to force men to withdraw from social and physical activity. For many men, extended periods of inactivity due to arthritis can have serious physical and psychological consequences. Depression, increased dependence, and an overall reduced quality of life appear to be quite prevalent when living with arthritis. It is very important to remember that having a social network of family, friends, or neighbors will be an important buffer when dealing with the pain and restricted mobility.

It is unfortunate that fully half of arthritis sufferers believe that the disease is simply a part of normal aging and therefore don't think that the symptoms can be alleviated. This is not the case.[26] It is generally recognized that a regular exercise regimen is an important strategy for maintaining physical function if you have arthritis. Recommended exercises include resistance training, fitness walking, aerobics, and Tai Chi, a series of movements and poses that together make up a meditative form of exercise that can offer physical and spiritual health benefits. Exercise can, in many cases, reduce the pain and stiffness associated with arthritis. In the later stages of osteoarthritis, joint replacement may be warranted.

GOUT

Gout is a medical condition characterized by attacks of acute inflammatory arthritis in the joints, most frequently between the metatarsal bones of the foot and the toes. It is the most common form of inflammatory arthritis affecting men. Gout is caused by elevated levels of uric acid in your body, either because you have prostate problems and your body has a difficult time ridding itself of uric acid, or because your body simply makes too much of it. When too much uric acid exists, it crystallizes, and the crystals are deposited in joints, causing the swelling and pain. Acute gout usually affects a single joint. Chronic gout may involve more than one joint (e.g., big toe, ankle, knee) during its repeated episodic flares, or perhaps continuous inflammation and pain. Men experiencing chronic gout report feelings of shame and embarrassment because of the way the illness is trivialized and because of their escalating pain and functional disability.[27]

The exact cause of gout is unknown; what is known is the discomfort, if not acute pain, which men describe as crushing and excruciating. The only treatment for gout is to reduce the factors that create uric acid. That's to say that men ought to drink less beer and reduce other purine-rich foods such as mushrooms, asparagus, meat gravies, and organ meat (liver, kidneys). NSAIDs such as ibuprofen are immediately recommended when gout flares up. Your physician will likely prescribe a urate-lowering drug and a stronger painkiller.[28] If persistent and/or recurring, you might also be treated with oral steroids or have a steroid injected into the inflamed joint.

JOINT SURGERY AND REPLACEMENT

Men with rheumatoid or other inflammatory arthritis should try physical therapy and medicines before considering surgery. The goal of joint surgery (or *arthroplasty*) is to restore the mobility of the joint and relieve pain by partially or completely resurfacing, reconstructing, or replacing a diseased joint. Perhaps the most common type of surgery is when the orthopedic surgeon removes a small portion of bone from an arthritic joint in order to recreate a gap in the socket. Sometimes a plastic or metal disk, or even a disk made of skin tissue, will be added between the two bones in a joint. This is a minimally invasive surgical procedure in which the surgeon uses a device called an *arthroscope* and repairs the damaged joint through small surgical incisions in the skin.

The emerging treatment of choice for end-stage arthritis of the knee or hip has become total joint replacement with an artificial knee or hip. Older age need not be a deterrent to undergoing this surgery. Even in the mid-1990s, three-quarters of the total knee replacements and two-thirds of the total hip replacements were performed on patients age 65 and older.[29]

You can expect that the average length of stay in a hospital after the surgery will range from 2 to 10 nights, depending on whether it was your knee or hip. Of course, there will be a longer recuperation period for rehabilitation and full recovery. Expect physical therapy to begin as soon as possible, and you will temporarily be using a walker, cane, or crutches for support. Rehab commonly includes exercises to improve range of motion (how far you can bend and straighten your knee, for example) and strengthen your leg muscles.

Physical Therapy—Why Do I Need It?

Physical therapists are trained to work with people experiencing injuries or disease. The function of physical therapy is to help decrease pain and increase mobility and health to the injured or debilitated joint. You can expect that your physical therapist will assess the severity of your injury or arthritis and then identify activities that you can engage in to help with your injury rehabilitation, such as massage, ultrasound treatment, stretching, and strengthening exercises to increase your endurance.[30] The fact is, however, that it is up to you to engage fully in your own therapy and rehabilitation by doing exercises as prescribed. Choosing to disregard recommended exercise, stretching, and strengthening regimens and neglecting to use prescribed equipment as directed will mean a longer healing period or possibly reinjury. Probably the worst thing that you can do is become passive during the course of the healing process. Do not cut back or give up.

FALLS: WATCH YOUR STEP

Do you have difficulty rising from a sitting position without using your hands to push off? Do you need to stand still immediately afterward? Do you walk slowly or with your legs spread wide apart to create a wide base of support? If you do, it is quite possible that you have a strength deficit or balance problem. Both are common as we get older and live with musculoskeletal changes. Both also increase our risk of falling. Believe it or not, according to the National Council on Aging, every minute of every day, at least three older adults are admitted to an emergency room for a fall. For older men, falling can be fatal; in fact, the CDC reports that falls are the leading cause of injury-related deaths among this age group, some 40 percent of older adults fall at least once each year, and every hour a fall results in the deaths of two older persons.[31] Falls are the main cause of emergency room admissions for older adults (15–30%).[32] Nonfatal fall-related injuries disproportionately affect women, probably because of sex differences in onset and severity of osteoporosis.[33] This statistic does not override the fact that many adult men fracture a bone when they fall; fractures that increase with men's aging include the pelvis (hip), vertebrae, and radius/ulna (arm).

> ### Break Your Fall
>
> One in three older adults fall each year, and at least a tenth of those falls result in serious injury. A fall can lead to loss of confidence, dependence on others, fear of falling, decreased activity levels, and deconditioned muscles, all of which can promote a sense of isolation and even depression.

Unfortunately, growing older increases our risk of and the severity of falls. Falls are caused by a multitude of factors, including declines in vision and hearing, muscle strength, coordination, and reflexes. If you have diabetes, heart disease, thyroid, or circulatory issues, your balance can also be affected.[34] Taking blood pressure medications, sedatives, antidepressants, and even herbal and over-the-counter medications can lead to unsteadiness of gait, which can, in turn, increase your risk of falling. If you also have osteoporosis, even minor falls can cause one or more bones to shatter.

Practical Steps to Take to Prevent Slips, Trips, and Falls

The CDC and National Institute on Aging offer good advice on a number of steps you can take to prevent falls by taking care of your overall health:[35]

> *Be physically active.* Maintaining a regular program of exercise strengthens your bones and muscles, improves balance, and will keep your tendons, joints, and ligaments flexible. Despite its reputation as a "jock" thing, strength training is important for everyone. Weight-bearing exercises are strongly recommended to slow bone loss from osteoporosis and increase muscle strength. Did you know that many senior-exclusive residential settings now include a weight room and a full-time exercise specialist?

> *Put your glasses on.* If your vision is dependent on wearing glasses, why add a risk to falling by not putting your glasses on when you wake up and leave your bed? Also, have your vision checked.

> *Remove the clutter.* Keep walking areas clear of loose rugs, cords, shoes, clothing, books, magazines, paper, and other clutter.

> *Name your medications.* Stay informed about the prescriptions you take, including their potential side effects, and review the meds regularly with your physician.

> *What's the hurry?* Avoid standing up too quickly after lying down or sitting in order to avoid feeling faint.

> *More than two legs.* If you have difficulty walking, consider using a cane, walking stick, or walker, especially when you are walking in unfamiliar and poorly lit places.

> *Slippery when icy.* Be especially cautious when walking on wet or icy surfaces—take it slow. Salt or sand entryways to your home.

> *Don't keep secrets.* Keep your physician informed of any falls you have taken, whether or not you were hurt.

Don't Forget to Make Your Home Safe

The majority of falls occur in our own home, many of which could have been avoided just by making a few small safety improvements. The National Institute on Aging offers some very practical recommendations[36] that can make your home a safe place to live:

> Handrails should be located on both sides of all stairs.

> All sets of stairs need to be well lit with switches available at the top and the bottom.

> Make sure all areas where you frequently walk are kept clear of cords and wires.

> Rugs should have nonslip liners underneath them to hold them in place.

> Install grab bars near toilets and in your tub and shower.

> Use night lights throughout your house, especially near your bed and the bathroom you use during the night.

> Keep a telephone near your bed with emergency numbers clearly posted at all times.

> You will also want to be sure that your sofas and chairs allow you to get in and out of them easily, that you are especially careful walking on wet floors, and that you never stand on chairs and unstable stools to reach for things (use "reach sticks" instead).

These recommendations aimed at preventing falls are not meant to create undue anxiety or fear but instead are meant to offer a reasonable degree of caution given the potential for very disruptive consequences should you fracture a hip or other bone. In fact, it is important that you not develop undue anxiety about the possibility of a fall, as there is some evidence that exaggerated anxiety about falling, even if tests have shown your risk to be low, may increase the probability that you could actually fall. Neuroscience researchers in Australia have found that people who are fearful to an extreme may become less active, which in turn results in physical deconditioning, a loss of strength and balance, and ultimately greater likelihood of falling.[37] Their message is to be cautious, but not to an extreme such that it diminishes your quality of life.

It Could Be Just a Matter of Balance

There are community training programs available if you are concerned about the possibility of falling. In addition to the Bone Builders program described earlier, you might want to consider a Matter of Balance class. A Matter of Balance is an award-winning program developed by Boston University's Roybal Center for the Enhancement of Late-Life Functioning and designed to manage falls and increase activity levels.[38] Taking these classes can help you learn to view falls as controllable, set goals for increasing activity, make changes to reduce fall risks at home, and exercise to increase strength and balance. The classes target anyone concerned about falls and interested in improving balance, flexibility, and strength. It is also meant for anyone who has fallen in the past or has restricted activities because of falling concerns. A Matter of Balance has received national awards from the American Society on Aging and the National Association of Area Agencies on Aging for innovation and quality in aging programs.

LIVING WITH CHRONIC PAIN

Living with the damage resulting from wear-and-tear or overuse injuries, arthritis, or other rheumatic disease can mean living with chronic pain. There are many medical and nonmedical ways of dealing with chronic pain. Medical treatments may include pharmaceutical approaches to decrease swelling and related pain such as acetaminophen, NSAIDs, or other pain medications. Physical therapy may help to strengthen injured areas and increase mobility while working to decrease pain. Activities such as swimming, yoga, or Tai Chi may provide health benefits and alleviate pain. Chiropractic or osteopathic care may be recommended. Surgery may be necessary to help resolve issues that otherwise would continue to cause pain. Alternative medicine practices such as massage, acupuncture, aromatherapy, or meditation may also greatly help some people live more successfully and comfortably with chronic pain conditions. There are other chapters that provide more information on alternative and holistic treatments that could benefit people living with arthritis or other musculoskeletal challenges.

Clearly, living with pain, let alone chronic pain, is cause for anyone to feel stress. This is especially true if you are experiencing interruptions in your regular routine or have had to give up work or other activities in order to deal with or receive treatment for your pain, illness, or injury. Depression and anxiety may accompany these life changes. Just remember that you have the ability to take control of the situation and avoid or even prevent many of the insults to your bones, muscles, and joints discussed in this chapter. The more informed we are, the more options we will have available when we are ready to decide what we want our destiny to be. So take control.

Dental and Oral Health

with Bethany O'Dell

Dental and oral health is not likely the first thing you think of when you think about men's health. Nor has dental health been one of the National Institutes of Health's priorities. If there was a report card for each dimension of men's health (e.g., heart, diabetes, hearing), dental health would certainly receive a low "grade" for most men's preventative efforts. Part of this too-close-to-failing grade reflects our individual efforts. Yet being able to afford to maintain the health of the mouth reveals the inequalities among men more than nearly any other type of health issue. We examine in this chapter the importance of oral health to a man's physical and social function, the most common dental diseases and their treatment, and the stark generational and socioeconomic differences evident in men's dental health.

> "I think, therefore I am" is the statement of an intellectual who underrates toothaches.
>
> —Milan Kundera

DENTAL HEALTH HISTORIES

A lot of media attention was drawn to the fact that more than 50 million Americans were without health insurance before the Affordable Care Act became law in 2010. Despite the historic health care reform legislation, the alarming fact is that about 40 percent of adults under age 65 in the United States will remain without a dental plan and affordable access to dental care. Don't think that older adults are better off. Once retired, 80 percent of older men are without dental insurance.[1] You probably did not know that most dentists do not participate in Medicaid, and Medicare does not offer dental coverage.[2] This leaves tens of millions of adult men unable to afford the essential dental health care they need because they may not be able to pay out of pocket and/or cannot find a provider who will treat them at reduced cost.[3]

As with general health, oral health tends to vary based on social factors, resulting in what amounts to "a silent epidemic" of dental and oral diseases for certain men.[4] As an example, men from different generations vary significantly in their experiences with, attitudes toward, and expectations of dental health and dental care. Many men born in the 1930s and early 1940s already suffered from poor dental health by the time they reached voting age. Nearly 45 percent of these men have lost six or more teeth due to tooth decay or gum disease before age 65, and 20 percent have lost all of their teeth (and are called "edentulous," meaning without any natural teeth).[5] Part of the explanation for this is because preventative and restorative dental care wasn't readily available until military service in World War II. The older generations did not visit dentists to *improve* their dental health; rather, extraction of a loose or decayed tooth was the usual "treatment." They also feared the dentist;[6] pain control had not yet been introduced when they were young. As one older man commented, "The injections they have today weren't there when we were young."[7] Further, this World War II / Korean War generation had not benefitted from water fluoridation or fluoride toothpastes, and it was the economically deprived men within this generation who ended up with the greatest number of pulled and missing teeth.[8]

For the baby boomer generation, the common view held by their fathers that losing teeth is a normal part of aging is no longer acceptable. Boomers' dental health education included television advertising when they were children which emphasized "brush, brush, brush" and encouraged regular dental checkups. Most boomers have some form of dental insurance. Owing to early self-care and preventive dental care, the boomer generation did not expect to lose teeth or endure painful dental infections. Many boomers retain their own teeth throughout their lives or have implants and/or caps to provide a full mouth of teeth. They have learned that the best thing they can do to avoid complicated and expensive dental work is to engage in regular dental visits, cleanings, and fixing small problems before they become big ones.

DENTAL HEALTH

What does "dental health" mean to men? For the older generation, the concept meant having enough teeth to chew and speak.[9] However, for boomers and younger men, they've learned that dental and oral health is important; they know that oral infections can lead to other health problems, and they've learned that periodontal (gum) disease contributes to stinky breath, lost teeth, and problems chewing, as well as doubling the risk of men suffering a fatal heart attack and tripling the risk of a stroke.[10]

Men also know that their teeth affect their well-being and social lives. The mouth is highly visible, and having missing teeth interferes with a person's speech, perception of himself, and social standing. Having visibly missing teeth and/or bad breath might stigmatize, given the increasing importance the boomer generation has placed on appearance. White, evenly shaped and straight teeth and quality of breath are criteria people use to make judgments about a man and can affect his ability to find (or keep) a good job. A spokesperson for the Academy of General Dentistry recently reported, "Many (men) have noticed the positive effects of a colleague's improved smile and . . . [how] a great smile has a lot of value in the business world."[11]

This chapter is titled "Dental and Oral Health" and not "Dental Problems" for good reason. Dental diseases are more often lifestyle diseases, no different from how smoking-related lung cancer is a lifestyle disease. Toothbrushes and flossing have replaced "chew sticks" and herbs, and studies show that most men are taking up other self-care practices.

The key word is *most* men. Researchers continue to find that men follow oral hygiene recommendations less conscientiously and draw upon less dental care than do their sisters and wives. Studies by the American Dental Association (ADA) have noted that barely half of men brush their teeth *twice* a day, much fewer floss daily, and more than half develop periodontal (gum) disease and will lose at least five teeth by their early seventies. Even when men actively engage in dental self-care at home, too few see a dentist or dental hygienist annually, and many live with undiagnosed problems.[12] Not every oral health problem is visible or results in the pain or discomfort that compels most men to seek dental care. Too many serious dental and oral problems are "silent."

SIMPLE WAYS TO CONTROL YOUR DENTAL/ORAL HEALTH

Brushing twice a day with a fluoride toothpaste, flossing daily, and regular dental checkups are the key factors in maintaining a healthy mouth and avoiding dental problems. The mouth includes more than the teeth and the gums (gingiva). There are the jaw bones and ligaments, the hard and soft palate, the soft tissue lining the mouth and throat, the tongue, the lips, the salivary glands, and the chewing muscles.

Stop the Tobacco Use

Men who smoke or chew tobacco are putting at risk not only their overall health but the health of their mouths as well. Cigars are not a safe alternative. Smokers are at increased risk for tooth abrasion from the grit in smoke, tooth discoloration (or staining of the teeth), hastened periodontal disease due to irritation of the gums, and the bad breath that comes from oral disease. Smokers routinely take longer to heal an oral wound, whether from an ordinary cut or following oral surgery.

Statistics show that chewing tobacco and snuff are less dangerous than cigarettes, but the smokeless products still raise the risk of oral cancer by 80 percent. The most frequent oral cancer sites are the tongue, floor of the mouth, soft palate, lips, and gums. It is very important for men who use tobacco to see a dentist frequently, not merely for cleanings but for an assessment of signs of an oral cancer. Most men do not recognize that when a dentist or hygienist begins your visit with a thorough look at your mouth, they are screening for oral cancer.

A Clean Mouth

It is important to control the growth of bacteria on the teeth, gums, and tongue. Removing the food particles from your mouth by brushing (or at least rinsing) as soon as possible prevents the development of bacteria, which cause bad breath, cavities, and other infections. First, drink plenty of water throughout the day. Water cleanses the mouth and removes food particles and bacteria that cause bad breath or other tooth and gum issues. Second, brushing your teeth and flossing are equal halves of the job of keeping a clean mouth, yet dentists report that most of their patients are not willing to floss. Fewer than 13 percent of the men in a recent study reported that they flossed daily.[13] Even though it may seem like a bother until you make it a habit, if you take just a minute to floss your teeth on a daily basis, you will be helping to prevent plaque and tartar buildup, gingivitis, and periodontal disease. Although not a substitute for flossing, an oral irrigator or water pick can help clean between teeth.

Equally important is a visit to the dentist two times a year for a professional cleaning. The cleaning will more than whiten your teeth; the hygienist removes the plaque from those hard-to-reach places your toothbrush didn't find. The dentist or hygienist will also be able to tell you how healthy your mouth is and what to do to improve your dental health.

These simple steps are the easiest way to keep control of your dental health. Much like the way flossing emerged as an added, valuable means of oral hygiene, dental professionals also recommend that we invest in an

Things Dentists Want Us to Know

- Use a soft-bristled toothbrush and reach every surface of each tooth.

- Brush your teeth and gums with fluoride toothpaste for 2–3 minutes each brushing. Choosing toothpaste with fluoride reduces tooth decay by as much as 40 percent.

- Brush your gums by positioning the toothbrush at a 45 degree angle where your gums and teeth meet.

- Change your toothbrush every 3 months. The bristles wear out.

- Rinse the toothbrush out with hot water after every use to help remove bacteria that collects in the bristles.

- Floss by using a back-and-forth motion, and curve the floss into a C shape against one tooth and then the other.

- Dental checkups and cleanings routinely screen for oral cancer.

- Men who smoke have a much greater risk of gum disease and oral cancer.

- Eating a nutritional diet with little sugar prevents periodontal disease and tooth decay.

- Bad breath is usually evidence of a dental problem, and mouth-wash only hides the problem temporarily.

- Dental problems do not go away untreated.

- Fear of pain from dental work is something to be discussed with your dentist and hygienist. Dental work can be made painless.

- Should you need it, choose the root canal, not a pulled tooth.

Sources: Academy of General Dentistry and the American Dental Association.

---

electric toothbrush and, if you need it, a tongue cleaner. The tongue tends to acquire a lot of bacteria, which is the main cause of bad breath, and cleaning your tongue will remove bacteria buildup that a brushing couldn't get off. An electric toothbrush does a much better job brushing, is a good tongue massager, and makes it much easier to position the brush at the recommended 90-degree angle to clean the spaces where the gums and teeth meet. You are also more likely to brush your teeth longer and better clean the areas where gums and teeth meet.

Nutrition Intake

The food we consume is directly associated with how healthy our mouths are. By having a meal plan of whole grains (breads, cereals), protein (fish, meat, beans), and dairy (milk, yogurt, cheese), we are giving our body the nutrients needed to maintain a healthy mouth. In contrast, practicing poor eating habits such as constant snacking, sipping on sodas, or even not eating at all will seriously harm your teeth and mouth. Constant snacking is detrimental simply because there are food particles being left on the surfaces of the teeth. The leftover food particles are fertilizer for bacteria. Drinking soda, even sugar-free soda, is equally harmful because the acid within the soda destroys the tooth's enamel. A sugary diet, especially one that includes bakery products and carbonated drinks, increases dental problems.

The worst thing for your teeth, however, would be to not eat much at all. It is critical that our body get food and needed nutrients. You can lower your risk for cavities, gum infections, losing teeth, and periodontal disease by simply getting an adequate amount of vitamin D and calcium into your body. Researchers have found that people who have a deficit in vitamin D and calcium are more likely to develop osteoporosis and tooth loss.[14] These two vitamins are essential for maintaining good bone to anchor the teeth and promoting overall oral health.

Vitamin D helps the body absorb the correct amounts of calcium and utilize it efficiently. Without enough vitamin D, the available calcium isn't absorbed, and the body then starts to take calcium away from teeth and bones.[15] Many adults, particularly men age 60 and older, have dietary intakes of calcium well below recommended levels.[16] Adult men are recommended to have 1,000–1,500 IU of vitamin D daily (or 10–15 micrograms). Sunshine and certain foods and drinks, such as milk, orange juice, cheese, eggs with the yolk, and salmon, have good amounts of vitamin D. Because many men spend too little time in the sun (with sunscreen) and no longer consume enough of these sources, vitamin D supplements are encouraged. A year's supply of a generic brand will cost little more than a case of beer. Men also need 1,000–1,500 mg of calcium daily in order to check the risk of bone loss and tooth loss. This level can be obtained by dietary intake or, if need be, from supplements. Dairy foods, bread, broccoli, and orange juice have large amounts of calcium. Low-fat and fat-free milk and dairy products (yogurt, cheeses) are especially good sources of both calcium and vitamin D.

Keeping the Mouth Moist

Have you ever woken up feeling parched, as if you've traveled the desert without water for days? You probably spent the night breathing through your mouth, perhaps as a result of chapped lips or congestion from a head cold, or you drank way too much alcohol the night before and woke dehydrated. Without adequate salivary flow *on a regular basis*, we are much more at risk of early oral health problems.

Good mouth care means keeping the mouth moist, and it is saliva (not gulping bottled water) that is the key ingredient to keeping your mouth healthy. Saliva contains antibacterial proteins, mucins (mucous), and ions that prevent oral infections and dental cavities. It helps neutralize acids from our stomachs, which protects our esophagus, and is vital to our ability to chew, swallow, and talk comfortably throughout the day.

The mucous layer in saliva that covers our teeth acts as a shield, protecting the teeth from decay, and fights the bacteria that cause gum disease. For men who have dentures, saliva is equally vital to help keep the dentures comfortable and fitting in the mouth. The recommendation is to stimulate saliva production by chewing sugarless gum (especially xylitol gum), sucking on a sugarless gum ball, or eating foods that require chewing, such as apples, carrots, celery, and hard bread.

Know Your Medications

Many medications, such as heart or blood pressure medications or antidepressants, reduce the natural production of saliva and cause dry mouth. Men who take saliva-inhibiting medications are at increased risk for cavities, periodontal disease, and other oral problems. Often the medications that are muscle relaxants, pain inhibitors, or sleeping aids (sedatives) or those that treat diabetes, allergies, colds (e.g., antihistamines), diarrhea, nausea, and hypertension (e.g., diuretics) will increase the risk of oral health problems.

Anatomy of a Tooth

A tooth is composed of several layers. The outermost layer, above the gum line, is called the *enamel*, and this is the hardest substance in the body. Beneath the gum line, a substance called *cementum* covers the tooth roots. Under the enamel and cementum is the *dentin*. The dentin is about as hard as bone, and it is the dentin that contains nerve endings. Beneath the dentin is the vascular tissue called the *dental pulp*.

DENTAL AND ORAL DISEASE

Healthy teeth are clean and have few cavities, healthy gums are pink and firm, and a healthy mouth is a window offering clues about your body's overall health. The enemy is bacteria. Plaque is a soft, colorless film of bacteria constantly forming on your teeth. It combines with sugar and other carbohydrates to form acids. Without brushing and flossing, the acids eat right through tooth enamel to cause cavities, and the plaque hardens into a porous, coarse tartar. The acids produced by the bacteria will cause your gums to become chronically infected (or inflamed), and the gum tissue next to the teeth breaks down and separates from the teeth. Plaque begins to accumulate on your teeth 20 minutes after eating, and if it isn't removed, you are at greater risk of tooth decay or gum inflammation. Together, plaque and tartar lead to a number of problems: gingivitis, periodontitis, bad breath (halitosis), tooth loss, and cavities. Before each of these dental problems is briefly reviewed, we discuss two other common problems: dry mouth and taste problems.

Dry Mouth

Adult men often suffer from dry mouth (known as *xerostomia*), especially as we get older. It is perhaps one of the most underappreciated, underdiagnosed, and undermanaged oral health conditions.[17] Dry mouth happens when the salivary glands are not working properly, resulting in decreased saliva production. Because saliva is the moisture that helps you talk, swallow, and digest your food, the sensation of dry mouth needs to be taken seriously. The amount of salivary tissue in the mouth decreases with aging, but it isn't physiological aging that causes dry mouth.[18] Rather, it is the prescription medications we are taking and/or the underlying medical conditions we have.

The uncomfortable, dry feeling can be a temporary problem or a chronic one. Your dry mouth may have started shortly after starting a new prescription or over-the-counter medication; dry mouth is a side effect of many medications, but especially the diuretics used to manage hypertension and the over-the-counter medications used for allergies and antidepressants. Two decades ago there were over 400 medications known to negatively affect salivary function.[19] Given that 50 percent of the adult male population in the United States is on at least one medication, most men will experience some change in how their salivary glands work.[20] The advice "Know your medications" is essential. Other times, it is the disease itself that decreases saliva functioning—diabetes, Parkinson's and Alzheimer's diseases, or more likely sleep apnea. Recent studies show that sleep-disordered breathing and snoring contribute to chronic dry mouth. Finally, radiation therapy and chemotherapy can cause damage to the salivary glands or make saliva thicker than normal.

There are plenty of ways to relieve the uncomfortable sensation of dry mouth. The absolute worst method is by sucking on sugared candies or lozenges. The key advice is to not ignore the problem and bring it to the attention of both your physician and dentist. If you are using medication and experiencing the discomfort of dry mouth, take control and ask your physician if there is an alternative medication. Below are a few tips to prevent dry mouth (at night) or help make your mouth a little more comfortable:

> Sip water often. A healthy mouth needs to be hydrated.

> Sip water at meals as well. This will help with the process of chewing and swallowing and circumvent the problem of dry mouth caused by illness or medical treatment.

> Just like sugar, caffeine can dry out the mouth. Put down that soda, and watch how much coffee or tea you drink.

> Keep sugarless gum or sugarless hard candy in your pocket. Chewing and sucking help to stimulate saliva flow in your mouth. Lemon and tart flavored are best to stimulate saliva.

> At night use a nasal strip to reduce snoring and sleeping with your mouth open. Snoring is a leading cause of experiencing dry mouth at night.

> If you mostly sleep with your mouth open and breathe through your mouth at night, it is a good idea to run a humidifier in the room to keep moisture in the air.

> Ask a dentist about oral moisturizers and gels that are designed to provide relief from dry mouth.

Taste Problems

Humans' taste palate falls into five basic groups: sweet, bitter, sour, salty, and umami (a Japanese word for "good" flavor, or savoriness). An anatomy professor would tell you that your sweet/salty taste buds are located near the front of your tongue, whereas the sour and bitter taste buds line the sides and very back of your tongue (see figure 17.1). As we age, our sense of taste changes, and

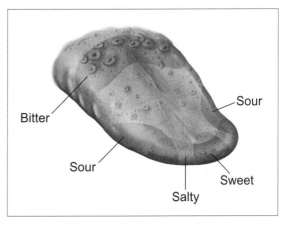

Figure 17.1. Tongue and taste regions. Illustration by Carlyn Iverson.

this is going to be certainly noticed by the baby boomer generation, which has grown up with sugars and salt. The order of "lost taste" begins with sweet and salty eroding first and sour last. Because 75 percent of what we "taste" actually comes from our sense of smell, and because the olfactory bulb in the brain responsible for processing smell becomes smaller as we age, both smell and taste become more blunted.

Aroma is what enhances our ability to taste our food, so when our sense of smell is decreased, many of us find that our food is bland. If your diet has long had a lot of salt (or sodium), as you get older you probably think whatever you are eating "needs a little more salt." It doesn't; you just think it does. Changes in tastes not only reduce the pleasure and comfort from food; they represent risks for nutritional deficiencies and challenge our willingness to adhere to a healthy diet. Don't pick up the salt shaker.

When food seems to have lost that taste that we enjoyed so much and sometimes crave, this can lead to a loss of appetite and a slow decrease in an older man's food intake, which eventually will make him more vulnerable to illnesses because of his lack of vitamins and nutrients. Alternatively, he might begin salting or sugaring up his food in order to get that flavor back, which puts him at further risk of obesity and hypertension.

We can be thankful that taste is one of the best senses we have and is not affected as drastically by aging as our other senses. Actual taste disorders are very rare, but over time we usually experience a gradual decrease in our ability to taste salty, sweet, sour/bitter, and pleasurable things such as the texture of chocolate, the hops in beer, or the zing in pepper-flavored Chinese food. Similar to dry mouth, our "loss of taste" is often caused by outside (exogenous) sources, not just aging. It might actually be caused by medicines you're taking, since both prescription and over-the-counter medications (including herbs) are chemicals that change your sense of taste. Many antibiotics and blood pressure pills can cause an unpleasant taste in our mouths. Viral infections—especially sinus infections and head colds—dull the sense of smell and then taste, and the problem can be chronic. Smoking damages the soft tissue inside the mouth and dulls the palate, as well as our sense of smell.

What can you do? First, check with your physician and/or dentist to see whether you are on any medications that alter smell and taste and, if so, whether the medication can be changed. Also, practice good oral hygiene to prevent gum disease and to retain your teeth. If you have a loss of appetite because food doesn't taste like you want it to, try to make your food appealing to the eye by using different colors and textures, or add herbs and spices instead of salt and sugar to provide a newer range of flavors.

Bad Breath (Halitosis)

Having bad breath is a dreadful, often embarrassing situation, if you know you have it. It is virtually impossible for people to find out if their own bad breath is an affront, simply because we become used to our odors and do not perceive whether our breath offends. Blowing into your hands and smelling your breath doesn't give you reliable feedback. That breath is from the lungs, whereas bad breath comes from the back of the mouth and is exhaled when we talk or sigh.

Bad breath is a common symptom of periodontal disease (discussed below) and can occur as a result of xerostomia. The primary cause is a dental problem, so don't rely on mouthwash or a breath freshener to "fix" your bad breath. They only mask the odor for a few minutes. A mouthwash kills some of the bacteria, but within a short time the remaining bacteria begin to multiply in an unrelenting, hard-hitting manner. Bad breath happens whenever the millions of bacteria in our mouths digest protein particles, which then produces sulfur gases.

Having a dry mouth sharply increases the chance of bad breath because the saliva that cleanses the mouth isn't in sufficient quantity. If you slept with your mouth open, your mouth has dried out. That dry environment is a perfect breeding ground for the anaerobic sulfur-producing bacteria that cause the morning's dragon breath. Whenever bad breath is caused by dry mouth, it stems from the back of the tongue, where there is too little saliva to cleanse that area. Typically, men age 65 or older will have to work a little harder to conquer their midday or continuous bad breath, since we have a higher probably of developing xerostomia as we age. Recall that it isn't aging itself that triggers the dry mouth and bad breath; it is most likely one of the medications you use. Your physician would know if there is an alternative medication that doesn't cause dry mouth as a side effect.

When that morning breath doesn't go away after brushing or when bad breath becomes an all-day fellow traveler, it is most likely a sign of gingivitis or periodontal disease. As troubling as the foul breath is, it is also a clear message to see a dentist and begin trying to manage the gum disease.

There are a number of easy things you can do to decrease the presence of bad breath while you and your dentist work to improve your overall dental health:

> Quick fixes: eat an orange, chew a handful of mini carrots, or eat an apple. Both the saliva flow caused by chewing and the coating these foods provide help cleanse the mouth.

> Eat yogurt (at least 6 ounces a day). Unsweetened yogurt contains two common bacteria called *streptococcus thermophilus* and *lactobacillus bulgaricus*. These bacteria battle the stink-causing bacteria; like a shield, the yogurt coats the mouth with the good bacteria to help prevent new stink-causing bacteria from forming.

> Chew sugarless, xylitol, or an antimicrobial gum. Chewing gum stimulates saliva flow, and it is the saliva that acts as a natural mouthwash, cleansing the teeth of bacteria. An antibacterial chewing gum can kill harmful mouth bacteria, such as the streptococcus mutants. There are different antimicrobial "agents" (additives to the gum), and several are digestible, benefiting the whole body.

> ⟩ Use peppermint oil. Because of its antiseptic properties, it can remove bad breath temporarily. Put a few drops in a glass of water and rinse before you have a social event or face-to-face meeting. It's no wonder that peppermint is added to many toothpastes and chewing gum.

> ⟩ Don't skip breakfast. Chewing food in the morning not only is nutritious but gets the saliva flowing. Do brush afterward to remove the microscopic particles of food that could become fertilizer for bacteria growth.

> ⟩ Brush the tongue. This is one of the easiest ways to fight halitosis, since it is the tongue surface that hosts millions of bacteria. Alternatively, have a tongue scraper handy and use once or twice a day to remove the layer of mucus on the top of the tongue, particularly toward the back. Don't let your tongue become a dirty carpet.

> ⟩ Use a natural oil toothpaste that contains fluoride. Even though you probably grew up using a minty toothpaste that left you feeling like you had a fresh mouth, mint has actually the least strength to mask bad breath. Many natural oils and herbs found across the world are concentrated within natural toothpastes and protect teeth, heal gums, and provide extended mouthwash-type freshness. However, ensure that your toothpaste has the ADA seal of approval and still contains fluoride.

> ⟩ It's not "girly" to use a straw. A straw can send sugary or sticky liquids past the teeth and tongue so they don't stay in the mouth and become home for bacteria.

> ⟩ Consuming plenty of water keeps your mouth moist and reduces the acidity of your mouth, creating a less friendly environment for bacteria.

Receding Gums

When the protective gum tissue around your teeth pulls away from the crown and moves downward toward the root, this is called *gingival recession*. Many times, we have no control over whether or not our gum tissue will recede; people who take care of their mouths on a daily basis may still experience this as they get older. One culprit is genetics. Because some people are born with teeth that crowd one another or with thin layers of gingival tissue, their gum tissue will most likely recede with time.

But there are causes of receding gum tissue that we are in control of. This includes harsh brushing of the gums, which can lead to their

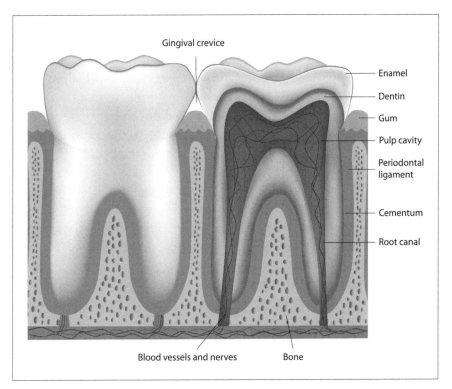

Figure 17.2. Anatomy of the tooth. Courtesy of Alila Sao Mai / Shutterstock.com.

deterioration. It is important to be gentle with your gums, change your toothbrush regularly, and floss on a daily basis in order to combat the potential receding of gingival tissue. Another common cause is inadequate oral hygiene, which eventually results in periodontal disease. If you are noticing that your gums are not where they used to be, notify your dentist to plan treatment options.

Gum Disease

Gingivitis is the earliest and reversible form of gum disease; *periodontitis* is the next and is subdivided into moderate and severe (or advanced) gum disease. Both gingivitis and periodontitis have decreased in prevalence since the early 1970s,[21] principally as a result of improved dental care, secondary to employer-based dental health insurance, which helps offset the cost of professional care. Both forms of gum disease remain more common among men, especially those with limited economic resources.[22]

Most men age 50 and older have given their gums quite the opportunity to become diseased, simply because we weren't encouraged to practice the rigorous oral habits that children are taught nowadays. More than half of all adult men, and nearly two-thirds of Hispanic men, have the gingivitis warning signs that include persistent bad breath, bleeding gums when brushing, and swollen, inflamed red gums.[23] Unfortunately, the more severe gum disease becomes, the more men report quality-of-life problems with eating, relaxing, feeling self-conscious, and avoiding going out.[24]

Gum disease is caused by plaque—the layer of bacteria that forms on our teeth when not properly cleansed. The gum tissue next to the teeth normally has a small "pocket" no more than 3 millimeters in depth. When the gum is chronically infected, the gingival tissue around the teeth decomposes and draws away from the teeth to cause deeper "pockets" between teeth and gum tissue. Bleeding of gum tissue when you brush or when the dentist probes the tissue is an indication that you already have gingivitis. Without conscious, active self-care and regular dental cleaning, the ride into periodontal disease becomes a free fall.

With periodontal disease, the pocket depth will increase to 5 millimeters or greater, becoming a virtual "pit" and breeding space for yet more aggressive bacteria to be produced, weakening tooth attachment to the bone. Eventually, if too much bone is lost, the teeth become loose and/or require removal. Most times gum disease causes us no pain, but there are other ways to self-diagnose. You will notice the persistent bad breath, even minutes after you've brushed and/or used a mouthwash. You find your gums tender (not necessarily painful or sore), and when you examine them in the mirror, most of the tissue looks redder rather than the expected salmon pink. You are witnessing periodontal disease. Should you find that your gums bleed while brushing or as you spit the toothpaste, the red flag is up. Changes in the way your teeth fit together and getting more food stuck in between your teeth are also warning signs.

Periodontal disease is treatable; however, the success rate depends on the progression of the disease before treatment and your commitment to self-care after therapy. As mentioned, severity is defined by the depth of the pockets—the spaces between the teeth and gums. If the disease isn't yet severe, the primary treatment includes root planing and scaling, along with medications to control the infections. When a dental hygienist does a "scaling" (or deep cleaning), the objective is to remove the plaque and tartar within the pockets under the gum line. Root planing entails the smoothing of the tooth's root surfaces, which makes it more difficult for plaque to build up and easier for the damaged gum tissue to heal. Traditionally, both procedures were done with a hand instrument (a scalar), which still may be the method of choice. The dental hygienist may want to use an ultrasonic cleaner or a diode laser to better remove the plaque-causing bacteria. The scaling and planing can be uncomfortable, and they are usually completed with a local anesthetic rubbed on or injected into the gums. The dentist also may prescribe some medication (usually a heavy-duty dose of ibuprofen) to help ease the posttreatment pain and induce a faster healing process. The scaling and root planing may be sufficient to stabilize the progression of the gum disease, and with ongoing dental visits for deep cleaning you can sustain your mouth's health.

For some men, scaling and planing are not sufficient; periodontal surgery becomes necessary when the gum tissue around your teeth is unhealthy and cannot be repaired with nonsurgical strategies. Rarely is this surgical procedure done by your general dentist. You are referred to a periodontal specialist, who will perform one or more types of periodontal surgery. One is pocket reduction surgery, which involves "folding back the gum tissue" and removing the disease-causing bacteria before securing the tissue back into place. More precisely, this surgery involves removal of the unhealthy gum tissue; it effectively reduces the pocket depth, and afterward there is less remaining gum surrounding the teeth. Another is a "regenerative procedure" to assist the bone supporting your teeth. When your bone loss is severe enough, the periodontist may prefer the latter method. Bone grafts or tissue-stimulating proteins can be used to encourage your body's natural ability to regenerate bone and tissue. A third type of surgery involves a soft tissue graft to cover exposed tooth roots and hopefully develop new gum tissue. All forms of periodontal surgery can be accomplished in one or more office visits. They require a few days of liquid or soft-food diets to give the gums time to heal. Each of the procedures is expensive, though often partially covered if you have dental insurance.

Tooth Decay (Cavities)

As we age, we may become more susceptible to tooth decay caused by periodontal disease, which exposes our teeth's roots to bacteria.[25] Cavities (also called *caries*) are decayed areas of your teeth that develop into tiny openings or holes. Untreated, the size of the cavity expands, and the decay usually causes a toothache if it reaches the pulp. In its early stages a cavity will not usually cause pain and can be treated by a simple filling; this is why regular dental checkups and early detection are so important. Otherwise, untreated cavities are the main cause for having to undergo a root canal and, sometimes, the need for a tooth implant or being fitted for dentures.

To avoid losing the ability to chew, swallow, and talk, it is worthwhile to understand how we get cavities. They develop when we eat food that contains carbohydrates (the starches and sugars from bread, grains, pasta, soda, beer, candy) but neglect to clean the teeth's surface afterward. The particles left behind feed the bacteria, and the acid produced by the bacteria is what destroys the tooth's enamel. The acid literally eats through the outside surface of the tooth, the enamel, and then exposes the root's protective coat, the cementum, which is more vulnerable than the enamel. When the bacteria and acid next invade the dentin, with its many nerve endings, we feel the pain.

RESCUING YOUR TEETH: ROOT CANALS AND CROWNS

Before resorting to pulling a tooth and hopefully replacing it with a permanent implant, saving the tooth is always the first line of defense. This might mean having a crown added—literally, capping the top of the tooth—or it might involve a root canal procedure. The benefit of both is a better quality of life compared with managing life with lost teeth.

A tooth needs to be treated when it is badly decayed or cracked, or when the tooth has already undergone several previous dental procedures. If your dentist tells you that you need a root canal, it is important to be informed on what the reasons are and what is going to happen. If you need a root canal, get it done. It is no longer the horror story that legends suggest. Your

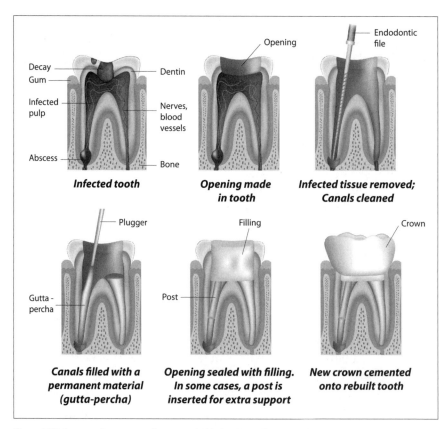

Figure 17.3. Root canal treatment. Courtesy of Alila Sao Mai / Shutterstock.com.

dentist will always first try to fill a decayed tooth and will only recommend a root canal procedure when the decay has infected the dental pulp.

You may wonder why it is called a "root canal" if the infected dental pulp is the part of the tooth that is being removed. Inside the root canals is the dental pulp, which contains blood vessels and nerves, and when the dental pulp becomes infected, the nerves in the canals are (electrically) charged and we experience nagging discomfort, often pain. This "sensation" demonstrates that the pulp is inflamed or infected and needs to be removed and then the area cleaned and sealed. Otherwise, bacteria will begin to fully colonize the dental pulp, and then there is risk for an abscess to be formed. An abscess is a pocket of pus that will fill at the ends of the tooth's roots, and if not taken care of promptly and correctly, it can cause worse damage, including significant bone loss and pain.

A root canal is called an *endodontic treatment*, which means that it treats the inside of the tooth. You can go to either your dentist or an endodontist, depending on the amount of damage to the tooth and level of difficulty. Much of the procedure parallels the experience of having a cavity filled. X-rays are used to examine the tooth and surrounding bone structures, the area of the jaw is numbed, and a hole is drilled into the tooth to access the internal canal, so that the entire inside of the tooth can be cleaned. If there is an infection active within the tooth, the endodontist usually puts medication inside the tooth, secures a temporary filling, and resumes the treatment a week later. More times than not, however, the root canal procedure is finished in the same appointment. The area of the dental pulp and the root's canal are filled with a rubber-based material, and the hole drilled into the tooth is sealed with a filling. After a procedure like this, the integrity of the tooth's structure is often weakened, and to avoid fracture the tooth will need to be restored with a cap or crown.

Each crown is original, built to fit the tooth. To make and apply a crown, the dentist first files down the sides and top of the natural tooth, intentionally reshaping it. An impression is made of the tooth using a Silly Putty type of molding compound, and this impression is then sent to a laboratory to construct a permanent crown that the dentist will insert in a follow-up appointment. Before concluding the initial visit, the dentist applies a temporary crown to protect the tooth.

There are a few different kinds of crowns, which look different, cost different amounts, and have different durability and lasting ability. It is important for you to choose the crown that will best fit your needs of appearance, functionality, and pocketbook. *Metal crowns* are made of different types of alloy (e.g., gold), and even though they are not truly appealing to the eye, they are known for being the most durable and lasting crown. They are also least likely to chip and do damage to other teeth that are nearby. The biggest downfall is that they make you look like you are in a rap music video, so keep the metal crowns for the back, out-of-sight teeth. *Porcelain-fused-to-metal crowns* have been the standard for many years. *All-ceramic* or *all-porcelain crowns* provide the best natural color, are preferred for the frontal teeth, and are the best choice when aesthetics are important, because they are the most able to replicate your normal teeth. Not only are they durable and long-lasting when properly maintained, but the development of new ceramic materials (referred to by such names as E-max, Laur, Bruxzir) has enabled dentists to dramatically improve the cosmetic appearance of the crowns. The new ceramics also permit the dentist to just cover that part of the tooth that is visible; this is known as a veneer and discussed later in the chapter. There are essentially no differences in the prices of ceramic and porcelain crowns; all-gold crowns are a little more expensive. Finally, *all-resin crowns* are made to match your teeth color and are the least expensive crown, but they are not used as a long-term solution, as they are prone to chipping.

TOOTH LOSS

Compared to earlier generations, fewer men are experiencing tooth loss. Adult men have 28 to 32 teeth to start. When a man has six or more teeth removed due to decay/disease, it is medically called *partial edentulism*. *Complete edentulism* is when no natural teeth remain. Tooth loss can be caused by tooth decay or periodontal disease. Whenever there is tooth loss, it affects the mouth's functionality (e.g., chewing), speaking, and the way a man perceives himself. The treatment for tooth loss depends on the number of teeth lost—ranging from permanent dental implants, to dental bridges, to the replacement of teeth with dentures, partial or full.

TOOTH REPLACEMENT

The replacement of missing teeth is very important. When teeth are lost, the remaining teeth tend to shift and fill some of the empty space created. The shifting leaves the remaining natural teeth leaning in odd directions, resulting in a crooked appearance. The basic types of tooth replacement are dental implants, fixed dental bridges, removable partial dentures, and removable complete dentures. All types of tooth replacement make a huge, positive impact on your life. They will increase your confidence with your appearance and enhance your ability to enjoy eating (biting and chewing), talking, laughing, and going out with family and friends.[26]

The cost-benefit analysis when considering one to several replacement teeth leans more favorably toward having dental implants. Implants can be used to replace one or several missing teeth. The result feels like a natural tooth. They do not rely on neighboring teeth for support, and each implant is designed to permanently fill the existing empty space. Within a short time you will not remember that you have a "false tooth" in your mouth. Implants involve titanium-threaded screws that are surgically placed into the jaw bone where the teeth are missing; the screws become the "roots" to hold a replacement tooth. If several adjacent teeth are missing, you do not have to place an implant for every tooth. An implant can hold one replacement (or prosthetic) tooth, and several implants can anchor a row of replacement teeth or an entire arch of teeth. The work is typically completed in stages. Most often you will be referred to a periodontist or oral surgeon for surgical implant(s), and then after you heal your dentist will attach a temporary cap. After you've healed for 1–2 months, your dentist will complete the procedure by adding the permanent crown or a row of crowns. Implants are quickly becoming the ideal way to replace teeth, since they will preserve the jaw bone and do not affect your adjacent teeth.

An alternative is a fixed bridge, which used to be a dentist's first choice in treating missing teeth, before implants came along. A bridge is a permanent restoration and will look stunningly similar to the natural teeth. For a fixed bridge, crowns are placed over the teeth residing next to the vacant spot and a "false tooth" is connected to these crowns. The adjacent teeth are what anchor the replacement tooth or teeth. Fixed bridges are sometimes preferred when the adjacent teeth are loose, because the bridge joins all these teeth together and provides greater strength. The cost of a fixed bridge is about the same as implants.

When dental implants or a fixed bridge are not affordable, partial dentures are a smart option. They are designed to keep the remaining teeth in their natural positions and fill empty tooth spaces to ensure proper biting and chewing, as well as a gap-free smile. A denture is a prosthesis that affixes false teeth to the existing natural teeth. The replacement teeth are traditionally attached to a pink or gum-colored plastic dental base that is held together by a metal structure. When inserted, there are small wire clasps that grip the surrounding natural teeth to secure the denture. All in all, a removable partial denture is the preferred option only if a fixed alternative is not affordable.

Complete dentures are used when there are no healthy teeth left in the mouth. If there are a few remaining teeth that are not salvageable, the dentist will pull them in order to make room for the complete denture. The conventional dentures are placed immediately after all the teeth are removed and then adjusted after 8–12 weeks. This is the time needed for the gums to shrink and for the fit to improve. Two common problems that many men have with their dentures is the adjustment needed to finally obtain the right fit and the need to have the dentures relined after a period of time. A small amount of denture adhesive may be applied to properly fit the denture.

Most men with a new denture are initially hesitant to bite and chew some foods, but after a while they get used to the feel and also learn to cut food into smaller pieces. Having dentures doesn't often interfere with maintaining a balanced nutritional diet, and dentists will often recommend that men with dentures take supplemental vitamins to assure their health.

COSMETIC DENTISTRY

It is clear that in today's society, image counts, and as a flood of advertising suggests, what better way is there to impress the person next to you than flashing a smile with perfectly white, straight teeth? Improving our image and in turn our self-esteem is becoming a key reason for middle-aged and older men to take care of their teeth. Even though brushing, flossing, and visiting the dentist are all part of the routine to keeping our mouths healthy, let's not kid ourselves—most men are as concerned with how our teeth and mouth appear. We can become embarrassed by the color of our teeth and go through great lengths not to show them. If you can afford it, is it time to stop hiding and start flashing those pearly whites? There are many ways to reverse all the coffee and food stains on the outside of our teeth, from getting our teeth professionally cleaned and examined for dental problems, to using whitening toothpastes or gels, to new professional cosmetic dentistry techniques.

Whitening/Bleaching

The means to obtain a white(r) smile differ in significant ways. They involve variations in cost, in the length of their effect, and in the amount of time needed for the procedure.

The first method includes over-the-counter whitening toothpaste, whitening strips, and/or whitening mouth guards. Each includes a very low level of whitening (or bleaching) agent, 3–6 percent hydrogen peroxide, and they are the most cost-efficient way of initially achieving a white(r) smile. The best part about *whitening toothpaste* is that you will not feel like you are going out of your way to whiten your teeth. It is necessary to be persistent in order to achieve the results you want, so you should brush with it at least twice a day. Over-the-counter *whitening strips* require a little more effort, but they can be worn as you go along with your everyday activities. Teeth-whitening strips are thin, clear, flexible pieces of plastic coated on one side with a thin film of hydrogen peroxide bleaching agent. The strips are positioned over the teeth and then gently pressed into place to stabilize them and maximize the contact between the whitening agent and the teeth. The process requires two sessions of roughly 30 minutes per day for 2 weeks before results are noticeable. If you are unable to find time or remember the white strips during the day, a great alternative is a *night whitening mouth guard*. Simply put the mouth guard on before bed, and within 2 weeks your teeth may look much brighter.

The next strategies involve making trips to the dentist and greater expense. As much as we like to avoid having a dentist scrape the plaque off our teeth, it is a fact that a regular professional cleaning whitens teeth. If you visit the dentist at least once a year for a cleaning, then you are already doing your appearance and teeth a favor. Your dentist is also able to provide you a whitening mouth guard sculpted specifically for your teeth. If you feel that your teeth need a dramatic change in color, another option is in-office bleaching. This method requires a high level of whitening agent being applied to the teeth, 25–35 percent hydrogen peroxide, and then use of heat or light to further increase the whitening effect. Results can be seen after only one appointment; however, maintaining the whiteness will require additional future appointments. This can also cause some tooth sensitivity, so you should discuss options with your dentist.

The lower the percentage of peroxide whitening agent, the more time is needed to whiten the teeth, but the less the expense. By comparison, if your teeth are already stained and have a darker baseline to start with, whitening methods will take longer to achieve the results you see advertised, and it is unlikely that you will ever mimic the "doctored" photos. Be careful: you can construct such a dazzlingly white set of teeth that the appearance effect is "unreal."

Veneers

Veneers are thin, custom-made porcelain moldings that are put over our teeth to hide cracks, gaps, and misshapen teeth. If you have been whitening and bleaching and not seeing results, veneers give a white smile that will not fade or discolor over the years. The process is much simpler than required to fit a cap or crown. First, the tooth (or teeth) is shaved down a bit by removing some of the existing enamel. This is done in order to keep the added thickness of the veneer from looking odd. Then, a mold is taken of the tooth (or teeth) for a lab to make the veneers custom fit your mouth. The last step is applying the veneers with an adhesive that binds to natural teeth.

The decision to invest in veneers pivots on the aesthetics versus costs. With veneers there is no need to be self-conscious about misshapen or cracked teeth anymore. Plus, they are stain-proof and retain the same whiteness from the day they are applied. This means that there is no need to use whitening or bleaching methods anymore, but it also means that you must studiously maintain the upkeep on your other teeth. Because there is no noticeable way to tell the difference between a natural tooth and a veneer, you would take care of veneers the same way that you would take care of natural teeth—by brushing and flossing regularly. Recognize, however, that the decision to get veneers is irreversible because of the enamel taken from natural teeth to fit the veneers.

Invisalign

Along with whitening and veneering, cosmetic dentistry also includes straightening teeth. If you believe that braces are too embarrassing for a middle-aged or older man, or simply not appropriate for a man your age, then there is a *clear* alternative: Invisalign. These clear "braces" are usually worn for 12 or 18 months, and during this time they can dramatically improve the straightness of your teeth and your bite without having an adolescent's "metal mouth." Much like a very thin mouth guard, the "braces" can be removed when eating, drinking, and for special occasions.

Another interesting advantage is that you can choose the way you want your smile to look. This is accomplished by the orthodontist showing you through computer technology how they can control the way your teeth shift to get that (perfect) smile. The Invisalign molds are changed every 2 weeks in order to keep your teeth and bite modification on track. However, Invisalign is expensive, equivalent to conventional metal braces, and depending on your dental insurance, the orthodontist visits could be costly. They cannot correct all problems, and a consultation with an orthodontist is necessary to determine if you are a candidate.

ORAL CANCER

Oral cancer is a scary topic to examine in the context of dental and oral health; however, it is important for men to understand that oral cancer is a growing risk. Public health agencies anticipate that the risk for oral or pharyngeal cancers is growing, affecting tens of thousands of men annually. Of men newly diagnosed, only half will be alive in 5 years. The high death rate is not because it is hard to diagnose, but because the cancer is routinely discovered very late in its development. Oral cancer commonly originates on tissue on the lips or tongue, but it can occur on cheek lining, gums, or either the roof or floor of the mouth. The tumors may resemble small ulcers or lumps, and men may initially disregard them as "cankerous sores." Symptoms include white (or mixed red and white) patches inside your mouth, a growing lump that is crusted and rough, and bleeding.

Oral and pharyngeal cancers have become the sixth most common type of cancer in men, mostly because men engage in high-risk behaviors and underrate the importance of routine dental cleanings and checkups. Early detection is crucial to increasing the survival rate for these cancers, but early signs of oral cancer are difficult for us to detect at home. Regular dental visits are your way to assure an early diagnosis.

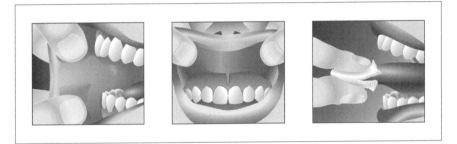

Figure 17.4. Routine oral cancer exam. Illustration by Jacqueline Schaffer.

The prominent cause is tobacco use. The decision to smoke—particularly cigarettes, but men who use cigars or a pipe are not immune—is a gamble against your health. Playing craps might have better Las Vegas odds than other types of gambling, yet the house nearly always wins. Smokers inevitably lose. "Smokeless" tobacco—whether called spit or spitting tobacco, dip, chew, or snuff—also leads to oral cancer. Men using snuff place a "pinch" between the cheek and gums or behind the upper or lower lip. Men who "chew" usually hold or "store" the tobacco toward the back of the mouth in the cheek, typically the lower cheek. By holding the tobacco against the cheek and gums, the nicotine and cancerous chemicals in tobacco are absorbed through the tissues lining the mouth, which can cause cancerous changes in the adjacent tissue.

The other prominent cause is the human papillomavirus (HPV), a sexually transmitted disease that men invisibly carry, rarely exhibiting symptoms.[27] Men are more likely to have an oral HPV infection than women, and a rise in oral sex may be driving up HPV infection rates in men. For men who smoke and reenter (or remain in) the dating marketplace, there is a near doubling of the risk of oral cancers. Sadly, the methods used to treat oral cancers (surgery, radiation, and chemotherapy) are disfiguring and costly.

IT IS A BIG DEAL

Men's motivation to participate in self-care and seek dental care has begun to shift from "doing nothing" to embracing oral health for life. The way we care for our teeth, gums, and mouth reflects and affects the way we view ourselves. Most of all, it affects our entire attitude toward how to live the second half of our lives. We now have the ability to make ourselves look and feel good about our mouth's appearance and ensure that our teeth and mouth retain their functionality. Struggling to chew, swallow, or talk diminishes your quality of life. Why should poor dental health be an accepted consequence of getting older, much as it marred our grandfathers' and fathers' well-being? We have the power to not be that guy grossing out others with his dragon breath. By taking up good dental health habits and, equally importantly, going to the dentist, we won't have to deal with the hassles of serious oral health problems. Any less distress is always a good thing. If you want to have strong and functional teeth, then take care of them. They are the only teeth you have.

CHAPTER 18

Vision and Hearing

with Cynthia Stuen

Think for 5 seconds and make a choice—if you had to lose your hearing or your vision, which one would you choose to keep? Many people who answer this question say "vision," probably because we live in such a visual society where we are constantly bombarded with information that is visual. However, it was Helen Keller who stated that her loss of vision cut her off from things, but that her loss of hearing cut her off from people. Put yourself right now in a restaurant with a friend and imagine you have no vision. You can still hear your waiter tell you what is on the menu, and you can eat your food and engage in conversation with your friend. If you had lost your hearing and your friend did not know sign language, you would probably dine in silence even though you could see everything around you.

This chapter is *not* about blindness or deafness. It is about the normal changes that occur with vision and our hearing as we age, and we summarize most of the eye disorders that older men might encounter. Many middle-aged and older men maintain normal or nearly normal sight and hearing well into late life; many of us (at least two-thirds) will face imperfect sight by age 60,[1] and 27 percent of men age 45 and older begin to have difficulty hearing.[2] Hearing loss and changes in our vision are too often accepted as a "normal" part of the aging process by men themselves, our long-term partners, and even health care providers. As a result, we tend not to actively seek or be referred to hearing and vision treatment services. Understanding what occurs, as well as what to become aware of and sensitive to, is a critical step toward preparing for what may be down the road.

NORMAL CHANGES TO VISION

Presbyopia

With 20/20 vision, the lens inside the eye can easily focus on distant and near objects. With age, the lens loses its ability to focus adequately. Somewhere in the fourth or fifth decade of life, the most common age-related vision change occurs and we become less able to focus on near tasks. It is called *presbyopia* (aging eye) and occurs when the lens of the eye becomes denser, more yellow, and less elastic. This change makes it harder to focus on tasks requiring near distance such as reading and/or intermediate tasks such as using the computer. We need to hold books, magazines, newspapers, menus, and other reading materials at arm's length in order to see and read the print. Presbyopia is correctable with a pair of reading glasses or eyeglasses with bifocal, trifocal, or progressive lenses. Unfortunately, many middle-aged and older men who require glasses choose not to use them; instead, they become those "guys" who always hold a memo or the newspaper at arm's length just to read it. This decision not to get and use reading glasses or a new lens prescription can get scary if you have trouble determining which medicine is in what orange bottle. Because the lens continues to change as you grow older, you can expect to occasionally need a stronger correction.

Accommodation

Another normal age-related vision change is a lag in *accommodation*, or the (re)focusing ability of the presbyopic eye. For example, going from a dark movie theatre to the outside on a sunny day illustrates the aging eye. The amount of time it takes for the adjustment from dark to light or vice versa increases as we grow older because of the increased thickness of the lens and the lesser flexibility of the (cilary) muscle that moves the iris. It is a modest inconvenience for most men.

Shrinking of the Pupil

The pupil of the eye becomes smaller as we age, allowing less light into the presbyopic eye. Actually beginning in about the third decade of life, you will need 10 percent more light with each passing decade to maintain the same level of visual function. When lighting is optimal for the task at hand, you can function very well with the normal age-related vision changes. However, night vision does become more problematic, since it is not as easy to get adequate light in the dark. This suggests that older men should not be surprised to find that seeing clearly in the dark while driving or working outside at night can become more challenging and will, in turn, require greater concentration and attention on their part, or giving up night driving.

Contrast Sensitivity

Contrast sensitivity is a vision-related capacity that also tends to diminish with age as the lens of the presbyopic eye becomes denser and more yellow over time. When you go to your sock drawer, you may well discover over the years that it becomes a bit harder to distinguish navy blue from black socks; colors become less vivid or faded, which is why having good color contrast in what you are looking at is important. To address diminished color sensitivity in your everyday life, you may want to pay special attention when approaching stairs and curbs, as the change in color between adjoining surfaces may become less apparent as you grow older. In your home you may want to make a special effort to create clearly contrasting color edges between floors and stairs.

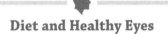

Diet and Healthy Eyes

These diet guidelines are suggested to improve your chance of healthy vision as you grow older:

- *Make sure you consume the healthy fats.* Fish, flaxseed oil, and canola oil have omega-3 healthy fats, which help to prevent dry eyes and can possibly help you avoid cataracts.

- *Try to eat whole grains and low-sugar cereals.* There is evidence to suggest that sugars and refined white flours may increase your chances of eye diseases.

- *Choose good sources of protein.* Remember to avoid saturated fats from red meats and dairy products because these may increase your risk of macular degeneration.

- *Avoid too much salt.* There is evidence that high sodium intake may add to your risk of forming cataracts. You will want to stay below 2,000 mg of sodium each day.

- *Keep your body hydrated.* Proper hydration may be helpful in reducing irritation from dry eyes.

Source: Jegtvig, S. (2010). *How diet and nutrition protect aging eyes.* San Diego, CA: All About Vision.

Increased Sensitivity

An increased sensitivity to glare is also a common vision complaint of men in their later years. Bright sunshine streaming in a window may need to be tempered with a blind or shade to control the glare, and shading the eyes when outdoors is advisable by wearing a hat or cap with a brim. Even highly waxed and polished floors can create a glare problem and cause visual discomfort. Increasing discomfort under bright lights or at night with oncoming car headlights may also be more pronounced.

Visual Acuity

There is some good news to report about men's vision in the second half of life, however. Visual acuity remains very well preserved throughout our life span, except, of course, for any eye disorder(s) that men might already have or acquire. A classic study of an entire town, the Framingham Heart Study, documented that 92 percent of individuals in the town between the ages of 65 and 74 and 70 percent between the ages of 75 and 85 retained corrected visual acuity of at least 20/25 in their better eye.[3] However, visual acuity is only one component of vision. The other components—contrast, accommodation, and glare—that affect your quality of life need to be taken into account.[4]

There are several things you can do to protect your vision. First of all, it is very important for all men to have a dilated eye exam every 1–2 years. If you have a family history of any eye disorder, it is also important to have an eye exam at least annually. For anyone with diabetes, it is very wise to have an annual dilated eye exam in order to detect leaking blood vessels in the eye and preserve as much vision as possible by early treatment. Wearing protective eyewear that blocks ultraviolet rays and protective eye gear when playing sports is also a smart thing to do. Good nutrition is also essential to maintaining healthy eyes (see boxed insert).

Increasing attention is being given to the role that the oxidation process has on our eyes. There are studies showing that cataracts and macular degeneration may be slowed by consuming foods rich in antioxidants, such as fruits and vegetables, particularly dark leafy green ones.[5]

Dry Eye

A healthy eye requires a constant flow of tears over the cornea to maintain comfort and to wash away any foreign matter that might enter the eye. With each blink, tears are spread across the front surface of the eye. However, our tear production often diminishes with age and as a side effect of certain medicines and some illnesses. Without enough tears washing over the eye to ward off the gritty, scratchy, or stinging feelings, dry eye can be uncomfortable.

Dry eye also can be caused by over-the-counter medications such as an antihistamine for allergies or a nasal decongestant, or by prescription medications for conditions such as the beta blockers and diuretics for high blood pressure and most antidepressants. Dry eye is associated with inflammatory rheumatoid arthritis,[6] as well as Parkinson's disease, which reduces eye blink.[7] Be sure to read all product information on any drugs being consumed to find out which ones may cause this uncomfortable condition. The National Eye Institute reports that older adults frequently experience dryness of the eyes, including over 1.5 million men 50 years of age and older.[8]

Seeing a doctor to determine the underlying cause of dry eye is the first step you should take. Using an over-the-counter gel, ointment, or artificial tears often solves the problem. If the problem is caused by a medication you are taking, your physician may be able to prescribe a different one that may not have this side effect. Using an air filter or humidifier in your home may also help to relieve the symptoms.

AGE-RELATED VISION DISORDERS

Common eye *disorders* such as cataracts, glaucoma, macular degeneration, and diabetic retinopathy are not particularly foreign terms to most of us, and they are the most common causes of vision impairment in American adults. They are age-related, but not the effects of aging itself. The simulations in figure 18.1 show normal vision and then how each of the various age-related eye disorders affects our field of vision.

Cataracts

Because we live longer than previous generations, we will likely get a cataract at some point. A cataract is a yellowing and clouding of the normally clear lens of the eye. When this occurs (see cataract simulation), everything looks hazy or blurry; there is a loss of contrast, and you may have trouble telling colors apart. Individuals with a cataract also complain that there is an increased sensitivity to glare. There are different types of cataracts, as well as different causes, but the impact is the same. No one is exactly sure of the cause, but it may result from prolonged exposure to ultraviolet light and is also correlated with diabetes, cigarette smoking, diet, alcohol consumption, and obesity.[9] Cataract removal is now done as an outpatient

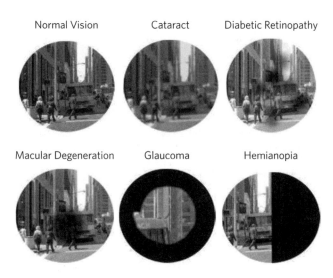

Normal Vision   Cataract   Diabetic Retinopathy

Macular Degeneration   Glaucoma   Hemianopia

Figure 18.1. Simulation of eye disorders. Lighthouse International.

procedure, in which a new ocular lens is implanted to restore clear vision. Oftentimes, following the lens implant, there is no longer a need for near or distance corrective lenses.

Macular Degeneration

Age-related macular degeneration (AMD) is a leading cause of vision impairment among older adults in the United States. As the cross-sectional diagram (figure 18.2) of the eye shows, the retina is the inside layer of the eye. The macula is the very central part at the back of the retina, and it is the part of our eye that we use for performing central vision tasks such as reading, writing, or driving. There is no cure for AMD.

There are two types of macular degeneration, with the dry (atrophic) form being the most common. When the light-sensitive cells in the macula slowly break down, there is a gradual blurring of central vision in the affected eye. While the changes are very subtle, it progresses, and you may come to see a more exaggerated blurred spot in the center of vision. Initially a person may keep rubbing

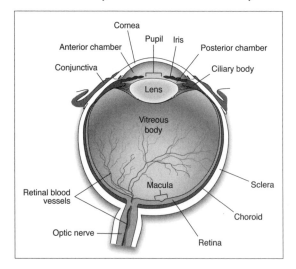

Figure 18.2. Anatomy of the eye. Illustration by Jacqueline Schaffer.

his eye to get the "spot" to go away. For example, when reading a word, parts of letters appear to be missing, or a straight line appears wavy. Dry AMD generally affects both eyes, but it may start out in only one.[10]

The Amsler grid, reproduced here (figure 18.3), is a convenient self-test to post at home and check your vision routinely. Check each eye separately, covering one eye and looking at the center of the grid with the other, and contact your eye doctor immediately if you see wavy lines.

A

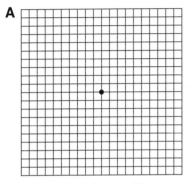

Normal Amsler grid

B

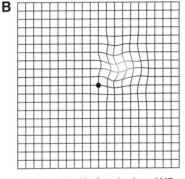

Amsler grid with distortion from AMD

C

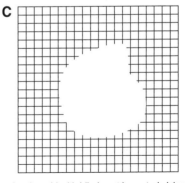

Amsler grid with blind spot in central vision

Figure 18.3. Illustration by Jacqueline Schaffer.

The "wet" (neovascular) form of AMD occurs more suddenly when abnormal blood vessels behind the retina start to grow in or under the macula. These new blood vessels tend to be fragile and often leak blood and fluid, which causes damage to the retina. A large dark spot appears in the center of vision, called a *scotoma*. With wet AMD, central vision loss can occur quickly, and you will need to be seen by an eye doctor immediately.

Treatment of the wet form has some promising new developments. For example, the National Eye Institute has funded 47 study centers throughout the United States to conduct randomized clinical trials comparing injections of Lucentis and Avastin, both of which have individually shown improvement for persons with wet AMD. Remember that these treatments are not cures; they may only slow its progression. Other treatments are on the horizon, but it is important to be under the care of an eye doctor when you have an eye disease.

Glaucoma

For many years, this eye condition was often called "the silent thief of sight." It is silent because it usually has no symptoms and its onset is so gradual that you don't realize it is occurring. Risk factors for glaucoma are age, African American ancestry, a family history of the condition, diabetes, and being extremely nearsighted. The effect of glaucoma is on your peripheral (or side) vision, and if untreated, it will progress so that all vision is lost except the very central "pinhole" vision (see simulation of glaucoma in figure 18.1). There are two major forms of glaucoma: open-angle glaucoma and angle-closure glaucoma. Your eye doctor will determine the type based on whether the fluid within the eye has access to the natural drain (trabecular meshwork), in which case it is open-angle glaucoma, or the drain is blocked by the iris (colored part of the eye), in which case it is angle-closure type. It is important to have your eye pressure checked as part of a routine eye exam; glaucoma is often identified because of elevated eye pressure. It is this pressure that damages the optic nerve, causing permanent loss to one's peripheral field of vision. It's also possible to have glaucoma even if your eye pressure is in the normal range, which is known as *normal tension glaucoma*.

If you have any of the risk factors, and even if no elevated eye pressure is noted, a field test can determine whether there is any loss to your visual field. The term *visual field* refers to the area of what you can see with your eyes fixed on one location. For example, while watching a stoplight, you might notice a car pulling up beside you in the next lane; this uses your peripheral vision. Remember that there are usually no warning signs for glaucoma and it happens very gradually, which is why you need to be alert and have routine eye exams.

Being under the care of an eye doctor to determine the best management of glaucoma is very critical to prevent vision loss from this disorder. Your doctor may prescribe eye drops, or in some cases laser treatments or surgery may be recommended.

Diabetic Retinopathy

One of the results of having diabetes for many years is diabetic retinopathy, which results in vision loss and blindness. Over time, the blood vessels of the retina break down and leak into the eye, causing retinal scars that distort vision or create blind spots. An ophthalmologist will often use laser treatment to seal off leaking blood vessels; however, a scar is present wherever a laser has sealed a vessel, and you cannot see through scar tissue. Roughly 40 percent of people with diabetes experience retinopathy,[11] and because African American, Hispanic, and Native American men have higher rates of diabetes, they are at higher risk for diabetic retinopathy (see the simulation in figure 18.1).

Given the nature of diabetes and the fluctuation in blood sugar levels, the diabetic man's vision may also fluctuate on a daily basis. He may find his vision better during one part of the day than another, but much depends on the overall management of diabetes. Depending on the degree of spotty vision and/or blurry, distorted vision caused by diabetic retinopathy, reading can be difficult. For men with more advanced diabetic retinopathy who may also be using insulin for diabetes control, magnification may be needed to see the syringe, and you can use a "talking glucose monitor" or other adaptive devices to manage medications. For diabetic men without much evidence of retinopathy, the progression of the disease can be slowed with close management of glucose levels, blood pressure, and serum lipids.[12]

Stroke / Brain Injury

Hemianopia occurs when there is damage to the optic pathways in the brain. It can result from a stroke, tumor, or trauma and causes vision loss in half of the visual field. The most common defect is right homonymous hemianopia, which occurs in corresponding halves of the right visual field. Hemianopia can also occur in corresponding left halves, or the upper or lower half of our visual field. This means that without awareness of the loss of half of our visual field, reading a page of text will appear to stop midway and not make any sense. Loss of vision in half of our visual field also means a high risk for bumping into or tripping over objects lying in the affected field of view. It is often missed by health care personnel following a stroke or other trauma to the brain, but it is important to check all four quadrants of the visual field to determine whether hemianopia has occurred, so that rehabilitation may begin.

LOW VISION AND VISION REHABILITATION

Most of the age-related eye disorders that men grapple with do not result in total loss of vision, but rather in low vision or partial sight. Diabetes can be the exception, where total blindness can occur if it is not controlled. Learning to live with low vision begins with a clinical low vision exam conducted by an ophthalmologist or optometrist who has specialized knowledge and focuses on your functional vision abilities. Low vision specialists may be in private practice or work in a not-for-profit vision rehabilitation organization or for a state office/division responsible for serving people who are blind or visually impaired.

It is unfortunate that many of the organizations that address visual impairment issues have in their name "for the Blind." Such language can be a turnoff to anyone who is not blind but just doesn't see very well. This is because fear of blindness is so palpable in our society that folks avoid anything related to blindness. Regardless of the names organizations use to identify themselves, it is critical that you ignore the labels, be brave, and cross the threshold to find help. A low vision specialist's unique training in maximizing your usable vision can help make a difficult task much easier to do, often with the prescription of an optical aid. To find a low vision specialist, contact a vision rehabilitation organization or call your state optometric or state ophthalmologic society and ask for listings for doctors specializing in low vision.

The low vision clinician will determine what tasks or activities your vision impairment is preventing you from doing and then prescribe the best low vision optical aid(s) for you. An array of optical and adaptive devices are available, which men have found useful to maintain their independence. They range from the simplest handheld magnifier to use when reading stock quotes or box scores or other small type, to a telescopic lens for playing golf, to high-powered telescopic lenses that might be used for driving (allowable in some states). Oftentimes the low vision specialist will loan you the device to practice with before making the investment to buy it.

More than recommending which optical aids are best for you, the low vision specialists will prescribe the appropriate power. This is why it is better to have your eye doctor assist you rather than depending on a trial-and-error approach with over-the-counter magnifiers. Also, the high-powered lenses are only available by prescription from an eye doctor. Different visual tasks—near distance (reading mail), intermediate distance (using a computer), or long distance (driving)—may require various adaptive optical enhancements. Just as all eye disorders do not manifest themselves in the same way, neither do their technological applications, which are changing almost daily. Be patient with yourself; learning to use the appropriate adaptive aid takes some time, practice, and adjustment.

Much more powerful magnification can be obtained with a closed-circuit television (CCTV) that can enlarge print up to 60 times. A CCTV can be a desk model or portable, can be in color, and also offers reverse polarity so print can be viewed in black on white or vice versa, depending on your individual preference.

In addition, there are other specialists on the vision rehabilitation team who can help you learn to do the usual visual tasks in alternate ways to maximize independence. Some simple adaptations of everyday, easily available items can make a big difference. Using a felt tip bold pen to write notes may be a very low-tech solution if using a regular pen is not sufficient. Any activity of daily living can be accommodated for a person with vision impairment; it will just take some time to master the vision rehabilitation strategies. How do you shave if you cannot see your face in the mirror, and how can you mow your lawn? All these activities have alternate means of accomplishment, but they take a little time to learn and a little more time to master. Occupational therapists with specialized preparation in low vision rehabilitation or vision rehabilitation therapists provide these services.

Safe mobility is a concern once your vision is impaired. Particularly for more advanced vision loss, an orientation and mobility instructor provides rehabilitation to teach you how to get around safely at home and in your community. Sometimes, having to give up the keys to the car is necessary. In more advanced vision loss or total blindness, learning to use a white cane can help a person walk independently, avoid obstacles on sidewalks/paths, and cross streets safely. Guide dogs are also an option to enhance independent travel, but only if you like dogs. Mastering the use of a white travel cane is a requirement before consideration of a guide dog.

Vision impairment in older adults is related to several health conditions, difficulty with activities of daily living and leisure participation, and increased risk for falls, related fractures, and nursing home placement.[13] Getting help early can make a tremendous difference in learning to adapt your life and how you conduct daily activities in new ways to ensure an ongoing good quality of life. Computers provide many options for enlarging print, changing the font size, and adjusting color contrast for easier reading with vision impairment. The newer handheld smartphones and tablets have various accessibility options that may ease their use depending on the type of vision loss you are experiencing. Increasingly, there are also voice output options for these devices which enable more independence for those who have difficulty reading print.

VISION LOSS AND EMOTIONAL WELLNESS

A variety of emotional responses are often present for a man experiencing vision impairment, such as embarrassment at needing to use a pocket magnifier in public, a sense of demoralization when not being able to drive in the evening or after dark, and the paramount concern that a man's vision loss will permanently strip him of his independence and put him in the passenger's seat. When visual impairment interferes with our ability to read, watch and enjoy television, sightsee, or engage the grandchildren, we may feel depressed and a deep sense of hopelessness. Be aware that for some men it can precipitate a crisis. Consider the airline pilot who can no longer keep his job and needs retooling for a midlife career change. This can result in anger, guilt, denial, and loss of self-esteem. Vision impairment negatively affects quality of life and is a major risk factor for depression.[14] In fact, depression is much more prevalent for persons with vision impairment than the general population.[15] Approximately one-third of older adults with impaired vision feel alienated and experience clinically significant depressive symptoms. As one 77-year-old widower said,

> If I was to lose [more of] my sight, I'd probably just as soon be dead, be finished with it. . . . Now I'm not being . . . I'm not suicidal or anything of that nature. Don't get me wrong. But . . . if you can't see . . . I'm not sure it would be worth living. I guess maybe it would be. . . . But I just feel that way now.[16]

You might think that the severity of the vision loss would be a factor in the severity of the depression, but it is not. Persons with even minimal vision loss are at no less risk for depression than those with more severe impairment.[17] It is very important to recognize the impact you may be feeling with vision loss and to not avoid seeking help. In addition to individual or group counseling, support groups have been found to be very helpful for most people coping with age-related vision impairments; however, the type of self-management group that shares information about novel coping strategies rather than dwelling on feelings will probably be more attractive. Don't judge all groups the same, especially if the first one you visit wasn't what you were looking for. Talking with others (even online) can provide you with helpful strategies for coping with vision loss. Knowing that you

Healthy Eyes

There are several ways men can maintain healthy vision:

- Wear a hat and sunglasses with ultraviolet (UV) protection whenever you are outdoors. The sun's UV rays increase the risk of developing cataracts and macular degeneration.

- Stop smoking. Smoking increases your risk of developing cataracts, macular degeneration, and many other diseases by increasing oxidative stress, narrowing blood vessels, and reducing blood flow to the eye.

- Maintain a healthy diet and adequate nutritional intake.

- Get regular, comprehensive eye examinations. Because many eye diseases have no symptoms until late in the disease, problems are not apparent until diagnosed during an eye examination.

are not alone can be calming; telling stories, laughing with others, and listening to other men's creative adaptations can be reassuring.

Involvement of family and friends is also important so that the significant people in your life can be supportive, if they know how to do so.[18] They can learn, and you can ask for specific support. Too often, well-meaning family or friends can be overprotective. Maintaining your independence as much as possible is good for emotional and physical health, but when the time comes, you need to be able to communicate to others when and how assistance is needed.

FUNCTIONAL VISION SCREENING QUESTIONNAIRE

Take a few moments to take the 15-item Functional Vision Screening Questionnaire.[19] It will help determine if you are having difficulty with visual tasks and need to see an eye doctor. Lighthouse International's Research Institute, the organization that developed this self-administered screening tool, advises that you wear your glasses or contact lenses, if you have them, when you answer the questions. Each question is answered with a "yes" or "no." Scoring is described at the end.

Notice that a score of 1 is applied to the vision problem related to each question. Even if you wanted to qualify some of your answers with "sometimes," you ought to go ahead and score your answer as a problem. A total score of 9 or more indicates that you really need to consult with an optometrist or ophthalmologist for a complete vision examination. Frankly, even a score of 1 is enough to consider making an eye exam appointment.

FUNCTIONAL VISION SCREENING QUESTIONNAIRE

Does the question describe you . . . ?	Yes	No
1. Do you ever feel that problems with your vision make it difficult for you to do the things you would like to do?	1	0
2. Can you see the large print headlines in the newspaper?	0	1
3. Can you see the regular print in newspapers, magazines, or books?	0	1
4. Can you see the numbers and names in a telephone directory?	0	1
5. When you are walking in the street, can you see the "walk" sign and street name signs?	0	1
6. When crossing the street, do cars seem to appear very suddenly?	1	0
7. Does trouble with your vision make it difficult for you to watch TV, play cards, do sewing, or any similar type of activity?	1	0
8. Does trouble with your vision make it difficult for you to see labels on medicine bottles?	1	0
9. Does trouble with your vision make it difficult for you to read prices when you shop?	1	0
10. Does trouble with your vision make it difficult for you to read your own mail?	1	0
11. Does trouble with your vision make it difficult for you to read your own handwriting?	1	0
12. Can you recognize the faces of family or friends when they are across an average-size room?	0	1
13. Do you have any particular difficulty seeing in dim light?	1	0
14. Do you tend to sit very close to the television?	1	0
15. Has a doctor ever told you that nothing more can be done for your vision?	1	0

Source: © The Lighthouse Inc., 1996.

HEARING LOSS

Think again about this chapter's beginning quote from Helen Keller, about her loss of vision cutting her off from things but her loss of hearing cutting her off from people. Claudia Dewane, writing about a day in the life of a hearing-impaired adult, helps to clarify Keller's statement by noting that each day may include being unaware when someone is talking, being unable to hear a normal voice across a room, not comprehending what is said when several people are talking, misunderstanding what is said on television or when someone's face is unseen, not hearing an alarm or telephone, or even missing out on hearing wind and the benefit of the "sweet nothings" softly spoken in a romantic situation.[20]

Sound Intensity: Decibel (dB) Levels

30 dB	Leaves rustling and quiet whisper
60–65 dB	Normal conversation
80 dB	Telephone dial tone
88 dB	Motorcycle (at 30 feet)
90 dB	Food blender
107 dB	Lawnmower
120 dB	Amplified music (rock)
140 dB	Gunshot or fire cracker

Source: American Hearing Research Foundation.

Different from an obvious physical disability, hearing loss is an invisible sensory disability. It is one of the most common health problems for men as we get older, far more common than vision loss, and is associated with getting older. Data from national surveys indicate that at least 20 percent of men older than age 20 have speech-related hearing impairment, and 45 percent have high-frequency related hearing loss.[21] When tested, more than two-thirds of men in the United States age 70 and older met the World Health Organization's criteria for hearing loss; however, barely one

Symptoms of Hearing Loss

- Phone conversations are hard to understand
- You struggle to hear above background noise
- It is difficult to follow a conversation when more than one person speaks at once
- You think people are not speaking clearly or are mumbling
- You misunderstand what people say and sometimes respond wrongly
- Your family complains that the car radio or the TV is too loud
- There is a ringing or hissing sound in your ears

in six men old enough to have Medicare supplement insurance will disclose that they have problems hearing normal conversations.[22] So many men have this slowly developing disability, but so few tell others or seek professional help. Men are five times more likely than women to have a hearing impairment, but we are not very likely to admit it. We might not even say "speak up," because to do so reveals a hearing impairment, and we avoid self-identifying as no longer "normal."

Hearing Loss: Decibel (dB) Levels

Hearing loss is measured by the quietest sounds you can hear:

- Normal hearing—down to 20 dB
- Mild hearing loss—25-40 dB
- Moderate hearing loss—40-70 dB
- Severe hearing loss—70-95 dB
- Profound hearing loss—nothing below 90 dB

Despite wanting someone to speak up, hearing impairment isn't always about volume. Much of the time, our difficulties are with words, accents, and types of sound. For example, an older "Yank" may have a harder time fully understanding a "Brit" with his distinctive British accent than a younger man, and as a man's hearing loss gradually progresses, he will have a harder time distinguishing what is said in conversations with children and some women. Often, words that sound similar, such as "flip" and "slip," cannot be distinguished. Our decreased hearing acuity for high-frequency sounds and decreased ability to discriminate sounds (and words) are the two primary ways we struggle with hearing.

There are different types of hearing troubles, but the hallmark is sensorineural, and it involves problems with the inner ear or auditory nerve dysfunction. Our hearing pathway is made up of the external ear, the middle ear, the inner ear, the nerve pathways, and the brain. Hearing loss is typically irreversible and has many causes that all contribute to the deterioration of the sensory and neural systems. What actually occurs is that the tiny, delicate hairs inside your inner ear (particularly, inside the snail-like structure of the organ of Corti in the cochlea[23]), which detect sound vibrations and convert the mechanical energy of sound waves into electrical signals for the brain to interpret, become damaged. The distressed hair cells supporting the delicate hairs gradually die, which is why most hearing loss is permanent. Alternatively, the nerve pathways (the cochlear nerve) from the inner ear to the brain can become damaged. Without sound activating the cochlear nerve, we do not hear.

Our ability to hear sound and speech gradually diminishes over time, resulting in common age-related hearing loss, also called *presbycusis* (aging ears). The Baltimore Longitudinal Study of Aging followed over 1,000 men for 30 years and found that the decline in hearing sensitivity begins to accelerate after age 20 in men and that the amount of decline in hearing

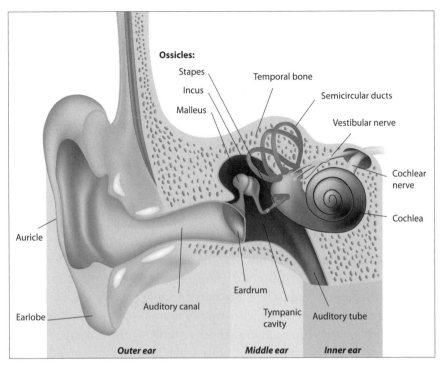

Figure 18.4. Ear anatomy. Courtesy of Alila Sao Mai / Shutterstock.com.

sensitivity to age 60 is twice as fast for men compared with women.[24] For men, the most important consequence of hearing loss is our difficulty in understanding speech, because over time it becomes more problematic to hear high-pitched sounds than to hear low-pitched sounds.[25] As a result, you will be able to hear thunder and a fishing boat but have difficulty hearing your young grandchildren and the mosquito hovering nearby. Speech begins to sound muffled or unclear because of our diminished ability to hear high-pitched sounds. Aside from normal aging, hearing loss can come from exposure to noise, certain drugs, and disease. Noise might be associated with your job, such as working around loud machinery or regularly working with a leaf blower without hearing safety earmuffs or earplugs. Exposure to loud music for long periods of time is also known to damage the hair cells in the inner ear. For some men it could be trauma, a family history of hearing loss, infections, or use of some medications that caused their hearing loss. For example, diuretics and chemotherapeutic drugs are ototoxic and can damage the auditory system. Recently reported in the *American Journal of Medicine*, the regular use of aspirin, acetaminophen, and nonsteroidal anti-inflammatory drugs has been found to increase the risk of men's hearing loss, particularly among men younger than the age of 60.[26] Also, men who use Viagra (sildenafil) or similar drugs for erectile dysfunction (ED) are twice as likely to report hearing impairment, and current warnings regarding the risk of hearing loss related to ED medication use seem to be justified.[27]

A doctor who specializes in problems of the ear, nose, and throat is called an *ENT specialist* or *otolaryngologist*. Once you disclose to your physician that your hearing has diminished, you can (or should) expect to undergo an audiological evaluation. That exam involves a referral to an audiologist, who first looks into your ears to check for anything in the ear canal that might affect the hearing test. Most often you participate in a "pure-tone" test to determine the faintest or softest tones you can hear at different pitches; wearing headphones, the audiologist will chart what you can and cannot hear on a line chart called an *audiogram* (figure 18.5). The most common kind of hearing loss results in a "ski slope" shape on the audiogram—it shows hardly any hearing problem in the low pitches but considerable loss in the high pitches. The degree of hearing loss is divided into five categories: normal, mild, moderate, severe, and profound. As noted on the sample audiogram, the normal aging process will eventually result in a severe loss of hearing sensitivity to high-pitched sounds.

Environmental accommodations such as limiting the immediately surrounding noise or the background noise when having a conversation will help some men. For example, you might need to avoid having conversations in large, open rooms, or you might need to stand a bit closer to the person you are listening to. For other men, enhancing the volume control on the telephone or using headphones when watching television may suffice. A hearing loss in the mild to moderate range may warrant the use of hearing aids to understand normally pitched conversation. If your diagnosis is an auditory processing issue, which could be caused by a stroke, mild cognitive impairment, or other illnesses, amplification will not help.

Four out of five Americans with hearing loss do *not* use hearing aids; this gap shrinks some with age—two out of three older adults do not use hearing aids. This is not because older men become less vain with age. Because the process of hearing loss is gradual, some men adapt to the loss and are not fully aware of how much their hearing is diminishing. Men who own hearing aids may recognize they need them, yet they say they get limited benefit using them and put them in the drawer. The men argue that they do not use the hearing aids because they are performing poorly—and they probably do, since researchers find that the unused hearing aids are the older models. Certainly, stigma remains an issue, and some men choose not to wear a hearing aid because they think they will get a negative reaction from those around them, such as "he's hard of hearing, he must also be dense."[28] There are many types of hearing aids that can be offered. Some fit in the ear; others fit over the earlobe. Your audiologist will review the pros and cons with you and make a professional recommendation.

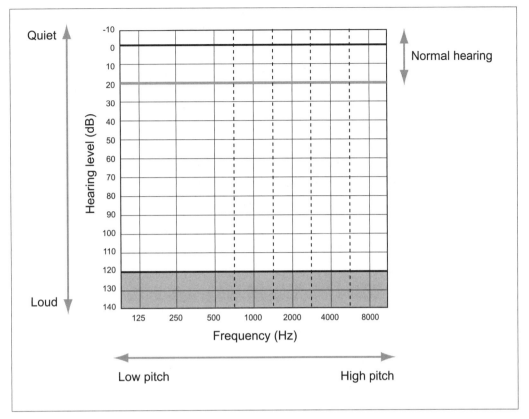

Figure 18.5. Audiogram. Image from the Ohio State University College of Medicine.

There are also assistive listening devices that can be utilized to enhance hearing function. Sometimes they provide an interim step before the purchase of a hearing aid. Increasing the amplification on telephones or using headsets for television or a sound system can increase your enjoyment of the listening experience and avoid annoying others around you who are not having difficulty with hearing. Increasingly, movie theaters and live performances in theaters offer hearing enhancement devices for audiences. If you are experiencing hearing loss, you should certainly ask what is available to make the "listening" environment more enjoyable when you go to the movies.

When a hearing aid is not enough, there are a host of other adaptive technologies, such as vibrating alarm clocks or fire alarms and doorbells that use flashing lights. There are also many text-based options such as closed captioned televisions and telephones. AT&T has a telephone device and service called CapTel that allows the telephone to display captions of everything your caller says. Other telephone service providers will probably also soon offer the same service. Every state also has a "relay" service for anyone who is profoundly hard of hearing and does not have a text phone to be able to directly communicate with a hearing person; your call can be relayed to a computer screen, a smartphone, or a wireless Bluetooth microphone. Newer technology, such as iPhones and iPads, supports voice recognition and can also produce captions for communication.

Just as with vision impairment, men with hearing loss are at increased risk for experiencing depression, anxiety, isolation, or grief. A common complaint from hearing-impaired persons is that they are "dismissed"; their loss is interpreted by others as diminished mental capacity. This can lead to a lot of frustration, especially for the spouse/partner and family and friends. Too often, since age-related hearing loss can be rather gradual, you may just think that people "mumble." Denial or avoidance of the reality will only prolong the agony. Given that so many men face hearing loss, we need to own up, get our hearing examined, and take charge by seeking help.

VISION AND HEARING LOSS—A DOUBLE WHAMMY

Much of the research literature focuses on a single sensory impairment; however, you should be aware that concurrent loss of hearing and vision can pose particular challenges for men. While loss in either vision or hearing may occur early in life as a result of accident, injury, disease, or genetic defect, most of the sensory assaults we face will occur in the second half of our life. Even though some sensory disorders affect certain populations differently, sensory loss knows no class, socioeconomic, or educational boundaries. No one is fully exempt.

The impairment of both vision and hearing function, often referred to as dual sensory loss, affects 22 percent of men age 70 and older, with an estimated 2 million new cases in this population group over the next 5 years.[29] Looking at the population bulge represented by the baby boomers (those born between 1946 and 1964), who are now retiring and joining the ranks of older adults, by 2030, it is estimated that 3.5 to 14 million can be expected to develop dual sensory loss.[30]

Most men will find ways to compensate for a loss of vision or hearing. For example, some men with diminished hearing will rely more heavily on visual cues by looking at closed captions on TV to verify their hearing comprehension, while someone with vision impairment may rely more heavily on auditory cues such as car traffic or use an audio book for easier reading.

Take a look back at the vision simulation examples presented earlier in this chapter and think about a man with macular degeneration (loss of central vision) who can no longer see his friend's facial expressions or read his lips and suddenly realizes that his hearing isn't very good anymore. The hearing was probably slowly deteriorating, but until the loss of central vision took place, he could get cues from the person's facial expression or mouth and could ferret out what was being said. Listening and speech reading, the two primary modes of communication, have been compromised—a double whammy indeed.

A person with vision impairment may appear timid or hesitant in a new situation; a person with a hearing impairment may appear confused, whereas, in reality, it is sensory deficit at work. Such misinterpretation of these behaviors can be very frustrating if an understanding of hearing and/or vision impairment is absent or inadequate. Unfortunately, vision rehabilitation and hearing (aural) rehabilitation are rarely offered in the same setting, and too often these rehabilitation specialists are not aware of each others' work. Keep that in mind should you need to seek professional help in response to any loss you may be experiencing in your vision or hearing.

Acknowledging the losses, taking control of our lives by seeking appropriate help from professionals, actively participating in either vision or aural rehabilitation, and learning about the adaptive techniques and technology that can enhance our lives are all critical ingredients in helping us move into the future with a vision and/or hearing loss with success. Having a vision, hearing, or a dual sensory impairment does *not* diminish us as people. Educate your spouse/partner, family, and friends about what is helpful and what is not.

Arriving at a social gathering and finding that the background music interferes with your ability to engage in conversation can be overcome simply by asking your host to turn the music down or off. Another alternative is to engage a person in conversation and ask to step to another room where it is quieter. "Take control, take charge" needs to be your mantra. Sensory loss will not kill you, but it will impact your quality of life unless you seek professional help and learn to do things in a new way.

You can use the self-administered questionnaire below to determine if your hearing sensitivity has diminished enough to consult an audiologist. If you are a hearing aid user, answer questions according to how you hear with the hearing aid. For each statement below, answer whether the situation describes you, does not describe you, or describes you sometimes. If the question does not apply, circle "no" as your response. For each question, circle the most appropriate response. If your total score is greater than 8, you would benefit from scheduling an exam with an audiologist.

HEARING HANDICAP INVENTORY FOR THE ELDERLY—SCREENING VERSION (HHIE-S)

Does the question describe you . . . ?	No	Sometimes	Yes
1. Does a hearing problem cause you to feel embarrassed when you meet new people?	0	2	4
2. Does a hearing problem cause you to feel frustrated when talking to members of your family?	0	2	4
3. Do you have difficulty hearing when someone speaks in a whisper?	0	2	4
4. Do you feel handicapped by a hearing problem?	0	2	4
5. Does a hearing problem cause you difficulty when visiting friends, relatives, or neighbors?	0	2	4
6. Does a hearing problem cause you to attend religious services less often than you would like?	0	2	4
7. Does a hearing problem cause you to have arguments with family members?	0	2	4
8. Does a hearing problem cause you difficulty when listening to TV or radio?	0	2	4
9. Do you feel that any difficulty with your hearing limits or hampers your personal or social life?	0	2	4
10. Does a hearing problem cause you difficulty when in a restaurant with relatives or friends?	0	2	4

Source: Ventry, I., & Weinstein, B. (1982). The Hearing Handicap Inventory for the Elderly: A new tool. *Ear and Hearing, 3,* 128–134. Lichtenstein, M. J., Bess, F. H., & Logan, S. A. (1988). Validation of screening tools for identifying impaired elderly in primary care. *Journal of the American Medical Association, 259,* 2875–2878.

CHAPTER 19

The Cancers

A cancer diagnosis will certainly trigger a range of powerful emotions—fear, despair, denial, stoic acceptance, anger. Unfortunately, too many men will experience prostate cancer, lung cancer, colon (bowel) cancer, or some other type. In contrast to the declining incidence of coronary heart diseases, with few exceptions the incidence of most cancers is increasing. With more than three-fourths of a million men diagnosed with cancer each year, over the course of our lifetime, half of all men will get cancer at least once. And each of us will be challenged to our core. The cancer diagnosis is a biographical disruption. Our sense of self before the diagnosis is no longer the reference point; we have a new identity. We are cancer patients or survivors. A cancer diagnosis affects our mind, spirit, and quality of life—rattling everything, from our spiritual side, to our psychological well-being, to relationships with family and friends.

Most Common Cancers in Men, All Races

- Skin
- Prostate
- Lung/bronchus
- Colon/rectal
- Urinary bladder
- Non-Hodgkin's lymphoma
- Kidney
- Leukemia
- Oral cavity and pharynx

Although cancers occur throughout the life span, the likelihood of men experiencing any of the common cancers increases as we get older. About 75 percent of all cancers are diagnosed in men age 55 and older. On average, African American men will get a cancer at an earlier age than white men;[1] half of their cancer diagnoses occur before age 64, compared to age 68 for white men. Information from the National Cancer Institute tells us that half of all malignancies among men are accounted for by three cancers: prostate, lung, and colorectal. Indeed, prostate cancer is normally diagnosed after the age of 65 and is the second most common cancer among men, accounting for 25 percent of new cancer diagnoses. The same age-related pattern is true for two of the most infrequent—Merkel cell carcinoma, a fast-growing skin cancer, and Waldenström's macroglobulinemia, a type of lymphoma, account for less than 0.5 percent of all cancers in men and occur most often among men older than 60.[2]

Age is not a causal risk; however, getting older increases the odds of experiencing a cancer. As a general rule, aging tissues and organs *may* be less capable of resisting the growth of cancer cells, because the body's immune system declines. Yet our cancer risk has much more to do with the cumulative effect of the thousands of lifestyle choices we make over time than our aging bodies. What is heartrending is that most cancer deaths are preventable. Scientific evidence suggests that a third of cancer deaths are related to men's lack of physical activity and/or poor diet, and another third are caused by smoking.

Because the likelihood of being diagnosed with an existing cancer increases once men become middle-aged, active surveillance of our bodies and regular checkups from a physician can help prevent most cancers from resulting in an early death. Surveillance and regular screening exams often lead to successful treatment when detected in the cancer's early stages. To emphasize the significance of active surveillance, the death rate associated with colon, skin, and oral cancers is high among men *not* because the cancers are hard to discover or diagnose, but because the cancer is too often discovered late in its development. Too many of us are notorious for ignoring symptoms, even ones that are deadly.

WHAT IS CANCER?

Our bodies are made up of many trillions of cells. Among adults, most cells regularly reproduce to repair injuries and damaged tissues. Cut yourself shaving, and within a few days the injured cells are replaced. Bump and bruise your leg, and within a week or so the damaged cells are replaced. Healthy cells divide and grow in a natural, orderly way, replacing the damaged or aging cells.

But sometimes cells mutate, and once they do, these cells are no longer naturally regulated—the mutant (cancer) cells divide and grow in a haphazard manner. And unlike healthy cells, they do not die. Consequently, the number of cancer cells may increase rapidly—but not always. Some cancers do not become evident until years after the first cancer cell is formed.

Whether fast growing or slow, cancer cells' unchecked growth usually results in a tumor. The tumor is the mass of cells that have the identical mutation within their genes, and the growing tumor is either benign (harmless, or precancerous) or malignant (cancerous).

Why these mutations occur is still not fully understood. Advances in genetics and molecular biology have increased reliable information about the inner workings of cells. Scientists know that cells evolve into cancer cells because the DNA (or gene) structure of the normal cell becomes damaged and the damaged DNA wasn't fully repaired. Damage to the DNA in our cells happens all the time, and typically, the cell detects the change and repairs it. If the DNA can't be repaired, the cell will get a signal from its control center, the nucleus, telling it to die. The nucleus contains the genetic blueprint that tells a cell what to do and when to grow and divide. But if the cell doesn't die and the mutation is not repaired, the mutant cell reproduces, and all of its offspring have the same damaged DNA as the original cell.

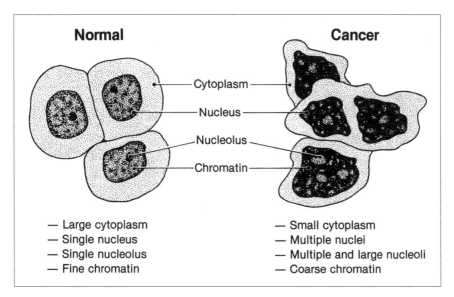

Figure 19.1. Normal and cancer cell structure. Courtesy of National Cancer Institute. Illustration by Pat Kenny.

Scientists are confident that the mutation of healthy cells into cancer cells most often begins as a result of our exposure to environmental carcinogens (or cancer-causing agents). Most cancers are caused by our decisions (e.g., overeating, alcohol misuse, overexposure to ultraviolet light, sexually transmitted infections) and toxic carcinogens found in cigarette smoking, dry cleaning chemicals, formaldehyde, radiation, asbestos, pesticides, and so on. But for many cancers, no specific cause has been found. The good (scientific-based) news is that an acquired cancerous mutation starts in one cell of the body and is found only in its offspring. Because very few cancer cells invade our reproductive cells, acquired mutations cannot be passed on to the next generation.

What are passed on by our families are genes that predispose the next generation to be adversely affected by environmental carcinogens. Our inherited genes either protect us from or put us at a greater risk for genetic mutations, and heredity is a factor in about 5–10 percent of all cancers. Only some cancers run in families. As an example, it is common among the 2,000 men annually diagnosed with breast cancer to have a family history of breast cancer (mother's or father's side) and inherit mutations in the BRCA2 gene. BRCA2 is usually one of several tumor suppressor genes, and like all genes of this type, it has the responsibility to regulate cell division (reproduction), repair DNA mistakes, and tell the cell when to die, which scientists call "programmed cell death." But when a tumor suppressor gene mutates and no longer functions predictably, that's when mutant cells reproduce and don't die. Should we inherit a mutation within a tumor suppressor gene, the risk of certain types of cancer is greater. Another example is the APC gene mutation that causes some people in affected families to develop hundreds or even thousands of colon polyps (or tumors growing on the inside wall of the colon). Too often, at least one of the polyps becomes cancerous.

Unlike the healthy cells in our bodies, cancer cells also may migrate or travel to almost any other part of the body and invade healthy organs and tissues, where they begin to grow and replace normal tissue. This process of cancer cells traveling from one location to another is called *metastasis*. This happens when cancer cells get into the bloodstream or the lymph vessels, which usually carry cells to fight infections. When this occurs, the cancer cells that grow in the new, metastatic site are the same as those in the original tumor—if lung cancer spreads to the spine, the cancer cells in the spine are lung cancer cells. Cancers also spread when a tumor in one part of the body touches neighboring tissue and begins to grow there. Spreading may never occur, or it may happen almost immediately as the first tumor begins to grow in the primary site.

RISKS AND PREVENTING CANCER

Cancer researchers and oncologists (physicians who treat cancer) use the word *risk* in two ways. *Lifetime risk* refers to the likelihood that a man will develop (or die from) cancer over the course of his lifetime. In the United States, for example, men have a one-in-six chance of being diagnosed with prostate cancer at some point during their lifetime. According to the

American Cancer Society, men have a bit less than a one-in-two lifetime risk of developing some form of cancer (45% of men develop cancer). *Relative risk* is a bit trickier. It compares the risk of developing cancer in men who have a specific exposure or trait to men without the same risk. For example, men who smoke are about 23 times more likely to develop lung cancer than nonsmokers; their relative risk is 23. Few relative risks are as large. As a comparison, men who are nonsmokers and married to a smoker are at 4 times greater risk of lung cancer than men who are partnered with nonsmokers.

Testicular Cancer Is Uncommon

A man's lifetime chance of getting testicular cancer is about 1 in 300, and 9 of 10 cases of testicular cancer are in men between the ages of 20 and 54.

The risk of developing most forms of cancer is related to our health habits. Although we can't control genetics, aging, and many unknowns, we certainly can control the choices we make every day to minimize the risk of most cancers. The epidemic rate of lifestyle-related cancers has compelled the National Cancer Institute to urge us to concentrate on what we have power over—our health behavior. There is no foolproof way to prevent cancer, but many of our decisions and health habits increase (or lower) the chance of getting cancer. You can be sure that making small changes within your everyday life will be worthwhile. Here are the seven most important:

1. *Do not use tobacco.* All forms of tobacco propel you toward becoming someone with cancer. The Centers for Disease Control and Prevention (CDC) estimates that men's tobacco use is and has been the leading cause of *preventable* death in the United States.[3] Compared to nonsmokers, men who smoke cigarettes are 20 times more likely to struggle with lung cancer; smoking causes 90 percent of lung cancers, and it also sharply increases the odds of getting cancer of the throat, esophagus, mouth, or voice box, as well as bladder and kidney cancer. Approximately 90 percent of those diagnosed with an oral cancer (including the mouth, tongue, lips, throat, parts of the nose, and larynx) are tobacco users. Don't despair. There are more ex-smokers than smokers in the United States—and most have quit "cold turkey." When a man finally decides to quit smoking, it may take several attempts because it is both a habit and part of the man's identity. Withdrawal symptoms from the physical addiction usually start within a few hours of the last cigarette and peak about 2–3 days later when most of the nicotine and its by-products are no longer in the body. So, symptoms last only a few days, and the physical addiction is entirely overcome within 10–14 days.

The real undoing has to do with seeing yourself as a nonsmoker. Quitting is hard because the habit is wrapped into your identity. Ex-smokers say that quitting was the hardest thing they ever did. After years of lighting up, smoking becomes part of your daily routine. You smoke when you are stressed, bored, angry, and relaxed. Here's some good news:[4]

> *Within 20 minutes* (of putting down a cigarette) you stop polluting the air, and your blood pressure and pulse decrease and read "normal."

> *Within 8 hours* the carbon monoxide level in the blood normalizes and oxygen levels increase.

> *Within 24 hours* your risk of heart attack starts to decline.

> *Within 2 days* nerve endings adjust to the absence of nicotine and your ability to taste food and smell things returns.

> *Within 3 days* your lung capacity improves to the point where you can actually breathe better.

> *Within days* your breath, clothes, and hair will smell better.

> *Within weeks* your fingers and fingernails will begin to appear less yellow.

> *Within 3 months* your circulation improves, your lung functioning is up by 30 percent, and walking becomes easier.

> *Within 9 months* your lungs are able to clean themselves again and your risk of infection goes down.

> *Within 1 year* your heart disease risk is now half that of a typical smoker's.

> *Within 5 years* your risk of stroke is close to that of a nonsmoker.

> *Within 10 years* your lung cancer death rate is similar to that of non-smokers and your risk of other cancers goes down as well.

> *Within 15 years* your heart disease risk is the same as that of a nonsmoker.

2. *Eat healthy foods.* Eating well and making smart choices while dining out lower your risk of several cancers, particularly the colorectal, esophagus, lung, and stomach cancers. A diet deficient in fresh fruits and vegetables and rich in salted or smoked fish or meats was common in the early twentieth century and was associated with many stomach cancer deaths. A leaner diet with less red meat and many fruits and vegetables reduces our risk of many cancers. Avoid as much as you can foods that are salted and/or high in sodium nitrites (found in lunch meats, pepperoni, and especially hot dogs). Nitrite additives in hot dogs are put there as preservatives, but

when the hot dog is cooked, the nitrites combine with the amines within meat to form carcinogens. The same goes for bacon, sausage, and spam.

3. *Stay active and at a healthy weight.* Remaining physically active and keeping a healthy weight also help prevent cancer. Physical activity reduces your risk of becoming overweight or obese, and by controlling your weight you reduce your lifetime risk of colon, stomach, kidney, and prostate cancer.[5] Colon cancer, for instance, has a much higher relative risk among men who are near or already obese. It is abdominal obesity that signals your risk.[6] Have you had to loosen your belt or buy new pants? Waist circumference may be your best warning sign that you're also adding a cancer risk.

4. *Regular screening and self-examination.* The best defense against cancer is early detection—finding the cancer while it is localized. Your self-examinations should include your mouth and skin; examine these areas, and consult a physician right away if you notice any odd changes or lumps (masses). Early detection certainly increases your chances of survival. Regular screening by your physician or a clinic will include your prostate and colon.

Men of color have not always been treated with respect when they sought medical care, and because of the legacy of perceived racism in health care,[7] some men end up delaying or avoiding routine medical visits and cancer screenings. Similarly, many mid- to late-life gay and bisexual men postpone routine medical visits because they prefer not to disclose their sexual orientation or have their sexuality affect the health care they receive. Don't let a (few) bad experience(s) deter you (or one of your friends)—find a *respectful* doctor or clinic.

5. *Protect yourself from the sun.* Don't avoid the sun, but limit your exposure and use sunscreen. We all need regular exposure to the sun for our bodies to produce vitamin D, but too much exposure jacks up the risk of skin cancer, which is our most preventable cancer.

6. *Reduce exposure to hazardous substances.* Limit your exposure to PVCs (e.g., cutting the plastic pipe made from polyvinyl chloride), oil paints and turpentine, fabric dyes, radon, photography chemicals, and creosote (e.g., the black tar deposit from the wood or coal smoke found on chimney walls, and the wood preservative on railroad ties and many other products). When you're using chemicals, work in a ventilated room and seriously consider wearing a ventilator mask. Many workplaces require men to wear masks, goggles, and gloves, for good reason.

7. *Know your family history.* If one of your parents, uncles, aunts, or grandparents had cancer, begin your own research and find out if more than one relative had the same cancer. If so, let your physician know your family history and be vigilant about having regular screening exams and

tests for that type of cancer. Most cancers have multiple causes, and a family history helps identify the risk factors.

SYMPTOMS, DIAGNOSIS, AND STAGING

Different cancers have different symptoms; however, the National Cancer Institute and the American Cancer Society have flagged a number of key warning signs: (1) *Persistent fatigue* is one of the most common cancer symptoms that is especially noticed when the cancer is more advanced, but it occurs in the early stages of some cancers. (2) *Bathroom routines* that involve conspicuous changes in bowel movements—constipation to diarrhea, blood in the stools, thinner stools, or just a general overall change in frequency of bowel habits—are warning signs. So too is having difficulties urinating or noticing blood in the urine. (3) *Unintentional weight loss* is a red flag for many illnesses, including cancer. (4) *A sore* that does not heal in the usual amount of time could be a sign of diabetes or skin cancer. (5) *Bleeding or discharge* from what you might first have thought was a mole, freckle, or "age spot" isn't normal, because these do not bleed or ooze. (6) *A lump* can be a benign cyst or a tumor, and it is too easy to think "cyst" and not have the lump examined. But consult your physician. (7) *A new cough or hoarseness* that is nagging, seems to be getting worse, and might be accompanied by blood or mucus needs to be evaluated by a physician. (8) *Chronic indigestion* and difficulty swallowing can be no more than acid reflux, or a signal of several cancers. (9) *A fever* that is persistent or one that comes and goes may be a signal of a bacterial infection common to prostatitis or a stressed immune system among men whose cancer has spread.

If you have one or two of these symptoms, do not panic. These symptoms are also associated with many noncancerous health concerns. But if you have one or more of these symptoms, they should be taken seriously by your doctor, who will (or ought to) run medical tests—blood and urine tests, imaging (such as X-rays or CT scans), and/or a biopsy. Your physician may refer you to a surgeon or other specialist for the biopsy. Typically this will involve a needle biopsy guided by an imaging technique to obtain a sample of cells or a laparoscopic procedure using a thin, flexible tube with a light on the end to see structures inside your body. Special tools can be passed through the tube to remove part or all of a tumor, allowing the tissue to be analyzed under a microscope to determine whether the growth is cancerous or noncancerous.

As a cancerous tumor grows in its original site, sometimes symptoms permit a diagnosis at an early stage. Other times, however, the growing cancer tumor remains asymptomatic. Even with aggressive and rapid growing cancers that double in size within 3 months, few men will actually notice anything unusual; in the case of prostate, lung, and colon cancers, for example, we cannot see the tumor's growth and have few symptoms to tell us that something is amiss. Before we know it, cancer cells may move from the original site to other parts of the body—through direct contact with neighboring tissues, or when the cancer is transported through the lymph vessels or the blood to other places in the body. Oncologists (cancer physicians) "stage" the growth of the cancer in our bodies as a way to estimate the extent of the disease. This information is vital to determine the best course of treatment.

Each type of cancer has its own staging criteria to reveal how widespread and advanced a cancer has become. Despite the variability in how different cancers are "staged," staging usually depends on cell type, tumor size, lymph node involvement, and metastasis. The tumor-node-metastasis (TNM) staging summarized below is used for most types of cancers; however, TNM staging does not apply to lymphomas (cancers of the blood or bone marrow):

Stage 0: Carcinoma in situ, or early cancer that is present only in the layer of cells in which it began and not deeper tissues. Other than skin cancer and a few others, rarely is a cancer found and staged 0.

Stage I: The cancer involves a small tumor, remains localized (not yet spreading to neighboring layers or structures), and is very treatable when found at this stage.

Stage II: The tumor is more advanced than stage I, and for some cancers the cells have traveled into nearby lymph nodes.

Stage III: The tumor is locally advanced (greater size), lymph nodes are involved, and the cancer cells may have already invaded nearby tissue or organs. The criteria differ according to the cancer.

Stage IV: Metastasis has occurred, and thus the original cancer has spread through the bloodstream or the lymph vessels to the bones, brain, or other parts of the body.

CANCER TREATMENT

Treatment must be individualized. You will work with your physician and oncologist to create a treatment plan based on the type of cancer, its stage and genetic features, your other co-morbidities (or concurrent illnesses such as heart disease) and overall health, your personal philosophy and fears, family interests, and your sense of autonomy. When faced with a cancer diagnosis, there are many treatment options, and each one needs to be discussed with your physician, a specialist whom you consult for a second opinion, and your partner. Options typically include one or more treatments, including surgery, chemotherapy, radiation therapy, or targeted drug therapy.

Some cancerous tumors can be effectively treated by surgery and radiation therapy. Other cancers necessitate whole-body chemotherapy, some can be best managed by "target therapies" (discussed below), and some are often too advanced to be cured. Treatment, however, usually will make living with an advanced cancer (e.g., lung or brain cancer) more comfortable until death occurs.

Surgery is the bedrock of cancer treatment. Surgery is intended to remove the cancerous tumor, neighboring tissue, and lymph nodes where the concentration of cancer cells exists. Depending on tumor size, your surgeon may remove part of an organ or the entire organ in an attempt to ensure that all the cancer has been removed. Most surgeries no longer require the surgeon to make large cuts into the body; there are less invasive procedures. Surgeons can place a long, flexible tube (laparoscope) through a small incision to perform the internal surgery that removes the tumor in pieces. When surgery is planned as treatment rather than diagnosis, it may be supplemented with other treatments because surgery alone is not enough to cure.

Radiation therapy (or radiotherapy) is administered on an outpatient basis at an oncology clinic or cancer center. It uses high-energy radiation, most commonly X-rays or radioactively charged particles, to burn (or shrink) tumors and kill the cancer cells. The radiation can be delivered by a machine outside the body, similar to a dentist's X-ray (*external-beam radiation therapy*), or it may come from radioactive material placed in the body near cancer cells (*internal radiation therapy*). Radiation usually has side effects similar to chemotherapy—nausea, diarrhea, fatigue, and sometimes burns (much like sunburn)—because it is designed to destroy the mutant cancer cells and can affect nearby healthy cells as well.

Cancer treatment drugs (*chemotherapy*) used for a whole-body approach include cisplatin, doxorubicin (Adriamycin), 5-fluorouracil (5-FU), and many others. These medications are used to manage many types of cancer. They often are successful in slowing the further spread of the cancer, and they provide some relief from symptoms. It is the only treatment method that has the capability to destroy cancer cells wherever they've migrated to. Because the chemicals are intentionally strong, they also affect other (healthy) cells, causing side effects such as a weakened immune system, hair loss, diarrhea, and nausea.

Clinical Trials (or Experimental Treatment Therapies)

Some treatments are "gold standard," or what is currently the "best" used treatment strategy. Other cancer treatments are being tested in clinical research trials, which are studies designed to (1) improve the current standard treatment or (2) gather information on new treatment. When clinical trials show that a new treatment is better than the standard treatment, that treatment usually becomes the new standard. Men are often asked to think about taking part in a clinical trial; you are assured that you will be informed of the potential benefits and costs. Be assured that no clinical trial is approved if the Human Subjects Review Board (a team of physicians and researchers from many different fields) thinks that there are insufficient benefits.

Targeted cancer therapies are distinct drugs and laboratory-produced antibodies designed to interfere with cell division, which blocks the growth and spread of a cancer. The targets are the specific molecules involved in tumor growth and progression. By zeroing in on the odd cellular and molecular expression of specific cancer cells, targeted therapies are sometimes more successful than other treatments. Targeted therapies might involve antibodies that carry toxins or radioactive material directly to a tumor, or they might involve a small-molecule drug that targets specific enzymes within some cancer cells. The aim is to interfere with cancer cell growth and proliferation, yet some therapies might target cell movement. Ask your cancer specialist about what FDA-approved targeted therapies might be available. They can be less harmful to normal cells than chemotherapy or radiotherapy.

Because of a cancer and/or its treatment, men very often need to modify their diet and follow *nutritional therapies* that include lots of fruits and vegetables, whole grain breads and cereals, and meat and milk products. The cancer and/or the side effects of treatment are draining, and there is a great need to eat well and keep up strength. To survive the cancer, usually there is a need to consume extra calories and protein—especially from milk, cheese, and eggs. Simply eating enough food is a challenge for some men, because chemotherapy may diminish appetite and change the taste or smell of foods. What were favorite foods may no longer be appetizing. The cancer center where you are treated ought to have nutritionists who can help you plan diets and solve eating problems.

Pain management is integral to cancer treatment, yet it too often remains undertreated.[8] One-third of men with solid tumors have pain at diagnosis, and at least two-thirds experience pain when their disease advances. Pain is rated by the sufferer on a scale of 0 to 10, and when a man rates his pain as 5 or higher, it is acknowledged as substantial pain and as interfering with his quality of life. In addition to being medically ill, men with cancer are distressed, and their distress can be heightened by existential challenges and worsened by social factors such as too few nearby friends or limited communication with their families.[9] For the vast majority of men with cancer, their pain and distress can be relieved through two basic approaches: primary disease-modifying treatment such as radiotherapy and analgesic therapy to alter the man's perception of pain by using opioid-based drugs, antidepressants, and/or nonpharmacologic approaches (acupuncture, massage, biofeedback, visualization/imagery, relaxation therapy).[10] Many nonpharmacological treatments improve pain control, distress, coping, and adaptation.

Prognosis means prediction. Think of it as an educated guess about the future course of the cancer. Physicians base prognosis on the type of cancer, evidence of gene mutation and protein expression, tumor size, location, and spreading (if any); the man's age; how long he has had symptoms before the diagnosis; how much the cancer has already affected his ability to function; types of treatment available to remove (or reduce) the tumor and kill off cancer cells that have spread; and treatment efficacy. When cancer cells are no longer found, a cancer is considered to be in *clinical remission*, meaning that the tumor disappears or the number of cancer cells diminishes and the person no longer experiences symptoms. Clinical remission, however, does not always mean that the cancer is eliminated or cured. Complete remission is when you have no symptoms and there is no evidence of the disease as assessed by biopsy or imaging, such as a CT or PET scan. Yet even when a man's cancer is in remission, there may be invisible collections of cancer cells that cannot be detected using current techniques. A *recurrence* is when the cancer comes back. It recurs because small amounts of cancer cells migrated from the original site and remain in the body after treatment.

LIVING WITH CANCER

Learning that you have cancer will change your life and the lives of everyone close to you. At the beginning, men have concerns such as, "How long will I live?" There are questions about the treatments that are recommended, the uncertainties of being hospitalized, how to live with treatment side effects, the medical bills, and their family's worries. Later, there is lingering doubt and much ill ease about whether changes you've had to make as a cancer patient were the best ones at the time.

Not all men are comfortable asking for help, but men with cancer tend to differ—they want to know their options, and nearly all are genuinely interested in others' support. If you suspect or know that you have a cancer, don't be the stereotypical man. Ask the physicians, nurses, and others that make up your health care team questions about your treatment or home care. Do not take this journey alone. Periods of anger, panic, grumpiness, sadness, and loneliness are going to occur, and it is okay to seek out a social worker, counselor, or clergy member when you want to talk about what you are feeling or about your worries. These people are professionals. They can provide you with practical contacts for transportation, help manage the financial costs, and just listen to your worries.

Questions You Ought to Discuss with Your Physicians

- What kind of cancer do I have?
- How far advanced is my cancer? (What stage is it?)
- Should I get a second opinion?
- What are all my treatment options? Are the treatment therapies new or experimental?
- What treatments are best for me?
- Will I have to stay in the hospital for treatment? If so, how long?
- Will treatment keep me from doing certain things I enjoy? What are the side effects of the treatment(s)?
- How often will I be checked after treatment?
- Will my insurance cover all the costs?
- What are the odds of survival, or cure?
- Can I go back to normal daily activities after treatment?
- Are there any clinical trials that might be beneficial?
- What has been your experience with cancer patients similar to me?
- Can you recommend any patient support groups for me?
- What materials can I read about my cancer?
- Who can I call when I have questions?
- Am I a good candidate for surgery? What are the chances that surgery will remove all the cancer?
- Should I consider chemotherapy? If so, how long will my chemotherapy treatments last? What experiences have other patients had with similar chemotherapy regimens?

Source: Adapted from CancerSurvivors.org and Yale–New Haven Hospital pamphlet "Questions to Ask Your Cancer Specialist."

Men's support groups can be a great resource, and they are rarely talky-feely. In groups such as "men surviving prostate cancer," the men and sometimes their families meet with other guys to exchange information and talk about what they have learned about coping with the cancer and the treatment. These groups aren't necessarily face-to-face; some are on the Internet.

> There are a couple of fellows there that didn't say a word all night. I could tell by just their posture that they have been just diagnosed and they were obviously terrified as I was when I was first diagnosed. (74-year-old)[11]

Researchers studying men with cancer find that a lot of men prefer to avoid disclosing their cancer whenever possible.[12] Some place a great deal of importance on sustaining a self-presentation that all is normal, and nearly all men look forward to hopefully returning to "normal" life (by "fighting" the cancer). In the past, men's decisions to limit who they told were too often based on a (false) perception that they had little need for others' support. At times a man wouldn't disclose his illness out of a fear of being stigmatized as a "cancer patient," still believing that other people might blame him.[13] Most often men worried about losing their job and simply wanted their cancer to remain *their* burden, hiding it even from children and close family. They did not wish to be dependent on their children for help, and they wanted to spare their family's disheartened feelings.

> I had asked my wife not to tell anybody. Don't tell my mother, don't tell my father, don't tell my children—don't tell anybody. So I didn't tell nobody. Uh, I know some people assumed that something was going on. (A 70-year-old with breast cancer)

There are many reasons men may still choose not to tell.

> I didn't tell my neighbors. Because I just felt—what can they do for you? Why go broadcasting it? Are they doctors? No, they can't help you. So why get into it? And I found, when I do tell someone, you have to go through the whole routine, explaining it. (Man with prostate cancer)[14]

There are dangers in thinking that it's best not to tell others. You may very well end up feeling isolated, even blaming yourself as a result of dumb things said by people who don't know why you might act differently. Recognize that you and many other men your age were encouraged to take health risks and were exposed to carcinogens at work. Those "real" man messages older men grew up with encouraged all kinds of bad health habits. Should you have cancer, look around—you are not alone. Over 100,000 men are diagnosed annually with lung cancer, and nearly 70,000 with colorectal cancer. If you are 60 or older, you probably lived the way you were encouraged. Find others like you; don't be the lone ranger.

We all know someone living with or who lived with a cancer. The remainder of the chapter describes some of the primary types of cancer that mature men confront.

SKIN CANCER / MELANOMA

Skin cancer affects men more often than women, because of the history of our health habits. Most often it is white men over age 50. Skin cancer is the most common type of cancer in the United States, even though it ranks lower in terms of the new cases diagnosed annually. What most people don't fully recognize is that skin cancer is the most preventable cancer. It also is highly curable, when treated early. Most skin cancer tumors are slow-growing, easy to identify, and almost always non-metastasizing—meaning that they do not spread from one part of the body to another.

There are three primary types of skin cancer: basal cell carcinoma, squamous cell carcinoma, and melanoma. The first two types are the least serious. They make up 95 percent of all skin cancers, and roughly 50 percent of American men will develop one of these skin cancers at least once by age 65. The tumors are located on the outer layer of the skin. They characteristically involve a small lump, spot, or bump that is shiny, smooth in texture, and/or pale in color. Some, however, involve a red lump, spot, or bump that is firm, and some others present as rough and scaly patches on the skin that are usually red or brown. Caused by the ultraviolet (UV) light within natural sunlight, or artificial sources like tanning beds, these skin cancers develop on UV-damaged areas. They are especially prevalent on the back of the neck, ears, face, or back of the hands.

The intensity of your UV exposure varies throughout the day, across the seasons, and by where you live geographically. You can get as much exposure from an hour in the sun in the middle of the day (10:00 a.m. to 2:00 p.m.) as from a longer period outdoors early in the morning or late in the afternoon. Men's exposure to an hour's worth of sun in Arizona or Florida is much more than 2 hours' worth of sunlight in Oregon or Vermont. Men who have an outdoor job, spend a lot of time outdoors, or live at higher elevations, where sunlight is the strongest, are at a greater risk. The sun's damaging UV light in the winter cannot be ignored either. Have you ever been sunburned while skiing?

The likelihood of being diagnosed with any of the three types of skin cancers increases with age, primarily because they are slow growing, often taking years for the tumor to become the size of a dime. Any man can get one or more of these skin cancers in his lifetime, but the risk is greater for men who have fair skin that burns easily, particularly men with freckles and naturally blond or red hair. Darker-skinned and darker-haired men are at lower risk. African American, Native American, Arabic, Asian, and Hispanic men sometimes falsely believe that they are not at risk because they are men of color. This false belief can lead to delayed diagnosis, sometimes well after the cancer has advanced and is life threatening. Despite a high concentration of the pigment melanin, no man is immune to skin cancer.

Sunscreen really is the best way to prevent skin cancer. The amount of protection from being burned by the UV rays in sunlight is called the *sun protection factor* (SPF). SPF 15 or higher is the gold standard. The sunscreen should be applied 15–30 minutes before spending time in the sun and re-applied 15–30 minutes after being in the sun. Wearing baseball hats (not backward), UV-protective sunglasses, and clothes that cover the skin and face are also first-rate ways to lower the risk of skin cancer.

Melanoma is the most dangerous type of skin cancer. The good news is that it is the least common—only about 5 percent of skin cancers are of this type—and if a melanoma is detected and treated early, its cure rate is very high. Recent statistics show that fewer than 5 out of 100 men are at risk of dying from melanoma. The bad news is that men often wait too long before consulting a physician about the mole or bump they noticed months earlier, and one man dies of melanoma every 93 minutes.[15] When men wait, they may not want to bother a physician with what they see as a minor problem, but a melanoma in its advanced state requires more extensive treatment. Unlike the other skin cancers, melanomas can rapidly spread (or metastasize) and affect internal organs. Should the melanoma tumor spread, a man's prognosis is poor. However, there have been important recent advances in melanoma target therapies that will likely begin altering the menacingly grim statistic.[16]

The melanoma tumor may resemble a normal mole or age spot, yet more often than not it appears as an irregular, colored patch or bump. Closely examine your skin (or have someone else do it), at least as often as you might get a haircut. Look for new moles or colored spots. The American Melanoma Foundation offered their ABCDs on recognizing a melanoma (see boxed insert).

A fourth type of skin cancer is known as Merkel cell carcinoma. Though it is very rare, it is as lethal as a melanoma. It is 40 times less common than a melanoma and usually develops on sun-exposed skin (e.g., head, neck, arms) as a painless, firm, fleshy-colored to red or blue bump. Because it grows rapidly, do not delay diagnosis or treatment.

Skin Cancer Treatment

Skin cancer is accurately diagnosed only through a biopsy. This involves a physician clipping away a small sample of the tissue and having the sample examined by a pathologist. Sometimes the biopsy can remove all of the cancer tissue, in which case no further treatment is needed. Treatment basically depends on the type of skin cancer and how large the lesion is. Topical chemotherapy can work on small tumors, and this form of chemotherapy only affects the treated skin and does not bring about the side effects associated with whole-body chemotherapy. Topical chemotherapy can cause some irritation and redness, because skin cells are killed. Surgery, however, is the most common treatment method, and there are different surgical methods based on the location and size of the skin cancer tumors:

ABCDs on Recognizing a Melanoma

Asymmetry: The shape of one half of the mole is different than the other half.

Border irregularity: The edges are ragged, notched, and/or blurred.

Color: A mole with more than one color—uneven shades of brown, tan, red, or black are present.

Diameter: If bigger than a pencil eraser, or if there is a considerable change in size, see a physician.

> *Cryosurgery*: This is not what most people think of as surgery, but it is. It involves the use of liquid nitrogen to literally freeze the surface tissue, "burning" away the cancer cells. It is used commonly to treat basal cell carcinoma and can be applied by your physician as part of your annual exam. Rarely is it used for melanomas.

> *Simple excision*: This method involves cutting away the tumor and a small amount of healthy tissue surrounding it. There are three common strategies. One involves "shaving" off the abnormal growth using a sterile razor. Another involves a special punch instrument that takes a very small plug of skin to remove skin tissue, including the tumor. The third is using a scalpel, usually reserved for larger lesions. All three are quick and quite painless, and the treating physician (a specialist) will offer you a local anesthesia.

> *Electrodessication and curettage*: This type of surgery involves the use of a surgical tool that first cuts (the curettage) and then burns (the electrocautery needle). The tumor is surgically removed with the spoon-shaped curette, and then a cauterizing needle is used to "burn away" the remaining cancer cells.

> *Laser surgery*: A laser (a beam of light of various frequencies) used at close range heats and vaporizes the targeted cancer cells.

Ignore the "manly" stereotypes and put on the sunscreen (SPF 15 or higher). It is the best way to prevent skin cancer, as well as to avoid wrinkled, leathery skin.

PROSTATE CANCER

Even though half of all men are treated for skin cancer, it is prostate cancer that we hear about more often. Chiefly because men are living longer, one in six men in the United States will develop and live with prostate cancer during their lifetime. It grows slowly, is most likely found when men are in their late sixties, and accounts for 25 percent of all cancers diagnosed annually among men.[17]

There is a scientific truism that more men eventually die *with* prostate cancer rather than *from* it. Researchers estimate that 60–90 percent of 80-year-olds live with prostate cancer, and neither they nor their physicians know that it is present.[18] Although prostate cancer can be slow growing, do not underestimate its potential threat, just because it is so common, or underestimate the disagreeable symptoms or side effects of treatment. Prostate cancer remains the second-leading cause of cancer deaths in American men.

Prostate cancer is as much a lifestyle-related cancer as it is an age-related cancer.[19] Like heart disease, prostate cancer seems to be the legacy

Prostate-Specific Antigen (PSA) Testing

There is controversy.

The good news: A study compared the profiles of newly diagnosed prostate cancer patients in 1988–1989 and 2004–2005 and found that the average age for detecting cancer decreased over the 15 years in between from age 72 to 67, and the number of men with advanced cancer also decreased from 52 per 100,000 to 8 per 100,000 among whites and from 91 per 100,000 to 13 per 100,000 among blacks. These numbers support the argument that regular PSA testing diagnosed more men with prostate cancer at a younger age and earlier stage.

The bad news: The U.S. Preventive Services Task Force released its 2008 decision that it no longer recommends routine PSA screening for seemingly healthy men and recommends against screening in men age 75 or older. This decision is because of the lack of health benefits—there are too many false-positive tests that cause short-term psychological harm, the false-positive tests result in unnecessary treatment (surgery, radiation therapy, or both), and it's not entirely clear whether the test actually leads to life-saving treatment.

of a sedentary Western lifestyle and our infamous unhealthy diet that is rich in red meat and processed fast foods and poor in fresh vegetables and fruits. Researchers have found that men of Japanese ancestry who were initially at a low risk of developing prostate cancer (because of their diet and less sedentary lives) but moved to Hawaii or California and adopted an American lifestyle show an escalated risk over time of developing prostate cancer.[20] Most cases of prostate cancer are found in men over the age of 65. And for reasons that are still unknown, African American men are one and a half to two times as likely as white men to develop prostate cancer and nearly three times more likely than men of Asian origin.[21] Only part of this can be attributable to differences in diet and lifestyle.

The risk of having prostate cancer is less than 2 percent while we are middle-aged and beginning to accept the need for an annual physical exam. This is the point at which, if you have a family history of prostate cancer, you ought to be discussing with a physician whether or not you should begin screening for prostate cancer. Too many men avoid annual physical exams, much less the digital (finger) rectal exam that can assess abnormalities of the prostate gland.

> It's one of those things that you just don't talk about. You know—men don't talk about prostate—we don't have problems down there. (A man in his sixties)[22]

Aside from lifestyle, family history is the strongest risk factor for prostate cancer. Having one or more close relatives with prostate cancer seems to increase our risk. A man with one close male relative (such as a father, uncle, or brother) with prostate cancer has twice the risk of developing prostate cancer as a man with no family history. Urologists and oncologists affiliated with the American Cancer Society continue to advocate that men need to be better informed about the meaning of the protein called *prostate-specific antigen* (PSA), the benefit/risk ratio of PSA testing, and the newer, more sensitive diagnostic tests that assess this enzyme (the AMARC and PCA3).

The PSA test measures an enzyme in the blood that's produced almost exclusively by the glandular cells of the prostate and often spikes when prostate cancer exists. Normally, only very small amounts of PSA are present in the blood. But an abnormality of the prostate is *thought* to disrupt the architecture of the gland and create a path for a greater amount of PSA to pass into the bloodstream. High blood levels of PSA are *thought* to indicate prostate problems, including cancer. However, there remains much debate about the usefulness of PSA testing—largely because there is no normal, absolute cutoff point to serve as a "gold standard." One man's normal PSA level might be another man's abnormal level. Unlike a ther-mometer and an absolute standard of a temperature of greater than 98.6 to define the onset of a fever, there is no absolute PSA metric. Because of this lack of a universal standard, the psychological worries that a false-positive number can trigger, and the hurried unnec-essary surgery some men have undergone, many researchers and physicians argue that we no longer ought to use single PSA mea-sures. Rather, attention has been refocused on how much the PSA level changes over a short time frame, known as *PSA velocity*. Nu-merous studies have shown that a high PSA velocity (for example, rapid doubling time of PSA or a rise of 0.2 ng/mL or more per year) more reliably signals a growing cancer than the absolute PSA level.[23]

PSA Screening or Not?

Serial PSA screening has at best a modest effect on prostate-cancer mortality during the first decade of follow-up. This benefit comes at the cost of substantial overdiag-nosis and overtreatment. It is important to remember that the key question is not whether PSA screening is effective but whether it does more good than harm.

Source: Barry, M. J. (2009). Editorial: Screening for prostate cancer—the controversy that refuses to die. *New England Journal of Medicine, 360,* 1351-1354.

There's another problem with serum PSA testing: when a greater level of the antigen is detected over a handful of years, such as an increase from 4 to 9.9 ng/ml, this change could be caused by a noncancerous enlargement of the prostate and not a cancer. Only a biopsy can determine whether or not it is a cancer. However, the absence of a clear metric for PSA testing could push a man toward an unneeded biopsy and, worse yet, unneeded surgery. In one study, only one-third of the men with a PSA level between 4.1 and 9.9 ng/ml had pros-tate cancer.[24] The side effects of worrying about needing a biopsy and/or unnecessary prostate surgery can be psychologically devastating and may outweigh the benefit of treatment.

A newer, more sensitive test (PCA3) uses urine rather than blood chem-istry to assess our risk of prostate cancer.[25] The specimen is collected after a digital rectal exam and has higher reliability in identifying prostate can-cer, but a biopsy is still needed to confirm a cancer diagnosis. These newer

Biopsy or Not?

The National Cancer Institute argues, "While it's important to make your own decision about cancer screening, everybody should consider getting a second opinion before getting something like a biopsy."

Source: National Cancer Institute (2009). Understand prostate cancer: A health guide for men. U.S. Department of Health and Human Services: National Institutes of Health. 09-4303.

screening tests will hopefully reduce the risk of unnecessary biopsies and surgical treatment. After prostate cancer has been diagnosed, tests are done to find out whether cancer cells have spread within the prostate or to other parts of the body.

Prostate cancer is now more often diagnosed before it involves a sizeable tumor or has spread, since more men are regularly having a rectal exam and/or PSA screening. Often, symptoms prompt further screening and a diagnosis. For example, the undiagnosed tumor can create some difficulty with having an erection and cause you to pass blood in the urine.

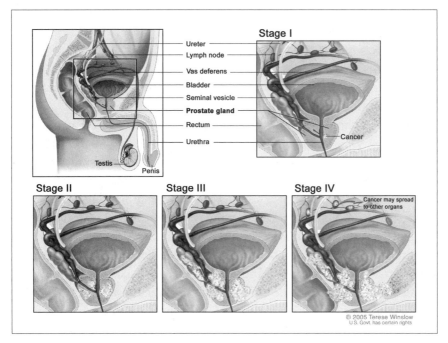

Figure 19.2. Prostate cancer, early tumor stages. © 2005 Terese Winslow LLC and the U.S. government.

Men diagnosed with localized prostate cancer will likely live for many years (even when diagnosed in stage T2, which means that prostate cancer can be felt during a digital rectal exam but is still only in the prostate). The treatment decisions you make will surely affect your life for a long time. It isn't uncommon for men with prostate cancer and their partners to experience considerable stress at this time, and consulting with a medical oncologist at a cancer clinic or a prostate survivor group can be most helpful. All that is needed is your willingness to ask; few men walk away from genitourinary cancer centers feeling that the consultation was unhelpful.[26] Consulting with other men who have faced a prostate cancer diagnosis is strongly advised as you need to weigh your worries, your fears, and the opinions of your partner.

Genitourinary cancer centers treat cancers of the urinary tract and male genital tract with the goals of controlling cancer and preserving quality of life after treatment. The right treatment for prostate cancer is not clear-cut, and the treatment options vary greatly based on the stage of the tumor. In its localized, early stage, you really need to weigh the costs of *any* invasive treatment, compared to the benefits of monitoring the cancer without active treatment. The "watchful waiting" applies to the early-stage cancer as much as to benign prostatic hyperplasia (BPH).

If the results of the diagnostic exams suggest prostate cancer, initially your physician will very often perform a transrectal ultrasound to better determine the size of the prostate and to identify the location of a tumor. (Similar assessment procedures are used for all cancers.) When the cancer is localized (confined to the prostate) or regional (spread only to local lymph nodes or tissue), there are a number of successful treatment options, now yielding a 5-year survival rate of nearly 100 percent, which is substantially better than the mid-60-percent survival rate in 1975.

However, should the cancer be localized and small, you may prefer to avoid surgery and its side effects and, instead, select radiation therapy to shrink the tumor. There are two types of radiation therapy: *prostate brachytherapy*, where radioactive seeds are injected inside the prostate, and *external beam radiation*, where you go to a cancer center to receive the radiation. The key feature of brachytherapy treatment is that it is a relatively straightforward, single treatment. By comparison, beam radiotherapy can involve 6–8 weeks of outpatient high-density radiation, but this might be the best option in some cases. There are side effects caused by the radiation therapies similar to the side effects of surgery (discussed below), such as the likelihood of erectile dysfunction (ED), urinary incontinence, diarrhea, skin irritations, swelling or bruising, red-brown urine or semen, and fatigue. Several newer treatment strategies are also available: cryotherapy, for example, involves injecting liquid nitrogen into the prostate and literally freezing to death the prostate cells.

In the rarer cases where the tumor is large, a radical prostatectomy is likely to be recommended. A radical prostatectomy is a surgical operation to remove the whole prostate gland and some surrounding tissue. In the past, the conventional prostatectomy procedure required a good-sized incision and a hospital stay of 2–4 days. One procedure (retropubic approach) entered from the front, with the incision between your navel and pubic bone. The other (perineal approach) involved an incision between the anus and scrotum. Both procedures are no longer the standard of care because of the surgery's invasiveness and the need to have a catheter left in your penis for several weeks to drain urine. Incontinence can also be an issue for a few months after the catheter is removed.

Fortunately, a prostatectomy can now be performed much less invasively by using laparoscopic surgery (or "keyhole surgery"). The surgeon makes several small incisions in the belly. One is used to insert a laparoscope (a long tube with a light on its tip), and then the surgeon uses surgical instruments to reach and remove the prostate and surrounding tissue through the other small incision. One recent study showed that men who experienced regular laparoscopic surgery tend to recover faster, but with more complications with incontinence and ED than men who have traditional, open surgery.[27] In addition, "robotic" technology now gives the surgeon greater precision, preserving continence and sexual function, as well as controlling the cancer and markedly reducing recurrence.[28]

Surgeons have also perfected a less troubling procedure called *nerve-sparing radical prostatectomy* for men with early prostate cancers. There are two bundles of nerves that help control erections which run alongside the prostate. Using robotic technology, if the surgeon cuts prostate tissue carefully away from the nerve bundles without damaging them, the man more likely can continue to have erections, though it will take a while. After the surgery, whether or not you regain erectile function is determined by your

Side Effects of a Prostatectomy

- *Erectile problems (dysfunction)*. Roughly three-fourths of men who have undergone a prostatectomy encounter problems in getting or sustaining an erection firm enough for penetration.

- *Urinary incontinence*. Roughly 20 percent of men have some minor problems and about 5 percent of men have major problems controlling the flow of urine (e.g., stress incontinence, where you can't control urine when coughing or sneezing, or overflow incontinence, where it takes a long time to urinate and the stream is weak). This occurs because of damage to the muscle that holds urine in your bladder.

- *Penis length*. Roughly 15 percent of men have a decrease in penis length. Physicians have no explanation for what causes this.

- *Infertility*. This isn't an issue for most men, because of their age and completed families. Yet all men will be infertile. No fluid is ejaculated during orgasm, because the seminal vesicle and prostate that would produce fluid have been removed.

- *Rectal injury*. Roughly 1–2 percent of men suffer a rectal injury, which may cause bowel incontinence—the inability to control bowel movements.

Source: Barry, M. J., Gallagher, P. M., Skinner, J. S., et al. (2012). Adverse effects of robotic-assisted laparoscopic versus open retropubic radical prostatectomy among a nationwide random sample of Medicare-age men. *Journal of Clinical Oncology, 30,* 513–518.

health and age: the younger you are, the better your chance of regaining an erection and experiencing an orgasm (without ejaculation). A recent study reports that over 80 percent of men were potent (able to have unassisted intercourse with or without the use of Viagra) 18 months after their nerve-sparing radical prostatectomy.[29]

Whether treatment is a prostatectomy, radiation, or hormone therapy, the treatment will inevitably strike at the heart of masculinity for many men, because it interferes with sexual performance on a permanent basis and can cause urinary incontinence and sometimes bowel problems. With regard to sex, older men with metastatic prostate cancer may have already begun to experience erectile difficulties, so this experience isn't new. Recent improvements in surgical procedures and the availability of oral ED medication are making permanent impotence less common. The temporary erectile problems after undergoing surgery may result in feeling ashamed and depressed, or "less a man."[30] Researchers report that men shift priorities away from the physical to the more relational aspects of sexual intimacy.[31] Discuss your concerns with your sexual partner and your physician. In one case, a near-80-year-old man who was diagnosed with stage IV prostate cancer talked over the consequences with his wife before deciding to have a prostatectomy, knowing that he was giving up sexual intercourse (but he refused chemotherapy because he did not want to lose his full head of hair). Though he and his wife missed intercourse, they have adopted other ways to express their sexual intimacy. Several advice books written by men with erectile problems are available for couples.[32]

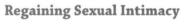

Regaining Sexual Intimacy

Because erectile problems remain common following prostate cancer surgery, clinicians recommend that as you start feeling better, you should again initiate being intimate with your partner to bring back your physical and emotional closeness and to reestablish your sexual libido.

New research suggests that inducing erections with medication soon after surgery—within 2 months—may help prevent further tissue damage and restore normal sexual function sooner.

You might want to start by trying the simplest method of treatment, the oral medications such as Viagra, Cialis, and Levitra. Don't anticipate too much.

When it comes to erectile problems, many men think you simply take the oral medication and boom, an erection occurs.

You need to be aware that these meds do nothing to increase sexual desire—they enhance performance once sexual desire has been aroused and sexual ability has been restored.

LUNG CANCER

A rare disease at the start of the twentieth century, lung cancer has now become the leading cause of cancer deaths for men. Epidemiologists (who study illness patterns) make the case that we are in an epidemic of lung cancer deaths. It had its beginnings following the production of manufactured cigarettes and their addictive additives.[33] Smoking cigarettes is by far the leading cause of lung cancer, accounting for 90 percent of cases. Put differently, before smoking was convenient, touted as fashionable and masculine, and symbolized by the rugged "Marlboro man," nine of every ten male lung cancer deaths were preventable.

The patterns of lung cancer reveal that it occurs about twice more frequently among African American men than men of European ancestry. The risk of the disease increases among smokers whose lifestyles and eating habits are unhealthy, as well as among men whose work environment contains exposure to radon, tar and soot, diesel exhaust, and asbestos. Interestingly, smokers who are physically active and eat well halve the risk of lung cancer, from 23 times greater risk than nonsmokers to 13 times greater risk; however, this "protective" shield that a healthy lifestyle and diet might have remains an unconvincing rationale to continue to smoke.[34]

There is strong evidence that the carcinogenic compounds in tobacco smoke also put at risk the nonsmokers who live and/or work with smokers

Your Lungs

The air we breathe passes from nose and mouth, through the throat, and into the larynx, where the vocal cords use the air we breathe in or out to form sounds. Connected below the larynx is the trachea (about where your Adam's apple is). It is a narrow tube that splits into an upside-down "Y," with the legs of the "Y" going into each lung; the tips of the "Y" which enter the two lungs are called the *bronchi*. The top of the lung area where the bronchi enter is the *hilum*, and this is where the key blood vessels also enter. Like an upside-down tree, the bronchi branch out into the smaller *lobar* and then *segmental* to carry air into the lung. Your right lung has three lobes, and the left has two. The air we breathe into the lungs eventually gets to the tiny air sacs (or *alveoli*). Surrounding the lungs is a membrane, the *pleura*, and it involves an inner (or *visceral*) and an outer (or *parietal*) lining.

The most common lung cancer starts from the mutated cells in the lining of the bronchi; the next most common lung cancer originates in the air sacs; both are non-small-cell carcinomas. The third most common are the small-cell carcinomas that begin in the lining of bronchi branches.

and breathe secondhand smoke. One 92-year-old Scottish grandfather who never smoked and was symptom-free died shortly after his stage IV lung cancer was diagnosed. His cancer was stumbled on in a routine chest X-ray and linked to his long-term exposure to secondhand cigarette smoke; he worked in a small shop for nearly 40 years with men who smoked all day. This man's symptom-free lung cancer death is not entirely uncommon; possible signs might include a cough that won't go away and shortness of breath.[35]

Most men, whether smokers or not, who develop lung cancer have few clinical symptoms suggesting that something is wrong. In fact, about 25 percent of men with lung cancer have no symptoms of their cancer when it is found,[36] and 40 percent of men at the time they are diagnosed have already progressed to stage IV lung cancer, where the cancer has spread to bones and other parts of the body. Had they had noticeable symptoms, they may have felt a shortness of breath; much later it would be wheezing, chest pain, and eventually coughing up blood.

When a lung cancer is diagnosed, the type of lung cancer cells present can be identified. The two primary types are small cell and non-small-cell lung cancer, and they are treated differently. Small cell (sometimes called oat cell) lung cancer affects about 20 percent of men with lung cancer. It is primarily caused by smoking. It usually begins in the larger airways (the bronchi, or breathing tubes) and grows very rapidly; the tumor becomes quite large, and it is almost always treated by both localized radiation and whole-body chemotherapy. By comparison, non-small-cell lung cancers are much more common, and because there are several variations, they collectively make up about 80 percent of the lung cancers. Biologically differing from one another, these cancers originate in more than one location within the lungs / respiratory system and grow more slowly than small cell carcinoma.

The stage of the cancer (the size of the tumor and whether the cancer remains in the lung or has spread to other places in the body) affects both prognosis and treatment options. Surgery is usually the first line of treatment when the tumor remains localized on the lung, and it may be recommended by an oncologist even after the cancer has spread to the lymph nodes. Radiation therapy is also a common course of treatment; it can be used alone for small tumors or administered after surgery and at the same time as chemotherapy. Chemotherapy is also used to treat lung cancer after surgery; it is highly individualized to the type of cancer and stage of the disease and may be the primary mode of treatment when the cancer has metastasized (stages III and IV). No one chemotherapeutic regimen seems more successful than another, and men are often asked to enroll in a clinical trial (a study) to assess the efficacy of a lung cancer treatment. When treatments offer little chance for clinical remission, your family and physician may recommend avoiding the harsh treatments and, instead, selecting supportive (or palliative) care. Men's median life expectancy for stage IV non-small-cell lung cancer (the time at which 50% of patients are alive and 50% have passed away) is only around 8 months. The 5-year survival rate is unfortunately less than 10 percent. Anyway you look at it, this is a nasty cancer. Treatment rarely cures, yet it can surely extend and improve quality of life for the remaining time.

COLORECTAL CANCER

Colon cancer is cancer of the longest part of the large intestine (colon), and rectal cancer is cancer of the last several inches of the colon. Together, they are referred to as *colorectal cancer*, which is the fourth most common cancer among men. Colorectal cancer is a later-life cancer; the median age at diagnosis is now age 70. The risk is greater for men than women, and greater for African American men than men of European ancestry, but the reasons are not well understood. The theory is that colorectal cancer is related to men's greater occurrence of abdominal obesity, smoking, and drinking, which are all more prevalent in African American men.

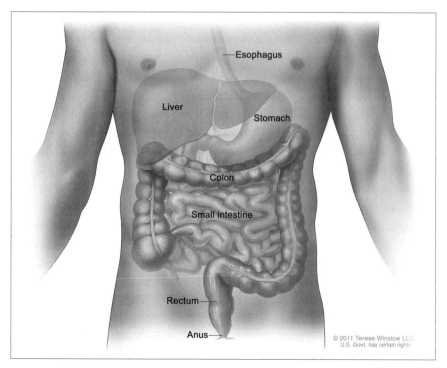

Figure 19.3. Colon and rectum. © 2011 Terese Winslow LLC and the U.S. government.

Most cases of colon cancer begin as small, noncancerous clumps of cells called *polyps*, and left untreated, some of these polyps become colon cancers. The benign polyps are typically small and rarely cause a man to experience symptoms, which, when present, may range from noticeable changes in bowel movements and/or regular abdominal discomfort, if not pain, to unexplained weight loss. Because of the near absence of symptoms, healthy men are encouraged to schedule a regular screening test (a colonoscopy) at least every 10 years starting at age 50.

In an outpatient visit, a gastroenterologist—a physician who specializes in the gastrointestinal system—uses a colonoscope (a long, thin, flexible tube with a tiny fiber-optic camera and cutting device included) to identify and remove the polyps that are in the colon. This procedure is simple and very rarely problematic. The "prep" for the procedure, however, can be quite challenging. Most often this involves drinking a powerful laxative to eliminate all fecal matter from the colon so that the physician doing the colonoscopy has a clear view of the walls of the colon. This is done the afternoon before, and you do not want to be too far from a toilet. Also, you eat nothing for the 12 hours before the procedure, again to keep the colon clear. Scheduling regular "scoping" every 3–5 years prevents benign polyps from becoming malignant.

Colostomy

Should you develop colorectal cancer and need surgery, the practice is to remove both the tumor and a portion of the neighboring bowel. Because a tumor in the colon often invades the wall of the bowel (large intestine) and surrounding tissue, it is necessary for the surgeon to remove the section of the colon containing the tumor. This is similar to snipping the middle section of a garden hose, and after the excision there are two options: stitch the remaining two ends together or use the shortened bowel. If the two ends of the remaining colon can be reconnected, this allows normal bowel function. However, a temporary (sometimes permanent) colostomy may be needed. Ostomy surgery is rare but sometimes a necessity as a result of colorectal cancer. When the cancer involves literally hundreds of small tumors and a significant amount of the colon has to be removed, a colostomy may be necessary. The need for this type of solution has become much less common as surgical treatment of colon cancer has improved over the years.

The colostomy procedure brings one end of the large intestine (colon) out through the abdominal wall. (If the procedure involves the small intestine, it is called an *ileostomy*.) The mouth of a section of the colon is stitched into the skin of the abdomen, usually close to one side, and a bag (called a *stoma* appliance) is secured around the new opening. Fecal matter normally discharged in a bowel movement through the rectum is redirected to the new intestinal drain and into a bag attached to the abdomen. When possible, a follow-up surgical procedure is scheduled to reconnect the remaining colon to the rectum.

Learning to live with the colostomy can be challenging. The stoma (or opening) and the bag represent quite a change in how you look nude and can make you feel self-conscious. As a 62-year-old man told us, "You're always aware that you have a bag of shit glued on to the side of your chest." Despite his self-consciousness, he knew that only he felt his pouch and no one saw it. Studies of men with a colostomy have affirmed that men's social and sex life can be as active as it was before surgery, but it takes some adjustment. Men with a permanent colostomy can enjoy all the things they did before, including eating at restaurants and sexual intimacy with their partner.

ANAL CANCER

Anal cancer is not the same as colon or rectal cancer. The anal canal is about an inch and a half long. Different tumors can develop, and not all are cancers. Some tumors are benign polyps, some are growths that started off as harmless but over time developed into cancer, some (called *condylomas*) are caused by infection from the human papillomavirus (HPV), and some are invasive squamous cell carcinomas or melanomas identical to the skin cancers. Anal cancer is fairly uncommon. It accounts for about 1–2 percent of gastrointestinal cancers. However, its incidence among men has increased 160 percent since the mid-1970s, probably because of increases in the prevalence of exposures such as anal intercourse, HPV infection, and a greater number of lifetime sexual partners. The American Cancer Society estimates that there are about 2,000 new cases of anal cancer among men each year (and 3,000 among women).[37] This cancer is more common among men who are not exclusively heterosexual. One study estimated that men who have more than 10 percent of their sex with other men were at five times greater risk of anal cancer,[38] and the CDC estimated that gay and bisexual men are about 17 times more likely to develop an HPV-caused anal cancer,[39] and this greater risk is because the men were not using a condom.

Anal warts and most (perhaps 90%) anal cancers are related to exposure to HPV, which is symptomless and unapparent.[40] One's HPV risk is increased by skin-to-skin contact with an infected area of the body, and this mostly happens during sex. Moving your finger from her vagina to the rim of your anus is one example of skin-to-skin contact. Men's risk is increased by having anal intercourse and/or different sex partners. It is important to recognize that a condom will not fully prevent your exposure to HPV, since the virus passes by skin-to-skin contact during oral sex or genital or anal contact not covered by the condom. Another key risk factor is a distressed immune system (only sometimes due to a preexisting HIV infection). Men can reduce their anal cancer risk by not smoking and limiting their number of sexual partners. Current smokers have at least twice the odds of anal cancer as nonsmokers.[41] The explanation for why smoking adds risk for anal cancer development remains unknown. Be conscious of rectal symptoms (bleeding, a lump near the anus, pain around the anus) and report any symptom to a physician right away; don't wait 6 months until your next annual physical. The annual rectal exam will find some cases of anal cancer early. Ask your physician about the anal Pap test, a fairly new test that can be done to screen for this cancer.

BREAST CANCER

Most men are unaware that men are capable of having breast cancer. As the story below discloses, the diagnosis of male breast cancer is nearly incomprehensible.

> And my physician says "Well, you have breast cancer." [long pause] And, then I was like speechless, and I asked, "Do you know this is Peter?" I was thinkin' he's got too many reports on his desk and he's looking at, instead of Peter, he's lookin' at Paula's report. And he says, "Yes, men get breast cancer and you have a very aggressive form." So, it was just, it was the ton of bricks—ah, you-have-got-to-be-fucking-kidding-me moment.

As rare as anal cancer is, male breast cancer isn't even on men's radar; however, roughly 2,000 men get breast cancer each year. Few knew it was even possible, and they are universally shocked. And because they had no idea, most end up consulting a physician when the tumor mass is sizeable (as big as a bite-size Snicker's bar, or half a ping-pong ball) and there is significant lymph node involvement at initial presentation. Men with breast cancer usually think that the lump is a cyst and ignore it.

The universal treatment is a mastectomy—often a "radical" mastectomy, where portions of the chest wall muscles and the lymph nodes near the arm pit are removed. Typical postsurgical treatment involves 5 years of estrogen-blocking hormonal therapy, which can have annoying side effects such as weight gain, hot flashes, lowered libido, and erectile difficulties. Despite all this, men with breast cancer fight to be recognized as breast cancer survivors, and they are not embarrassed by the site of their cancer.[42]

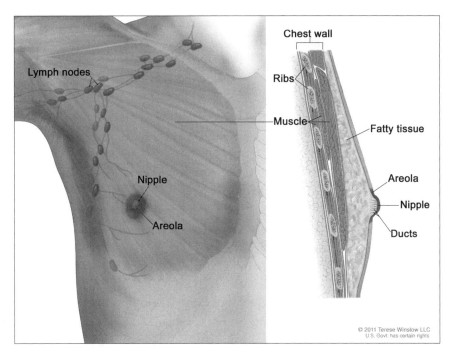

Figure 19.4. Anatomy of the male breast. © 2011 Terese Winslow LLC and the U.S. government.

BLADDER CANCER

Another malignancy among men is (urinary) bladder cancer, affecting 55,000 men annually. The National Cancer Institute estimates that at least 400,000 men are alive who have had a history of bladder cancer. It is mostly caused by smoking cigarettes,[43] yet studies also show that men exposed to high levels of hydrocarbons and petroleum chemicals are at greater risk.[44] The bladder is a hollow, muscular organ located in the pelvis which stores urine produced by the kidneys. Typical of our body's construction, each organ has a number of distinct cells. Bladder cancer nearly always originates in the (transitional epithelial) cells that make up the innermost lining of the bladder, which explains why it is also called *transitional cell carcinoma*. It is the fourth most common newly diagnosed malignancy among men (ranked eighth among women), and twice as prevalent among white men as either African American or Hispanic men. Not surprisingly, because it is an environmentally caused cancer and takes years of exposure to toxins to grow to a diagnosable size, it is more likely diagnosed among men in their sixties and seventies.

Bladder cancer will cause blood in the urine, and other possible symptoms include pain while urinating, frequent urination, and/or feeling the need to urinate without voiding. It can be detected through a routine screening of a urine specimen. Once bladder cancer is suspected, a definitive diagnosis can be determined by CT scan and then a biopsy. The most widely used therapies are surgery, radiation, and chemotherapy, either alone or in combination.

PANCREATIC CANCER

The pancreas is a pear-shaped, 6-inch gland near the stomach which produces both fluids to help in digestion and insulin to help control blood sugars. Pancreatic cancer is the fourth leading cause of cancer-related death among men in the United States (behind lung, prostate, and colorectal). However, it isn't the fourth most frequently diagnosed cancer. It is relatively rare and more often fatal. Only 20–25 new cases are diagnosed annually per 100,000 men (compared to 240 or more new prostate cancer cases per 100,000 men). The 1-year survival rate is only 24 percent, and the 5-year survival rate is less than 5 percent. Typically, pancreatic cancer remains symptom-free for years. The first signs are weight loss, painless jaundice, and perhaps abdominal pain that feels like constipation. It is the jaundice that alerts a man that something is not right, yet it is the increasing abdominal and/or back pain that spurs him to see his physician. By the point of diagnosis, however, the cancer has ordinarily spread, metastasizing first to the regional lymph nodes and then to the liver, which causes the jaundice. Pancreatic cancer can also metastasize to any surface in the abdomen, including the stomach, colon, and lungs. There is a greater incidence of pancreatic cancer among black men and an increased incidence as men get older. The median age at diagnosis is mid- to late sixties.

Curative treatment isn't really possible at this point, particularly if this cancer has already spread. Surgery is only recommended if the tumor is small, and many physicians question whether an elderly man in poor health ought to be a candidate for invasive surgery, given the likelihood of complications. Men undergoing aggressive chemotherapy often experience a sharp deterioration in their quality of life as a result of their treatment. Researchers have found that depression is often associated with this cancer, and a number of cancer centers offer complementary therapies such as nutritional and spiritual support. Palliative treatments, which are intended to provide adequate symptom relief, are encouraged.

ORAL CANCER

Oral cancers manifest as a wound (lesion) or abnormal growth in the lining of the mouth. Discussed in more detail in chapter 17, oral cancers are diagnosed in about 1 percent of men annually, or more than 28,000 new cases, and most are age 60 and older at diagnosis. The cellular compositions of all mouth cancers are all very similar and involve the flat squamous cells that cover the surfaces of the lips, mouth, and tongue—the same cells as "common" skin cancers. But in the mouth they are malignant and spread rapidly. If the tumors are diagnosed by your dentist or physician in their early stage, the 5-year survival rate is greater than 80 percent. But, sadly, the majority of men with mouth cancer wait and do not get diagnosed until the cancer is late stage, resulting in a high death rate of nearly 45 percent within 5 years of the cancer being found.

Smoking and other tobacco use cause 70–80 percent of mouth cancers; it is both the smoke and heat from cigarettes, cigars, and pipes which irritate the tissues in the mouth and cause healthy cells to mutate. Use of chewing tobacco or snuff equally causes inflammation. The other major risk is the HPV infection, which is passed from person to person through sexual contact. Two lesser risk factors are poor dental and mouth hygiene and lip blistering from exposure to the sun.

Like most other cancers, treatment in the early stages consists of surgery to remove the tumor and/or localized radiation. If the mouth cancer has metastasized, chemotherapy with or without radiotherapy is usually recommended. Do consider a second opinion before you initiate your treatment; opinions differ.

LYMPHOMA AND OTHER CANCERS

Although not restricted to older men, the median age of a non-Hodgkin's lymphoma diagnosis is early sixties, and it is the sixth most frequently diagnosed cancer in the United States.[45] Lymphoma is actually a very diverse group of cancers that affect cells within the lymphatic system, such as our marrow, spleen, white blood cells, and lymph nodes. These cancers are not staged in terms of TNM; rather, since they eventually involve enlarged, painless lymph nodes in the neck, under an arm, or in the groin and not tumors, they are staged by what is called the Ann Arbor staging system. Similar to TNM, the greater the stage, the more severe the cancer. Other than the swollen lumps, symptoms are nonspecific and include fever for no known reason, fatigue, night sweats, and weight loss. Treatment for lymphoma depends on the type and stage and most often involves chemotherapy and/or radiation therapy.

There are many other types of cancers, such as of the digestive system (e.g., stomach, esophagus), urinary system (e.g., kidney), and brain, that have not been summarized in this chapter. However, they are just as important. For a man living with one of these "other" cancers, his experiences with symptoms, diagnosis, treatment, and hopes for clinical remission and a satisfactory quality of life are equal to the way men with lung or prostate cancer cope with decisions and their disease. The goal isn't always the same: sometimes it is treatment and eventual remission, whereas other times the objective becomes palliative, in which case improving the man's quality of life with supportive care is the prime objective.[46]

MEN MANAGING THEIR CANCER

Mentioned in the opening of the chapter, conversations with cancer patients and survivors tell us that a cancer diagnosis is a biography disrupter. It's an awakening that we are mortal and may soon face death. A cancer has the potential to undermine a man's sense of his independence and obliges him to seek medical help, as well as support and comfort from others. The diagnosis becomes a spiritual "calling" that challenges men to step back, rethink, and step up. For more than 30 years, medical sociologists and psychologists have studied the ways men live with chronic illness, especially cancer. The most common finding is that before the cancer diagnosis, men were not attentive to their bodies or engaged in healthy self-care. We chose to be "guys"—to eat and drink a lot, work ungodly hours, and ignore the unusual changes on and in our bodies, those signs (e.g., lumps, sores) and symptoms (e.g., fatigue, pain) that signify that a cancer is growing.

Researchers studying men's experiences with cancer discovered that once men are told their cancer diagnosis, there is a "mind shift" that occurs. For most men, neither the diagnosis nor the cancer strikes hard enough to wound their sense of themselves as men. They will embody the cancer, step up, and "take it on." As one man undergoing treatment commented, "Cancer has the word *can* in it." Men living with cancer reformulate their life plan and even abandon the tendency to refuse help. When our priorities shift from ignoring the body to taking control of the cancer, men openly rely on partners and close friends for emotional support; their physicians and cancer center for advice, guidance, and palliative care; and their spiritual sense for resiliency. Treatments are never pleasant, but they're experienced as a means to an end—to survive.

> Just because they define that you're a Stage-IV, doesn't mean you're not going to live for the next twenty years. (62-year-old man with prostate cancer)

Men seem to recover quickly from the setback of the diagnosis and re-frame their life to conquer the mutant cells. They're motivated by a well-established masculine way of thinking that deals with "bumps in the road."

> It's kind of my philosophy of my life. You know, it's another hurdle that's been put in front of me. What are you going to do with it? You gonna jump over it and keep going, or you gonna stand behind and say "Oh god, it's too tall, I can't get over it"? Hey, God throws you another hurdle, keep going. (63-year-old man with coronary heart disease and lung cancer)

> This is just another hill to climb, so you just make peace with it, then don't go over it a thousand times. Just, "Okay, this is my situation, my percent-ages are . . . you gotta do what you gotta do." (69-year-old man with breast cancer)

Living with cancer, even among men with stage IV lung cancer or pan-creatic cancer and a very limited life expectancy, is something most men make peace with. A 64-year-old retired colonel who died in the early 1980s of lung cancer, having been diagnosed 5 months before his death, calmly said, "Things happen." He took control, entered chemotherapy and radi-ation treatment, and assured himself (and his family) a good 5 months. Researchers studying men's cancer experiences regularly notice that once men are told their cancer diagnosis, the mind shift that occurs is one of "taking control," focusing on the positives, and getting their end-of-life matters in order. Surely sadness, or depression, is commonplace, but there often remains the hope to survive.

PART IV

LIVING WITH OTHERS

CHAPTER 20

Sexual Intimacy

with Amanda Barusch

In this chapter we consider aspects of men's sexual intimacy and sexuality from several perspectives, including physical, psychological, emotional, and social. We begin by exploring the meaning of intimacy and then move to what is unique about middle-aged and older men's sexuality. The ways in which our quality of life—our physical and mental health—is both impacted by and can affect our sexual lives are reviewed, as are the options available to take on the sexual challenges that men can experience as they grow older.

WHAT IS INTIMACY?

Of all the topics addressed in this book, intimacy is one of the most difficult to define. The word itself derives from two Latin words, *intimus* and *intimare*.[1] *Intimus* was an adjective describing something "innermost, profound, or secret," while *intimare* was a verb meaning "make familiar, to disclose." Contemporary definitions of intimacy run along the lines of "close or warm friendship" or "a euphemism for sexual relations." An anonymous poet described the profound connectedness of intimacy this way: "Henceforth there will be such a oneness between us—that when one weeps the other will taste salt."

Many people might say that while intimacy is difficult to define, you know it when you feel it. In an intimate relationship with another person, we share things that are deeply private. The hallmarks of intimate relationships are the emotional and physical experiences occurring inside the relationship that become couple secrets and barred from the public—the private rituals, verbal and nonverbal codes of the "we," defining moments and memories, personal weaknesses and desires. The result is deep knowledge of the other person. Our partner and lover also can know us to our very core, perhaps even better than we understand ourselves. Being sexually involved, of course, can be and usually is central to intimate love relationships. On top of good sex, satisfying intimate relationships rest on trust, open and honest communication, shared goals and expectations, and mutual respect and concern. The essence of intimacy is the shared experiences that are deeply personal, and in practice intimacy ranges from empathy to sex. The biblical Hebrew term for "to know" is *Yada*, a term that refers to a multifaceted experience that encompasses love, mercy, and justice.

Intimate moments are not always defined in terms of relationships established with other individuals. They can also occur and be satisfied by the nonhuman relationships we establish and the trust that evolves between ourselves and a beloved pet, as well as in vicarious fashion through connections we have via the characters in a book or movie, or more generally in the lives of others. The hermit may have chosen the life he leads because it represents the level of human intimacy he desires.

Intimacy can also extend far beyond what's found in our most important, one-on-one relationship. We experience deep understanding and connectedness in a wide range of circumstances, even short-term relations. We can even experience bonding moments when we exchange glances of exasperation with strangers in an airport security line. When we work together with colleagues for many years, we often develop deep knowledge of each other and are able to anticipate each other's comments or complete one another's sentences. While these may not represent "intimate moments" in the literal sense, they are examples in which we "connect," even briefly, with another person and share a secret experience that is often meaningless outside the moment or relationship.

Intimate relations most commonly take place within close relationships between two lovers. Indeed, the norms of romantic love that became an integral part of Western culture foster the notion that long-term love relationships are the best (or even the only) venues for intimate contact.[2] The implication is that only one relationship—our primary love relationship—ought to be the "home" of all our secrets and meaningful experiences. But every man has more than one core relationship that both defines him and bolsters his quality of life. Recent research even suggests that sexual monogamy does not come naturally, and therefore only one primary, sexually exclusive love relationship may not be certain.[3] In addition, we have brothers and/or sisters, close buddies, and work associates who also define us and share some of our "secrets." The good news is that research on the emotional lives of older adults suggests that, like many other complex abilities, our capacity for intimacy improves with age.[4]

GENDER DIFFERENCES IN INTIMACY: MARS, VENUS, OR BOTH?

By now, you've heard the popular psychology shtick that men *so* differ from women when it comes to intimacy and sexual intimacy that we "guys" are on a different planet.[5] By the way, the implication is that we are on the wrong planet. Maybe you also have heard that men's late life is sometimes described as utterly unlike our younger years: there is supposedly an androgynous drift as we age,[6] when the rigid masculine versus feminine expectations that valorized youth in our earlier years blur and as adult men we are no longer expected to be one-dimensional, defining ourselves by our toughness and breadwinning. The older man (who is passing 60), in this view, may be less stoic, more nurturing and emotionally vulnerable, and receptive to deeper intimacy than he was in his youth. The values within postmodernity, the era we are currently in, also have been described as a time of less gender separateness[7] and less ageism,[8] freeing middle-aged men from the misconceptions that being intimate isn't masculine and getting old means becoming unattractive and disadvantaged. Changing times and the lengthening of the individual life course would seem to be "granting permission" to men to explore more fully emotional closeness and let go of the (sexual) performance anxieties that dominated our youth.[9]

> Gender (masculinity and femininity) is an accomplishment. It is social, not biological.

Ageism and sexism are still prevalent in popular culture, casting heterosexual men as if they are on a war planet and stupid when it comes to their feelings or understanding the feelings of others.[10] It is likely that the same can be said for gay men as they ponder their aging and the mind-set of their middle-aged and older partners.[11] As much as this view and its stereotypes have been discredited, middle-aged and older men do operate in a gendered world. Consistent with our gendered past, there is continuity in how we see ourselves as we get older, and a primary focus of older men's lives is instrumental (making things happen), but these characteristics do *not* mean that men's lives are unemotional and unnurturing.

Men are stereotyped as clods, but in real life we are interested in making our friends and lovers feel good. Some have argued that women express their love by communicating feelings, whereas men express love not by talking but by doing things or engaging in physical acts.[12] This popular thesis has been around for at least the past 30 years and suggests that men think about close relationships such as romances and marriage in fundamentally different ways than women do.[13] This is partly true. Yet both academic scholars and popular press authors have called attention to "sex differences," which unavoidably homogenizes men into stereotyped characters and frankly ignores what men really feel and do. An alternative view is that both men and women regard close relationships similarly; men also seek intimacy from close relationships and look upon trust and empathy as the core features of these relationships.[14] Amanda Barusch, who interviewed older adults to write *Love Stories in Later Life*, commented that one of her great lessons was how irrelevant gender could be to the emotional experience of romance. Men do have feelings, can love and care about their partner, and, unlike the stereotypes, do not single-mindedly equate intimacy with sex. Maybe men tend to be doers, and maybe women are better at expressing feelings. Even so, men are not inexpressive doers, as stereotyped.[15] Both women and men can be (and are) nurturing, aggressive, task focused, and sentimental.

COMMUNICATION STYLE

People in intimate relationships need to be aware of *all* of the factors influencing how the other person will hear what they have to say. What we say (the content) often is less important than how we say it and what the other person "hears."[16] The quality of intimate moments with a partner is enhanced significantly by physical and visual factors, including tone and volume of voice, posture, eye contact, standing position, "air" of confidence, and body position. And these all affect listening. Put simply, the language of intimacy (and love) is not only heard; it is seen and felt as well.

The Opportunity for Personal Development

Intimacy transforms us. It opens us to powerful lessons and insights. We come to know ourselves better. This enhances our ability to know others. Intimacy calls on us to develop new skills for communication and disclosure. These translate into other settings, improving our effectiveness in other types of relationships. As a vehicle for self-discovery, intimacy is essential to our personal development. Leo Buscaglia explained in his 1996 book *Love*,

> As soon as the love relationship does not lead me to me, as soon as I in a love relationship do not lead another person to himself, this love, even if it seems to be the most secure and ecstatic attachment I have ever experienced, is not true love . . . real love is dedicated to continual becoming.[17]

Herbert Wong, a sociologist, concurs and argues that relationships stagnate (and some people have affairs) because self-discovery ends.[18]

SOCIAL CONTEXT OF LATE-LIFE INTIMACY

Even men's most intimate relationships take place in a social context. A match may be made in heaven, but its fate is determined on earth by people who have feet of clay. The importance of community is reflected in the rituals around marriage and civil commitments, in which our loved ones are invited to witness, validate, and support intimate relationships. New suitors around the world know that the judgments of family and friends can be deal breakers. This is also true in later life, though the cast of characters may be different. Parents are replaced by adult children, and some friends may be replaced by professional caregivers. These supporting actors are typically influenced by ethnic traditions and may hold ageist attitudes.

Later-life intimacy is an intergenerational affair. Children, both young and adult, look to their parents for lessons in intimacy. Some use their parents as lessons in what not to do, but more commonly adult children's relationships echo the experiences of the previous generation.[19] Two sociologists from Pennsylvania State University, Paul Amato and Alan Booth, did a fascinating study of the relationship between parents' marital relationships and those of their adult children. They surveyed a national sample of parents and their married offspring, collecting data for 18 years. They found that discord in the parents' marriages is reflected in the relationships of their adult children. Even more intriguing was the finding that change in parental marriages was reflected as well. When parents experienced greater harmony or less conflict, their adult children tended to report a similar change in their own marriages.[20]

When parents find new romantic partners in old age, some children react from their "inner ageism." As Robert Butler explained, "Many adult children continue to be bound by a primitive childhood need to deny their parents a sex life."[21] Several of the people interviewed by Barusch for *Love Stories in Later Life* restricted their romantic involvements out of concern for their children. Some pursued relationships that are now described as "living apart together," in which they were committed to each other and spent "quality time" together but maintained separate households. Others decided not to marry. Still others could not even consider entering into a new relationship for fear that their children would be upset. Time and again Barusch confesses that she found herself aching to tell a respondent to ignore the children and live the life he or she dreamt of.[22] But, as we know, adult children cannot be ignored. They are vital in the lives of older men (and women), giving emotional support, opportunities to reminisce, and a link to the future.

Men also can discover that the quality of the relationship that exists with children will change over time based on the developmental needs of the latter, consequently altering the degree to which you can share facets of your life with them. Children moving through adolescence and young adulthood tend to have strong urges to express their emerging sense of independence by distancing themselves from their parents. During that period, a son or daughter may show little interest in your life generally, much less the relationship you have established with a new partner. By middle age, they may tend to be more accepting of your behaviors and actions, including relationships you have established with others.

AN EMPTY NEST CAN BE A GOOD THING

While the departure of grown children from the home can put additional pressure on a married couple or partners to relate more directly and continuously with each other, it does not often put the relationship at risk. The quality of a marital or partnered relationship can actually improve at this time in your life. University of California at Berkeley researchers found that marital satisfaction actually tends to increase after children have left home, and it's not because married couples and partners spend more time together, but rather because the quality of the time they spend together improves.[23] Gail Saltz, a psychiatrist, describes this particular life transition as creating the time and opportunity for men and their spouses to embark on second honeymoons in which their time alone can really boost their sex drives.[24] This happens, in part, because the couple has more time to rediscover why they fell in love with each other in the first place, resulting in a rekindled romance that might have been thought to be long gone. An empty house can also allow the freedom and spontaneity to engage in romantic behavior and sexual activity without the worry of being unexpectedly interrupted by a child who wakes up crying because of a bad dream or needs help with their math homework.

Separating Your Work and Personal Worlds

For some middle-aged and older men, their allegiance to their jobs regularly impacts on their private lives, and not necessarily in a good way. All too often, these men are so heavily enmeshed in their careers in order to make more money, get ahead, or avoid receiving the dreaded pink slip that they have little time and energy left at home to devote to meaningful romance, intimacy, and sex play with their spouse or partner. The stress and strain associated with our jobs can have a major influence on our capacity for intimacy at home, especially for those of us who consider ourselves workaholics. This does not have to be the case. There are steps you can take to reverse the trend. Consider the following relatively straightforward action steps that Pepper Schwartz has suggested to alter the pattern:[25]

> Cut down on your hours at work to a level that puts your work and personal lives in better balance.

> Don't bring your work home—stop answering work-related phone calls and e-mails when you are with your spouse or partner.

> Spend quality time with the person you care about—focus on that individual completely over a glass of wine and romantic music.

> Create a separation between the mind-set of your work and personal worlds when you get home by doing things such as taking a shower, changing your clothes, or taking a walk.

Intimacy in Other Relationships

Intimacy can be realized in a variety of relationships that don't involve having a spouse or partner. For many older men, a great deal of satisfaction is found in time spent with children and grandchildren, as well as with close friends and confidants. Serving as a mentor for a student or as a Big Brother or Big Sister can also be very gratifying. And don't forget the joy that can come from caring for an animal, which then rewards you in return with their love, affection, and companionship.

SEXUAL INTIMACY

According to traditional heterosexual stereotypes, men pursued women who resisted sexual advances as long as they possibly could. Traditionally, it was assumed that women didn't enjoy sex at all, and men were just out to "get their rocks off." Modern times have brought more open recognition that women also want to have pleasurable orgasms.[26] For some couples, sex took on a new goal, the "simultaneous orgasm," and when all was said and done, couples asked each other, "Did you come?"

But, as recent research on human sexuality has demonstrated, "good sex" is not only about orgasms. In a recent study,[27] Australian men were asked what made sex good. A 21-year-old said,

> Um, good sex is a feeling that you get when you're really into the other person and, it doesn't really matter what you do, it's just how it feels between the two of you . . . getting to know each other's bodies, and things like that, laughter during sex, spending the whole day in bed. It doesn't matter how many times you come.

Likewise, a 42-year-old said,

> Oh, kissing and cuddling . . . and also, um, seeing the passion in a [part-ner's] face. . . . Oh, it's the intimacy. It's feeling loved, I think, yeah. It's a celebration, you know.

In a different study, a 62-year-old Native American who was interviewed said,[28]

> If you truly love someone and you have sex with them, oh boy there is a difference! . . . because you love that person. You just feel them. And they feel you.

These comments—the first from a gay man, the rest from heterosexual men—are characteristic of men's sexual intimacy. Gender stereotypes aside, it is important to understand that men (and women) want a connection that feels good. As sex therapist Bernie Zilbergeld explains,

> It is not his job to give her an orgasm, but it is in his interest to understand her desires and to fulfill them to the best of his abilities. . . . A good lover is attentive to his partner's breath, sounds, and movements, and notices what works and doesn't work for her.[29]

Vera's experience of her husband's sexuality is probably typical.[30] In her midsixties her husband had health problems that affected his erectile ability. As Vera explained, "There's other ways to have sex—oral sex—and I just love to be held and told that I'm loved. I like it when I'm out with him. He puts his arm around me and makes me feel like I'm number one in his life."

As these narratives suggest, sexual intimacy for men does not revolve simply around penetrative sex. Sexuality is about intimacy; sex also can be recreational and pleasurable without orgasm or intercourse. Typically, the longer the duration of our primary relationship, the greater our relationship happiness and sexual satisfaction will be.[31] The importance of sex in maintaining a good relationship persists as we get older. For men between age 65 and 75, more than half (53%) are sexually active and having intercourse.[32] Indeed, 15–40 percent of men in their eighties report having intercourse at least once a month.[33]

The sexual activity of men in partnered relationships predictably declines with age—from 73 percent among men 57–64, to 53 percent among men 65–74, to 26 percent among men 75–85.[34] The simple explanation for changes in sexual activity is the health of the men and/or their partner.

Within long-term relationships, sexual activity often involves a shift from the primacy of sexual intercourse to other forms of sexual intimacy.

Among older men who remain sexually active, the activity may eventually shift entirely to kissing, hugging, sexual touching, and oral sex.[35] Sexual intimacy for men in partnered relationships emphasizes relaxing, gentle sex, and mutual enjoyment, and sexual intimacy plays a vital part in most men's sense of self throughout their middle and later years. A study by the American Association of Retired Persons (AARP), "Sexuality at Midlife and Beyond," reported that 60 percent of respondents agree that sexual activity is a critical part of a good relationship, and 63 percent of men and women described themselves as extremely satisfied or somewhat satisfied with their sex lives.[36] The results from a global study involving 29 countries discovered that it's the 40- to 80-year-olds who have the best time during sex,[37] and sex for a man in his fifties is better than for a man in his thirties and forties. Why? The theory is simple: middle-aged and older men are less concerned about sexual performance than younger men; for them, sex is about intimacy.

Sex Has Many Health Benefits

- Improves your immune system
- Releases endorphins to enhance your mood
- Provides cardiac exercise
- Has lasting positive psychological effects
- Relieves physical and mental stress
- Increases blood flow and improves skin appearance

GADGETS, GIZMOS, AND AGING BODIES

The advertising media often go to great lengths to persuade older adults that aged bodies are not sexually attractive. But age will not be erased, and the pernicious ageism in the advertising industry can lead many older adults to develop body image problems and lose confidence in their physical attractiveness. Women seem to be particularly vulnerable to this, and this, in turn, can erode their interest in sexual activity. Nor are men immune to the same pressures, as evidenced by the market success of erection-enhancing drugs.[38]

Most of us actually place our partner's changing physical appearance relatively low on our list of concerns with our partner. But—if we let them—the physical changes associated with normal aging can interfere with our sex lives. Given the inevitability of age-related changes in our appearance, how can we help each other pay less attention to how our bodies have changed physically and more attention to enjoying them? Those men who love older women (or older men) would do well to remind them that they are attractive by finding creative ways to offer a kind word, a smile, an honest compliment, or an appreciative touch.

The Facts about Sexuality and Aging

- Sexuality is normal and natural in old age.

- As you age, the amount of sexual activity generally decreases, but the amount of sexual interest and ability remains fairly constant.

- If your sexuality is constant throughout life, the physical and biological changes associated with aging are less pronounced and sexuality is usually less affected.

- Sexual health can be beneficial to overall health.

- Sexual activity is possible and takes place through the seventies and beyond.

- There is more to sexuality than just intercourse. There are many other forms of intimate expression that can enhance your experience, including spending time together, holding hands, hugging, touching, kissing, masturbation, and oral sex.

- The physical exertion associated with sex is roughly equivalent to walking up two flights of stairs. Sex for a person with heart disease is rarely dangerous (it is recommended that you consult a physician concerning the risks associated with sex and heart disease).

Age also brings subtle changes in the sexual experience itself. Some of these changes can encourage older lovers to take more time in their lovemaking, identify new erogenous zones, and experiment. For instance, while older men (and women) can take longer to be aroused, and older women may experience decreased vaginal elasticity and lubrication, both of these changes can (and usually do) result in extended foreplay and use of different kinds of the available personal lubricants. In his midsixties, one of the men interviewed by Barusch explained gleefully, "Now that the kids are gone, foreplay can last all day!"[39]

Some men also find that accessories and sexual aids come in handy. Today, companies like the Sinclair Institute include an advisory panel of professional counselors and sex therapists. Sinclair describes itself as "the leading source of sexual health products for adults who want to improve the quality of intimacy and sex in their relationships."[40] A range of aids, from explicit educational videos and personal lubricants to vibrators, masturbation sleeves, penile pumps, and sex position aids, is available to adventuresome men, as well as those seeking to adapt to a disability.

More Foreplay Can Be a Good Thing

Older men may need more and more stimulation to become aroused, maintain an erection, and achieve an orgasm. Strategies for dealing with this are not limited to the use of medications but include having more foreplay before sex and masturbation.

THERE ARE EMOTIONAL RISKS

Emotional intimacy can make us feel vulnerable, and couple satisfaction may be the most perilous aspect of our sexual involvement. What of jealousy and betrayal? How to manage ugly emotions? Should we share these feelings with our partner? Are we allowed no secrets? Many men understand sexual intimacy to include good feelings: closeness, warmth, acceptance, or caring. But it is important to remember that our sexual lives and histories also may include painful feelings like embarrassment, resentment, and even rage.

Couples make decisions about what fits into their private world and what does not—what experiences they will keep secret, and what experiences and feelings they will share. The emotional intimacy boundaries are constantly in flux as we establish and renegotiate agreements with our partner, sometimes explicit and sometimes not. When one partner breaks the rules, the other partner may feel betrayed. We see this most often in relation to sexual exclusivity, but betrayal can also include a wide range of misbehavior from revealing couple secrets to an outsider, failing to disclose information to a partner, or responding with an emotion considered inappropriate. As most lovers know all too well, painful feelings large and small are almost always part of the package.

A fascinating body of work suggests that age improves our ability to manage interpersonal conflict. Kira Birditt, at the University of Michigan, suggests that when faced with conflict, older adults are more likely to use what she calls "loyalty strategies" (remain calm and wait for the situation to blow over, or do nice things to improve the emotional atmosphere); when we were younger adults, we were more likely to argue, end the relationship, leave, call the person names, or yell, practices she terms "exit strategies."[41] Further, the theory of "socioemotional selectivity," coined by Laura Carstensen at Stanford, suggests that in later life we learn to more consciously manage our emotional lives, avoiding experiences that hurt or irritate us. Taken together, these skills can improve the quality of our loving relationships.[42]

When men spend most of their lives in settings that call for competition and achievement, intimate relationships are the only relational space where they can be vulnerable. After talking with men about their experiences of intimacy, Shawn Patrick and John Bechenback suggested that this heightens the risks for men. Because of the emotional exclusivity of our love relationship, we may be particularly sensitive to judgments from our intimate partner.[43]

THERE ARE PHYSICAL RISKS

Late-life sexual intimacy is not risk-free. For example, 10–15 percent of new AIDS cases in the United States are people 50 and over, and in the United Kingdom the rate of sexually transmitted infections (STIs) more than doubled for men older than 55 from the late 1990s to the early 2000s.[44] Neither heterosexual nor gay men are exempt from infection with HIV/AIDS or developing chlamydia, herpes, or HPV (for more details, see chapter 15). Partners in intimate long-term relationships often engage in unprotected sex; this behavior says they trust their partners. However, men who are having sex with new or multiple partners need to protect themselves, because they cannot afford to put their partner(s) at risk of a sexually transmitted illness.

Tips for Good Sex in Later Life

A variety of disabilities, illnesses, surgeries, and medications can have a negative impact on your capacity to engage in and enjoy sex:

- Arthritis
- Chronic pain
- Diabetes
- Heart disease
- Incontinence

- Stroke
- Dementia
- Surgery
- Medications
- Alcohol

However, there are a wide range of treatments and procedures available that can enable you to still have a fulfilling sex life. Sometimes, simply modifying certain behaviors is all you need to do. This is often the case for all the conditions listed above. Talk to your physician and learn about what options are available to help you enjoy sex more.

Source: National Institute on Aging (2010, Apr. 20). *Age page: Sexuality in later life.* Bethesda, MD: National Institute on Aging.

Regardless of sexual orientation, the guidelines offered by the Mayo Clinic for protecting oneself from HIV/AIDS are instructive.[45] These include both partners getting tested and not engaging in unprotected sex unless they remain monogamous and are absolutely certain they are disease-free. Otherwise, using a condom is essential. Mayo Clinic staff recommend limiting the amount of alcohol you consume and refraining from using drugs (both of which can increase the likelihood of taking sexual risks), as well as avoiding sexual venues like sex parties, bathhouses, and the Internet, where multiple, anonymous, and risky sexual behaviors are more likely to occur. And finally, getting vaccinated can provide an added degree of protection from serious liver infections such as hepatitis A and B arising from unprotected sex. Of course, the safest practice is to remain monogamous with a partner who has tested negative for HIV and other STIs.

ERECTILE DYSFUNCTION AND INTIMACY

Illness, disability, and medications may change the way we experience sex. As many as one in five men over 25 in the United States experience erectile dysfunction (ED).[46] That figure increases to 70 percent among men older than 70. The pervasiveness of ED is largely because of the health of the nation's aging male population. ED is often caused by other conditions, including benign prostate enlargement, cardiovascular disease, diabetes, obesity, and prostate cancer. It can be a side effect of many of the medications used to manage chronic conditions, as well as a side effect of heavy alcohol and tobacco use.[47] Sedentary lifestyles and overeating are also risk factors for ED.[48] (See chapter 15 for a full discussion of ED.)

Despite these challenges, older adults can still enjoy a satisfying sex life. In recent years one of the first lines of defense for ED has become the use of phosphodiesterase type 5 inhibitors such as Viagra (sildenafil), Levitra (vardenafil), and Cialis (tadalafil). As a rule, these extremely popular medications are effective and are accompanied by few side effects, although they are not recommended for men taking nitrate medications. All of these drugs increase the amount of the chemical nitric oxide in the body, which opens and relaxes the blood vessels in the penis, thereby enabling a man to achieve and maintain an erection. However, because these medications do not stimulate your sex drive, you must be sexually aroused for the drugs to work.

Caution is advised in taking these medications if you have heart problems, high or low blood pressure, a history of stroke, certain eye problems, leukemia, or sickle cell anemia. You should always inform your physician about other medications you are taking, especially those known to interact with ED drugs, including antibiotics, blood thinners, certain heart medications, antiseizure drugs, and alpha blockers. ED drugs should never be taken in combination with nitrate drugs used to treat angina (heart pain) such as nitroglycerin, isosorbide, and illegal drugs like amyl nitrite.

AGEISM IN RESIDENTIAL CARE

Nowhere are ageism and its negative impact on older men's sexuality and opportunity for intimacy more apparent than in the residential care facilities that serve the needs of older men, especially those men who have experienced significant functional impairment.[49] Entering a nursing home means subjecting yourself to a new set of rules, most of which are designed for the convenience of management. Sexuality among older adults is a difficult topic for the nursing care staff and their administrators, and restrictive policies are not uncommon. This is even more likely to be true for gay men, who are often forced to "reenter the closet" when they go into institutional care to avoid being bullied. Even heterosexuals are usually invited to check their sexuality at the door.[50]

Consider the story of two older adults we will call Dorothy and Bob, both of whom suffered from dementia.[51] Dorothy and Bob met in the nursing home. In time they became close, and then physically intimate. Of necessity, nursing homes don't offer much privacy, so perhaps it was inevitable that someone would walk in on them. Unfortunately, that person was Bob's son. Shocked by what he saw, the son insisted that nursing home staff keep Bob and Dorothy apart. Dorothy stopped eating. She lost 21 pounds, was treated for depression, and eventually went into a hospital for dehydration. Bob's family moved him to another facility. Dorothy sat by the window waiting for him until her memory slipped away. Her doctor suggested that if she didn't have Alzheimer's, the loss might have killed her. Published on Slate.com, this story drew an interesting response. One commentator hit the nail on the head: "The idea of geriatrics [sic] having sex freaks people out."

It is important to know that federal regulations require nursing homes to allow married couples to share a room if they wish. But, like many Americans, staff and managers in residential care facilities can maintain cruel ageist stereotypes that make it hard to tolerate—let alone celebrate—physical intimacy among the very old.[52] This must contribute to the loneliness experienced frequently by at least one in four nursing home residents.[53] Acknowledging a constitutional right to privacy, the American Medical Directors Association (AMDA) has offered a model policy for "making reasonable and appropriate accommodations for residents who choose to engage in consensual sexual activity with others."[54] Generally these policies support "age- and gender-appropriate" interactions among people who are legally able to consent to sexual activity. But therein lies the complication. First of all, who is to say what "gender-appropriate" means? Second, over half of nursing home residents suffer from some form of dementia, which means they are legally not able to consent.[55] Anyone who works with dementia knows that there is no distinct line between competent and incompetent, and many times dementia patients are able to clearly express their desires. But, sadly, a diagnosis of dementia means that the person who holds the durable power of attorney for the nursing home resident may well be the one who decides whether or not that individual can have a love life in the nursing home. Some will be fortunate, while others, like Bob, may lose the love of their later lives to their families' ageist prejudices.

DON'T BE AFRAID TO TALK TO YOUR DOCTOR

Health care professionals are not likely to raise the issue of sexuality themselves or feel totally comfortable talking about matters of intimacy and sexual concerns with their aging adult patients. Even so, it is very important that you not be afraid to talk with your doctor if you are having a problem that is affecting your sex life. While doctors commonly suggest treatments for ED, they can also be helpful in identifying and correcting a drug interaction that is adversely affecting your sexual experience or suggest ways in which to reduce the negative impacts of chronic health conditions you are experiencing. Your doctor can also refer you to a therapist or counselor who has special training in helping with intimacy and sex issues of an emotional nature.

Unfortunately, too many of us are hesitant to discuss our concerns, especially issues regarding our sexual lives, with our physician. We might not really know the physician. We may feel that it is a betrayal of our partner's confidence. We may feel that the physician will see our sexual worries as representing "impotence" and other signs of weakness. In any case, by not addressing the issues undermining your quality of life, you are keeping yourself from potentially feeling better and enjoying a more fulfilling life.

CLOSING THOUGHT

A definition of intimacy has been offered that is based on the etymology of the word: disclosure or sharing of that which is deeply personal. Sex and emotional intimacy are interpreted in these contexts: sex as an exchange of sensations, and emotional intimacy as a process of shared meaning making. We have suggested that social context shapes and complicates men's intimate relationships and sexual lives. The impact of ageism within our adult children's and professional caregivers' responses to our sexual and love relationships in later life is something to think about.

Intimacy in late life can be different, richer, and more intense than it was in younger years. Some think the intensity of late-life intimacy stems in part from death's proximity. "If not now, when?" becomes a major theme when death could be breathing down our necks. Our intimate relationships call on us to know ourselves and to share ourselves with our partners; both are fairly tall orders. Fortunately, the cognitive and emotional maturity developed over a lifetime has equipped most of us to handle these challenges. That may be why so many late-life lovers comment that love, like wine, improves with age.

CHAPTER 21

Retirement

Setting a retirement date is no longer a question of age; it's a matter of the size of your retirement nest egg, your general health, how you feel about your job, and what you want to do when you leave the workforce. Thanks to healthier lifestyles and breakthroughs in medical technology, our life expectancy has increased significantly during the past half century. While it's good news that you can expect to live longer in retirement and have a better quality of life, it also means we need to make sense of the next 25 years or more, which could represent as much as one-third of your life.

THE OPTION TO RETIRE

Retirement has increasingly become a life phase that men can begin while healthy and active. This was not the case for the majority of our grandfathers and great-grandfathers. In 1900 the average age of retirement was 74, but roughly two-thirds of men age 65 and older never exited the labor force. Working mostly in farming or nonagricultural manual labor, men worked until their death or "retired" because of ill health or disability.[1] By midcentury, about half of the older men retired because they could; they typically left blue-collar and white-collar jobs with small pensions and Social Security benefits.[2] Even when forced to retire because of a mandatory retirement age, existing pension plans and welfare policies (e.g., Social Security beginning in 1935, Medicare beginning in 1965) provided our fathers and grandfathers with the financial security and health insurance necessary to leave behind their work careers.

Forecasted in the lyrics of Bob Dylan's 1964 title song "The Times They Are a-Changin,'" we now view retirement as a norm, an expectation, and a right.[3] Public attitudes toward men choosing to exit the labor force and adopt a "leisure lifestyle" shifted to guarded approval during the 1960s.[4] By 1967 the Age Discrimination and Employment Act (ADEA) prohibited the use of age as a criterion in personnel policies, and the 1986 ADEA amendments prohibited mandatory retirement in all but a few occupations. Corporations responded by introducing early retirement incentive programs (ERIPs) to help downsize their older work force, and new opportunities to choose early retirement (or voluntary redundancy[5]) became available and enviable.[6] "Phased," or gradual, retirement has replaced the traditional "cliff" retirement pattern.

But the age-old expectation for us men to remain productive throughout our lives does not end when we retire. So long as each retired man maintains a high level of activity and is "busy," his status as retired is no problem. He continues to need to "do things" to be a man, and this expectation is a moral imperative. David Ekerdt, a sociologist who studies retirement, commented, "Just as there is a work ethic that holds industriousness and self-reliance as virtues, so, too, there is a 'busy ethic' for retirement that honors an active life."[7] Cutting out paper dolls for our granddaughters isn't good enough; volunteering in a kindergarten is okay. Better yet, participating in voter registration efforts, volunteering with your town's Department of Public Works effort to create a nature trail, or working in behalf of a food pantry affirms our industriousness and masculinity, legitimizes our other "leisure" time, and lets us explore untapped skills and interests.

> The question isn't at what age I want to retire, it's at what income.
>
> —George Foreman

THE DECISIONS

Retirement is more than an event with a ceremonial dinner and round of handshakes. It is better thought of as a life project that slowly unfolds, beginning well before and continuing long after the "event." There's a long preretirement phase (or at least there should be) where we begin saving for retirement. The advice from one retirement planning advisor after another is to start early (at least by our early thirties) and consistently invest in our future. During preretirement, we also begin imagining what we're going to do once we stop working. Early retirement is something many American men dream about—whether it's financially realistic or not. Most of us develop a reasonable target date for retiring, but it is a moving target.[8]

Three to five years before our target date, it is very common that many of us become hesitant about retiring, mostly because of the gap between our anticipated lifestyle in retirement and having not set aside enough money to enjoy it.[9] Once retired, there's the risk of inflation and rising health care costs. We spend a lifetime saving for retirement, and as we approach retirement age we begin to weigh the actual risk of outliving those savings. An American man retiring at age 65 can expect to live an average of 13 more years, and he has a 40 percent chance of living to age 85. If he is married, there is a 75 percent chance that the man or his wife will live into their mideighties. Recognizing this, what do we typically do? Scale back on the imagined "leisure years." And of course there are the regrets that we should have done more to prepare, even when doing more wasn't at all possible. Planning for the future has become our *individual responsibility*, and we accept it, despite how economic recessions have eroded savings and other forms of assets.

The Financial Implications of a Long Life

The biggest risk that future retirees face is running out of money and losing financial independence. Among married couples who are age 65, some 75–80 percent can expect one of the partners to live until at least age 85.

The more we wisely sock away savings at a young age, the more likely we can ride out market turbulence and arrive better funded in retirement.

By retiring at age 70 instead of 62, a typical man could almost double his annual retirement income.

Reaching the decision to retire is affected by a blizzard of choices. The creation of early retirement incentives and phased retirement as options, the decision whether to begin receiving Social Security benefits at age 62 while employed or to wait until age 70 when the benefit is larger, and the fear of outliving our savings and investments have stretched the "normal" retirement age to reveal much greater individuation on when men exit the labor force.[10] One trend is the normalcy of early retirement for those who can afford it. For several decades (1970–1990) the national median retirement age for men hovered at age 62, which means one-half of men had retired by age 62 and more than 40 percent of those retirees had started collecting Social Security. But recently, many older men have decided to continue to work, and the national median retirement age has risen. You continue to work either because you have to financially, given your predicted life span and rising health care costs,[11] or because you like the social interaction or pleasure of the work—or maybe both.

The new norm is that 50 percent of men who retire do not end their work careers until sometime after their sixty-fifth birthday and often well after their sixty-seventh or seventieth birthday. Why? A key issue is our precarious financial preparation versus our projected longer life span. As one 45-year-old man mused,

> I did some calculation [on] how much money I will have when I retire. Then I have to guess my retirement age, the annual growth rate of my funds, and so on. Given the recent swings in the economy, I don't even know what to put in. I am not even sure when I will retire. With all these layoffs going on, I am not even sure if I will still have a job tomorrow.[12]

This man's worries are not unusual. A recent national survey by the Transamerica Center for Retirement Studies uncovered a genuine lack of confidence that people will meet their retirement needs: about 45 percent of the men were certain that they were not building a large enough nest egg, and 70 percent of the boomers who were still working didn't believe they could save enough money to retire at age 65. Many of the men in this study plan to work past age 70 or never retire.[13] A different study by the Employee Benefits Research Institute found that only 14 percent of the people were "very confident" they would have enough money to live comfortably in retirement.[14] Working longer can certainly improve our financial security.[15]

THE DECISION ABOUT WHEN

Despite doom and gloom, for about half of the middle-aged and older men, the question will not be "Can I afford to retire?" Most men will eventually retire with a relatively stable three-legged stool of economic security: personal savings, social insurance programs, and "pension plans" that now most often are our individualized 401(k)/IRA and 403(b) plans. One 50-year-old commented,

> I have a friend who just passed away suddenly, and his family was affected financially. I have two children, and I want to make sure they will be protected if anything happens to me now or in the future. So my wife and I started consulting some financial experts about wills and trusts and all that stuff. And also retirement planning. I guess as I get older and more financially stable, it is time to think about all these things.[16]

Even if the economic stool remains wobbly and our retirement security isn't completely certain, the decision making about when to begin retirement really is not explained by an economic calculus. Nor is it solely an individual matter: it routinely involves a joint decision between the man and his wife (or partner), as well as the options employers may offer.

Should You Delay Retirement?

For men very near retirement (less than 3 years away), the decision to postpone the beginning of retirement is more often than not based on financial well-being.

- *Your 403(b) or 401(k)/IRA tanked.* Has your retirement nest egg lost value? With market turmoil occurring virtually every third year, your retirement portfolio might not have enough money for you to retire. Is it worth waiting a few years longer for the market to (hopefully) recover? Is it time to consult a financial planner?

- *You've got debts.* If you started a home equity line of credit to pay tuitions, or if you have a five-figure credit card debt at 14 percent interest, you might think about holding off on retirement and clearing up the debt first.

- *Your retirement fund is anorexic.* Maybe you began contributing to your retirement fund late, or you tapped it and withdrew funds sometime back to pay for a wedding. Working a couple more years and contributing heavily to the fund may provide you the security you need.

- *Health insurance.* Leaving behind your employer-supported insurance for Medicare often results in things not covered. Your wife needs on-and-off private nursing care for another 9 months to recover from her accident, and Medicare doesn't cover this. Nor does Medicare cover routine eye exams, dental care, and most other preventive care.

Factored into each man's decision making—to stay in the labor force or exit it and begin his retirement—are multiple reasons, and chief among them are feelings about our work and our partner's opinions. If we take pleasure in the ways work structures our days and our family's way of life, we stay longer. If work is enjoyable enough and we want the income, we stay longer. If we feel indispensible, we stay longer. But if a man feels "redundant" and no longer required,[17] if he has flagging energy because his work has lost enough of its attraction,[18] if he was cut loose when his employer downsized and he is weighing early retiring rather than looking for new employment in an unwelcoming economy—these "ifs" and many others are the layers on the onion revealing how retirement decisions are not strictly based on our financial health.

It's equally important for pre-retirees to consider the psychological adjustments they and their partners will need to make once they've retired. There are the issues of

> organizing your day-to-day life without the structure and purpose of a work schedule;

> finding purpose or meaning once your primary career has ceased being a major feature in your life—especially for men very attached to their career identity; and

> considering what effect your decision to end your primary career and begin claiming Social Security will have on your partner.

For most men, retirement has become a joint decision with their partner and in consideration of other family matters.

Diversity amid Uniformity

The proportion of men approaching age 65 who decide to deter retirement and remain in the labor force began to surge in the mid-1980s, when the early-1980's recession sapped men's confidence about their retirement savings and Social Security slowly began raising the full retirement age to 67 from 65.[19] Some men simply will not ever be able to afford to retire; they are the men at the economic bottom—those who worked seamlessly with many employers while being paid poorly, often in cash and without their employers offering pension options and/or without contributing to Social Security. They also do not qualify for Medicare because they do not have 40 quarters of contributions to Social Security. These are the men whose meals depend on their earnings, and they continue working as long as their health permits.

For other men, staying longer in the labor force is calculated as a short-term necessity to be able to afford a decent retirement lifestyle. These men often have competing economic needs (e.g., paying off tuition loans, daughters' weddings) and have not saved enough for the lifestyle they want. Their retirement income is not a guaranteed pension; rather, they are dependent on what they put away in their 403(b) or 401(k)/IRA plan to assure their retirement security, and for nearly half of the men over the age of 50, they haven't put away enough. The Center for Retirement Research estimated that more than 40 percent of the older boomers and nearly one-half of younger boomers fit this category; they are "at risk" of retirement insecurity.[20]

For many men who continue to work into their late sixties and seventies, their retirement decision does not orbit around personal finances.

Rather, for these men there's no life without work. The men chose to stay because they enjoy their careers, social connections, and the rhythms of work weeks, weekends, and vacationing.[21] Some of these men eventually opt for a phased retirement, in which the transition from full-time employment to not working at all is gradual. Their decision eliminates the "cliff" retirement leap. Among the men participating in Robert Weiss's study of *The Experience of Retirement*, a former businessman retired after his heart attack, but a year later he began a part-time second career for a firm that had been his major competitor, and he commented, "So I'm back working again, because I love working. I think my hobby, my pleasure, and my total enjoyment outside of my family is working."[22] Continuing to work isn't uncommon among men in professions:

> I am retired except for one day a week. On Thursdays I see private patients. I don't have a huge patient load, but I have some patients that I have been seeing for a long time. . . . I don't know whether I would have more difficulty separating from them or they from me.[23]

Recently, rather than going cold turkey from work to retirement, a majority of older men retire and then begin a "bridge job" or "encore career," which serves as another chapter in the postretirement process.[24] Indeed, continuing to work after retirement is more common when men retire early—one study reported that roughly three-fourths of retired men age 59–64 who are in very good health take up a bridge job, and even 50 percent of the retired men whose health was poor to good also chose to work.[25] Men enjoy working—it's an affirmation of our sense of masculinity, and it

Benefits of a Phased Retirement

- *Social interaction*. A phased-retirement job is a perfect environment for forming new friendships and maintaining a social life.

- *Sense of purpose*. Being employed, even part-time, will provide a sense of routine, reasons to get out of the house, and a feeling of value.

- *Sense of worth*. Looking back to your career of 30 or more years, your work contributed to more than how a paycheck helped provide you with a life. Finding a new "job" in a nonprofit organization or working in a new field is psychologically gratifying.

- *Extra income*. A bridge job can produce enough income to enjoy 4-day weekends, not spend down retirement savings, and perhaps provide health insurance coverage.

adds income, structures time, and helps us feel socially involved. In addition, paying for health insurance out of pocket can be a major expense once we retire, but working longer allows you to keep your employers' group health insurance coverage.

Encore Careers

Marc Freedman, founder and CEO of Civic Ventures, has an optimistic vision that other boomers are very likely to share. For this generation, challenging traditional ways of doing things has never been an issue. There is a good chance that this generation is going to reinvent "retirement." Among the half that can afford to "retire" are the men who choose to become social entrepreneurs and tackle social challenges, for pay or not. They start "encore" careers[26] after their income-producing career ends. For example, Senator Edward Kennedy's Serve America Act (2011) created a series of programs that direct retirees into new roles in nonprofit and public service, such as providing free golf lessons and classes to middle schoolers, joining a construction team or a venture capital team that builds homes to reduce poorer families' homelessness, or becoming a volunteer research assistant in a medical center assisting older men caregivers who need skills to continue to care for their wives.

DESIGNING YOUR RETIREMENT

Many men nearing retirement aren't so much ready to quit working as they are ready for change. Planning for this phase of your life involves exciting choices and challenging decisions. Retirement begs for thorough planning, or the personal guts to wing it and go with the surprises. Both paths translate into active retirement—someone with a bucket list of interests and commitments versus someone freewheeling it, much as a pachinko ball might bounce its way down through a dense forest of pins. Each pathway, which Savishinsky distinguished as the "master planners" and the "Zen masters,"[27] will transport you into a new identity and life phase.

In retirement, we have the opportunity to redefine our masculinities outside the workplace and breadwinner box, take up new interests, and recognize that there is life beyond work. We have options when we retire: Is later life a long-awaited "do list" you can systematically work through—being an active grandpa, taking up kayaking and fly-fishing, learning Spanish or French? Is it a natural frontier, one that you intend to map as you go along? To avoid your retirement becoming a slow boat to shrinking social networks and looming social isolation, as many men fear, take up the opportunities to reinvent yourself. For example, establish yourself as a cabinet refinisher or an unpaid electrician apprentice and help remodel other people's homes, or become a YWCA antiviolence speaker and advocate.

Our "retirement years" (also called "later life") can become the stereotypical lifestyle that's supposedly associated with leisure and its "busy ethic"—adventures with the grandkids, traveling, and hobby-filled days. Though stereotypic, even this lifestyle requires us to think through the gains and losses. Later life involves a large amount of unstructured time. Research studies regularly find that to be happily retired, your later life needs purpose and structure at the same time that it provides you with a sense of identity and meaning.

Advantages

Studying both pre-retirees' and retirees' attitudes, both groups think that having more control over their time is the best thing about retirement.[28] Men typically report that retirement frees them from an awful daily commute, on-the-job stresses, and the depressing tedium of 30+ years of work. When retired, you don't have to work through lunch. Sleep-disturbed nights and work-related anxiety are much less common. There's recognition that where you live needn't be dictated by your employment. Of course, there are new emotional stresses when no longer working, but these rarely outweigh the feelings of liberation that come with no longer struggling to balance work with family and personal time. Later life has the advantage of being one of the very few times in our biographies when we can freely arrange our priorities.

One study[29] unraveled the impact of retirement versus aging on life satisfaction in later life and found that the small decline in personal satisfaction over time is the result of age-associated declines in health and physical ability, not retirement. Another study[30] finds that older men interpret their stressors and hassles as less troubling, no matter the type of stressor they encounter; this seems to reflect changes in our postretirement perspective on life. We no longer have to be always on our toes or wary of being wounded.

Part of the stress reduction is because we have more time to sleep, exercise, and eat healthful foods—making retirement an opportunity to actually improve overall health. What's interesting is that most men actually report an improvement in their health once they retire. Many retired men take up something athletic, such as daily walking or regular golf or tennis several times a week, which carries over to promote being and *feeling* healthy. Equally important, the opportunity to relax is typically cited as one of the best things about retirement. Men still in the labor force know how very difficult it is to carve out just 10–15 minutes during the workday for an opportunity to relax (and not feel guilty).

Challenges

With very few exceptions, wherever we worked before our retirement, our workplace and occupation provided us the playing field to present ourselves as men and put bread on the table. Entering retirement is nothing but a staggering changeover from what we knew as normal, and it tests the way we feel about ourselves. Whether we talk about it or not, there is a hidden inverse correlation between masculinity and retirement. We grew up being coached on how not working was evidence of troubled or failed masculinity. Not surprisingly, it is the loss of the context of work and the way employment configures our opportunities to do what it takes to be a man that most men soon miss when they retire.

> I don't know whether I can put it into words, because it's a new feeling. . . . It's sort of a vague feeling of unease, I guess, not easy to define. I am no longer doing something I was trained to do. . . . [There's] sort of a vague feeling of discontinuity—suddenly not doing something that I've been doing eight hours a day for thirty-five years.[31]

Studies have consistently found that the men who adjust better to retirement are the men who developed interests outside of work. You might think about signing up for a beginning photography course and learning about f-stops and lighting, or start going to a gym and alternate an elliptical workout with yoga (yes, yoga) and its mind-cleansing, body-centered consciousness. Regardless how we imagine spending our retirement, post-employment roles will provide us meaningful time with others, new identities, and structured weeks.

Another obvious challenge is the likelihood of spending too much of our day at home and alone. It's not only the rhythms and meaningfulness of work that we leave behind; it is the community of people—colleagues, customers, and competitors. Social isolation is a risk, especially for men who depended on their work to provide them with a social life (which is the case for a substantial number of older men). Feeling the isolation can sneak up without a man knowing something is wrong, and it can become venomous. If your routine is another evening reading or turning on the television for company, you might want to reach out to a local political party organizing committee, join an investment club, or start a book club. Later life becomes empty unless we take control of our time and lives.

Men do not often anticipate that we may feel socially marginal or lonely as a result of our retirement. But as reported in the Ameriprise Financial *New Retirement Mindscape II* study (see figure 21.2), retirees identified the loss of social connections as one of the core challenges when they first retired, and it was far more troublesome than feeling bored.[32] But don't jump to a false conclusion. Some of the downsizing of our social lives isn't a direct effect of our retirement; as we get older, some of our social connections fade away as people our age move or die.

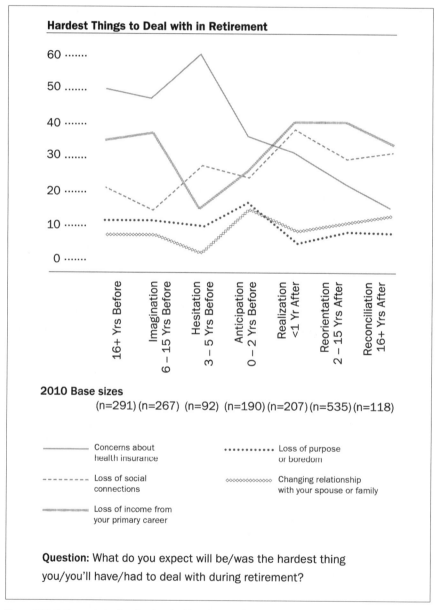

Figure 21.2. Retirement worries. Reprinted with permission from Ameriprise Financial, Inc., from its *New Retirement Mindscape II* study. All rights reserved.

For the vast majority of retired men and their partners, there will be a need to be frugal, maybe even clipping coupons. Living off of our retirement savings and no longer earning a yearly income, our lifestyles can become crimped as our budget is squeezed by inflation and rising medical care expenses. There are, however, a number of strategies that we can take up to survive on a fixed income:

> *A retirement emergency fund.* Income from your 401K, Social Security benefits, and/or pension is hopefully adequate to cover routine expenses and vacations. We also need to plan ahead for replacing a car, having the house painted, or a major health event. To draw down on our retirement nest egg will affect our entire future retirement income. Set aside money in a retirement emergency fund for the out-of-the-ordinary expenses.

> *Retire without big debts.* Making monthly debt payments for a vacation home, second car, or even your primary home will wallop you when you are on a fixed income. Pay down your debts as much as possible before you start drawing on your retirement savings. Monthly loan payments can become a retirement killer.

> *Consider renting rather than owning.* Tired of yard work, painting, and large utility bills for a nearly empty house? Renting is an option that eliminates the time hog and many expenses inherent to home ownership. Even the property tax bill disappears.

> *Push your children off the payroll.* A *U.S. News and World Report* columnist recommended that when our children are gainfully employed, it is time to cut the financial feeding tube and stop paying for their auto insurance, cell phone, and other expenses. Certainly do not take on debt to help your adult children. They are your children, yet they are no longer children, and there comes a time to be politely and firmly selfish about your money.[33] Remind yourself: they can inherit whatever is left.

Another key challenge interrupting the retirement experience is the impending decline in a man's health (or his partner's health). This type of worry isn't because we retire. Concerns about some deterioration in our health rise up with the recognition that we are moving into later life, and retirement is a pretty clear marker that we've begun that journey.

> I tell you what hit me more than anything, and it [retirement] makes you think more about your health than I did when I was working . . . am I going to get this, am I going to get that? (age 62)[34]

What's fundamentally at issue is the way men's retirement and later-life opportunities can be interrupted by health problems.

During middle age, we look forward to the pot-of-gold retirement promises, yet once we retire, we have to face up to the constraints our budgets and physical health can place on the 25 years or more that later life may bring. Don't wait until you retire to carve out some leisure time and interests outside of work. As men, we have a proclivity to compartmentalize, and we ought not segment our mature lives into work years and retirement years. Merging the gains anticipated when retired with the gains and stresses of employment brings forward a commitment not to wait for the elusive pot of gold, which exists only in fables and fiction.

Three Retirement Rules of Thumb

1. *Get to know yourself.* Sit down and have a conversation with yourself. Ask yourself, do I want to travel? Or how about, I hated skiing when I was a kid, but should I give it another try? The point is, don't assume anything at this point in your life. Give yourself the freedom to try everything all over again as if it were the first time or determine that you are going to embark on experiences yet to be tried.

2. *Be adventurous.* Finding out who you are as a nonworking person does not mean that you need to take a round-the-world trip that costs tens of thousands of dollars. You can find new and interesting things to do right in your own backyard. It is great if you have a friend or partner to share in these new adventures, but if you don't, that is OK too. Part of this phase of life may be finding out that you are OK with trying things on your own. Meeting new people and establishing friendships along the way are surely skills that are great to become more proficient in at any age.

3. *Allow yourself to make mistakes.* If you remember back to the first time that you learned to parallel park a car, you probably will admit that you did not succeed in fitting perfectly into that parking space. You should view retirement no differently than learning to parallel park. You will have to practice to get it right. Sometimes you will make the right choices, and sometimes you will have missteps. But just like parallel parking, you can always take another shot. Don't be discouraged if you have a hard time finding your way in the beginning. It's a long journey: it probably took you many years to feel comfortable in your career, and you should allow yourself the same latitude now in this phase of life.

Sources: Excerpted and reprinted with permission from Kaye, L. (2012, Spring). Standing on the threshold of retirement: Three rules of thumb. *Silverwire: Newsletter from the UMaine Center on Aging, 8* (3), 2–4.

CHAPTER 22

Caregiving

HELPING OTHERS THROUGH DIFFICULT TIMES

The vast majority of families take care of their own during times of need. Years ago, certainly because of the lack of alternatives, families relied on one another as first-line supporters. Even now, we rely on our family well before we turn to health professionals or other service providers for assistance. The eventual call from our families to provide assistance has increased quite a bit in the past few decades, and it is certain to continue to grow simply because we are all living much longer. As men's and women's life spans have increased, we are now living with disabling illnesses that people never had before (such as dementia, osteoporosis, postmenopausal breast cancer, cardiovascular disease). With longevity comes a greater number of older individuals who have chronic health problems and need some measure of care—and the call has gone out to men to be caregivers. Nearly everyone will become a caregiver at some point in life—it's natural, expected, and virtuous. More men are taking on this responsibility.

> There are only four kinds of people in this world. Those who have been caregivers, those who are caregivers, those who will be caregivers, and those who will need caregivers.
>
> —Rosalynn Carter, former First Lady

Traditionally, women shouldered the lion's share of responsibility of caring for family and neighbors. When relatives have asked "Who will care for me?" the answer has most likely been wives, daughters, granddaughters, and other women who came forward and lent a hand. Although women still provide 60–66 percent of the aid, being male and helping someone in need of assistance are not contradictory terms. Each and every day, millions of husbands, gay partners, sons, sons-in-law, uncles, brothers, male friends, and other men take care of family, friends, and other older adults who are frail or not well. The math is simple—if 60–66 percent of caregivers are women, then 34–40 percent are men.[1]

According to an estimate by the National Alliance for Caregiving, more than 65 million people in the United States provided unpaid care to a friend or member of their family who was chronically ill, disabled, or frail.[2] On any given day, there are almost 22 million men who have taken on the responsibility of providing some assistance for a relative, friend, or neighbor who is having difficulties managing alone. The average man who finds himself helping someone in need will do it for approximately 4 years (just as long as a woman), is 47 years of age, is caring for someone who is 77 years of age, and is likely caring for a parent, usually his mom. Beyond the call for the natural "horizontal caregiving" that husbands and gay partners provide to someone of their same generation, there has been a 600 percent increase in the number of sons who provided care to a parent since the mid-1990s, and now one in six adult sons are caregivers.[3]

Men quite commonly come to the aid of their spouses and partners. These men tend to be older (most likely in their fifties or older) and transition into caregiving. It is what you do for your wife or partner when you have been in a long-term relationship—in that sense, caregiving is an extension of living together and sharing a home. You slowly and incrementally increase your hours per week preparing meals, cleaning, shopping,

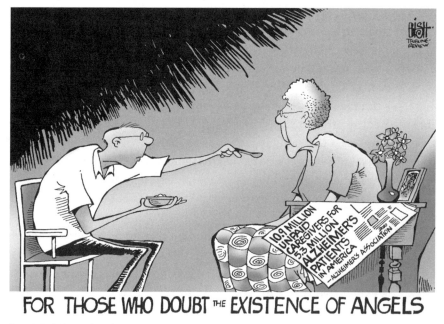

FOR THOSE WHO DOUBT ᴛʜᴇ EXISTENCE OF ANGELS

From R. Bish (2010, Oct. 7). Caring for Alzheimer's patients. *Pittsburgh Tribune-Review.*

doing laundry, and eventually assisting with some of the "body work" such as bathing and dressing. You might not even perceive yourself as a caregiver, but you are. Spousal caregivers are more likely retired; however, a sizeable number, perhaps as many as 25 percent of men caring for their wives, tackle the responsibilities of caregiving while simultaneously dealing with the demands of part-time or full-time employment. These men are commonly caring for a spouse or partner suffering from a disabling disorder such as chronic heart failure or Alzheimer's disease and have to deal with the special challenges that accompany helping someone gradually deteriorating physically and cognitively. If you are one of these caregivers, the demands placed on you can be especially great.

As an example, there are nearly 15 million Alzheimer's and dementia caregivers providing 17 billion hours of unpaid care annually. At least 40 percent are men.[4] Because Alzheimer's disease is more commonly diagnosed in women and requires high levels of care, and because the majority of women with dementia live in the community, many men find themselves stepping up and performing the role of caregiver, something they never anticipated.[5] You need to know that men who are caregivers generally, and particularly those who are Alzheimer's caregivers, suffer enough emotionally and physically to be called the "silent victims," because caregiving is extended in duration, sometimes 24/7, and the person being cared for slowly ceases to exist—their personality, behavior, and memory change dramatically and they become increasingly dependent on someone else to care for them. Men may well be less distressed than the women who embodied care work (at least on the various ways social scientists measure caregiving stress and burden); however, while husbands providing care for Alzheimer's wives view the symptoms of this disease to be a less problematic condition and normalize their wife's deterioration,[6] they still report high levels of distress and symptoms of depression.[7]

What is a caregiver (for example, to a wife)? There are two dimensions: First, you are actually providing her with the help needed to remain as healthy as possible, which means you are providing food, getting her to take her medications, and perhaps bathing and dressing her. You also are "being there" and providing her the emotional TLC she needs. Second, you take on full responsibility for all the household chores and other things she used to do—from changing the sheets and doing the laundry, to writing notes in birthday cards to children and friends, to shopping, cooking, and managing all the financial matters.

Men who are caring for a parent may not provide 24/7 care, but they provide help an average of 17–18 hours a week while at the same time usually holding down a full-time job. These so-called vertical caregiving relationships that cross generations are no longer unusual. Some sons (or sons-in-law) appear to make caregiving a second career, committing 30, 40, and 50 hours or more a week to these efforts. These younger caregiving men tend to live farther away from the person they are helping and, as a result, have to travel farther and spend more time organizing care that is provided when they are not on hand. Men who provide care from a distance find using outside services particularly helpful, especially when it comes to meeting the transportation needs of loved ones and handling their personal care needs (help with dressing, bathing, personal hygiene). Long-distance caregiving sons generally also make heavy use of the Internet as a source for finding resources they may need to help them in their responsibilities as the caregiver.[8] As Eleanor Ginzler reminds us, what is perhaps most important is that while the men who become caregivers are fewer in number, they are equal to women in terms of their dedication to the task.[9] In the rest of this chapter we consider the experiences and responsibilities of middle-aged and older men helping others, or caregiving, as it will be termed here.

A CARING MAN IS NOT AN OXYMORON

So what does it mean to be a caregiver? It is likely that many men who are reading this chapter have already assumed the role of informal caregiver to some degree. If married or partnered, you have roughly a 50-50 chance of performing some, if not all, of the functions of a caregiver during your lifetime. So why do news analysts, some academic researchers, and so many relatives and friends assume that men are not the caregiving kind? Well, likely that can be traced back to traditional gender stereotypes, namely, the tendency to characterize men as rough brutes, unwilling and unable to express themselves as loving and caring individuals.[10] That perception is longstanding, widespread, and an extremely difficult mentality to alter. Yet men who are caregivers prove the stereotype wrong, day in and day out. They might adopt more of the instrumental approach that can segment the nuts and bolts of care work into "work" from the enjoyable time providing "care," yet as caregivers men readily do the expected care work and they care.[11]

BALANCING WORK AND CARE

Don't be surprised if one day you need to consider discussing your caregiving responsibilities with your employer and perhaps agree on certain adjustments in your work pattern such as changing your hourly schedule or shifting from full- to part-time employment. It could mean that you need to leave work early on occasion or arrive late. These can be difficult discussions to have with your supervisor or manager, especially if you think that they may not be particularly understanding or willing to accommodate your needs. Employers very often do not comprehend that their male employees need "family time." Other men, because of "male pride," may not want to admit that they are finding it difficult to juggle the competing demands that exist in their work and personal lives and elect instead to hide this from their work colleagues. Either way, there is little to be gained by not making the effort to negotiate a healthier balance between work and your caregiving responsibilities.

Stoic pride and/or hesitation to make every effort to plan a more manageable work/family arrangement can easily backfire on you, leading to consequences that include poor performance, lower productivity, and more distress over the caregiving responsibilities awaiting you at home. These two-pronged, snake-bite consequences could ultimately lead to a negative performance evaluation at work and premature burnout as a caregiver at home. The majority of men who make the effort to adjust aspects of their work life to meet the demands of caregiving are able to do that.

Over 8 in 10 men caregivers in the United States were employed full- or part-time when they were caregiving in 2009, and among these employed caregivers, two-thirds report that they have gone in late, left early, or taken time off during the day to deal with caregiving issues; one in three have altered their work-related travel, and one in five indicate they needed to take a leave of absence.[12] These employed caregivers are older and more likely to perform blue-collar work.[13] What policies and resources are available to those men who are employed and carry caregiving responsibilities at the same time?

In 1993 an important piece of federal legislation was enacted that supports the efforts of family caregivers. The Family and Medical Leave Act (FMLA) requires that covered employers provide up to 12 weeks of unpaid leave for eligible employees who have family and medical obligations requiring that they devote time at home to care for a family member in need, be with them during a medical emergency, or arrange for services provided by others. The U.S. Department of Labor website (www.dol.gov /whd/fmla/) provides you with full details about the FMLA, including all the regulations and eligibility rules and a variety of fact sheets. States have also enacted similar such laws extending the coverage to a more broad range of employees, as well as, in some cases, allowing for partial paid leave for family-related needs.

You should inquire into what caregiver information and resources might be available through your employer's human resources or employee assistance departments. Some employers will also work with you to modify your work schedule in order that you can more easily tend to the needs of those you are helping at home. You can find information on workplace programs, legal/financial issues, online discussion groups, and more from the Work and Elder Care section of the Family Caregiver Alliance's National Center on Caregiving.

CAREGIVING IS HARD WORK— REMEMBER TO TAKE CARE OF YOURSELF

Caregiving can be taxing work—physically, mentally, and financially. It is not unusual for men who are caregivers to report significantly lower levels of life satisfaction and losses of freedom to take a walk or drive or pursue social activities with friends. And these men caregivers are likely to feel that their care work is unappreciated by other family members. This appears to be especially the case for those men who are the sole or primary caregiver rather than a secondary caregiver. That is to say, for those men who are the only one providing help or the one providing the lion's share of the help, being the caregiver can be expected to be more demanding. Men who are the sole or primary caregiver are also more likely to rate their overall health (physical, functional, mental, and emotional) lower. It is also not particularly unusual for these men to say that their lesser health curtails some of the care they are able to provide. This appears to be especially the case for caregivers who are older, have serious health problems, survive on lower incomes, perform more caregiving tasks, and care for more severely disabled persons.[14]

Describing the physical and emotional demands of caregiving is done not to dissuade you from carrying out the responsibilities of being a caregiver. Rather, it is done to encourage men generally, and spousal/partner caregivers in particular, to make a concerted and continuing effort to take care of themselves. You will ultimately be of little benefit to those in need of your help if your own health needlessly suffers. Too many caregivers find themselves sleep deprived, saddened if not depressed, using more

Take Care of Yourself

- Learn to use stress-reduction techniques
- Attend to your own health care needs
- Get proper rest and nutrition
- Exercise regularly
- Take time off without feeling guilty
- Participate in enjoyable activities
- Get help from others
- Seek supportive counseling when you need it
- Identify and fess up to your feelings
- Try to be positive
- Set goals for yourself

Source: Family Caregiver Alliance, National Center on Caregiving.

medications, psychologically distressed, and suffering from new physical health problems because they did not tend to their own needs in a timely fashion. Still others suffer premature caregiver burnout because they did not seek help early enough. Warning signs of caregiver burnout include loss of energy, lowered resistance to colds and the flu, constantly feeling exhausted, neglecting your own needs, not finding satisfaction in the help you are providing, finding yourself unable to relax, feeling impatient and irritable, and feeling overwhelmed, helpless, and even hopeless.

It is important to remember that the vast majority of men who care for others do it well. Most men who are caregivers approach their tasks with an attitude that caregiving is their responsibility and brings them considerable emotional gratification. These men do it regardless of how much strain it can add to their own personal and professional lives. However, while not unusual statistically, caregiving can be a precarious situation. It might lead others to question whether you are taking advantage of the person you care for; there is also the potential for unintentionally mistreating the person you are responsible for. Skeptics might think that sons are caring for a parent in hopes of collecting inheritance, or if a son moves back to his parents' home to care for his frail mother, people may assume he is just "sponging" off the parent.

Alzheimer's Caregiving

For ten years, A.B. shepherded his wife, Frances, through the dark maze of Alzheimer's disease. . . . He was there through the early stages, when they laughed over Frances' locking her keys in her car, or forgetting a friend's name. But slowly the signs became unavoidable. Always the trusted copilot on their frequent road trips, Frances could no longer read a map. Once a master gardener, Frances slowly abandoned the hobby. The landscaping on their Grant, FL home soon deteriorated to bland, basic upkeep. . . .

All the responsibilities Frances had maintained through nearly 60 years of marriage—paying bills, making appointments, housekeeping, cooking—fell to A.B., now 82. He accepted his new role without complaint, even as he found himself feeling less like a partner in a marriage and more like a father parenting a child.

Source: Ramnarance, C. (2010, Sept. 13). Till dementia do us part? As a spouse is stricken with Alzheimer's disease, more caregivers seek out a new love. *AARP Bulletin.*

There are just enough cases where care recipients are subject to instances of mistreatment in the form of exploitation, neglect, and abuse. Whether you are a husband, partner, son, brother, or other male relative, the person you care for is, by definition, vulnerable. Because her capacity is necessarily compromised, if you take her out for a drive, stopping to run in the grocery store and letting her stay in the (hot) car, you might return to find a police officer wanting to know why you left this older person locked in the car. Worse yet, she may have Alzheimer's disease and wander off on her own. Both scenarios put you in the position of being judged by others for neglecting her. Unfortunately, the facts support others' wariness—the vast majority of those who abuse, neglect, or exploit care recipients are relatives rather than strangers.

Periodically a well-known personality brings to light the disturbing consequences of elder abuse. During spring 2011, veteran actor Mickey Rooney disclosed his experience of being emotionally blackmailed and financially exploited by his stepson. Ninety-year-old Rooney, in testimony before the Senate's Special Committee on Aging, pointed out that "if elder abuse happened to me, Mickey Rooney, it can happen to anyone."[15] He described being intimidated and bullied, having his access to mail blocked, being deprived of food and medications, having his money taken and misused, and not being allowed access to information about his finances.

Cases like this reveal the too-frequent reality about some men caregivers' horrific behavior, and what they do tarnishes the reputation of all men who unwaveringly provide care and love to a dependent older adult.

If you occasionally find your stress or anger reaching dangerous levels, call someone. Remove yourself from the situation if only temporarily, by finding respite. If you raised children, you know that it is better to walk away from a situation and cool off. Should others think that you are mistreating the person you are caring for, they are obliged to report it.

THERE IS HELP OUT THERE—DON'T GO IT ALONE

The most significant struggle men caregivers face is coping with the isolation.[16] A seemingly obvious step to ease the isolation and the demands of caregiving is for you to enlist help from other members of your family and your friends and neighbors. The responsibilities of caregiving are much more manageable when you are not the sole caregiver and share the tasks with others. When sharing caregiving tasks with one or more other people, it is advisable for those involved to determine who is best prepared to perform particular responsibilities.

As obvious as asking for help may seem, you might find it difficult to do. Often men's drive toward self-sufficiency blocks the logic of asking others to help. Research shows that some men caregivers are considerably less likely to ask for assistance from family or friends and from community organizations. They were raised to "tough it out" and handle things on their own no matter how difficult the situation might be.[17] Unfortunately, this stiff-upper-lip mentality can be injurious to your well-being.

Men need time with friends (and more than e-mail time) to receive the emotional support we can get "hanging out" together over breakfast or a card game.[18] Family team work and reaching out to your local Area Agency on Aging (AAA) for in-home services will make the tasks of caregiving much more manageable and less stressful for everyone concerned. A successful family caregiving team needs to agree in advance who will do what. Whenever possible, the assignment of tasks should be based on the abilities and interests of each member of the family team, as well as a realistic appraisal of how much time each person has available to volunteer to help.

Quiz for Caregivers

Knowing your and other caregiving team members' strengths and limits cannot be captured any better than the questions suggested by the National Institute on Aging.

When reflecting on your strengths, consider the following:

- Are you good at finding information, keeping people up-to-date on changing conditions, and offering cheer, whether on the phone or with a computer?
- Are you good at supervising and leading others?
- Are you comfortable speaking with medical staff and interpreting what they say to others?
- Is your strongest suit doing the numbers—paying bills, keeping track of bank statements, and reviewing insurance policies and reimbursement reports?
- Are you the one in the family who can fix anything, while no one else knows the difference between pliers and a wrench?

When reflecting on your limits, consider the following:

- How often, both mentally and financially, can you afford to travel?
- Are you emotionally prepared to take on what may feel like a reversal of roles between you and your parent—taking care of your parent instead of your parent taking care of you? Can you continue to respect your parent's independence?
- Can you be both calm and assertive when communicating from a distance?
- How will your decision to take on caregiving responsibilities affect your work and home life?

Source: National Institute on Aging (2010, Aug.). *So far away: Twenty questions and answers about long-distance caregiving* (NIH Publication No. 10-5496), p. 9.

If you live an hour or more from the person who needs care, you are considered to be a long-distance caregiver. There are 7 million or more long-distance caregivers across the country. Caring from a distance can be particularly challenging. You may feel like you are not doing enough or that what you are doing is not particularly important. Yet long-distance caregivers, in particular, may be able to provide important emotional support and periodic relief for others who are the primary caregivers.[19] They can also be helpful by staying in touch with the person in need of help by phone or e-mail and by researching online sources of support, managing finances, paying bills, and arranging for services. Another way they can help is with the cost of care.

TAKE ADVANTAGE OF COMMUNITY SERVICES

The National Family Caregiver Support Program (NFCSP), established in 2000 and funded through the U.S. Administration on Aging, provides a range of services to support you if you are a caregiver of someone 60 or older. Their goal is to relieve some of the financial and emotional hardships that are inherent in care work. The services are delivered through the network of AAAs. Contacting your local AAA, you can get the information you need to identify what free and pay-as-you-go services are available in your community. The agency also usually provides caregiver training, can identify men's caregiver support groups, and offers individual counseling and respite care services on a limited basis. Other services available in most communities can be invaluable added sources of support:

> In-home services include homemakers, home health aides, and home attendants who can provide a wide variety of non-medical-related help, such as assisting with a person's bathing, dressing, or using the toilet; preparing meals; providing transportation; offering companionship; and escorting to doctors' appointments.

> There are meals that can be delivered to the home (frequently by the local AAA) or offered at a group (congregate) nutrition site in some churches, senior centers, senior housing facilities, and community buildings.

Examples of Home- and Community-Based Services

- Adult day care programs
- Case managers / geriatric care managers
- Emergency response systems
- Friendly visitor / companion services

- Home health care / home care
- Homemaker/chore services
- Meal programs
- Senior centers
- Respite
- Transportation services

For husbands, sons, and gay men who live with the person they are caring for, there are "respite services" that give you temporary relief and time off from your caregiving. Many men find these services exceptionally important, for it gives them the opportunity to do things without worrying about the care of their wife, parent, or partner. They also provide you with a critical respite, if only temporarily, from the stress and strain of being the caregiver.

Adult Day Care

Other than a "friendly visitor" coming to your home to be the temporary, substitute caregiver, there is another type of respite service for men caring for an adult who is cognitively impaired (with a dementia) or functionally impaired: adult day care. There are increasing numbers of adult day care programs across the United States (more than 4,600 currently). They represent an important source of temporary relief for caregivers. These programs offer a set of services in a community setting, ranging from some health services to supervised care in a safe environment. Meals and snacks are usually provided, as well as door-to-door transportation. Adult day care centers are generally open Monday through Friday during the day—check out the options in your community. Some programs offer more intensive health and therapeutic services, and some specialize and only serve adults with dementias or other specific disabilities. If you are in a rural community, without readily available community services, be prepared for your caregiving to be more challenging since there will probably not be as many community services available to you.

Support Groups for Men

Watching a loved one battle cancer, dementia, or any other devastating illness can be very difficult. From the fear of losing your loved one, to family worries, to financial concerns, caring can be overwhelming at times. You may find joining groups of other men caregivers to be an agreeable way of seeking companionship and/or help. Caregivers have voices of experience. You all share a common lifestyle, and you can also gain some satisfaction from helping other men. Getting together over a breakfast or lunch, you may be able to gain insight on ways to solve your own problems.[20]

There are an increasing number of caregiver support groups available to men in communities throughout the United States. These groups may include both men and women or operate exclusively to serve men; some groups are exclusive to men caring for women with breast cancer, or cancer more generally, or to men whose wives and partners have a dementia.

Regardless, these groups meet to provide encouragement and an opportunity for members to share their experiences. Typically no referral is required. Groups can be found through local AAAs, disease associations, or online. Online bulletin boards and chat rooms may be perfect for men who have demanding schedules and who want anonymity.

If you are caring for someone with Alzheimer's disease or a related disorder, the Alzheimer's Association offers peer or professionally led groups for caregivers. These groups are all facilitated by trained individuals. Many communities offer specialized groups for adult children, men caring for younger-onset or early-stage Alzheimer's, and husband caregivers with specific needs. The Alzheimer's Association's online message boards and chat rooms offer a forum in which to ask your questions and, if you feel so inclined, to share your experiences. Their message boards have thousands of members from around the United States and many more people who simply browse men's stories and the information that is offered 24 hours a day.

A Geriatric Care Manager Could Be Just What the Doctor Ordered

Geriatric care managers are commonly social workers with a master's degree or professionals in nursing who have demonstrated competencies in helping families who are caring for older relatives. These professionals can help you and the person you are caring for and are often affiliated with a professional care management association. Geriatric care managers are able to help you find needed services and resources in the community which can make your work as a caregiver easier. They can also provide counseling aimed at resolving issues that may be causing difficulties or arguments between you and the person you are helping. Ultimately, the care manager, who is usually paid by the hour for the services they provide, aims to assist older adults with chronic needs, including individuals suffering from Alzheimer's disease and related disorders, and persons with disabilities in attaining their maximum functional potential. It is recommended that you check to see if the geriatric care manager you want to contract with is a member of the National Association of Professional Geriatric Care Managers (NAPGCM) because they are then guided by an established Pledge of

---

Contracting a Professional Geriatric Care Manager: Questions You Should Ask

1. Are they a licensed geriatric care manager?

2. Are they a member of the National Association of Professional Geriatric Care Managers?

3. How much experience do they have?

4. Are they available during emergencies, evenings, and weekends?

5. What are their fees?

6. Do they have references?

Source: National Institute on Aging (2010, Aug.). *So far away: Twenty questions and answers about long-distance caregiving* (NIH Publication No. 10-5496), p. 11.

Ethics and Standards of Practice that charge them to act only in the best interests of the person you are caring for.

If You Have Legal Issues, Consider an Elder Law Attorney

Elder law attorneys have special expertise in planning, counseling, educating, and advocating for you and/or the person you may be caring for. They commonly deal with personal care planning, including powers of attorney, living wills, wills and trusts, estate planning and tax matters (see chapter 23), and how to protect assets for the caregiver when his loved one requires long-term care.

Caregiver Tax Breaks

While the availability of tax breaks is not likely to be the driving force behind why you might become involved in caring for another person, you should know that the help you provide an older adult may qualify as a tax deduction. On average, caregivers spend approximately $5,500 a year providing care,[21] and currently there are deductions available to help defray some of those costs.[22] Some men may be able to claim the recipient of their care as a dependent and therefore an exemption, which would have reduced their taxable income by $3,800 in the 2012 tax year. To be eligible, you must have provided more than half of the financial support for that person over the past year (this could be a relative living with you or on their own, or a nonrelative who resides in your home). You can still potentially claim the deduction if you are one of multiple individuals who provided the support, as long as your share of the support was at least 10 percent of the care recipient's annual expenses. In addition, you may be eligible for a dependent care credit as long as the person you care for is unable to physically and mentally care for him- or herself. You may also be able to deduct medical and dental expenses that you paid for the individual if, together with your medical expenses, they exceed 7.5 percent of your adjusted gross income. If you are a single caregiver, you may be able to change your filing status to "head of household," which will lower your rate of taxation and increase your standard deduction by several thousand dollars.[23]

There are also federal and state programs that may be able to provide help with the various costs associated with caring for someone at home. Agencies to consult with include the Centers for Medicare & Medicaid Services (CMS), which administers Medicare and Medicaid (for people with limited resources); the Program for All-Inclusive Care for the Elderly (PACE); and the State Health Insurance Counseling and Assistance Program (SHIP).

LGBT CAREGIVING

While many of the challenges are the same for caregivers regardless of their sexual preference, there are issues of special significance to gay, bisexual, and transgender caregiving men. Gay and transgendered men often do not have the same familial supports to help them construct a caregiving team as they provide care for their partner or a friend. However, many of these men have developed social networks of friends, coworkers, and neighbors, often referred to as "families of choice," who can assist.[24] You might well be one of those friends. Don't wait to be asked for help; volunteer.

What's different about LGBT caregiving? Actually, there are more similarities between LGBT and non-LGBT caregivers than differences.[25] The differences pivot on heterosexual men not having to confront discrimination. It is important to note that certain policies are beneficial to heterosexual married couples and not supportive of gay (or lesbian) couples or unmarried heterosexual elder couples who live together. The FMLA does not cover same-sex partners; however, some states have FMLA-type regulations that do support taking a leave from work to care for a sick partner. Also, spousal impoverishment policies within Medicaid tend to be financially beneficial to married heterosexual couples but not others, and many state laws deny LGBT caregivers the medical decision-making authority automatically provided to married (heterosexual) couples. It is important for gay, bisexual, and transgendered men to be aware of the local services in their areas, as well as the laws and regulations in their cities and/or states to ensure that they and their loved ones are protected. The National Resource Center on LGBT Aging has launched an interactive, multimedia, Internet portal focused on caregiving resources for LGBT caregivers, including legal and financial issues, HIV/AIDS, and housing and health care access.

THE CHALLENGES OF CARING FOR AN ADULT CHILD WITH MENTAL ILLNESS

For those men who have been involved in caring for a child with serious mental illness such as bipolar disorder or schizophrenia, you are no doubt aware that the challenges can be great. The demands associated with caring for this family member in fact grow as the child enters adulthood because these men caregivers are growing older themselves and facing their own age-related problems. What is known about fathers' experiences caring for an adult child with mental illness remains sketchy, since most studies continue to study "parents" and do not distinguish fathers' experiences from mothers'. In an early study, Jan Greenberg did investigate the differences between fathers and mothers, and he found that fathers saw themselves very involved in the care of their son or daughter, provided a similar amount of caregiving assistance as mothers, yet were not as engulfed or burdened by their care responsibilities as mothers.[26] There are good resources available to assist these parents, especially from the National Alliance on Mental Illness and one of its 1,000 or more local affiliates.

RAISING GRANDCHILDREN AND OTHER RELATIVES

A growing number of grandfathers are stepping forward to care for and even raise their grandchildren. Unfortunately, many kinship caregivers, as they are called, do not know others who are in similar situations. Nor are they necessarily aware of the available resources to help make the responsibilities of raising a grandchild easier. This can lead to feelings of isolation and frustration. Even when some support services are available, kinship caregivers often face prohibitive barriers to participation in those programs; as a result, they lack substitute child care.

There is no "typical" grandparent-headed household, other than that two-thirds of the grandparents raising grandchildren are married couples. There are over 1 million grandfathers who are responsible for most of the basic needs of a grandchild.[27] Men of all different races report being responsible for grandchildren: 47 percent of these grandparents are white, 29 percent are African American, 17 percent are Hispanic or Latino, 3 percent are Asian, and 2 percent are American Indian or Alaskan Native. One estimate finds that nearly 40 percent of these families live at or below the poverty line, even though close to half have at least one caregiver who is employed.[28]

When older men find themselves parenting again and doing what is neither typical nor expected for their age, the reality is stressful. These grandfathers are understandably going to have to make some adjustments. There are the schools that must be dealt with, as well as the teachers and guidance counselors who may treat you like a temporary parent, rather than who you've become. The men very likely face new health challenges of their own as they adapt to parenting again.

If your grandchild(ren) are staying with you, you need to have a document granting you power of attorney to care for the children. The document authorizes you to make medical decisions and avoid delays in timely medical care. AARP offers a number of helpful resources for kinship caregivers. The Grandcare Support Locator allows kinship caregivers to search for specific types of groups and services in their state or community. Using the free online search form, users are able to search in English or Spanish within their zip code to find services and programs (e.g., child care, health care, respite care, newsletters) or support groups (in-person, telephone support, or online), and they can restrict the search to information most relevant to grandparents raising grandchildren or to grandparents experiencing visitation issues.

THE TIME MAY COME TO MAKE OTHER ARRANGEMENTS

This chapter began by emphasizing how supportive and helpful relatives, partners, friends, and neighbors have traditionally been when someone is in need of assistance. Yet the time may come when the level of care needed extends beyond what can be provided by the most caring of men at home, even with the assistance of others and available community services. In those cases, relocating someone you care deeply about to a long-term care facility (e.g., a nursing home or assisted living facility) may need to be considered. This is obviously an extremely difficult decision for everyone concerned and requires thoughtful planning. Arriving at such a decision should involve the person receiving care, to the degree that this person is able to participate in the discussion, and all other people providing you support. Having a professional intermediary, such as a geriatric care manager (discussed earlier in this chapter), can make those discussions easier to manage and ensure that all possible options or alternatives are taken into consideration. Whatever the decision, many men will discover that their caregiving experience does not end when a relative, partner, or friend is admitted into a long-term care facility. In fact, your ongoing caregiving can continue to serve a critical role in easing the potential trauma associated with transition into an institutional setting. Not only will the person you've been caring for have that continued contact, but so will you. Your responsibilities change from doing all the care work by yourself to becoming an ombudsman for your loved one—you supervise the care the facility provides, continue to take walks (even if a wheelchair is needed), have frequent or occasional meals together, and enjoy a few moments holding hands while watching a favorite television program. The type of long-term care needed can range from adult foster care settings, where the care work is provided in someone else's home, to assisted living and continuing care retirement communities.

A TRANSFORMING EXPERIENCE

Serving as a caregiver to an ill or incapacitated relative can represent an important opportunity for you to role model caring behavior for the next generation of caring men. Men interviewed by Kaye and Applegate have suggested that those who served as caregivers were more likely to have other men in the family (e.g., sons) assisting them in their caregiving tasks than women.[29] The researchers speculate that men who accept the responsibilities of caregiving have the ability to teach the next generation of potential men caregivers that helping others can be included among the adult responsibilities they assume as members of their family network grow older and less able to manage independently. Maybe this is already happening: in the Asian communities in the United States, 48 percent of people over age 50 are being cared for by men, most often sons, and in other ethnic communities one-third of these caregivers also are men.[30]

For Louis Colbert, a son and person of color, caring for his mother in her home was a privileged and empowering experience.[31] Was it difficult? Extremely so, given her advancing dementia and her worsening physical health. It also caught Louis, as it does many men, by surprise. He was not prepared, and he was fearful and ignorant as to what was expected of him. He didn't know how to transfer her from the bed to the wheelchair or from the wheelchair to the toilet. The first few months were rough—in his words, "I was a big mess." He didn't even think of himself as a caregiver for the first 2 years. But years later, Louis recognizes that he is surprised at what he can do. He has learned self-care techniques and when to ask for help, which is his immediate advice to his fellow caregivers on what they can do to make the experience more manageable.

Whether you become a supportive friend providing just a little care work—driving a friend or relative to chemotherapy, stopping by for coffee and conversation—or a full-time caregiver of a spouse or partner, you will learn a lot about yourself and become well versed in tasks that you may never have been particularly skilled in. You already may be skilled to varying degrees in home maintenance and managing household finances. But don't be surprised if you learn to be a more informed shopper and consumer, or how to prepare meals for two (not huge ones with too many leftovers) and literally feed your dinner partner what you've prepared. While helping someone with their personal care needs (bathing, toileting, dressing) is likely to be particularly difficult, over time men discover that they become more capable and confident in these tasks as well. In addition, men who care for others often discover that they become better listeners and problem solvers—in other words, they tap into their "feminine side" and are both affective and sensitive. That is not a bad thing.

CHAPTER 23

End-of-Life Matters

with Stefanie Tedesco

The preventative measures discussed throughout the book are invaluable to maximize our physical and emotional well-being well into later life. In spite of everything we might do, there are no guarantees of either an easy late life or a good death. Our death is inevitable. What this chapter addresses is how to approach end-of-life matters with purposeful preparation. When facing head-on what may initially feel terrorizing, why not use options that give you greater personal control over *your* future? Asserting your preferences sooner rather than later is undoubtedly one of the best ways to take hold of your end-of-life decisions; the goal is to eliminate the unwanted uncertainties that you and/or your family may be required to face. A common mistake too many men make is putting off the "legal stuff" until it's too late. There is a right time to talk about your decisions concerning later life, and that time is now.

What you need to think (and talk) about may not be easy, but it is important. Issues related to the end of one's life include estate planning and what to do with pets, as well as who you want to make decisions for you if you are not able to make them on your own, particularly regarding financial matters and your health care. The same person may not be right for both. Have you privately weighed what medical treatments and types of care are and are not acceptable to you, and have you thought about where you prefer to be cared for if you become terminally ill—in a hospital, at home, or somewhere else? What would you like done with your body when you die? Because of the extraordinary financial costs of end-of-life care, have you considered how your care will be paid for?

Thinking about and actually planning end-of-life matters might provoke procrastination for a multitude of reasons: perhaps it strikes you as menacing, complicated, time-consuming, expensive, or just dismal. But do not follow Mark Twain's advice to "never put off until tomorrow what you can do the day after tomorrow." If you haven't begun planning ahead, you are not atypical. But do not forfeit your choices. Making sure you have wishes written down will give you a sense of security and alleviate future worries that you and your loved ones will certainly later face. There are several virtually pain-free steps you can take in the process of planning your "estate," long-term care decisions, and death. This chapter is a basic guide to taking control of late life and death, on your own or with an attorney and/or spiritual guide. With legal documentation and direct communication of your wishes, you can better assure that your own interests are known and preserved.

CREATING AN ESTATE PLAN

It's not just the rich who need an estate plan. The primary goal of an estate plan is to establish a legal guide for others, so that they can honor your wishes regarding health care (through your advance directive) and financial affairs in late life and after your death. No matter your net worth, the benefits of having a basic plan are significant. Estate planning documents cover three phases of your life: while you're alive and well, if you become disabled, and after you die. Apart from being the only way to assure that your decisions will be honored and your assets will go where you want them to, "estate planning" is a practical way to get relationships and financial affairs in order, saves on future legal hassles, and helps avoid probate court when issues arise later on.

Many men assume that they do not have "assets" significant enough to be planned for; however, it is invaluable for you to select certain individuals to protect your rights and requests in the event of unexpected incapacity or an early, unanticipated death. There are several easy steps to establishing an estate plan, and there are numerous resources available to help you begin planning on your own (see Appendix). The basic documents that make up an estate plan are a will, durable power of attorney, and health care proxy with advance directives. In some states, a living will and trust(s) are also basic documents. As a guide for familiarizing yourself with estate planning, the following is a brief description of each of these key documents.

THE WILL

In the simplest terms, the last will and testament is a document that only takes effect after death and directs another individual, who is named as executor, to collect your assets, pay any debts, and distribute remaining assets to the named beneficiaries. Drafting and signing a will in the presence of witnesses allows you to divide your physical and monetary property as you want. It is a chance to specifically state who should receive what and who should be responsible for ensuring the will's implementation. The executor of your will acts as your personal representative when distributing the components of your estate. The executor can be a person or an organization.

THE TRUST

In the most basic terms, this is a legal arrangement between three people: grantor, trustee, and beneficiary. In establishing a trust, you are the grantor, the trustee is the person you authorize to oversee and control the trust, and the beneficiary is the person who receives the "equitable title" and the benefits of the property held in the trust. To clarify, *legal title* to a house refers to the duties and responsibilities of maintaining and controlling that property. Insurance needs to be maintained, taxes have to be paid, and there is the upkeep of the property itself. By comparison, *equitable title* refers to the benefits and enjoyment of that property. At the heart of a trust is the splitting of the legal title and equitable title, such that the trustees have the legal title and control the property while the beneficiaries own the equitable title and the use and enjoyment of the property. Assume that you have a vacation cottage and want your adult children and grandchildren to all enjoy its use. You can appoint an organization to be the trustee and to hold the legal title (for a small annual maintenance fee), and then you give your three adult children equally the equitable title. Or, assume that you ask your younger sister and brother-in-law to serve as trustees for your money and financial assets until your grandchildren are 25, at which time each grandchild receives a share of the money (an inheritance). Both examples split legal title and equitable title. The property in a trust can be any kind of real or personal property, including money, real estate, stocks, bonds, collections, business interests, personal possessions, and cars. Trusts can be revocable or irrevocable.

A trust is commonly used to transfer assets to your heirs without going through probate, which saves time and money. By not establishing a trust and leaving all your assets to your spouse and/or children, you do not use your estate tax exemption and, instead, you increase their taxable estate. That means your wife or partner and children are likely to pay more in estate taxes. A trust is very appropriate even if you have a very modest estate but would like to have your property managed in the event of your incapacity or disability. Though it may sound quite similar to a last will, a trust can do a number of things a will cannot, including managing assets efficiently if you should die and your beneficiaries are minor children, or if you think the heirs are not up to the responsibility of managing the estate. Additionally, unlike a will, a trust is confidential so it also protects your privacy, along with reducing taxes on your assets and speeding transfers of your assets to beneficiaries after your death.

Creating a trust is especially advantageous if (1) you want to avoid the need for a court hearing in the event of becoming incapacitated, (2) you wish to provide for grandchildren, minor children, or relatives with a disability that makes it difficult for them to manage money, or (3) your property is difficult to divide. Trusts also come in handy when issues of long-term care arise. When facing costs of nursing homes or other medical facilities needed for long-term care in later life, most individuals need to "spend down" their assets in order to qualify for public benefits such as Medicaid. While spend-down requirements vary for each state, some trusts can be used to transfer assets, as if they are spent. For instance, a special needs trust might be used in some states to protect assets for you or your spouse when the other eventually goes into a care facility, and with limitations, one could be set up to preserve assets for your children as well. But federal rules impose a 5-year look-back on the transfer of assets if you seek to qualify for Medicaid. If you plan to develop a "special needs" trust, do it early. One type of special needs trust is described as a "self-settled" trust, which allows the assets to be used only as supplemental needs beyond what the government benefits pay for; however, this trust must be irrevocable to be exempt from the eligibility calculation.

ADVANCE DIRECTIVES

In anticipation of medical and health-care decisions toward the end of life, you need to think about your wishes, write those preferences down, and share them with your family or whomever you are appointing to serve as your health care proxy. Make sure the people you've appointed to act on your behalf know what you want and where to find your documents, so that in a moment of crisis they can be reassured that they are following your preferences, not theirs.

The Health Care Proxy

The health care proxy (or health care power of attorney) is a legal document that assigns an individual to be your health care agent, empowering the person to make any and all health care decisions when you are unable to do so yourself. Physicians and other health care providers commonly look to family members for advice, and they can convey what they think your preferences are related to a particular treatment. However, in most states, only the health care agent you appoint has the legal authority to make treatment decisions if you are unable to decide for yourself.

In many ways, the health care proxy is quite similar to the power of attorney (discussed below), but strictly with regard to health care issues. The health care proxy takes effect only when you are incapable of communicating your choices regarding medical treatment, even if the situation is temporary. This document usually expects that you will name at least one alternative health care agent along with the primary person you choose, in case your first choice is not willing, able, or reasonably available to make decisions for you. It grants these individuals the power to make your decisions, stating in advance whom an attending physician should consult about treatment decisions if you are unable to speak for yourself. The health care proxy document rarely lists your specific medical requests or decisions; living wills do that (see below). The document simply ensures that the people you choose will serve as your decision maker(s), rather than whoever happens to be the physician on duty. The agents should be individuals you trust to respect and honor your wishes above their own. In most states this document authorizes your agent the right and responsibility to approve or disapprove any diagnostic test, surgical procedure, or medication; select or discharge health care providers and institutions; and direct the provision, withholding, or withdrawal of artificial nutrition and hydration and all other forms of health care, including cardiopulmonary resuscitation. Remember, you have to be unable to make your own decisions before the designated health care agent is consulted.

Many hospitals and other health care providers make available the forms free of charge. Beyond signing a health care proxy, communicating your preferences to your health care agent is vital. Imagine that an event occurs requiring a major action to be taken, perhaps a blood transfusion, the insertion of a feeding tube, or a life-saving measure in response to a heart attack or stroke, and you simultaneously have advanced dementia. These may be frightening hypothetical situations for your representative to have to make decisions, but when your doctor turns to your health care agent and asks what should be done, you want them to confidently know they are responding as you would want them to. The right answer is only up to you.

The Durable Power of Attorney

The *durable* power of attorney document declares a trusted individual as your "attorney-in-fact" and becomes effective as soon as it is signed in front of witnesses, extending the authority from you to your selected attorney-in-fact to manage your financial affairs and legal responsibilities, even after you become incapacitated. As a rule, a durable power of attorney authorizes someone to serve as your conservator and guardian—to make financial and personal decisions on your behalf. It is unlike the more limited power of attorney document that authorizes a person or organization to handle all of your affairs should you be unavailable or temporarily unable to do so. It is important to construct the durable power of attorney to reflect the scope of power the attorney-in-fact may need to have to perform on your behalf. You can assign this person the authority to make decisions with respect to your property and financial affairs, but not those matters that fall under the authority of your health care agent. In some states, however, the durable power of attorney can also be the health care proxy agent.

There is a "springing" power of attorney document that only becomes effective when the grantor (you) lacks capacity. However, a physician must determine when the grantor lacks capacity and present evidence to the court for approval, much like a guardianship or conservatorship.

You can choose more than one attorney-in-fact, and, often, it is wise to select a successor in case the original agent(s) cannot serve for some reason. If you do choose two people to serve as your attorney-in-fact, they have to act jointly. Both people must agree and act together on every decision.

Signing a durable power of attorney gives a good amount of power to the individual you choose; they will have the authority to manage your money, real property, and other matters such as life insurance and retirement accounts. This being so, it is important to choose your representative wisely. Your spouse is a good first choice, as their understanding and handling of affairs probably closely aligns with your own. When appointing others, even children, you will need someone who is responsible and lives relatively close to you. You should pay attention to their ability to deal with stress and willingness to honor *your* wishes, not their own interests. It is helpful to remind yourself that in making these seemingly intimidating decisions, you are not relinquishing control, but taking control over who will help you and who will not.

The Living Will

Common law recognizes that a competent adult has the right to determine what will be done to his person or body, and this includes the right to accept or decline medical treatment. Unless you explicitly instruct your physicians and caregivers otherwise, whenever you are admitted to a hospital, you are assumed to be "a full code" and everything will be and must be done to keep you alive. That's what medical care is about—curing, at all cost. Given our legal (and moral) right of self-determination, an advance directive is a legal document that makes known what medical treatment you desire near the end of life or in a situation following a near-fatal accident where you are unable to communicate your treatment preferences. This living will document is at times referred to as a health care or physician's directive for end-of-life care. Federal law now requires all hospitals to provide information about advance directives, and most states also have specific laws.

The point of an advance directive is to inform health care providers (and your family and designated health care agent) about your request for or decision to waive particular medical treatments, should you be unable to speak for yourself.[1] This document is most useful for people who are imminently facing death and who have strong and specific beliefs about what they prefer. It is a document that will affirm any directive you may have provided one physician before you became incapable of communicating your preferences, at which time another physician or caregiver may become responsible for your care.

There are many decisions that can be made regarding possible end-of-life situations: the major ones include breathing and feeding tubes, last-chance surgeries, or any life-saving measures if you have advanced dementia. While some of these considerations may seem perplexing or morbid, the process of thinking through your preferences is important to comfort your family and perhaps even offer you some peace of mind. There are formal living wills widely available to you. There also are national organizations, such as Five Wishes (www.agingwithdignity.org), that encourage family discussions about end-of-life matters and help people plan for their end-of-life care. Five Wishes offers a comprehensive document legally recognized in 42 states and useful in the other 8 to help identify your health care agent, the kind of medical treatment you do or do not want, how comfortable you want to be, how you want people to treat you, and what you want your family and friends to know.

Generally, the living will provides end-of-life treatment directives for your health care providers and caregivers. It may include your request not to be hospitalized; it may forbid the use of various kinds of medical treatment; or it may directly request cardiac resuscitation, mechanical breathing, and/or tube feeding. If you have specific preferences as to medical treatment under certain circumstances, it is important to spell them out in the document itself. We cannot assume that physicians and family members know what we want. Living wills can provide the following specific directives:

> *Do not resuscitate (DNR) order*. This is a request not to have cardio-pulmonary resuscitation (CPR) performed if your heart stops or if you stop breathing. Your living will doesn't have to include a DNR order, nor do you have to have a living will to initiate a DNR order. Your attending physician can put a DNR order in your medical chart, and in most hospitals a DNR medical bracelet is available. But when you enter a hospital or nursing home, you may not be able to communicate your DNR request. A living will becomes effective when you are incapacitated, and it is in your best interests to disclose your preferences well before there is a need.

> *Do not intubate (DNI) order*. This is a similar request. You are refusing mechanical breathing (respiration and ventilation) in a situation where continued treatment will inevitably cause more discomfort and/or prolong the dying process, as may be the case when difficult breathing comes with end-stage pneumonia. Your living will doesn't have to include a DNI order. If you are able to decide to activate a DNI order while hospitalized, you will have a medical bracelet saying so.

Living wills have not been very successful.[2] The document is often unavailable when decisions need to be made. It is tucked away in your "important papers," and you may have forgotten to tell someone where to find it. Even when it is available, too often your preferences end up being too general or way too specific to assist the physician or caregiver with an issue that needs to be decided. Someone might write in their living will "Do whatever is necessary for my comfort, but nothing further." That's too open for interpretation. Someone else might prefer a DNR when hospitalized and at the end of life, but his request "Do not call a 'Code Blue' and try to revive me should my heart stop" lacks clarity for when decision makers should apply these instructions, and he mistakenly thought he did not need to discuss his preference with his attending physician.

Despite the limitations of living wills, researchers who have studied older adults' end-of-life decisions and experiences conclude that it is better to have a living will than not to have one.[3] It is meant to be viewed as a guide for part of your end-of-life planning. It creates opportunities for conversations, especially with the people you designate as your health care agent. The most important thing is informing your health care agent, your close friends and family, your doctor, and perhaps your lawyer of your decisions to ensure that you will still maintain control until the end. The medical community concurs: there is renewed interest among physicians to start a discussion with each patient about preferences and to translate those preferences into medical orders that protect their wishes.[4]

It is strongly advised that you keep your living will current, updating it annually and signing it each time. This will show that it reflects your most current thinking and wishes. You should also post it in several locations, to avoid it getting misplaced, and give copies of it to designated relatives.

As a final caution, this document's authority is effective only after your doctor *and* another doctor certify that you are either suffering from a terminal illness or permanently unconscious. This means that should you suffer a heart attack at age 60 but do not have a terminal illness and are not expected to be permanently unconscious, your living will is *not* the guide physicians will use. EMTs and the ER physicians will try to resuscitate you.

Organ Donation

How do you feel about organ donation? This issue is at times addressed in a living will, but it need not be included. A man with a neurological disease might feel that studying his brain could be educational for medical students. Medical schools need bodies to teach medical students about anatomy, and he contacts a medical school several years before his death to donate his entire body. Another man, by contrast, is adamant that he will not be an organ donor, because his faith regards a dead body as spiritually powerful and the act of donating is equivalent to injuring the dead. Most religious faiths, however, recognize the life-giving benefits of donating organs and tissue for transplant purposes. Many individuals also recognize the social value of donating tissue, organs, or body parts for medical scientific research or for helping another person survive. Research facilities are in need of diseased organs and whole bodies to study disease processes so they can develop cures. The decision to donate all or part of your body is one that requires planning ahead; your family and friends would need to be advised of your plans, especially if you elect to donate your body to a medical school, as there would be no body for a funeral.

THE FUNERAL

What do you want to occur at your funeral? Funeral planning is something nearly all of us will have to do at some point, and your decisions will be influenced by cultural and religious traditions, personal preferences, and costs. Given that the events following your death will be a very emotional time for your family members, planning ahead will reduce their distress and significantly relieve them of the need to make unpleasant financial decisions while they are grieving. It also gives your family the ability to make arrangements according to your preferences. You may be daunted at first by the myriad of choices and even upset by the commercial funeral industry, but planning ahead will help you manage these issues.

Every family member is different, and not everyone will want the same type of funeral for you. Your children might hold differing opinions about what they think you would have wanted. Therefore, ask yourself, what do you want? You might not even know where to begin, or what questions to ask. Your taste, beliefs, and budget should dictate the type of funeral you arrange. First of all, do you want your body to be cremated or buried? More people are choosing cremation, partly because of its simplicity, people's personal philosophies, and the raw fact that families are often no longer geographically located near one another. If you prefer to be cremated, do you want your ashes in a columbarium (a place for the storage of your cremated remains, such as an urn or vault) or scattered some place?

If your preference is to be buried, do you want a "traditional" full-service funeral—with embalming and hand-crafted brass casket, religious service, hearse, and formal burial site service—or a direct burial shortly after death in a simple container? Do you want a traditional religious service in a place of worship or a secular memorial celebration? If you served in the military, do you want an honor guard to participate in your funeral and present your family with a flag? Do you prefer calling hours (or a viewing) at a mortuary and a wake to follow? Open casket or closed? If you want to be buried, do you have preferences on who ought to be pallbearers? Is there something you want said in your obituary, and are there things not to be mentioned? What about memorial contributions? If you decide to donate your body to a medical school and a traditional funeral is no longer at issue or a cost, what type of family gathering and memorial service would you think your family might want?

Whether your preference is a funeral (with the body present) or a memorial service (without the body), it is the coming together of your family and friends that is most important. The funeral or memorial service is sort of a reunion for them. Recognize that the typical (or "traditional" and expensive) American funeral has no roots in Christianity, Judaism, Islam, or any other religion. But if this type of funeral brings you peace of mind and you can afford it, arrange one. A funeral is almost guaranteed to be used—the question is *when* to plan for *what* you want.

Funeral costs seem rather crass to discuss. But the cost must be dealt with. Expenses include a funeral home's transportation and care of the body, the purchase of a casket or burial container, and the purchase of a cemetery plot or crypt or a location for your ashes. If you choose to be buried and have a traditional graveside service, funeral homes and cemeteries usually charge basic service fees such as the costs of embalming and the grave liner or vault. But if you prefer a simpler "green" burial, there is a growing interest in green cemeteries, and they do not accept embalming, metal caskets, vaults, and conventional upright markers; it is a return to simplicity. Finally, there is the expense of the gathering of family and friends at a hall or a home after the memorial service or funeral.

If you give thought to these matters ahead of time, you can preplan your funeral and burial expenses. These arrangements are commonly referred to as "preneed funeral arrangements" or "prepaid funeral agreements." There are many honest and reputable funeral services that offer preneed funeral arrangements, and funeral directors are required to give you itemized prices and, in most states, provide a statement of the exact goods and services you are purchasing. Your preneed funds may be placed in an interest-bearing funeral trust account with a local bank, to be paid to a funeral home after your death, or in a funeral insurance policy, either of which must be placed in your name. The purchase of a preneed funeral is an acceptable spend-down for Medicaid, though states vary regarding the allowable cost of the preneed funeral.

LATE-LIFE CARE ARRANGEMENTS

Close to one in every three older men will require some 24/7 long-term care services at some point in their lives. It may be the extended rehabilitation you need following a fall and hip replacement, or it could be the care needed in late-stage dementia. Long-term care decisions are part of what comes with planning for late life. Some men will only need home health assistance, and others will require more extensive care, and ordinary health insurance generally does not cover the care provided by skilled nursing facilities.

Continuing Care Communities

Continuing care retirement communities have become a first choice for older couples who decide they no longer want to maintain their own home or downsize into a condominium and pay the condo fees. As a rule, a continuing care community is on a "campus" that provides different types of housing, community dining options, health care, and social services. The housing on the campus may range from separate (or single-family) duplexes to apartments within a large facility, and joining one of these communities gives you access to long-term care services. Continuing care communities give you the option to live in one location for the duration of your life, with much of the future care you may need already in place. Typically, you move into the community as an independent resident, and months or years later when you want or need temporary nursing services, they are readily available. When you need more care or become unable to live independently, you can move from your independent housing into an assisted living unit or into the on-site or affiliated skilled nursing home.

Costs typically include a sizeable entrance fee and then a monthly fee (similar to a condo fee) based on the type and size of your independent living unit and any prepaid services. In some communities, after the first year the initial entrance fee can become a down payment on assisted living and/or nursing home services. In other communities, your monthly fee is all-inclusive and does not increase even if you move to a different setting on the campus. The monthly payments and contracts vary widely and can be quite costly.

Home Health Care

Largely because of people's aversion to the idea of going to a skilled nursing facility and their preference to stay in their own home, as well as health insurers' interest in reducing costs, home health care alternatives to help older adults live independently at home have become readily available. Between 80 and 90 percent of older men (and women) indicate they would prefer to remain in their own homes as long as possible. Think of home health care as paid caregivers taking over for family members who can no longer provide (free) care because of their own health needs or geographic distance.

Some standard health insurance policies provide limited coverage, and most long-term care insurance policies support many home health care services. A widowed older man, for example, can live alone longer when home nursing and housekeeping services are contracted occasionally in his home. The cost of home health aides who cook meals, shop for groceries, or help with bathing can vary considerably, ranging from $40/hr in one city to $10/hr in another 100 miles away. The registered nurses (RNs) who provide more skilled medical services, such as wound and incision care, IV administration, or inserting and changing a Foley catheter, may cost $100/hr. If a man wanted a "live-in" home health aide who will be with him 24 hours a day, most of the time two different aides would be contracted to cover the week—e.g., one who works for 4 days and another who works the remaining 3 days, at a monthly cost near $7,500, which can be less than the cost of a nursing home in some states. Nonetheless, it might be what you want and can afford. One 81-year-old man who decided to reverse mortgage his home to stay in it commented,

> I know I'm not gonna be around forever. But I told my kids I was going nowhere! I want to be in my own place. Me and the dog. My son lives here

in town and my daughter is only a few miles west. We worked it out so the house can help pay for care if and when I need it and then it's theirs when I'm gone. I don't want to be a burden to no one . . . they're good kids and this way I get to see the grandkids too. They mow the lawn. This house has important memories for me, but once I'm gone, the kids already have their own places; they don't need or want this house, so I like the idea of putting the home's value to work for me![5]

Take caution, however: geriatric care managers have told us that they have had clients who have initiated a reverse mortgage and, sometimes within 2 years, depending on the value of the house, had the mortgage depleted. Their clients then had to move to a nursing home to keep up the necessary medical care services. Plan ahead—the decision to initiate a reverse mortgage is a decision to stay in your home as long as you can. It is not a sure bet that the funds are an insurance policy to cover all future costs.

Long-Term Care

Long-term care is designed to meet health and personal care needs over an extended period of time. Most long-term care involves helping you with the activities of daily living (ADLs), which are bathing, dressing, eating, using the toilet, and moving to and from a bed or chair. The goal of long-term care services is to help you maximize your independence at a time when you are unable to be fully independent.

Traditionally, the responsibility of long-term care belonged to the family, and care work was the work of the women in men's lives—their wives, daughters, sisters, and sisters-in-law. However, this is no longer our culture's expectation. Rather, older men and women foresee the limits of what their families can do and should be expected to do. While considering a long-term stay at any medical facility in your future is not the brightest daydream, planning ahead for such things will help in a very big way. Because no one really wants to think forward to a time when they might need long-term care, planning for this possibility gets put off. Frankly, most of us prefer to avoid thinking about becoming dependent on others to bathe and to eat. But thinking through the options will make future decisions less stressful emotionally and financially.

The costs of long-term care are significant, and most people misunderstand how it is paid for. Nursing homes charge a basic daily or monthly fee. At the beginning of 2010 the national median cost for a private room in a nursing home was roughly $200 a day, and a semiprivate room shared with one other person was no bargain—$185 a day on average, ranging from $47,000 to $126,000 annually.[6] Cost (and quality) also can vary markedly within a state. Recognize that these estimates do not include the cost of any medication, physician visits and dental care, podiatry services, or hair care.

Moving into assisted living will cost at least $3,000 monthly, and this type of care is basically the hands-off, don't-touch-the-body type of care.[7] Assisted living does provide social and recreational opportunities, a "club" environment of men and women who want to remain independent and socially active, and communal dining as options. You can usually purchase and receive "hands-on" services in your housing unit.

There are three basic planning trajectories to fund long-term care costs. One is paying *out of pocket*, and on average nearly 20 percent of long-term care costs are paid this way. For most men, paying for long-term care with personal savings and assets will be challenging, particularly if you end up needing multiple years of nursing home care. The average is 1.75 years for men over age 65.

The second is applying for government benefits. When you become eligible for Medicare at age 65, your actual out-of-pocket costs can be lessened. Medicare is, however, not comprehensive. Medicare (Parts A and B) will pay for several weeks of care in a skilled nursing facility or hospice and home care, but too often several weeks of coverage is not enough. It is important to remember that Medicare, which is a public insurance plan for the older population, can only cover short-term care along with physician, rehab, and drug costs. Part A is a Social Security entitlement. Part B must be purchased; it is the insurance to pay for medically necessary services and supplies provided by Medicare, to include outpatient care, doctor's services, physical or occupational therapists, and additional home health care. An alternative is a Medicare Advantage (Part C) plan, which is the combination of Part A (hospital insurance) and Part B (medical insurance). The main difference in a Part C plan is that coverage is provided through private insurance companies approved by Medicare, rather than through the Social Security Administration (SSA). Opting for "Part C," you may have lower out-of-pocket costs and receive extra benefits. There are several different types of Medicare Advantage (Part C) plans, including membership in a health maintenance organization (HMO) or a preferred provider organization (PPO), as well as the less common options of HMO point-of-service plans and medical savings accounts.

If you are 65 or older and do not have a Medicare Advantage plan or private medical insurance that provides prescription drug coverage, you also ought to consider adding Medicare Part D, which is a stand-alone prescription drug coverage insurance that you purchase from the SSA. Like other prescription drug insurance plans, Medicare Part D requires most people to pay a monthly premium to the SSA, and all medically necessary drugs are typically covered.

To assure more thorough coverage than provided by Medicare, it is wise to purchase a "Medigap" policy. You do not need and cannot buy a Medigap insurance policy (or Medicare Supplemental Insurance) if you have a Medicare Advantage plan. The Medigap insurance policy must be purchased *before* needing services and is sold by private insurance companies to fill the "gaps" in original Medicare (Part A) coverage. As of 2010, all Medigap policies, in every plan type, pay the Medicare Part A hospital coinsurance amounts, plus the full cost up to 365 additional hospital days after Medicare coverage runs out. And, if you are transferred from a hospital to a skilled nursing facility, the policy kicks in with a 50 or 75 percent co-pay of the costs after you pay out of pocket for several months of care. If you do not have a Medicare Advantage plan, purchasing a Medigap policy is something you will want to seriously consider. The coverage provided by competing insurers is virtually identical, even though the policy costs can differ markedly. Between Medicare (Parts A and B) and your Medigap policy, most of the health care costs are covered. Yet most people pay a deductible, as well as the monthly or annual expense of their coinsurance.

Medicaid is responsible for covering long-term care costs for people with few assets. Ownership of even modest amounts of property or income can disqualify you from Medicaid eligibility. This is where "spending down" assets becomes necessary for many people. Spend-down restrictions are expansive, and a good alternative to address the asset problem is to set up a special trust to preserve and manage your assets in a way that lets you (or your loved one) qualify for government assistance. A special needs trust (or supplemental needs trust) can be initiated at the last minute in most states. It is a legal document designed for a person who becomes "disabled" as a result of, for instance, an acquired illness, a stroke, or a progressive dementia. The special needs trust enables you to have held in trust for your benefit an unlimited amount of assets. In a properly drafted special needs trust, those assets are not considered countable assets for purposes of qualification for certain governmental benefits.

The third option, *long-term care insurance*, is now the strategic alternative most men will follow to take control of long-term care costs. It helps you avoid the difficult process of "spending down" to become Medicaid eligible and spending all your savings paying out of pocket for your care. Current long-term care insurance policies have choices for care, including home care, adult day care, and assisted care, in addition to nursing homes. There are also flexible options for benefit and waiting periods. Most long-term care insurance policies guarantee monthly cash payments if you come to require long-term care, while you, the insured, would pay a form of co-pay along with your benefits. The benefits usually kick in when you demonstrate need, by either physical inability to perform daily living tasks or severe cognitive incapacity. Unlike life insurance, very few long-term care policies have the option of returning a portion of the premiums you paid should you not need the benefits. For this reason, it can be wise to purchase a life insurance policy with a long-term care rider, which generates a sum of money that can be used to pay for care needs, but when you do not end up needing any or all of the money, it is automatically added to the death benefit, giving much of your money back to your beneficiary. To take control of your options, investigate the alternatives and determine what best fits your own financial situation. Be aware that long-term care policies are costly and their cost increases based on the age at which you initiate coverage.

Palliative Care

Palliative care is both a philosophy and a medical specialty that aims to improve the overall quality of life for seriously ill patients and their families. Surgeons, urologists, and many other health care providers can provide palliative (as well as curative) care. Members of a palliative care team typically include professionals from surgery, medicine, nursing, and social work, with additional support from clergy and professionals in nutrition, rehabilitation, and pharmacy. Unlike in the past, palliative care is no longer segregated as a different "service" within hospitals, as you might still find for urology services, oncology, and cardiac care. Palliative care is the philosophy of care brought into a wide range of health care settings (including your home), emphasizing quality of life. Nor is it only for people who are terminally ill.

Palliative care emphasizes the importance of open communication and an equal relationship between patient and professional caregivers, pain and symptom management, and coordination of care. It tries to relieve the suffering that an illness and the exhausting treatment side effects jointly cause, whether it be pain, fatigue, shortness of breath, nausea, loss of appetite, or difficulty sleeping. It aims to help all seriously ill people at any stage of their illness gain the strength to carry on with their daily life, and it is provided by a team of professionals working to offer collaborative and seamless care. Researchers have found that palliative care is appropriate at any point once a serious illness is diagnosed; it can be provided at the same time as other treatment is meant to cure, and the sooner initiated when someone is seriously ill, the better the person's mood and quality of life.[8] Yet researchers also find that use of palliative care services remains disturbingly low, partly because some physicians continue to see palliative care services as an "alternative" rather than a complementary form of care that ought to begin with diagnosis,[9] and partly because those who might benefit from it either do not know about or choose not to avail themselves of the services.

Hospice Care

Most men do not die traumatically. More than half of all deaths are caused by chronic heart disease or cancer, and the last weeks of most men's lives are usually spent in a hospital or nursing home. Knowing these facts, improving end-of-life care and helping individuals achieve a "good death" has become the mission of many organizations and individuals. As one group of medical ethicists argues,

> Too many Americans die unnecessarily bad deaths—deaths with inadequate palliative support, inadequate compassion, and inadequate human presence and witness. Deaths preceded by a dying marked by fear, anxiety, loneliness, and isolation. Deaths that efface dignity and deny individual self-control and choice.[10]

There are care opportunities available to better assure a "good death," which usually includes feeling a sense of control, not being alone, adequate pain control and symptom management, maintaining a sense of dignity, avoiding an unnecessarily prolonged dying process, and finding an emotional and/or spiritual sense of completion.[11]

One route to a "good death" is hospice care, and one in three men now choose this option. While most people have heard of hospice, few know that it is not a place. Fewer men know how it works, and even fewer know that every American is entitled to hospice benefits through Medicare and most health insurance policies. Hospice care is a special concept of care. It provides a holistic approach to end-of-life care, bringing together a multifaceted "team" of nurses and physicians, social workers, clergy, and other professionals, including massage therapists and counselors to provide emotional support for family members. It does not prolong life, nor does it hasten death. A hospice team emphasizes pain control, symptom management, natural death, and quality of life to comfort both the person's body and their emotional/spiritual well-being. Hospice begins with an individually designed, end-of-life plan to minister to what each person specifically needs and wishes wherever he lives, and when he has been given only a short time to live. Hospice care can be brought into a health care facility or nursing home, and it can be arranged to provide the support for someone to remain at home. Hospice care can provide services over the last 6 months of life; however, one study[12] found that the median length of time someone is actually involved with hospice care is 26 days, and nearly one-third of the people in the study were enrolled in the last 7 days of life. Because hospice is actually about *taking control* of an inevitable situation, it shouldn't be thought of as all about dying. It is about continuing to live as the person you are and to make the best choices for yourself at the end of life.

AVOIDING THE LAST OPTIONS:
GUARDIANSHIP AND CONSERVATORSHIP

Unfortunately, there are times when the real advantages of planning ahead only can be seen in hindsight. This is when procrastination overruled planning ahead. When an individual becomes unable to take care of his own basic needs or make his own decisions, whether because he is "mentally incompetent" as a result of his dementia or slips into unconsciousness following a stroke, someone needs to speak in his behalf. People who have not established the durable power of attorney and/or health care proxy agent ahead of time will require a guardian and conservator. Guardianship and conservatorship are the only remaining options to protect the person's welfare and best interests when no prior legal arrangement was initiated. Both involve a judicial procedure. In front of a judge, someone is appointed to take charge of the incapacitated man's legal, financial, medical, and personal affairs.

A legal guardian is appointed by a probate court judge to have the right and responsibility to assure that food, housing, health care, and other necessities of life are provided. This legal guardian is often a spouse or close relative who has petitioned the court to become the after-the-fact health care agent and attorney-in-fact. However, for men who lived alone and/or have no nearby relative who is able to become a guardian, guardianship is likely to be assigned by the court to a geriatric social worker who specializes in guardianship, an administrator for a nursing home, or an interested law office. The petitioner who wishes to become the guardian typically must present medical affidavits that demonstrate your incapacity, since the court is essentially stripping a man of his self-determination rights and defining him as legally "incapacitated."

In recent years laws and regulations in most jurisdictions have maximized the ill person's autonomy and limited the rights and responsibilities of the legal guardian. There are now limited guardianships that offer the greatest autonomy, compared to the general guardianships. In both cases, the guardian is directed by the court to monitor the "ward's" welfare and make sure that he lives in the most appropriate, least restrictive environment possible and is provided social opportunities and medical care. Some older men might worry that a family member or health care administrator will take over making decisions too early. Though laws vary, most states aim to keep an individual in charge of his own care as long as he is able.

Guardianship can be easily avoided by an earlier selection of advocates to serve as your health care agent and attorney-in-fact, and it *should* be avoided because of the difficulties guardianship causes and the cost and probate necessities that accompany it. Guardianship appointments burden your surviving family members, because they will be forced to choose the person to represent you, go through the cumbersome process of retrieving a time-limited clinical diagnosis to prove your incapacity (which sometimes expires before the guardianship petition is approved), report to the court annually concerning your condition, and accept full responsibility over your health, support, care, and welfare, often without even knowing what *you* would have wanted. All of this too commonly happens in a moment of crisis, such as following a myocardial infarction that starved the brain of oxygen. Though children can be appointed co-guardians, this alternative is not advisable because in many states it may be necessary for each co-guardian to approve every decision, even in an emergency situation.

Conservatorships place one or more individuals in charge of your financial affairs, if you have not properly appointed someone to serve as your attorney-in-fact. The conservator has to manage your "estate" (property and assets) without the direction of an estate plan; additionally, both the conservator and guardian will be forced to file bonds to be appointed to these critical positions. It is evident that having an estate plan and advance directives ahead of time will avoid many emotionally strenuous procedures for others, while simultaneously preserving your wishes.

CONSULTING A PROFESSIONAL

While establishing an estate plan and end-of-life care plan is relatively easy and can be done on your own, there is always the alternative of hiring a lawyer or financial consultant to guide you through this process. You may save time and money by using workbooks or online sources, but there are certainly benefits to having a lawyer and long-term care financial consultant at your disposal. An attorney who specializes in elder law and estate planning can be a precious resource for unbiased advice and help in determining the course of action that best suits your specific circumstances. You are "hiring" someone who can provide an analysis of the elder laws and regulations and has experience in advocating for clients and preserving the older adult's autonomy. If you have family members that might disagree with your decisions and your care, a lawyer can act as a positive mediator. On the flip side, if you don't have other individuals to confide in, a lawyer is a first-rate option for communicating your future decisions, and you can often appoint the law firm as a trustee of your estate. Beyond simple estate planning, an elder law attorney would be familiar with the guidelines for long-term care concerns, including Medicaid, long-term care insurance, and Supplemental Security Income (SSI) eligibility and application processes, which are important elements of end-of-life planning. Hiring an elder law attorney is often the smartest way to ensure that your decisions and affairs are in proper order, so do not be held back simply by the intimidation of fees or dealing with law firms.

You also have the option of hiring a geriatric care manager who takes on many tasks to alleviate stress for yourself and your family. They will assess *your* needs, guide *your* care planning, coordinate services, and act as a mediator between you and other professionals, such as doctors, lawyers, and finance experts. Geriatric care managers are very sensitive to aging issues, and they bring a combination of compassion and practicality to their work. Care managers can develop a very close relationship with you and your family, as their professional responsibility demands intensive, personal involvement with their client. Hiring a geriatric care manager is a wise decision if you need the extra help of a professional advocate and resource. They become the go-to person for any and all developing concerns.

If you choose to take immediate control by hiring an attorney or a care manager, do your research. Look for individuals you feel comfortable around and with whom you can easily communicate. Choose an attorney who demonstrates an interest in your attorney-client relationship and has experience in several areas of elder law. While it may sound strange to look for compassionate and friendly qualities in an attorney, you need to feel as if you can trust and confide in this individual in order to take the best control of your needs. A great source for finding information on local elder services, legal and care resources, and qualified elder law attorneys is the National Academy of Elder Law Attorneys, whose website alone will set you on the right path toward finding professional guidance.

DON'T WAIT

While we are all aware that aging and death aren't easy subjects to talk about, this reality makes the end of life even more pertinent to discuss. There will never be a perfect moment to broach the subject with your family or friends; even if you are comfortable with your own mortality, they may not be. But by thinking, talking, and writing before it is too late, you can save them from knowing the distress that many will face. By planning ahead you ensure that *you* are still the one deciding your future and that others know exactly what your wishes demand. Fear of old age and death is commonplace, but do not let this lead to procrastination. Take charge: establish an estate plan, communicate your end-of-life wishes, and consider the future before it is the present. Assert your authority now so as to avoid limitations and unnecessary crisis later. Guarantee your dignity.

Places to Turn for More Information

with Jennifer A. Crittenden, Elisha M. Foss, and Lindsay Day

This appendix provides additional resources that may be helpful in your search for solid and reliable health information. As a disclaimer, we do not endorse the resources listed in this chapter. Information gathered from these resources should not take the place of advice from your own health care provider or other support personnel with whom you are working. Resources are listed by topic.

AGING AND HEALTH RESOURCES

American Society on Aging (ASA)
1-800-537-9728
www.asaging.org

The ASA is a professional organization that offers publications and online information. The primary publications are *Aging Today*, a bimonthly newspaper, which covers news, advances and controversies in research, practice, and policy; and *Generations,* a scholarly quarterly journal, with in-depth articles on best practice, policy, research, and model programs.

Centers for Disease Control and Prevention (CDC)
1600 Clifton Road
Atlanta, GA 30333
1-800-CDC-INFO (1-800-232-4636)
cdcinfo@cdc.gov
www.cdc.gov

The mission of the CDC is "to collaborate to create the expertise, information, and tools that people and communities need to protect their health—through health promotion, prevention of disease, injury and disability, and preparedness for new health threats." The CDC offers a wealth of trusted resources on various health topics, including emergency preparedness, healthy living, workplace safety, and most specific health challenges (e.g., arthritis, gout). The CDC website provides a searchable format for finding the health resources you need.

Healthy Aging: Over 50

www.mayoclinic.com/health/healthy-aging/MY00374/

The Healthy Aging: Over 50 webpage was developed by the Mayo Clinic to provide tips for maintaining a healthy and active lifestyle. The site features a wealth of resources and searchable health topics such as healthy eating, sexuality, exercise, healthy retirement, and caring for others.

Men: Stay Healthy at 50+

www.ahrq.gov/ppip/men50.htm
Agency for Healthcare Research and Quality
Office of Communications and Knowledge Transfer
540 Gaither Road, Suite 2000
Rockville, MD 20850
301-427-1364

Or write to AHRQ and request a copy of Publication No. 08-IP002, which is an easy-to-read checklist for maintaining good health produced by the Agency for Healthcare Research and Quality.

My HealthEVet

www.myhealthevet.va.gov

This site is an online health tool, designed for veterans and their families, that allows beneficiaries to access a health library, information about their benefits, health care coverage, prescriptions, and other self-assessment tools.

National Council on Aging (NCOA)

1901 L Street, NW, 4th Floor
Washington, DC 20036
202-479-1200
www.ncoa.org

NCOA is a service and advocacy organization that helps to improve the lives of older adults. They work with many organizations to help individuals find jobs, seek benefits, improve their health, live independently, and remain active in their communities.

National Hospice & Palliative Care Organization (NHPCO)
1731 King Street, Suite 100
Alexandria, VA 22314
703-837-1500
nhpco_info@nhpco.org
www.nhpco.org

NHPCO is a national membership organization devoted to improving end-of-life care through advocacy and education. This organization can provide you with important resources on end-of-life care and assistance in locating local end-of-life care options.

National Institute on Aging Publications and Age Pages
National Institute on Aging
Building 31, Room 5C27
31 Center Drive, MSC 2292
Bethesda, MD 20892
1-800-222-2225
niaic@nia.nih.gov
www.nia.nih.gov/HealthInformation/Publications/
www.nia.nih.gov

The National Institute on Aging has an extensive list of publications covering various health topics. The publications are easy to read, and most are available free of charge. You can view publications online or have them delivered to your home. Topics include diet and exercise, caregiving, sexuality, how to read and understand your health care information, alcohol use, sleep, and many more.

National Institutes of Health (NIH), Health Topics A–Z
http://health.nih.gov

This is a searchable website with links to articles and other national organizations that address general health topics, including African American health, Native American health, Asian American health, and Hispanic American health.

U.S. Food and Drug Administration (FDA)
10903 New Hampshire Avenue
Silver Spring, MD 20993-0002
1-888-INFO-FDA (1-888-463-6332)
www.fda.gov

The FDA works to protect "public health by assuring the safety, efficacy and security of human and veterinary drugs, biological products, medical devices, our nation's food supply, cosmetics, and products that emit radiation." To that end, the FDA provides important consumer resources on topics such as medications, medical equipment, vaccinations, and food, along with cutting-edge information on recent developments that relate to health and well-being.

United States Government Senior Citizens' Resources Page
www.usa.gov/Topics/Seniors.shtml

This is a one-stop shop for all government information that is of interest to older adults. Resources available on this website include information on caregiving, consumer protection, housing, retirement, government benefits, travel, taxes, and more.

World Health Organization (WHO)
Avenue Appia 20
1211 Geneva 27
Switzerland
+41-22-791-21-11
info@who.int
www.who.int

WHO is the leading organization in international health matters and is responsible for coordinating control of infectious disease and treating such diseases as AIDS, tuberculosis, and swine flu. Their evidence-based research focuses on monitoring and assessing health trends. Visit their Health Topics webpage to find practical information about common health conditions.

COMPLEMENTARY AND ALTERNATIVE MEDICINE

American Holistic Medical Association (AHMA)
27629 Chagrin Boulevard, Suite 123
Woodmere, OH 44122
info@holisticmedicine.org
www.holisticmedicine.org

The AHMA works to increase understanding of natural healing and the integration of holistic medicine with conventional medicine. Their work is focused on prevention and addressing contributing factors to illness.

National Center for Complementary and Alternative Medicine (NCCAM)
NCCAM Clearinghouse
PO Box 7923
Gaithersburg, MD 20898
1-888-644-6226
1-866-464-3615
www.nccam.nih.gov

NCCAM is the federal government's lead agency for scientific research on the diverse medical and health care systems, practices, and products that are not generally considered part of conventional medicine. The website features an array of health topics (from A to Z) supported by evidenced-based treatments and conditions for most health challenges (e.g., sleep, eczema, bone health).

SPECIFIC HEALTH RESOURCES

Bones, Joints, and Muscles

Arthritis Foundation National Office
1330 W. Peachtree Street, Suite 100
Atlanta, GA 30309-0669
1-800-283-7800
www.arthritis.org

The foundation works to educate, control, and cure over 100 types of arthritis and associated conditions. They have several service locations throughout the country which help individuals take control of their arthritis and improve their quality of life.

National Institute of Arthritis and Musculoskeletal and Skin Diseases (NIAMS)
Office of Communications and Public Liaison
National Institutes of Health
1 AMS Circle
Bethesda, MD 20892-3675
1-877-22-NIAMS (1-877-226-4267)
NIAMSinfo@mail.nih.gov
www.niams.nih.gov

This institute serves as a national clearinghouse of information on arthritis, musculoskeletal disease, and skin diseases. The institute features resources for professionals, patients, and the public on a variety of diseases and conditions.

National Osteoporosis Foundation
1150 17th Street NW, Suite 850
Washington, DC 20036
1-800-231-4222
www.nof.org

The foundation is dedicated to the prevention of osteoporosis and broken bones through offering a wide range of educational resources and programs related to changing one's lifestyle behaviors and appropriate treatment options. Think osteoporosis is just a women's issue? Visit their "Just for Men" resource page to learn more about men and osteoporosis and download "The Man's Guide to Osteoporosis" at http://nof.org/articles/236.

National Resource Center on Osteoporosis and Related Bone Diseases
2 AMS Circle
Bethesda, MD 20892-3676
1-800-624-BONE (1-800-624-2663)
202-466-4315
NIHBoneInfo@mail.nih.gov
www.bones.nih.gov

This national resource center, situated within the NIH, works to increase awareness among professionals, patients, and the public of a variety of bone disorders. The center provides access to online and printed resources on prevention, detection, treatment, and management of bone-related disorders. The center's website features a section devoted to men's health which includes information on osteoporosis and men, as well as on bone health for prostate cancer survivors.

Cancer

American Cancer Society (ACS)
1-800-227-2345
1-866-228-4327
www.cancer.org

The ACS works to help people stay well and get well, by finding cures and by fighting various forms of cancer. It is a nationwide, community-based health organization dedicated to eliminating cancer as a major health problem. The ACS is headquartered in Atlanta, Georgia, and hosts 12 chartered divisions with more than 900 local offices nationwide and a presence in more than 5,100 communities. The ACS provides helpful resources on a wide variety of cancers and can help you connect with local resources.

National Cancer Institute
NCI Office of Communications and Education
Public Inquiries Office
6116 Executive Boulevard, Suite 300
Bethesda, MD 20892-8322
1-800-4-CANCER (1-800-422-6237)
cancergovstaff@mail.nih.gov
www.cancer.gov

The National Cancer Institute, housed within the NIH, is tasked with researching and supporting cancer diagnosis, prevention, treatment, and rehabilitation. The institute funds cancer studies, in addition to providing cancer-related resources specifically for professionals, patients, and the public. The institute's website features a live chat function that allows you to connect with resources and support regarding this issue.

Prostate Cancer Foundation
1250 Fourth Street
Santa Monica, CA 90401
1-800-757-CURE (1-800-757-2873)
info@pcf.org
www.pcf.org

The Prostate Cancer Foundation was established to develop treatment and cures for prostate cancer. As the largest source of support for prostate cancer research, the foundation provides information on prostate cancer to both health care professionals and patients.

The Skin Cancer Foundation
149 Madison Avenue, Suite 901
New York, NY 10016
212-725-5176
www.skincancer.org

The Skin Cancer Foundation has set the standard for educating the public and medical professionals about skin cancer. The foundation teaches prevention and protection strategies, detection, and effective treatment. It is the only international organization devoted solely to combating the world's most common cancer, now occurring at epidemic levels.

Dental

American Dental Association (ADA)
211 East Chicago Avenue
Chicago, IL 60611-2678
312-440-2500
www.ada.org

The ADA is the oldest and largest national dental society in the world and the leading source of oral health information for dentists and the general public. The ADA can help you locate a dentist near you and provide you with the latest information on dental health and dental disorders.

Diabetes and Kidney Disease

American Diabetes Association
ATTN: Center for Information
1701 North Beauregard Street
Alexandria, VA 22311
1-800-DIABETES (1-800-342-2383)
AskADA@diabetes.org
www.diabetes.org

The mission of the American Diabetes Association is to prevent and cure diabetes and improve the lives of all people affected by diabetes through research, advocacy, informational resources, and support services. Visit their website for resources, information, and to find support for those with diabetes.

National Kidney Foundation, Inc.
30 East 33rd Street
New York, NY 10016
1-800-622-9010
www.kidney.org

The National Kidney Foundation works to prevent kidney and urinary tract diseases while improving the lives of those affected by kidney disease. They provide community service, education, and advocacy and support research for new treatments.

Hearing Loss and Vision Loss

American Academy of Otolaryngology—Head and Neck Surgery (AAO-HNS)
1650 Diagonal Road
Alexandria, VA 22314-2857
703-836-4444
www.entnet.org

AAO-HNS is the world's largest organization representing specialists who treat the ear, nose, throat, and related structures of the head and neck. AAO-HNS's website provides a wealth of health information pertaining to issues of the ear, nose, and throat.

American Council of the Blind
2200 Wilson Boulevard, Suite 650
Arlington, VA 22201
1-800-424-8666
info@acb.org
www.acb.org

The council works to improve education, rehabilitation facilities, and opportunities for those who are blind. The council engages in public education and collaborates with public and private institutions that serve the blind in order to both encourage and assist individuals who are blind or visually impaired.

Hearing Loss Association of America (HLAA)
7910 Woodmont Avenue, Suite 1200
Bethesda, MD 20814
301-657-2248
www.hearingloss.org

The HLAA is the nation's leading organization focused on supporting individuals affected by hearing loss. The HLAA carries out this mission by providing resources on hearing loss prevention, treatment, screening, and support. The website for the HLAA features online articles on hearing loss topics, an online support community, and a search tool to assist in locating a local hearing loss professional.

Lighthouse International
111 East 59th Street
New York, NY 10022-1202
1-800-829-0500
www.lighthouse.org

Lighthouse International is the leading organization dedicated to preserving vision and helping people of all ages overcome the challenges of vision loss by providing clinical services, education, research, and advocacy. Their website will help connect you to local resources and providers who can assist with vision loss.

National Eye Institute (NEI)
31 Center Drive
Bethesda, MD 20892-2510
301-496-5248
www.nei.nih.gov

The NEI, part of the NIH, is the federal government's lead agency for vision research. The NIH is an agency of the U.S. Department of Health and Human Services (HHS). NEI's website provides a plethora of information on eye health, as well as up-to-date news and events surrounding vision care.

National Institute on Deafness and Other Communication Disorders (NIDCD)
National Institutes of Health
31 Center Drive, MSC 2510
Bethesda, MD 20892-2510
301-496-7243
nidcdinfo@nidcd.nih.gov
www.nidcd.nih.gov

The NIDCD is a subdivision of the NIH focusing on researching and providing public resources on deafness and communication disorders. The NIDCD website features resources on disorders impacting hearing, balance, smell and taste, voice, speech, and language. NIDCD provides you with the ability to view online articles and resources or order printed materials to be delivered to your home.

Heart Conditions

American Heart Association (AHA)
National Center

7272 Greenville Avenue
Dallas, TX 75231
1-800-242-8721
www.heart.org

American Stroke Association (ASA): A Division of AHA

7272 Greenville Avenue
Dallas, TX 75231-4596
1-888-4STROKE (1-800-478-7653)
214-706-5231
strokeinfo@heart.org
www.strokeassociation.org

The AHA and ASA have a wealth of information on heart health and work to support appropriate cardiac care through education and research with the goal of reducing disability and death. They are widely known for their education in CPR and first aid.

Division for Heart Disease and Stroke Prevention

1600 Clifton Road
Atlanta, GA 30333
1-800-CDC-INFO (1-800-232-4636)
1-888-232-6348
cdcinfo@cdc.gov
www.cdc.gov

Through research and action the Division for Heart Disease and Stroke Prevention focuses on improving cardiovascular health for everyone. They educate on risk and protective factors, detection and treatment, and decreasing reoccurrence of heart attacks and strokes.

Mental Health

Geriatric Mental Health Foundation

7910 Woodmont Avenue, Suite 1050
Bethesda, MD 20814
301-654-7850
web@GMHFonline.org
www.gmhfonline.org

The Geriatric Mental Health Foundation works to raise awareness of geriatric mental health issues, reduce the stigma that surrounds mental illness, increase access to mental health treatment options, and support healthy aging. The consumer/patient section of their website provides information on a variety of mental health topics, including Alzheimer's, caregiving, anxiety, depression, and substance abuse. Their website also features a geriatric psychiatrist locator tool. Printed brochures on geriatric mental health topics are also available through the foundation.

National Alliance on Mental Illness (NAMI)
3803 North Fairfax Drive, Suite 100
Arlington, VA 22203
1-800-950-NAMI (1-800-950-6264)
info@nami.org
www.nami.org

NAMI is a grassroots advocacy organization dedicated to improving the lives of those affected by mental illness. NAMI can help you learn more about national advocacy around mental illness, as well as help you connect with mental health resources, treatment, and support both through their website and through their help line.

National Institute of Mental Health (NIMH)
Science Writing, Press, and Dissemination Branch
6001 Executive Boulevard
Room 6200, MSC 9663
Bethesda, MD 20892-9663
www.nimh.nih.gov

NIMH centers their work on understanding the treatment of mental illness through research that promotes prevention, recovery, and cures. Their research has examined the role of genetics, neuroscience, and psychiatric medications in the causation and treatment of mental illness. The Health Info page of their website provides valuable information about getting help, understanding mental illness, and other items of interest.

Neurological Diseases and Conditions

Alzheimer's Association
225 North Michigan Avenue, Floor 17
Chicago, IL 60601-7633
312-335-8700
1-800-272-3900
312-335-5886
www.alz.org

The Alzheimer's Association offers a toll-free, 24/7 Helpline for Alzheimer information, referrals, and support in multiple languages. Community-based Alzheimer's Association chapters provide services to families and professionals, including information and referrals, support groups, care consultation, education, and safety services.

National Institute of Neurological Disorders and Stroke (NINDS)

PO Box 5801
Bethesda, MD 20824
1-800-352-9424
301-468-5981
www.ninds.nih.gov

The goals of NINDS are to conduct and coordinate research on the causes, prevention, diagnosis, and treatment of neurological disorders and stroke to support those suffering or caring for someone with a neurological disease.

Sleep

American Academy of Sleep Medicine (AASM)

2510 North Frontage Road
Darien, IL 60561
webmaster@aasmnet.org
www.sleepeducation.com

The AASM membership consists of more than 8,000 physicians, researchers, and other health care professionals who are working to set standards in health care, education, and research. The members specialize in studying, diagnosing, and treating disorders of sleep and daytime alertness such as insomnia, narcolepsy, and obstructive sleep apnea. AASM's sleep education website provides a wealth of helpful articles about various sleep disorders.

American Sleep Association (ASA)

www.sleepassociation.org

The ASA increases awareness of the importance of sleep health and the impact of sleep disorders in the community and provides information on symptoms of sleep disorders, treatment, and how to locate a sleep doctor or support group near you.

National Sleep Foundation (NSF)
1010 N. Glebe Road, Suite 310
Arlington, VA 22201
202-347-3471
nsf@sleepfoundation.org
www.sleepfoundation.org

NSF works to educate the public about the importance of adequate sleep and improve the quality of life for those with sleep disorders. NSF promotes proper diagnosis and early detection to maximize the benefits of sleep disorder treatment.

Urologic Conditions

American Urological Association
1000 Corporate Boulevard
Linthicum, MD 21090
1-866-746-4282
info@urologycarefoundation.org
www.urologyhealth.org

The American Urological Association supports and promotes research, patient/public education, and advocacy to improve the prevention, detection, treatment, and cure of urologic diseases. The association provides information for caregivers, patients, researchers, and medical professionals. It also offers a urologist locator service.

The Male Health Center
Dr. Ken Goldberg
541 W. Main Street
Lewisville, TX 75057
www.malehealthcenter.com

The Male Health Center was founded by Dr. Kenneth A. Goldberg, a board-certified urologist. The center's webpage features a range of topics pertaining to issues related to men, including information and tips on sexual health.

National Association for Continence (NAFC)
PO Box 1019
Charleston, SC 29402-1019
1-800-BLADDER (1-800-252-3337)
memberservices@nafc.org
www.nafc.org

The NAFC is a nonprofit dedicated to improving the quality of life of people with incontinence, voiding dysfunction, and related pelvic floor disorders. They offer several helpful publications and services related to treatment, prevention, and advocacy.

SUPPORT SERVICES

Abuse and Violence Resources

National Center on Elder Abuse (NCEA)
c/o University of California–Irvine
Program in Geriatric Medicine
101 The City Drive South
200 Building
Orange, CA 92868
ncea-info@aoa.hhs.gov
www.ncea.aoa.gov

The NCEA is a national resource for elder rights, law enforcement and legal professionals, public policy leaders, researchers, and the public on the issue of elder abuse. The center works to promote understanding, knowledge sharing, and action on elder abuse, neglect, and exploitation. The center's website features resources on identifying, treating, and preventing elder abuse, in addition to providing state-specific resources that can assist you in finding local assistance.

National Domestic Violence Hotline
1-800-799-SAFE (1-800-799-7233)
1-800-787-3224
www.thehotline.org

The National Domestic Violence Hotline provides assistance to anyone involved in a domestic violence situation, including those in same-sex relationships, male survivors, those with disabilities, and immigrant victims of domestic violence. All calls to the National Domestic Violence Hotline are confidential. The hotline website features helpful resources about domestic violence.

Caregiving and Grandparenting

American Association of Retired Persons (AARP) Grandcare Support Locator

www.giclocalsupport.org

The AARP Grandcare Support Locator is a new online database that assists grandparents and other relatives who are raising kin children in finding support and services. The AARP Foundation has launched the Grandcare Support Locator, which allows kinship caregivers to search for specific types of groups and services within their state or jurisdiction. Using the online search form, users can search within their zip code to find services (e.g., child care, health care, respite care, newsletters) or support groups (in-person, telephone support, or online). Users can limit the search to Spanish- or English-language results, and they can restrict the search to items relevant to grandparents raising grandchildren or to grandparents experiencing visitation issues.

AARP Grandparenting Website

www.aarp.org/relationships/grandparenting/

This website, dedicated specifically to grandparenting issues, provides articles on fun activities to do with grandchildren, as well as articles that discuss specific grandparenting issues such as visitation rights and maintaining relationships with your grandchildren.

Generations United (GU)

1331 H Street NW, Suite 900
Washington, DC 20005
202-289-3979
gu@gu.org
www.gu.org

GU is a national organization that works to improve the lives of children, youth, and older people through intergenerational strategies, programs, and public policies. Visit their website to find resources about grandfamilies, intergenerational activities and programs, and intergenerational policy news.

National Alliance for Caregiving

4720 Montgomery Lane, 2nd Floor
Bethesda, MD 20814
info@caregiving.org
www.caregiving.org

The alliance was created to conduct research and policy analysis, develop national programs, increase public awareness of family caregiving issues, strengthen state and local caregiving coalitions, and represent the U.S. caregiving community internationally. The alliance serves as a national resource that works to improve the lives of those who are caring for loved ones.

National Family Caregivers Association (NFCA)
10400 Connecticut Avenue, Suite 500
Kensington, MD 20895-3944
1-800-896-3650
info@thefamilycaregiver.org
www.thefamilycaregiver.org

The NFCA educates, supports, empowers, and serves as a voice for the more than 65 million Americans who are caring for a loved one with a chronic illness or disability. Its website features a variety of helpful features such as practical information about caregiving, books and other resources, and information on how to connect with online caregiver communities and support groups.

Community Services

Aging with Dignity
PO Box 1661
Tallahassee, FL 32302-1661
850-681-2010
1-888-5WISHES (1-888-594-7437)
fivewishes@agingwithdignity.org
www.agingwithdignity.org

Aging with Dignity is a nonprofit dedicated to supporting the ability of individuals to age with dignity, particularly as they approach the end of life. Aging with Dignity fulfills this mission by providing education and advocacy around end-of-life care. You can request a copy of their Five Wishes guide, which is a document that can be used to communicate end-of-life wishes with family members and health care providers.

Benefits CheckUp

www.benefitscheckup.org

This site is a free service of the National Council on Aging designed to help older adults and professionals working with older adults explore public and private benefits available to them. Benefits CheckUp can access information on both local and federal benefits and programs for which an older adult may be eligible. This website also features their Medicare Rx Extra Help Online service for saving money on prescription medications.

Consumer's Guide to Legal Help

www.abanet.org/legalservices/findlegalhelp/home.cfm

This online tool hosted by the American Bar Association assists the public in locating legal help. The guide provides state-by-state options for legal assistance, including legal self-help guides, free local legal assistance, and other legal resources of interest.

Eldercare Locator

www.eldercare.gov
1-800-677-1116

The Eldercare Locator is a free service of the U.S. Administration on Aging which connects older adults and caregivers to information on available services and resources.

Government Benefits Website

www.govbenefits.gov

This website was created to streamline and simplify the process of obtaining benefits information from the federal government. It serves as an online tool that assists in locating the government benefits for which you may qualify.

Hospice Foundation of America

1710 Rhode Island Avenue, NW, Suite 400
Washington, DC 20036
1-800-854-3402
hfaoffice@hospicefoundation.org
www.hospicefoundation.org

Hospice Foundation of America is a national organization working to improve the role of hospice within health care. The foundation provides patient and family education materials about death, dying, bereavement, and hospice care options.

LeadingAge
2519 Connecticut Avenue, NW
Washington, DC 20008-1520
202-783-2242
info@leadingage.org
www.leadingage.org

LeadingAge's 6,000 member organizations work to connect individuals with services all over the country. LeadingAge can provide information about available adult day services, home health, community services, senior housing, assisted living residences, continuing care retirement communities, and nursing homes in your local area.

Medicare Rights Center (MRC)
1224 M Street NW, Suite 100
Washington, DC 20005
202-637-0961
info@medicarerights.org
www.medicarerights.org

MRC is a large independent source of Medicare information for Medicare beneficiaries and professionals who work with beneficiaries. The MRC engages in public policy making, advocacy, technical assistance, direct service through their HMO and Medicare Part D appeals hotlines, education efforts, and public awareness coordinated with media outlets. The MRC website features information and tools for consumers and professionals, as well as publications.

Medicare Website
www.medicare.gov

This is the official website for those with Medicare, profiling Medicare benefits, including a Medicare benefits tool, and also providing information pertaining to local nursing facilities and home health and chronic care services.

National Academy of Elder Law Attorneys
www.naela.org

The National Academy of Elder Law Attorneys is a national organization of attorneys who specialize in the legal issues of older adults and individuals with special needs. The website for this organization can help you connect with a local elder law attorney, in addition to providing access to informational resources about some of the common legal issues faced by older adults and their families.

Social Security Administration (SSA)
Office of Public Inquiries
Windsor Park Building
6401 Security Boulevard
Baltimore, MD 21235
1-800-772-1213
1-800-325-0778
www.ssa.gov

The SSA has information about social security benefits, disability, retirement planning, and Medicare, as well as information specifically for widows and widowers. The SSA also provides a useful 1-800 number and website for more information pertaining to benefits and local SSA offices. Both the SSA phone line and website allow you to apply for benefits or request benefits statements.

USDA Food and Nutrition Service
3101 Park Center Drive, Suite 808
Alexandria, VA 22302
301-504-5414
www.fns.usda.gov/snap/

The USDA Food and Nutrition Service oversees the food stamp program (also known as the Supplemental Nutrition Assistance Program or SNAP) for low-income families and individuals in the United States. The website provides a prescreening tool that provides information on eligibility for the program in addition to a step-by-step guide for consumers on how to apply for food stamps and a locator tool for finding a nearby food stamp program office.

Disability Resources

American Association on Intellectual and Developmental Disabilities (AAIDD)
501 3rd Street, NW, Suite 200
Washington, DC 20001
1-800-424-3688
www.aamr.org

This association promotes universal rights for all people with intellectual disabilities through progressive policies, effective practice, and research. The AAIDD meets this mission through establishing partnerships with other organizations, advocacy, public education, professional development, and taking a multidisciplinary approach. Their website contains resources pertaining to various intellectual and developmental disabilities.

Americans with Disabilities Act

www.ada.gov

This website is the government's link to information about the Americans with Disabilities Act, including links, publications, and information on other agencies of the government which deal with its enforcement.

Disability Information Website

www.disabilityinfo.gov

The government's disability information page includes resources pertaining to independent living, health, housing, civil rights, employment, and education.

Relationships, Sexuality, and Sexual Identity

AARP Love & Sex Website

www.aarp.org/relationships/love-sex/

This is a website set up by AARP to provide information about relationships, love, and sex after 50. AARP provides a wealth of resources that are both engaging to read and easy to understand.

American Social Health Association (ASHA)

PO Box 13827
Research Triangle Park, NC 27709
919-361-8400
919-361-8488
www.ashastd.org

ASHA is recognized for developing and delivering accurate, medically reliable information about sexually transmitted infections. This is where you will find facts, support, resources, questions and answers, and thorough information on sexually transmitted diseases.

National Healthy Marriage Resource Center (NHMRC)

1950 W. Littleton Boulevard #306
Littleton, CO 80120
1-866-916-4672
http://healthymarriageinfo.org

The NHMRC is a clearinghouse for quality, balanced, and timely information and resources on healthy marriage. The NHMRC provides information, resources, and training to a wide variety of audiences, including individuals and couples.

National Resource Center on LGBT Aging
c/o Services & Advocacy for GLBT Elders (SAGE)
305 Seventh Avenue, 6th Floor
New York, NY 10001
212-741-2247
info@lgbtagingcenter.org
www.lgbtagingcenter.org

The National Resource Center on LGBT Aging, the country's first and only technical assistance resource center working to improve the quality of services and support offered to lesbian, gay, bisexual, and transgender (LGBT) older adults, was established in 2010. The center is led by Services & Advocacy for GLBT Elders (SAGE) in partnership with 10 other leading organizations from around the country.

Senior Sex: Tips for Older Men
www.mayoclinic.com/health/senior-sex/MC00057

The Senior Sex webpage was developed by the Mayo Clinic to provide tips for maintaining a healthy and satisfying sex life as you get older.

Resources and Support in Times of Crisis

National Suicide Prevention Lifeline
1-800-273-TALK (1-800-273-8255)
www.suicidepreventionlifeline.org

The National Suicide Prevention Lifeline is a 24-hour, toll-free, confidential suicide prevention hotline available to anyone in crisis or emotional distress. Calls received on the lifeline are routed to the nearest crisis center in a national network of more than 140 crisis centers, which provide crisis counseling and mental health referrals day and night.

Veterans Crisis Line
1-800-273-8255 and Press 1
www.veteranscrisisline.net

This free and confidential crisis line provides support to veterans and their family members who are in crisis or just in need of support. The service is provided 24 hours a day, 7 days a week. In addition to the hotline, the VA provides a free confidential chat via the crisis line website, where you can get support and connect with resources.

Retirement

American Association of Retired Persons (AARP)
601 East Street, NW
Washington, DC 20049
1-888-OUR-AARP (1-888-687-2277)
1-877-434-7589
1-877-MAS-DE50 (1-877-627-3350)
www.aarp.org

AARP serves people 50 and older to enhance the quality of life for all by leading positive social change and delivering value to members through information, advocacy, and service.

Center for Retirement Research
Hovey House
258 Hammond Street
Chestnut Hill, MA 02467
617-552-1762
crr@bc.edu
http://crr.bc.edu

As a facility within Boston College, the Center for Retirement Research's goal is to conduct research on retirement issues and disseminate findings to researchers, policy makers, and the public. The website for the center provides publications on retirement-related issues, benefits, and trends.

Corporation for National and Community Service
1201 New York Avenue, NW
Washington, DC 20525
202-606-5000
1-800-833-3722
info@cns.gov
www.nationalservice.gov

The role of the Corporation for National and Community Service is to engage Americans in service by administering volunteer initiatives such as AmeriCorps and Senior Corps programs. The corporation can help you find volunteer activities of interest to you and connect with local volunteer resources.

Encore Careers

www.encore.org

The Encore Careers website hosted by Civic Ventures is a premier source for information on launching into your own encore career. Encore careers are careers that are taken up later on in life "that combine personal meaning, income, and social impact." Learn more about encore careers, how to find or build one, and read inspiring stories of other baby boomers and older adults who have found careers that are personally meaningful to them.

Substance Abuse Resources

Alcoholics Anonymous (AA)

PO Box 459

New York, NY 10163

212-870-3400

www.aa.org

AA provides support and resources to individuals and families affected by alcohol addiction. The AA model is one that brings together those affected by alcohol addiction to share with one another and support one another so that they may recover from their addiction. The AA site has a locator page that can help you find local meetings and AA chapters.

AA World Services, Inc.

Grand Central Station

PO Box 459

New York, NY 10163

212-870-3400

Al-Anon (for families of alcoholics)

1-888-425-2666

www.al-anon.org

National Clearing House for Alcohol and Drug Information

1-877-726-4727

www.ncadi.samhsa.gov

National Institute on Alcohol Abuse and Alcoholism

301-443-3860

www.niaaa.nih.gov

Substance Abuse and Mental Health Services Administration (SAMHSA)

SAMHSA's Health Information Network
PO Box 2345
Rockville, MD 20847-2345
1-877-SAMHSA-7 (1-877-726-4727)
SAMHSAInfo@samhsa.hhs.gov
www.samhsa.gov

SAMHSA works "to reduce the impact of substance abuse and mental illness on America's communities" by providing information, research, and resources to professionals, researchers, and community members. SAMHSA can provide you with online and printed resources about the latest research, treatment options, and support available to address substance abuse and mental illness.

Notes

CHAPTER 1. MEN'S HEALTH AND HEALTHY AGING

1. Lindau, S. T., & Gavrilova, N. (2010). Sex, health, and years of sexually active life gained due to good health: Evidence from two US population based cross sectional surveys of ageing. *British Medical Journal*, *340*, doi:10.1136/bmj.c810. Cahill, K., Giandrea, M., & Quinn, J. (2006). Retirement patterns from career employment. *Gerontologist*, *46*, 514–523. Merrill Lynch & AgeWave (2005, Feb.). *The Merrill Lynch new retirement survey: A perspective from the baby boomer generation*. Retrieved from http://askmerrill.ml.com /pdf/RetirementSurveyReport.pdf. SunAmerica & AgeWave (2011, July). *The SunAmerica retirement re-set study*. Retrieved from http://retirementreset.com/wp-content/uploads /2011/07/M5124RPT_07111.pdf. Grusky, D. B., Western, B., & Winer C. (2011). *The Great Recession*. New York: Russell Sage Foundation.

2. Charles Schwab & AgeWave (2008, July). *Rethinking retirement: Four generations of Americans share their views on life's third act*. Retrieved from www.agewave.com/research /SummaryReport071108.pdf. American Financial & AgeWave (2006, Jan.). *The new retirement mindscape study*. Retrieved from www.ameriprise.com/global/docs/mindscape-study -0106.pdf. American Financial (2010, Sept.). *The new retirement mindscape II study*. Retrieved from www.ameriprise.com/global/docs/mindscape-ii-study.pdf.

3. Drummond, M. (2003). Retired men, retired bodies. *International Journal of Men's Health*, *2*, 183–199, p. 192.

4. Fischer, D. (1978). *Growing old in America*. New York: Oxford University Press.

5. Butler, R. (1969). Age-ism: Another form of bigotry. *Gerontologist*, *9*, 243–246.

6. Levy, B. R. (2004). Mind matters: Cognitive and physical effects of aging self-stereotypes. *Journal of Gerontology: Psychological Sciences*, *58B*, P203–P211.

7. Hewitt, R. (2012, Spring). New aged. *UMaine Today*, *12* (1), 2–5, p. 3.

8. Snyder, M., & Miene, P. (1994). On the functions of stereotypes and prejudice. In M. P. Zanda & J. M. Olsen (eds.), *The psychology of prejudice: The Ontario symposium*, vol. 7 (pp. 33–54). Hillsdale, NJ: Lawrence Erlbaum.

9. Miner-Rubino, K., Winter, D. G., & Stewart, A. J. (2004). Gender, social class, and the subjective experience of aging: Self-perceived personality change from early adulthood to late midlife. *Personality and Social Psychology Bulletin*, *30*, 1599–1610.

10. Nolan, J., & Scott, J. (2009). Experiences of age and gender: Narratives of progress and decline. *International Journal of Aging and Human Development*, *68*, 133–158.

11. Bureau of the Census (1995). *Sixty-five plus in the United States*. Washington, DC: U.S. Department of Commerce, SB/95-8.

12. National Center for Health Statistics (2010). *Health, United States, 2009: With special feature on medical technology*. Hyattsville, MD.

13. Arias, E., Rostron, B. L., & Tejada-Vera, B. (2010). United States Life Tables, 2005. *National Vital Statistics Reports*, *58* (10). Hyattsville, MD: National Center for Health Statistics.

14. Crescioni, M., Gorina, Y., Bilheimer, L., et al. (2010, Apr. 21). Trends in health status and health care use among older men. *National Health Statistics Reports*, no. 24. Hyattsville, MD: National Center for Health Statistics.

15. Valliant, G. E. (2003). *Aging well: Surprising guidepost to a happier life from the landmark Harvard Study of Adult Development*. New York: Little, Brown.

16. Courtenay, W. H. (2000). Constructions of masculinity and their influence on men's well-being: A theory of gender and health. *Social Science and Medicine, 50,* 1385–1401.

17. Courtenay, W. H. (2000). Engendering health: A social constructionist examination of men's health beliefs and behaviors. *Psychology of Men and Masculinity, 1,* 4–15.

18. Bandura, A. (2004). Health promotion by social cognitive means. *Health Education and Behavior, 31,* 143–164.

19. Reed, D. M., Foley, D. J., White, L. R., et al. (1998). Predictors of healthy aging in men with high life expectancies. *American Journal of Public Health, 88,* 1463–1468.

CHAPTER 2. STAYING ACTIVE

1. Sheffield-Moore, M., Paddon-Jones, D., Cree, M. G., et al. (2005). Effects of androgens on muscle, bone, and hair in men. In R. S. Tan (ed.), *Aging men's health: A case-based approach* (pp. 83–92). New York: Thieme.

2. LaCroix, A. Z., Leveille, S. G., Hecht, J. A., et al. (1996). Does walking decrease the risk of cardiovascular disease hospitalizations and death in older adults? *Journal of the American Geriatrics Society, 44,* 113–120. Ettinger, W. H. (1996). Physical activity and older people: A walk a day keeps the doctor away. *Journal of the American Geriatrics Society, 44,* 207–208.

3. Haskell, W. L., Lee, I., Pate, R. R., et al. (2007). Physical activity and public health: Updated recommendation from the American College of Sports Medicine and the American Heart Association. *Journal of the American College of Sports Medicine, 39,* 1423–1434.

4. Andrew Jackson, Oct. 26 issue of *Archives of Internal Medicine.* Frisard, M. I., Fabre, J. M., Russell, R. D., et al. (2007). Physical activity level and physical functionality in nonagenarians compared to individuals aged 60–74 years. *Journal of Gerontology: Biological Science, 62,* 783–788.

5. Johannsen, D. L., DeLany, J. P., Frisard, M. L., et al. (2008). Physical activity in aging: Comparison among young, aged, and nonagenarian individuals. *Journal of Applied Physiology, 105,* 495–501.

6. Larson, E. B., Wang, L., Bowen, J. D., et al. (2006). Exercise is associated with reduced risk of incident dementia among persons aged 65 and older. *Annals of Internal Medicine, 144,* 73–81.

7. Allender, S., Foster, C., Scarborough, P., et al. (2007). The burden of physical-activity ill health in the U.K. *Journal of Epidemiology and Community Health, 61,* 344–348. Allender, S., Foster, C., & Boxer, A. (2008). Occupational and non-occupational physical activity and the social determinants of physical activity: Results from the Health Survey for England. *Journal of Physical Activity and Health, 5,* 104–116.

8. Centers for Disease Control and Prevention (2003). Prevalence of physical activity, including lifestyle activities among adults—United States, 2000–2001. *Morbidity and Mortality Weekly Report, 52,* 764–768.

9. Drummond, M. (2003). Retired men, retired bodies. *International Journal of Men's Health, 2,* 183–199, p. 193.

10. Allender, S., Cowburn, G., & Foster, C. (2006). Understanding participation in sport and physical activity among children and adults: A review of qualitative studies. *Health Education Research, 21,* 826–835.

11. National Center for Health Statistics (2010). Health, United States, 2009 (Table 72). Hyattsville, MD: U.S. Department of Health and Human Services.

12. Kruger, J., Yore, M. M., & Kohl, H. W. (2008). Physical activity levels and weight control status by body mass index, among adults—National Health and Nutrition Examination Survey 1999–2004. *International Journal of Behavioral Nutrition and Physical Activity*, 5, 5–25.

13. Duncan, G. E., Anton, S. D., Sydeman, S. J., et al. (2005). Prescribing exercise at varied levels of intensity and frequency. *Archives of Internal Medicine*, 165, 2362–2369.

14. Pluim, B. M., Staal, J. B., Marks, B. L., et al. (2007). Health benefits of tennis. *British Journal of Sports Medicine*, 41, 760–768.

15. Aniansson, A., Grimby, G., Rundgren, A., et al. (1980). Physical training in old men. *Age and Ageing*, 9, 186–187. Latham, N. K., Bennett, D. A., Stretlong, C. M., et al. (2004). Systematic review of progressive resistance training in older adults. *Journal of Gerontology: Medical Sciences*, 59, M48–M61.

CHAPTER 3. EATING WELL AND LESS

1. Davidson, K., Aber, S., & Marshall, H. (2008). Gender and food in later life: Shifting roles and relationships. In M. M. Raats, C. P. G. M. De Groot, & W. A. Van Staveren (eds.), *Food for the ageing population* (pp. 110–127). Cambridge, UK: Woodhead.

2. Drummon, M., & Smith, J. (2006). Ageing men's understanding of nutrition: Implications for health. *Journal of Men's Health and Gender*, 3, 55–60.

3. Davidson, K., Aber, S., & Marshall, H. (2008). Gender and food in later life: Shifting roles and relationships. In M. M. Raats, C. P. G. M. De Groot, & W. A. Van Staveren (eds.), *Food for the ageing population* (pp. 110–127). Cambridge, UK: Woodhead.

4. Gough, B., & Conner, M. T. (2006). Barriers to healthy eating amongst men: A qualitative analysis. *Social Science and Medicine*, 62, 387–395.

5. Melanson, K. J. (2008). Promoting nutrition for men's health. *American Journal of Lifestyle Medicine*, 2, 488–492.

6. De Souza, P., & Ciclitira, K. E. (2005). Men and dieting: A qualitative analysis. *Journal of Health Psychology*, 10, 793–804, p. 798.

7. U.S. Department of Health and Human Services. (2000). *Healthy People 2010: Understanding and improving health*. Washington, DC: Government Printing Office.

8. van Dam, R. M., Rimm, E. B., Willet, W. C., et al. (2002). Dietary patterns and risks of Type 2 diabetes mellitus in U.S. men. *Annals of Internal Medicine*, 136, 201–209.

9. Erber, E., Hopping, B. N., Grandinetti, A., et al. (2010). Dietary patterns and risk of diabetes: The multiethnic cohort. *Diabetes Care*, 33, 532–538. Lloyd-Jones, D., Adams, R. J., Brown, T. M., et al. (2010). Heart disease and stroke statistics 2010 update: A report from the American Heart Association. *Circulation*, 121, e46–e215.

10. National Center for Health Statistics (2010). Health, United States, 2009 (Table 72). Hyattsville, MD: U.S. Department of Health and Human Services.

11. Wansink, W., & Payne, C. R. (2008). Eating behavior and obesity at Chinese restaurants. *Obesity*, 16, 1957–1960.

12. Steinert, R. W., Frey, F., Topfer, A., et al. (2011). Effects of carbohydrate sugars and artificial sweeteners on appetite and the secretion of gastrointestinal satiety peptides. *British Journal of Nutrition*, 105, 1320–1328.

13. Butt, M. S., & Sultan, M. T. (2011). Coffee and its consumption: Benefits and risks. *Critical Reviews in Food Science and Nutrition*, 51, 363–373.

14. Cannell, J. J., Hollis, B. W., Zasloff, M., et al. (2008). Diagnosis and treatment of vitamin D deficiency. *Expert Opinion on Pharmacotherapy*, 9, 107–118.

15. Endoy, M. P. (2005). Anorexia among older adults. *American Journal for Nurse Practitioners*, *9* (5), 31–38.

16. Davidson, K., Aber, S., & Marshall, H. (2008). Gender and food in later life: Shifting roles and relationships. In M. M. Raats, C. P. G. M. De Groot, & W. A. Van Staveren (eds.), *Food for the ageing population* (pp. 110–127). Cambridge, UK: Woodhead.

17. Bennett, K., Hughes, G., & Smith, P. (2003). "I think a woman can take it": Widowed men's views and experiences of gender differences in bereavement. *Ageing International*, *28*, 408–424.

CHAPTER 4. PSYCHOLOGY OF HEALTHY AGING

1. Valliant, G. E. (2003). *Aging well: Surprising guidepost to a happier life from the landmark Harvard Study of Adult Development*. New York: Little, Brown. Valliant G. E., & Mulamal, K. (2001). Successful aging. *American Journal of Psychiatry*, *158*, 839–847.

2. Grewal, R. P., & Finch, C. E. (1997). Normal brain aging and Alzheimer's disease pathology. In Brioni, J. D., & Decker, M. W. (eds.), *Pharmacological treatment of Alzheimer's disease: Molecular and neurobiological foundations* (pp. 179–192). New York: Wiley-Liss.

3. Bartzokis G., Lu, P. H, Tingus, K., et al. (2010). Lifespan trajectory of myelin integrity and maximum motor speed. *Neurobiology of Aging*, *31*, 1554–1562.

4. Fjell, A. M., & Walhovd, K. B. (2010). Structural brain changes in aging: Courses, causes and cognitive consequences. *Reviews in the Neurosciences*, *21*, 187–221.

5. Gage F. H., & Van Praag, H. (2008). Neurogenesis in the adult brain. In K. L. Davis, D. Charney, J. T. Coyle, et al. (eds.), *Neuropharmacology: 5th Generation of Progress* (pp. 109–117). Philadelphia: Lippincott, Williams, & Wilkins.

6. Kempermann, G., Gast, D., & Gage, F. H. (2002). Neuroplasticity in old age: Sustained fivefold induction of hippocampal neurogenesis by long-term environmental enrichment. *Annals of Neurology*, *52*, 135–143.

7. Mahncke, H. W., Connor, B. B., Appelman, J., et al. (2006). Memory enhancement in healthy older adults using a brain plasticity-based training program: A randomized, controlled study. *Proceedings of the National Academy of Sciences of the U.S.A.*, *103*, 12523–12528.

8. Brannon, R. (1976). The male sex role: Our culture's blueprint of manhood, and what it's done for us lately. In D. David & R. Brannon (eds.), *The forty-nine percent majority: The male sex role* (pp. 1–45). Reading, MA: Addison-Wesley.

9. Mayr, U., Wozniak, D., Davidson, C., et al. (2012). Competitiveness across the life span: The feisty fifties. *Psychology and Aging*, *27* (2), 278–285.

10. Erikson, E. H. (1959). Identity and the life cycle. *Psychological Issues*, *1*, 18–164. Erikson, E. H. (1982). *The life cycle completed: A review*. New York. W. W. Norton.

11. Erikson, E. H., Erikson, J. M., & Kivnick, H. Q. (1986). *Vital involvement in old age*. New York: W. W. Norton.

12. Cohen, S. (2004). Social relationships and health. *American Psychologist*, *59*, 676–684.

13. Atchley, R. C. (1999). *Continuity and adaptation in aging*. Baltimore, MD: Johns Hopkins University Press.

14. Bosse, R., Aldwin, C. M., Levenson, M. R., et al. (1991). How stressful is retirement? Findings from the Normative Aging Study. *Journal of Gerontology: Psychological Sciences*, *46*, 9–14.

15. Orth, U., Trzeniewski, K. H., & Robins, R. W. (2010). Self-esteem development

from young adulthood to old age: A cohort-sequential longitudinal study. *Journal of Personality and Social Psychology*, *98*, 645–658.

16. Tannenbaum, C. (2011). Effect of age, education and health status on community dwelling older men's health concerns. *Aging Male*. Published ahead of print, doi:10.3109/13685538.2011.626819.

17. Maimaris, W., Hogan, H., & Lock, K. (2010). The impact of working beyond traditional retirement ages on mental health: Implications for public health and welfare policy. *Public Health Reviews*, *32*, 532–548.

18. Myers, J. B., & Meacham, R. B. (2003). Androgen replacement therapy in the aging male. *Reviews in Urology*, *5*, 216–226.

19. Buvat, J., & Lemaire, A. (1997). Endocrine screening in 1,022 men with erectile dysfunction: Clinical significance and cost-effective strategy. *Journal of Urology*, *158*, 1764–1767.

20. Tannenbaum, C. (2011). Effect of age, education and health status on community dwelling older men's health concerns. *Aging Male*. Published ahead of print, doi:10.3109/13685538.2011.626819.

21. Idler, E. L. (2003). Discussion: Gender differences in self-rated health, in mortality, and in the relationship between the two. *Gerontologist*, *43*, 372–375.

22. Deeg, D. J. H., & Kriegsman, D. M. W. (2003). Concepts of self-rated health: Specifying the gender difference in mortality risk. *Gerontologist*, *43*, 376–386.

23. Levy, B. R., Slade, M. D., & Kasl, S. V. (2002). Longitudinal benefit of positive self-perceptions of aging on functional health. *Journal of Gerontology: Psychological Sciences*, *57*, P409–P417. Levy, B. R., Slade, M. D., Kunkel, S. R., et al. (2003). Longevity increased by positive self-perceptions of aging. *Journal of Personality and Social Psychology*, *83*, 261–270.

24. Caserta, M. S. (2003). Widowers. In R. Kastenbaum (ed.), *Macmillan encyclopedia of death and dying* (pp. 933–938). New York: Macmillan. Glick, I. O., Weiss, R. O., & Parkes, C. M. (1974). *The first year of bereavement*. New York: John Wiley & Sons. Lund, D. A., & Caserta, M.S. (2001). When the unexpected happens: Husbands coping with the deaths of their wives. In D. Lund (ed.), *Men coping with grief* (pp. 147–167). Amityville, NY: Baywood. Richardson, V. E., & Balaswamy, S. (2001). Coping with bereavement among elderly widowers. *Omega: Journal of Death and Dying*, *43*, 129–144.

25. Bennett, K. (2005). "Was life worth living?" Older widowers and their explicit discourses of the decision to live. *Mortality*, *10*, 144–154. Bennett, K. (2007). "No sissy stuff": Towards a theory of masculinity and emotional expression in older widowed men. *Journal of Aging Studies*, *21*, 347–356.

26. Addis, M. E. (2008). Gender and depression in men. *Clinical Psychology: Science and Practice*, *15*, 153–168.

27. Magovcevic, M., & Addis, M. E. (2008). The Masculine Depression Scale: Development and psychometric evaluation. *Psychology of Men and Masculinity*, *9*, 117–132.

28. Cochran, S. V., & Rabinowitz, R. E. (2000). *Men and depression: Clinical and empirical perspectives*. San Diego: Academic Press. Real, T. (1998). *I don't want to talk about it: Overcoming the secret legacy of male depression*. New York: Simon & Schuster. Addis, M. E. (2011). *Invisible men: Men's inner lives and the consequences of silence*. New York: Times Books.

29. Addis, M. E., & Mahalik, J. R. (2003). Men, masculinity, and the contexts of help-seeking. *American Psychologist*, *58*, 5–14.

30. Kessler, R. C., McGonagle, K. A., Swartz, M., et al. (1993). Sex and depression in the National Comorbidity Survey I: Lifetime prevalence, chronicity, and recurrence. *Journal of Affective Disorders*, *29*, 85–96.

31. Davidson, J. R. T., & Meltzer-Brody, S. E. (1999). The under-recognition and under-treatment of depression: What is the breadth and depth of the problem? *Journal of Clinical Psychiatry, 60* (suppl. 7), 4–9.

32. Bruce, M. L. (2002). Psychosocial risk factors for depressive disorders in late life. *Biological Psychiatry, 52,* 175–184.

33. Alexopoulos, G. S., Buckwalter, K., Olin, J., et al. (2002). Co-morbidity of late life depression: An opportunity for research in mechanisms and treatment. *Biological Psychiatry, 52,* 543–558.

34. Shenk, J. W. (2005). *Lincoln's melancholy: How depression challenged a president and fueled his greatness.* Boston: Houghton Mifflin.

35. Flint, A. J. (2002). The complexity and challenge of non-major depression in late life. *American Journal of Geriatric Psychiatry, 10* (3), 229–232.

36. Kessler, R. C., Chiu, W. T., Demler, O., et al. (2005). Prevalence, severity, and comorbidity of twelve-month DSM-IV disorders in the National Comorbidity Survey Replication (NCS-R). *Archives of General Psychiatry, 62,* 617–627.

37. Kessler, R. C., Tubinow, D. R., Holmes, C., et al. (1997). The epidemiology of DSM-III-R bipolar I disorder in a general population survey. *Psychological Medicine, 27,* 1079–1089. Arnold, L. M. (2003). Gender differences in bipolar disorder. *Psychiatric Clinics of North America, 26,* 595–620.

38. Gildengers, A. G., Butters, M. A., Seligman, K., et al. (2004). Cognitive functioning in late life: Bipolar disorder. *American Journal of Psychiatry, 161,* 736–738.

39. Charles, S. T., & Carstensen, L. L. (2010). Social and emotional aging. *Annual Review of Psychology, 61,* 383–409.

40. Cozolino, L. (2008). *The healthy aging brain.* New York: W. W. Norton.

CHAPTER 5. MEN'S STRESS AND HEALTH

1. Marmot, M. (2005). *The status syndrome: How social standing affects our health and longevity.* New York: Holt.

2. Kiecolt-Glaser, J. K., & Galser, R. (1989). Psychoneuroimmunology: Past, present, and future. *Health Psychology, 8,* 677–682.

3. Real, T. (1997). *I don't want to talk about it: Overcoming the secret legacy of male depression.* New York: Fireside.

4. Matthews, K. A., Weiss, S. M., Detre, T., et al. (1986). *Handbook of stress, reactivity, and cardiovascular disease.* New York: Wiley.

5. Dienstbier, R. A. (1989). Arousal and physiological toughness: Implications for mental and physical health. *Psychological Review, 96,* 84–100.

6. Courtenay, W. H. (2000). Constructions of masculinity and their influence on men's well-being: A theory of gender and health. *Social Science and Medicine, 50,* 1385–1401.

7. Folkman, S., & Lazarus, R. S. (1985). If it changes it must be a process: Study of emotion and coping during three stages of a college examination. *Journal of Personality and Social Psychology, 48,* 150–170.

8. Eisler, R. M., & Skidmore, J. R. (1987). Masculine gender role stress: Scale development and component factors in the appraisal of stressful situations. *Behavior Modification, 11,* 123–136. O'Neil, J. M. (2008). Summarizing twenty-five years of research on men's gender role conflict using the Gender Role Conflict Scale: New research paradigms and clinical implications. *Counseling Psychologist, 36,* 358–445.

9. Taylor, S. E., Burklund, L. J., Eisenberger, N. I., et al. (2008). Neural bases of

moderation of cortisol stress responses by psychosocial resources. *Journal of Personality and Social Psychology, 95,* 197–211.

10. Levesque, K., Moskowitz, D. S., Tardif, J., et al. (2010). Physical stress responses in defensive individuals: Age and sex matter. *Psychophysiology, 47,* 332–341.

11. Thoits, P. A. (2010). Stress and health: Major findings and policy implications. *Journal of Health and Social Behavior, 51* (suppl.), S41–S53.

12. Scully, J. A., Tosi, H., & Banning, K. (2000). Life events checklist: Revisiting the Social Readjustment Rating Scale after 30 years. *Educational and Pyschological Measurement, 60,* 864–876.

13. Fiske, A., Gatz, M., & Pedersen, N. L. (2003). Depressive symptoms and aging: The effects of illness and non-health-related events. *Journal of Gerontology: Psychological Science, 58,* P320–P328.

14. Kivimaki, M., Vahtera, J., Elovainio, M., et al. (2002). Death or illness of a family member, violence, interpersonal conflict, and financial difficulties as predictors of sickness absence: Longitudinal cohort study on psychological and behavioral links. *Psychosomatic Medicine, 64,* 817–825.

15. Marmot, M. (2005). *The status syndrome: How social standing affects our health and longevity.* New York: Holt.

16. Todorava, I. L. G., Falcon, L. M., Lincoln, A. K., et al. (2010). Perceived discrimination, psychological distress, and health. *Sociology of Health and Illness, 32,* 843–861. Pieterse, A. L., & Carter, R. T. (2007). An examination of the relationship between general life stress, racism-related stress, and psychological health among black men. *Journal of Counseling Psychology, 54,* 101–109.

17. Sapolsky, R. M. (1990). Stress in the wild. *Scientific American, 252,* 116–123.

18. Williams, D. R. (2003). The health of men: Structured inequalities and opportunities. *American Journal of Public Health, 93,* 724–731.

19. Cannon, W. B. (1932). *The wisdom of the body.* New York: W. W. Norton.

20. Seyle, H. (1956). *The stress of life.* New York: McGraw-Hill. Seyle, H. (1974). *Stress without distress.* Philadelphia: Lippincott.

21. Lazarus, R. S. (1968). Emotions and adaptation: Conceptual and empirical relations. In W. J. Arnold (ed.), *Nebraska symposium on motivation,* vol. 16 (pp. 175–266). Lincoln: University of Nebraska Press. Lazarus, R. S., & Folkman, S. (1984). *Stress, appraisal and coping.* New York: Springer.

22. Folkman, S. (1984). Personal control and stress and coping processes: A theoretical analysis. *Journal of Personality and Social Psychology, 46,* 839–852.

23. Ming, E. E., Adler, G. K., Kessler, R. C., et al. (2004). Cardiovascular reactivity to work stress predicts subsequent onset of hypertension: The Air Traffic Controller Health Change Study. *Psychosomatic Medicine, 66,* 459–465.

24. Lundberg, U. (2005). Stress hormones in health and illness: The roles of work and gender. *Psychoeuroendocrinology, 10,* 1017–1021.

25. Levenstein, S. (1998). Stress and peptic ulcer: Life beyond helicobacter. *British Medical Journal, 316,* 538–541.

26. Kiecolt-Glaser, J. K., & Glaser, R. (1999). Psychoneuroimmunology and cancer: Fact or fiction? *European Journal of Cancer, 35,* 1603–1607.

27. Block, J. P., He, Y., Zaslavsky, A. M., et al. (2009). Psychosocial stress and change in weight among US adults. *American Journal of Epidemiology, 170,* 181–192. Kivmaki, M., Head, J., Ferrie, J. E., et al. (2006). Work stress, weight gain and weight loss: Evidence for bidirectional effects of job strain on body mass index in the Whitehall II study. *International Journal of Obesity, 30,* 982–987.

28. Chandola, T., Brunner, E., & Marmot, M. (2006, Jan. 20). Chronic stress at work and the metabolic syndrome: Prospective study. *British Medical Journal, 332,* 521–525.

29. Newcomer, J. W., Selke, G., Melson, A. K., et al. (1999). Decreased memory performance in healthy humans induced by stress-level cortisol treatment. *Archives of General Psychiatry, 56,* 527–533.

30. Maslach, C., Schaufeli, W. B., & Lieter, M. P. (2001). Job burn out. *Annual Review of Psychology, 52,* 397–422.

31. Zapf, D., Seifert, C., Schmutte, B., et al. (2001). Emotion work and job stressors and their effects on burnout. *Psychology and Health, 16,* 527–545.

32. Flint, A. J. (1994). Epidemiology and comorbidity of anxiety disorders in the elderly. *American Journal of Psychiatry, 151,* 640–649. Flint, A. J. (1995). Anxiety and its disorders in later life: Moving the field forward. *American Journal of Geriatric Psychiatry, 13,* 3–6.

33. Flint, A. J. (1999). Epidemiology and comorbidity of anxiety disorders in later life: Implications for treatment. *Clinical Neuroscience, 4,* 31–36.

34. Kessler, R. C., Sonnega, A., Bromet, E., et al. (1995). Posttraumatic stress disorder in the National Comorbidity Survey. *Archives of General Psychiatry, 52,* 1048–1060.

35. Kessler, R. C., Sonnega, A., Bromet, E., et al. (1995). Posttraumatic stress disorder in the National Comorbidity Survey. *Archives of General Psychiatry, 52,* 1048–1060.

36. Prins, A., Ouimette, P., Kimerling, R., et al. (2003). The primary care PTSD screen (PC-PTSD): Development and operating characteristics. *Primary Care Psychiatry, 9,* 9–14.

37. Buunk, B. P., Collins, R. L., Taylor, S. E., et al. (1990). The affect consequences of social comparison: Either direction has its ups and downs. *Journal of Personality and Social Psychology, 59,* 1238–1249.

38. Cosley, B. J., McCoy, S. K., Saslow, L. R., et al. 2010. Is compassion for others stress buffering? Consequences of compassion and social support for physiological reactivity to stress. *Journal of Experimental Social Psychology, 46,* 816–823.

39. Taylor, S. E., Klein, L. C., Lewis, B. P., et al. (2000). Biobehavioral responses to stress in females: Tend-and-befriend, not fight-or-flight. *Psychological Review, 107,* 411–429.

40. Glynn, L. M., Christenfeld, N., & Gerin, W. (1999). Social support, gender, and cardiovascular responses to stress. *Psychosomatic Medicine, 61,* 234–242.

CHAPTER 6. SOCIAL HEALTH: VITAL RELATIONSHIPS

1. Russell, R. D. (1973). Social health: An attempt to clarify this dimension of well-being. *International Journal of Health Education, 16,* 74–82.

2. Smith, K. P., & Christakis, N. A. (2008). Social networks and health. *Annual Review of Sociology, 34,* 405–429.

3. Lillard, L. A., & Panis, C. W. A. (1996). Marital status and mortality: The role of health. *Demography, 33,* 313–327.

4. Durkheim, E. (1951). *Suicide: A study in sociology.* New York: Free Press.

5. Schmutte, T., O'Connell, M., Weiland, M., et al. (2009). Stemming the tide of suicide in older white men: A call to action. *American Journal of Men's Health, 3,* 189–200.

6. Rosenthal, C. J. (1985). Kinkeeping in the familiar division of labor. *Journal of Marriage and the Family, 47,* 965–974.

7. Swain, S. (1989). Covert intimacy: Closeness in men's friendships. In B. J. Risman & P. Schwartz (eds.), *Gender in intimate relationships* (pp. 71–86). Belmont, CA: Wadsworth. Walker, K. (1995). Men, women, and friendship: What they say; what they do.

Gender & Society, *8*, 246–265. Walker, K. (1994). "I'm not friends the way she's friends": Ideological and behavioral constructions of masculinity in men's friendships. *Masculinities*, 2 (2), 38–55.

8. Zaslow, J. (2010, Apr. 7). Friendship for guys (No tears!). *Wall Street Journal*, D1.

9. Garfinkel, P. (2011, July 25). Men in grief seek others who mourn as they do. *New York Times*, D5.

10. Swain, S. O. (1989). Covert intimacy: Closeness in men's friendships. In B. J. Risman & P. Schwartz (eds.), *Gender in intimate relationships: A microstructural approach* (pp. 71–86). Belmont, CA: Wadsworth.

11. Strate, L. C. (2001). Beer commercials: A manual on masculinity. In S. Craig (ed.), *Men, masculinity and the media* (pp. 78–92). Newbury Park, CA: Sage.

12. Matthews, S. H. (1986). *Friendships through the life course: Oral biographies in old age*. Beverly Hills, CA: Sage.

13. Plath, D. W. (1980). *Long engagements: Maturity in modern Japan*. Stanford, CA: Stanford University Press. Kahn, R. L., & Antonucci, T. C. (1980). Convoys over the life course. Attachment, roles, and social support. In P. B. Baltes & O. G. Brim (eds.), *Life-span development and behavior* (pp. 254–283). New York: Academic Press.

14. Field, D. (1999). Continuity and change in friendships in advanced old age: Findings from the Berkeley Older Generation Study. *International Journal of Aging and Human Development*, *48*, 325–346.

15. Stevens, N. L., & Van Tilburg, T. G. (2010). Cohort differences in having and retaining friends in personal networks in later life. *Journal of Personal and Social Relationships*, *28*, 24–43.

16. Matthews, S. H. (1986). *Friendships through the life course*. Beverly Hills, CA: Sage. Matthews, S. H., Delaney, P. J., and Adamek, M. E. (1989). Male kinship ties: Bonds between adult brothers. *American Behavioral Scientist*, *33*, 58–69. Matthews, S. H. (1994). Men's ties to siblings in old age: Contributing factors to availability and quality. In E. H. Thompson Jr. (ed.), *Older men's lives* (pp. 178–196). Newbury Park, CA: Sage. Bedford, V. H., & Avioli, P. S. (2006). "Shooting the bull": Cohort comparisons of fraternal intimacy in midlife and old age. In V. H. Bedford & B. F. Turner (eds.), *Men in relationships: A new look from a life course perspective* (pp. 81–101). New York: Springer.

17. Thomas, D. (1985). *A child's Christmas in Wales*. New York: Holiday House.

18. Mason, J., May, V., & Clarke, L. (2007). Ambivalence and the paradoxes of grandparenting. *Sociological Review*, *55*, 687–706.

19. Sorensen, P., & Cooper, N. J. (2010). Reshaping the family man: A grounded theory study of the meaning of grandfatherhood. *Journal of Men's Studies*, *18*, 117–136, p. 128.

20. Waldrop, D., Weber, J., Herald, S., et al. (1999). Wisdom and life experience: How grandfathers mentor their grandchildren. *Journal of Aging and Identity*, *4*, 33–46.

21. Szinovacz, M. (1998). Grandparents today: A demographic profile. *Gerontologist*, *38*, 37–52.

22. Dellmann-Jenkins, M., Papalia, D., & Lopez, M. (1985). Teenagers' reported interaction with grandparents: Exploring the extent of alienation. *Journal of Family and Economic Issues*, *8* (3/4), 35–46. van Ranst, N., Verschueren, K., & Marcoen, A. (1995). The meaning of grandparents as viewed by adolescent grandchildren: An empirical study in Belgium. *International Journal of Aging and Human Development*, *41*, 311–324.

23. Townsend, N. W. (2002). *The package deal: Marriage, work and fatherhood in men's lives*. Philadelphia, PA: Temple University Press.

24. Cherlin, A. (1992). *Marriage, divorce, remarriage* (3rd ed.). Cambridge, MA: Harvard University Press.

25. Brown, S. L., & Lin, I. F. (2010). *Divorced in middle life and later life: New estimates from the 2009 American Community Survey*. The Center for Family and Demographic Research at Bowling Green State University.

26. Montenegro, X. P. (2004). *The divorce experience: A study of divorce at midlife and beyond*. Washington, DC: American Association of Retired People.

27. Gerson, K. (2009). *The unfinished revolution: How a generation is reshaping family, work, and gender in America*. New York: Vintage Books.

28. Vaughn, D. (1990). *Uncoupling: Turning points in intimate relationships*. New York: Vintage Books.

29. Stevenson, B., & Wolfers, J. (2007). Marriage and divorce: Changes and their driving forces. PSC Working Paper Series PSC 07–04. Lin, I., & Brown, S. L. (2012). Unmarried boomers confront old age: A national portrait. *Gerontologist, 52*, 153–165.

30. Kreider, R. M. (2005). Number, time, and duration of marriages and divorces: 2001. Current Population Reports, P70-97. Washington, DC: U.S. Census Bureau.

31. Parkes, C. M., Benjamin, B., & Fitzgerald, R. G. (1969). Broken heart: A statistical study of increased mortality among widowers. *British Medical Journal, 1*, 740–743.

32. Koren, C., & Eisikovits, Z. (2010). Life beyond the planned script: Accounts and secrecy of older persons living in second couplehood in old age in a society in transition. *Journal of Social and Personal Relationships, 28*, 44–63.

33. Moore, A., & Stratton, D. 2003. *Resilient widowers: Older men adjusting to a new life*. New York: Prometheus Books.

34. Bennett, K. M. (2007). "No sissy stuff": Towards a theory of masculinity and emotional expression in older widowed men. *Journal of Aging Studies*, 21, 347–356. Bennett, K. M. (2010). How to achieve resilience as an older widower: Turning points or gradual change? *Ageing & Society*, 30, 369–382.

35. Klinenberg, E. (2012). *Going solo. The extraordinary rise and surprising appeal of living alone*. New York: Penguin. Caserta, M. S. (2003). Widowers. In R. Kastenbaum (ed.), *Macmillan encyclopedia of death and dying* (pp. 933–938). New York: Macmillan.

36. Mahay, J., & Lewin, A. C. (2007). Age and the desire to marry. *Journal of Family Issues, 28*, 706–723.

37. Calasanti, T., & Kiecolt, K. J. (2007). Diversity among late-life couples. *Generations, 31* (3), 10–17.

38. Glick, I. O., Weiss, R. O., & Parkes, C. M. (1974). *The first year of bereavement*. New York: John Wiley & Sons.

39. Reissman, C. K. (1990). *Divorce talk: Women and men make sense of personal relationships*. Piscataway, NJ: Rutgers University Press.

40. Davidson, K. (2001). Late life widowhood, selfishness and new partnership choices: A gendered perspective. *Ageing and Society, 21*, 297–317, p. 313.

41. Carr, D. (2004). The desire to date and remarry among older widows and widowers. *Journal of Marriage and Family, 66*, 1051–1068.

42. Laumann, E. O., Gagnon, J. H., Michael, R. T., et al. (2007). A study of sexuality and health among older adults in the United States. *New England Journal of Medicine, 357*, 762–777.

43. Sweeney, M. M. (2010). Remarriage and stepfamilies: Strategic sites for family scholarship in the 21st century. *Journal of Marriage and Family, 72*, 667–684.

44. de Jong Gierveld, J. (2004). Remarriage, unmarried cohabitation, living apart together: Partner relationships following bereavement or divorce. *Journal of Marriage and Family, 66*, 236–243.

45. AARP (2005). *Sex at midlife and beyond: 2004 update on attitudes and behavior*. Washington, DC: American Association of Retired Persons, table 15a.

46. Madden, M. (2010). Older adults and social media. Social networking use among those age 50 and older nearly doubled over the past year. Washington, DC: Pew Research Center. Retrieved July 22, 2011, from http://pewinternet.org/Reports/2010/Older -Adults-and-Social-Media.aspx.

47. Schwalbe, R. (2008). *Sixty, sexy, and successful*. Westport, CT: Praeger, pp. 129–131.

48. Leslie, B., & Morgan, M. (2011). Soulmates, compatibility and intimacy: Allied discursive resources in the struggle for relationship satisfaction in the new millennium. *New Ideas in Psychology, 29*, 10–23. Baker, A. J. (2005). *Double click: Romance and commitment among online couples*. Cresskill, NJ: Hampton.

49. van den Hoonaard, D. (2010). *By himself: The older man's experience of widowhood*. Toronto: University of Toronto Press.

50. Caradec, V. (1997). Forms of conjugal life among the "young elderly." *Population: An English Selection, 9*, 47–73, p. 55.

51. Strohm, C. Q., Seltzer, J. A., Cochran, S. D., et al. (2009). "Living apart together" relationships in the United States. *Demographic Research, 21*, 177–214.

52. House, J. S., Robbins, C., & Metzner, H. L. (1982). The association of social relationships and activities with mortality: Prospective evidence from the Tecumseh Community Health Study. *American Journal of Epidemiology, 116*, 123–140.

53. Shippy, R. A., Cantor, M. H., & Brennan, M. (2004). Social networks of aging gay men. *Journal of Men's Studies, 13*, 107–120.

54. Simons, T., & O'Connell, M. (2003). Married-couple and unmarried partner households: 2000. Washington, DC: U.S. Census Bureau. Retrieved June 14, 2011, from www.census.gov/prod/2003pubs/censr-5.pdf.

55. Kimmel, D. C. (1978). Adult development and aging: A gay perspective. *Journal of Social Issues, 34* (3), 113–130.

56. Nardi, P. (1992). That's what friends are for: Friends as family in the lesbian and gay community. In K. Plummer (ed.), *Modern homosexualities: Fragments of lesbian and gay experience* (pp. 108–120). New York: Routledge.

57. Heaphy, B., Yip, A. K. T., & Thompson, D. (2004). Ageing in a non-heterosexual context. *Ageing & Society, 24*, 881–902, p. 889.

58. Bergling, T. (2004). *Reeling in the years: Gay men's perspectives on age and ageism*. Binghamton, NY: Harrington Park.

59. Metlife Mature Market Institute & the Lesbian and Gay Aging Issues Network of the American Society on Aging (2010). Out and aging: The MetLife study of lesbian and gay baby boomers. *Journal of GLBT Family Studies, 6*, 40–57.

60. McLaughlin, K. A., Hatzenbuehler, M. L., & Keyes, K. M. (2010). Responses to discrimination and psychiatric disorders among black, Hispanic, female, and lesbian, gay, and bisexual individuals. *American Journal of Public Health, 100*, 1477–1484.

61. Stein, G. L., Beckerman, N. L., & Sherman, P. A. (2010). Lesbian and gay elders and long-term care: Identifying the unique psychosocial perspectives and challenges. *Journal of Gerontological Social Work, 53*, 421–435, p. 429.

62. Cahill, S., South, K., & Spade, J. (2000). *Outing age: Public policy issues affecting gay, lesbian, bisexual and transgender elders*. Washington, DC: Policy Institute of the National Gay and Lesbian Task Force Foundation.

63. Wagner, J. F. (2012, June 19). Hurt and dismayed by marriage inequality. Letter, *Plain Dealer*, A7.

64. Putnam, R. D. (2000). *Bowling alone: The collapse and revival of American community*. New York: Simon & Schuster.

65. Rozario, P. A. (2006). Volunteering among current cohorts of older adults and baby boomers. *Generations, 30* (4), 31–36.

CHAPTER 7. SLEEP: A NECESSITY OF LIFE

1. Unruh, M. L. (2008). Subjective and objective sleep quality and aging in the sleep heart health study. *American Geriatrics Society Journal, 56*, 1218–1227.

2. The American Heritage® Medical Dictionary (2007). New York: Houghton Mifflin.

3. Moore-Ede, M. C., Sulszman, F. M., & Fuller, C. A. (1982). *The clocks that time us: Physiology of the circadian timing system.* Cambridge, MA: Harvard University Press.

4. Arendt, J. (2005). Melatonin: Characteristics, concerns, and prospects. *Journal of Biological Rhythms, 20*, 291–303.

5. Borbély, A. (1982). A two process model of sleep regulation. *Human Neurobiology, 1*, 195–204.

6. Pace-Schott, E. F., & Spencer, R. M. (2011). Age-related changes in the cognitive function of sleep. *Progress in Brain Research, 191*, 75–89. Harand, C., Bertran, F., Doidy, F., et al. (2012, Feb.). How aging affects sleep-dependent memory consolidation? *Frontiers in Neurology.* Epub ahead of print, doi:10.3389fneuro.2012.00008.

7. Sassin, J. F., Parker, D. C., Mace, J. W., et al. (1969). Human growth hormone release: Relation to slow-wave sleep and sleep-waking cycles. *Science, 165*, 513–515.

8. Meadows, R., Arber, S., Venn, S., et al. (2008). Engaging with sleep: Male definitions, understandings and attitudes. *Sociology of Health and Illness, 30*, 696–710.

9. Sainz, R. M., Mayo, J. C., Tan, D. X., et al. (2005). Melatonin reduces prostate cancer cell growth leading to neuroendocrine differentiation via a receptor and PKA independent mechanism. *Prostate, 63*, 29–43.

10. Mongrain, V., Carrier, J., & Dumont, M. (2006). Circadian and homeostatic sleep regulation in morningness-eveningness. *Journal of Sleep Research, 15*, 162–166.

11. Dijk, D. J., Groeger, J. A., Stanley, N., et al. (2010). Age-related reduction in daytime sleep propensity and nocturnal slow wave sleep. *Sleep, 33*, 211–223. Klerman, E. B., & Dijk, D. J. (2008). Age-related reduction in the maximal capacity for sleep: Implications for insomnia. *Current Biology, 18*, 1118–1123.

12. Biss, R. K., & Hasher, L. (2012). Happy as a lark: Morning-type younger and older adults are higher in positive affect. *Emotion, 12*, 437–441.

13. *International classification of sleep disorders, revised: Diagnostic and coding manual,* 2nd ed. (2005). Darien, IL: American Academy of Sleep Medicine.

14. Sack, R. L. (2010). Jet lag. *New England Journal of Medicine, 362*, 440–447. Yanni, E. A. (2012). Jet lag. In G. W. Brunette, P. E. Kozarsky, & A. J. Magill (eds.), *CDC health information for international travel 2012: The yellow book* (pp. 65–67). Atlanta, GA: Centers for Disease Control and Prevention.

15. National Sleep Foundation (2011). *Annual sleep in America poll exploring connections with communications technology use and sleep.* Arlington, VA: National Sleep Foundation.

16. Maher, S. (2005). Sleep in the older adult. *Nursing Older People, 16* (9), 30–35.

17. Ohayon, M. M. (2002). Epidemiology of insomnia: What we know and what we still need to learn. *Sleep Medicine Reviews, 6*, 97–111. Calen, M., Bisla, J., Dewey, M., et al. (2012). Increased prevalence of insomnia and changes in hypnotics used in England over 15 years: Analysis of the 1993, 2007, and 2007 National Psychiatric Morbidity Surveys. *Sleep, 35*, 377–384.

18. Perlis, M. L., McCall, W. V., Jungquist, C. R., et al. (2005). Placebo effects in primary insomnia. *Sleep Medicine Reviews, 9*, 381–389.

19. Jordan, A., & McEnvoy, R. D. (2003). Gender differences in sleep apnea: Epidemiology, clinical presentation and pathogenic mechanisms. *Sleep Medicine Reviews, 7*, 377–389.

20. Young, T., Palta, M., Dempsey, J., et al. (1993). The occurrence of sleep-disordered breathing among middle-aged adults. *New England Journal of Medicine, 328*, 1230–1235.

21. National Institutes of Health (2005, Mar. 16). *Sleep and aging*. Bethesda, MD: National Institutes of Health.

22. Postuma, R. B., Gagnon, J. F., Vendette, M., et al. (2009). Quantifying the risk of neurodegenerative disease in idiopathic REM sleep behavior disorder. *Neurology*, *72*, 1296–1300.

23. National Sleep Foundation (2009). *Sleep in America poll*. Washington, DC: National Sleep Foundation.

24. Johns, M. W. (1991). A new method for measuring daytime sleepiness: The Epworth Sleepiness Scale. *Sleep*, *14*, 540–545. Johns, M. W. (1993). Daytime sleepiness, snoring, and obstructive sleep apnea. The Epworth Sleepiness Scale. *Chest*, *103*, 30–36.

25. Murck, H., Nickel, T., Kunzel, H., et al. (2003). State markers of depression in sleep EEG: Dependency on drug and gender in patients treated with tianeptine or paroxetine. *Neuropsychopharmacology*, *28*, 348–358.

26. Ancoli-Israel, S. (2004). Sleep disorders in older adults: A primary care guide to assessing 4 common sleep problems in geriatric patients. *Geriatrics*, *59* (1), 37–40.

27. Lamberg, L. (2010). Sleep treatments improve PTSD symptoms in vets. *Psychiatric News*, *45* (18), 5–23.

28. Tanaka, H., Taira, K., & Arakawa, M. (2002). Short naps and exercise improve sleep quality and mental health in the elderly. *Psychiatry and Clinical Neurosciences*, *56*, 233–234.

29. Li, F., Fisher, J., & Harmer, P. (2004). Tai Chi and self-rated quality of sleep and daytime sleepiness in older adults: A randomized controlled trial. *Journal of the American Geriatrics Society*, *52* (6), 892–900.

30. Reid, K. J., Baron, K. G., Lu, B., et al. (2010). Aerobic exercise improves self-reported sleep and quality of life in older adults with insomnia. *Sleep Medicine*, *11* (9), 934–940.

31. Buysse, D. J., Browman, K. E., Monk, T. H., et al. (1992). Napping and 24-hour sleep/wake patterns in healthy elderly and young adults. *Journal of the American Geriatrics Society*, *40*, 779–786.

32. USA Weekend Extra (2010, Oct. 25–28). Be the best you can be, p. 15.

CHAPTER 8. APPEARANCES: OUR BODIES, HEAD TO TOE

1. Algars, M., Santtila, P., Varjone, M., et al. (2009). The adult body: How age, gender and body mass index are related to body image. *Journal of Aging and Health*, *21*, 1112–1132.

2. Tiggemann M. (1992). Body-size dissatisfaction: Individual differences in age and gender, and relationship with self-esteem. *Personality and Individual Differences*, *13*, 39–43.

3. Davidson, T. E., & McCabe, M. P. (2005). Relationships between men's and women's body image and their psychological, social, and sexual functioning. *Sex Roles*, *54*, 463–475.

4. Baker, L., & Gringart, E. (2009). Body image and self-esteem in older adulthood. *Ageing & Society*, *29*, 977–995.

5. McCabe, M. P., & McGreevy, S. (2010). The role of partners in shaping the body image and body change strategies in adult men. *Health*, *2*, 1002–1009.

6. Stough, D., Stenn, K., Haber, R., et al. (2005). Psychological effect, pathophysiology, and management of androgenic alopecia in men. *Mayo Clinic Proceedings*, *80*, 1316–1322. Hunt, N., & McHale, S. (2005). The psychological impact of alopecia. *British Medical Journal*, *331*, 951–953.

7. Wells, P. A., Willmoth, T., & Russell, R. J. H. (1995). Does fortune favour the bald? Psychological correlates of hair loss in males. *British Journal of Psychology, 86,* 337–344.

8. Severi, G., Sinclair, J. L., Hopper, R., et al. (2003). Androgenetic alopecia in men aged 40–69 years: Prevalence and risk factors. *British Journal of Dermatology, 149,* 1207–1213. Rhodes, T., Girman, C. J., Salvin, R. C., et al. (1998). Prevalence of male pattern hair loss in 18–49 year old men. *Dermatologic Surgery, 12,* 1330–1332.

9. Hamilton, J. B. (1951). Pattern of hair loss in men: Types and incidence. *Annals of the New York Academy of Science, 53,* 708–728.

10. Cash, T. F. (2009). Attitudes, behaviors, and expectations of men seeking medical treatment for male pattern hair loss: Results from a multinational study. *Current Medical Research and Opinion, 25,* 1811–1820.

11. Budd, D., Himmelberger, D., Rhodes, T., et al. (2000). The effects of hair loss in European men: A survey of four countries. *European Journal of Dermatology, 10,* 122–127.

12. Hummert, M. L., Garstka, T. A., Shaner, J. L., et al. (1994). Stereotypes of the elderly held by young, middle-aged, and elderly adults. *Journal of Gerontology, 49,* 240–249.

13. Donofrio, L. M. (2000). Fat distribution: A morphologic study of the aging face. *Dermatological Surgery, 26,* 1107–1112.

14. Kalmovich, L. M., Elad, D., Zaretsky, U., et al. (2005). Endonasal geometry changes in elderly people: Acoustic rhinometry measurements. *Journal of Gerontology: Medical Sciences, 60A,* 396–398. Heathcote, J. A. (1995). Why do old men have big ears? *British Medical Journal, 311,* 1668.

15. Rexbye, H., Petersen, I., Johansens, M., et al. (2006). Influence of environmental factors on facial aging. *Age and Ageing, 35,* 110–115.

16. Branchet, M. C., Boisnic, S., Frances, C., et al. (1990). Skin thickness changes in normal aging skin. *Gerontology, 36,* 28–35.

17. Farage, M. A., Miller, K. W., Berardesca, E., et al. (2009). Clinical implications of aging skin: Cutaneous disorders of the elderly. *American Journal of Clinical Dermatology, 10,* 73–86.

18. May, A. K. (2009). Skin and soft tissue infections. *Surgical Clinics of North America, 89,* 402–420.

19. Davies, A. (2008). Management of dry skin conditions in older people. *British Journal of Community Nursing, 13,* 254–257.

20. Yosipovitch, G., & Tang, M. B. Y. (2002). Practical management of psoriasis in the elderly. *Drugs & Aging, 19,* 847–863.

21. Lowes, M. A., Bowcock, A. M., & Krueger, J. G. (2007). Pathogenesis and treatment of psoriasis. *Nature, 445,* 866–873.

22. Chau, J. V., & Chen, W. H. (2010). Herpes zoster vaccine for the elderly: Boosting immunity. *Aging Health, 6,* 169–176. U.S. Department of Health and Human Services, Centers for Disease Control and Prevention (2009, Oct. 6). *Shingles vaccine: What you need to know.* Atlanta, GA: DHHS, CDC.

23. Flegal, K. M., Carroll, M. D., Ogden, C. L., et al. (2010). Prevalence and trends in obesity among US adults, 1999–2008. *JAMA, 303,* 235–241.

24. Gruson, E., Montaye, M., Kee, F., et al. (2010). Anthropometric assessment of abdominal obesity and coronary heart disease risk in men: The PRIME study. *Heart, 96,* 136–140. Mason, C., Craig, C. L., & Katzmarzyk, P. T. (2008). Influence of central and extremity circumferences on all-cause mortality in men and women. *Obesity, 16,* 2690–2695.

25. Janiszewski, P., Janssen, I., & Ross, R. (2007). Does waist circumference predict diabetes and cardiovascular disease beyond commonly evaluated cardiometabolic risk factors? *Diabetes Care, 30,* 3105–3109.

26. Carroll, J. (2005, Apr. 9). Who's worried about their weight? Gallop 2005 Consumption Habits Survey. Retrieved Nov. 6, 2010, from www.gallup.com/poll/17752/Whos -Worried-About-Their-Weight.aspx. Mendes, E. (2010, Nov. 10). In U.S., 62% exceed ideal weight, 19% at their goal. Gallop 2010 Health and Healthcare Survey. Retrieved Jan. 14, 2011, from www.gallup.com/poll/144941/Exceed-Ideal-Weight-Goal.aspx.

27. Gough, B. (2005). Barriers to healthy eating among men: A qualitative analysis. *Social Science & Medicine, 62*, 387–395.

28. Carroll, J. (2005, Aug. 16). Six in 10 Americans have attempted to lose weight. Gallop 2005 Consumption Habits Survey. Retrieved Nov. 6, 2010, from www.gallup.com /poll/17890/six-americans-attempted-lose-weight.aspx.

29. Ristovski-Slijepcevic, S., Bell, K., Chapman, G. E., et al. (2010). Being "thick" indicates you are eating, you are healthy and you have an attractive body shape: Perspectives on fatness and food choice among Black and White men and women in Canada. *Health Sociology Review, 19*, 317–329.

30. De Souza, P., & Ciclitira, K. E. (2005). Men and dieting: A qualitative analysis. *Journal of Health Psychology, 10*, 793–804.

31. Robertson, L., Evans, C., & Fowkes, F. G. (2008). Epidemiology of chronic venous disease. *Phleobology, 23*, 103–11. Evans, C. J., Fowkes, F. G., Ruckley, C. V., et al. (1999). Prevalence of varicose veins and chronic venous insufficiency in men and women in the general population: Edinburg Vein Study. *Journal of Epidemiology and Community Health, 53*, 149–153.

32. Sobel, E., Levitz, S. J., Caselli, M. A., et al. (2001). The effect of customized insoles on the reduction of postwork discomfort. *Journal of the American Podiatry Medical Association, 91*, 515–520.

33. Nixon, B. P., Armstrong, D. G., Wendell, C., et al. (2006). Do US veterans wear appropriately sized shoes? *Journal of the American Podiatric Medical Association, 96*, 290–292.

34. Menz, H. B., Roddy, E., Thomas, E., et al. (2011). Impact of hallux valgus severity on general and foot-specific health-related quality of life. *Arthritis Care & Research, 63*, 396–404.

35. Gilheany, M. F., Landorf, K. B., & Robinson, P. (2008). Hallux valgus and hallux rigidus: A comparison of impact on health-related quality of life in patients presenting to foot surgeons in Australia. *Journal of Foot and Ankle, 1*, 1–14.

36. Paoloni, J. A., Milne, C., Orchard, J., et al. (2009). Non-steroidal anti-inflammatory drugs in sports medicine: Guidelines for practical but sensible use. *British Journal of Sports Medicine, 43*, 863–865.

37. Drake, L. A., Scher, R. K., Smith, E. B., et al. (1998). Effect of onychomycosis on quality of life. *Journal of the American Academy of Dermatology, 38*, 702–704.

38. Rodgers, P., & Bassler, M. (2001). Treating onychomycosis. *American Family Physician, 15*, 663–673.

39. Ara, K., Hama, M., Akiba, S., et al. (2006). Foot odor due to microbial metabolism and its control. *Canadian Journal of Microbiology, 52*, 357–364.

CHAPTER 9. GETTING IN TOUCH WITH YOUR SPIRITUAL SELF

1. Idler, E. (1987). Religious involvement and the health of the elderly: Some hypotheses and an initial test. *Social Forces, 66*, 226–238. Ellison, C. G., & Levin, J. S. (1998). The religion-health connection: Evidence, theory and future directions. *Health Education & Behavior, 25*, 700–720. Levin, J. S., & Chatters, L. M. (1998). Religion, health, and

psychological well-being in older adults: Findings from three national surveys. *Journal of Aging and Health*, *10*, 504–531.

2. Black, H. K. (1995). "Wasted lives" and the hero grown old: Personal perspectives of spirituality by aging men. *Journal of Religious Gerontology*, *9*, 35–48. Black, H. K. (2001). Jake's story: A middle-aged, working-class man's physical and spiritual journey toward death. *Qualitative Health Research*, *11*, 293–307. Wallace, M. (2003). Uncertainty and quality of life of older men who undergo watchful waiting for prostate cancer. *Oncology Nursing Forum*, *30*, 303–309. Johnson, M. (2008). Our guest editors: Talk about religion, spirituality, and meaning in later life. *Generations*, *32* (2), 4–5.

3. Ainlay, S. C., & Smith, D. R. (1984). Aging and religious participation. *Journal of Gerontology*, *39*, 357–363. Atchley, R. C. (2009). *Spirituality and aging*. Baltimore: Johns Hopkins University Press. McFadden, S. H. (1996). Religion, spirituality, and aging. In J. E. Birren et al. (eds.), *Handbook of the psychology of aging*, 4th ed. (pp. 162–177). San Diego: Academic Press.

4. Fowler, J. W. (1981). Stages of faith: The psychology of human development and the quest for meaning. San Francisco: Harper & Row. Aldwin, C. M., Spiro, A., III, & Park, C. L. (2006). Health, behavior, and optimal aging: A life span developmental perspective. In J. E. Birren & K. W. Schaie (eds.), *Handbook of the psychology of aging* (pp. 85–104). Burlington, MA: Elsevier Academic Press.

5. Tornstam, L. (1999). Gerotranscendence: The contemplative dimension of aging. *Journal of Aging Studies*, *11*, 143–154. Thoresen, C. E. (1999). Spirituality and health: Is there a relationship? *Journal of Health Psychology*, *4*, 291–300. George, L. K., Larson, D. B., Koenig, H. G., et al. (2000). Spirituality and health: What we know, what we need to know. *Journal of Social and Clinical Psychology*, *19*, 102–116.

6. Snowden, D. A. (2001). *Aging with grace: What the Nun Study teaches us about leading longer, healthier, and more meaningful lives*. New York: Bantam.

7. Levin, J. F. (1996). How religion influences morbidity and health: Reflections on natural history, salutogenesis, and host resistance. *Social Science and Medicine*, *43*, 849–864.

8. McFadden, S., & Kozberg, C. (2008). Religious and spiritual supports for late-life meaning. *Generations*, *32* (2), 6–11.

9. Atchley, R. C. (2008). Spirituality, Meaning, and the experience of aging. *Generations*, *32* (2), 12–16. Doka, K. J., & Martin, T. L. (2010). *Grieving beyond gender: Understanding the ways men and women mourn*, rev. ed. New York: Routledge.

10. Frankl, V. E. (2006). *Man's search for meaning*. Boston: Beacon Press [originally published 1959].

11. Zinnbauer, B. J., Pargament, K. I., Cole, B. C., et al. (1997). Religion and spirituality: Unfuzzing the fuzzy. *Journal for the Scientific Study of Religion*, *36*, 549–564. Spilka, B. (1993). Spirituality: Problems and directions in operationalizing a fuzzy concept. Paper presented at the annual meeting of the American Psychological Association, Toronto.

12. Gallup, G. H., Jr., & Lindsay, D. M. (2000). *Surveying the religious landscape: Trends in U.S. beliefs*. New York: Morehouse. Gallup, G. H., Jr. (2003, Feb. 3). Americans' spiritual searches turn inward. Princeton, NJ: Gallup Organization. Retrieved from www.gallup.com/poll/7759/americans-spiritual-searches-turn-inward.aspx.

13. Bianchi, E. (2005). Living with elder wisdom. *Journal of Gerontological Social Work*, *45*, 319–329. Roof, C. W. (1999). *The spiritual marketplace: Baby boomers and the remaking of American religion*. Princeton, NJ: Princeton University Press.

14. Roof, C. W. (1999). *The spiritual marketplace: Baby boomers and the remaking of American religion*. Princeton, NJ: Princeton University Press.

15. Sadler, E., & Biggs, S. (2006). Exploring the links between spirituality and "successful ageing." *Journal of Social Work Practice, 20* (3), 270.

16. Harris, I. (1997). The ten tenants of male spirituality. *Journal of Men's Studies, 6,* 29–53, p. 32.

17. Atchley, R. C. (2009). *Spirituality and aging.* Baltimore: Johns Hopkins University Press, p. 13.

18. Young, C., & Koopsen, C. (2011). *Spirituality, health, and healing.* Sudbury: Jones & Bartlett, p. 15.

19. Atchley, R. C. (2008). Spirituality, meaning, and the experience of aging. *Generations, 32* (2), 12–16, pp. 12–13.

20. Stanczak, G. C. (2006). *Engaged spirituality: Social change and American religion.* New Brunswick, NJ: Rutgers University Press, p. 20.

21. Harris, I. (1997). The ten tenants of male spirituality, *Journal of Men's Studies, 6,* 29–53, pp. 42–43.

22. Wink, P., & Dillon, M. (2002). Spiritual development across the adult life course: Findings from a longitudinal study. *Journal of Adult Development, 9,* 79–94, p. 80.

23. Ramsey, J. L. (2008). Forgiveness and healing in later life. *Generations, 32* (2), 51–54.

24. Chiesa, A., & Serretti, A. (2010). A systematic review of neurobiological and clinical features of mindfulness meditations. *Psychological Medicine, 40,* 1239–1252. Ludwig, D. S., & Kabat-Zinn, J. (2008). Mindfulness in medicine. *Journal of the American Medical Association, 300,* 1350–1352. Park, C. L. (2007). Religiousness/spirituality and health: A meaning systems perspective. *Journal of Behavior Medicine, 30,* 319–328.

25. Newberg, A. B., d'Aquili, E. G., & Rause, V. (2001). *Why God won't go away: Brain science and the biology of belief.* New York: Ballantine Books, p. 8.

26. Paulson, S. (2006, Sept. 20). Divining the brain. *Salon.* San Francisco, CA: Salon. com. Retrieved June 5, 2012, from www.salon.com/2006/09/20/newberg/.

27. Koenig, H. G. (2010). Spirituality and mental health. *International Journal of Applied Psychoanalytic Studies, 7,* 116–122.

28. Sloan, R. P., Bagiella, E., & Powell, T. (1999). Religion, spirituality, and medicine. *Lancet, 353,* 667.

29. Bianchi, E. (2005). Living with elder wisdom. *Journal of Gerontological Social Work, 45,* 319–329.

30. Connell, R. W. (1995). *Masculinities.* Berkeley: University of California Press. Katz, J. (2006). *The macho paradox: Why some men hurt women and how all men can help.* Naperville, IL: Sourcebooks.

31. Gelfer, J. (2009). *Numen, old men: Contemporary masculine spiritualities and the problem of patriarchy.* London: Equinox.

32. Atchley, R. C. (1997). Everyday mysticism: Spiritual development in later adulthood. *Journal of Adult Development, 4,* 123–134. Moody, H. R. (1995). Mysticism. In M. A. Kimble, S. H. McFadden, J. Ellor, et al. (eds.), *Aging, spirituality, and religion: A handbook* (pp. 87–101). Minneapolis, MN: Fortress Press.

33. Bianchi, E. (2005). Living with elder wisdom. In H. R. Mood (ed.), *Religion, spirituality, and aging* (p. 321). Binghamton, NY: Haworth Social Work Practice Press.

34. National Center for Complementary and Alternative Medicine (2010). *Meditation: An introduction.* Bethesda, MD: NCCAM.

35. Ibid.

36. Newhouse, M. (2010, May/June). Legacy: A powerful rite of passage. *Social Work Today, 10* (3), 6. Retreived June 2, 2012, from www.socialworktoday.com/archive/052010 p6.shtml.

37. Fritsch, T., Kwak, J., Grant, S., et al. (2009). Impact of TimeSlips, a creative expression intervention program, on nursing home residents with dementia and their caregivers. *Gerontologist, 49*, 117–127. Basting, A. D. (2006). Arts in dementia care: "This is not the end . . . it's the end of this chapter." *Generations, 30*, 16–20.

38. Schachter-Shalomi, Z., & Miller, R. S. (1997). *From age-ing to sage-ing: A profound new vision of growing older.* New York: Grand Central.

39. Leider, R., & Spears, L. (2009). *Savoring life through servant-leadership.* Indianapolis: Spears Center.

CHAPTER 10. ALCOHOL AND DRUGS

1. Kirchner, J. E., Zubritsky, C., Cody, M., et al. (2007). Alcohol consumption among older adults in primary care. *Journal of General Internal Medicine, 22*, 92–97. Blow, F. C., Walton, M. A., Barry, K. L., et al. (2000). The relationships between alcohol problems and health functioning of older adults in primary care settings. *Journal of the American Geriatrics Society, 48*, 769–774.

2. National Institutes of Health (2010). *Rethinking drinking: Alcohol and your health* (NIH Publication No. 10–3770). Rockville, MD: National Institute on Alcohol Abuse and Alcoholism.

3. Fillmore, K. M., Stockwell, T., Chikritzhs, T., et al. (2006). Moderate alcohol use and reduced mortality risk: Systematic error in prospective studies and new hypotheses. *Annals of Epidemiology, 17* (suppl.), S16–S23.

4. Office of Applied Studies (2008). *Results from the 2007 National Survey on Drug Use and Health: National findings* (DHHS Publication No. SMA 08–4343). Rockville, MD: Substance Abuse and Mental Health Services Administration.

5. Lin, J. C., Guerrieri, J. G., & Moore, A. A. (2011). Drinking patterns and the development of functional limitations in older adults: Longitudinal analyses of the Health and Retirement Survey. *Journal of Aging and Health, 23*, 806–821.

6. Mozaffarian, D., Kamineni, A., Carnethon, M., et al. (2009). Lifestyle risk factors and new-onset diabetes mellitus in older adults: The Cardiovascular Health Study. *Archives of Internal Medicine, 169*, 798–807.

7. Lang, I., Wallace, R., Huppert, F., et al. (2007). Moderate alcohol consumption in older adults is associated with better cognition and well-being than abstinence. *Age and Ageing, 36*, 256–261.

8. Cheng, J. Y. W., Ng, E. M. L., & Ko, J. S. N. (2007). Alcohol consumption and erectile dysfunction: Meta-analysis of population-based studies. *International Journal of Impotence Research, 19*, 343–352. Kim, L. W., Lee, D. Y., Lee, B. C., et al. (2012). Alcohol and cognition in the elderly: A review. *Psychiatric Investigation, 9*, 8–16. Saitz, R. (2005). Unhealthy alcohol use. *New England Journal of Medicine, 352*, 596–607.

9. Spencer, R. L., & Hutchinson, K. E. (1999). Alcohol, aging, and the stress response. *Alcohol Research and Health, 23*, 272–283.

10. Bernstein, L., Folkman, S., & Lazarus, R. (1989). Characterization of the use and misuse of medications by an elderly, ambulatory population. *Medical Care, 27* (6), 654–663.

11. National Institute on Alcohol Abuse and Alcoholism (2007). *Harmful interactions: Mixing alcohol with medications* (NIH Publication No. 03–5329). Washington, DC: US Government Printing Office.

12. Anderson, P., & Baumberg, B. (2006). *Alcohol in Europe: A public health perspective.* London: Institute of Alcohol Studies.

13. American Psychiatric Association (2012). *Diagnostic and statistical manual of mental disorders*. 5th ed. Washington, DC: American Psychiatric Association.

14. Simoni-Wastila, L., & Yang, H. (2006). Psychoactive drug abuse in older adults. *American Journal of Geriatric Pharmacotherapy, 4*, 380–394.

15. Substance Abuse and Mental Health Services Administration (2010). *Substance abuse among older adults: A guide for social service providers* (DHHS Publication No. SMA 04–3971). Washington, DC: US Government Printing Office.

16. Widlitz, M., & Marin, D. (2002). Substance abuse in older adults: An overview. *Geriatrics, 57* (12), 29–34.

17. McGrath, A., Crome, P., & Crome, I. (2005). Substance misuse in the older population. *Postgraduate Medical Journal, 81*, 228–231.

18. Moos, R. H., Brennan, P. L., Schutte, K. K., et al. (2010). Older adults' health and late-life drinking patterns: A 20-year perspective. *Aging & Mental Health, 14*, 33–43.

19. Choi, N. G., & Dinitto, D. M. (2011). Heavy/binge drinking and depressive symptoms in older adults: Gender differences. *International Journal of Geriatric Psychiatry, 26*, 860–868.

20. Widlitz, M., & Marin, D. (2002). Substance abuse in older adults: An overview. *CME Geriatrics, 57* (12), 29–34.

21. Office of Applied Studies (2008). *Substance use among older adults: 2002 and 2003 update*. Rockville, MD: Substance Abuse and Mental Health Services Administration.

22. Patterson, T., & Jeste, D. (1999). The potential impact of the baby-boom generation on substance abuse among elderly persons. *Psychiatric Services, 59*, 1184–1188.

23. Widlitz, M., & Marin, D. (2002). Substance abuse in older adults: An overview. *CME Geriatrics, 57* (12), 29–34.

24. Helpguide.org (2011). Depression in older adults and the elderly: Recognizing the signs and getting help.

25. AAA Foundation for Traffic Safety (2009). *2009 older adults knowledge about medications that can impact driving*. Washington, DC: AAA Foundation for Traffic Safety.

26. Kaye, L., Crittenden, J., & Gressitt, S. (2010). *Executive summary: Reducing prescription drug misuse through the use of a citizen mail-back program in Maine*. Washington, DC: Environmental Protection Agency. Retrieved from www.epa.gov/aging/RX-report -Exe-Sum/.

27. Bernstein, L., Folkman, S., & Lazarus, R. (1989). Characterization of the use and misuse of medications by an elderly, ambulatory population. *Medical Care, 27*, 654–663.

28. Ives, T. J., Chelminski, P. R., Hammett-Stabler, C. A., et al. (2006). Predictors of opioid misuse in patients with chronic pain: A prospective cohort study. *BMC Health Services Research, 6*, 46.

CHAPTER 11. HOLISTIC MEDICINE

1. National Center for Complementary and Alternative Medicine (2010). *What is complementary and alternative medicine?* Bethesda, MD: NCCAM.

2. Ibid.

3. Hasler, C. (1998). Functional foods: Their role in disease prevention and health promotion. *Food Technology, 52* (2), 57–62.

4. Zonis, S. (2007, Apr.). Which foods contain probiotics? Part III: What is probiotic food? *The Nibble*. Retrieved Nov. 8, 2010, from www.thenibble.com/reviews/nutri/pro biotic-food3.asp.

5. Reid, G. (2012). Microbiology: Categorize probiotics to speed research. *Nature*, *485*, 446.

6. Reid, G., Jass, J., Sebulsky, M. T., et al. (2003). Potential uses of probiotics in clinical practice. *Clinical Microbiology Reviews*, *16*, 658–672. National Center for Complementary and Alternative Medicine (2008). *An introduction to probiotics*. Bethesda, MD: NCCAM.

7. Lobo, V., Patil, A., Phatak, A., et al. (2010). Free radicals, antioxidants and functional foods: Impact on human health. *Pharmacognosy Review*, *4*, 118–126. Diplock, A. T., Charleux, J. L., Crozier-Willi, G., et al. (1998). Functional food science and defense against reactive oxidative species. *British Journal of Nutrition*, *80* (suppl. 1), S77–S112.

8. Age-Related Eye Disease Study Research Group (2001). A randomized, placebo-controlled, clinical trial of high-dose supplementation with vitamins C and E, beta carotene, and zinc for age-related macular degeneration and vision loss: AREDS report no. 8. *Archives of Ophthalmology*, 119, 1417–1436.

9. Johns Hopkins Medicine Health Alerts (2009). *Dietary supplements: Yea or nay?* New York: Remedy Health Media, LLC.

10. Choi, H. K., Gao, X., & Curhan, G. (2009). Vitamin C intake and the risk of gout in men: A prospective study. *Archives of Internal Medicine*, *169*, 502–507.

11. Nippoldt, T. B. (2008). *Calcium supplements: Do men need them too?* Rochester, MN: Mayo Foundation for Medical Education and Research (MFMER).

12. Melhus, J., Michaelsson, K., Kindmark, A., et al. (1998). Excessive dietary intake of vitamin A is associated with reduced bone mineral density and increased risk for hip fracture. *Annals of Internal Medicine*, *129*, 770–778.

13. Balk, E. M., Lichtenstein, A. H., Chung, M., et al. (2006). Effects of omega-3 fatty acids on serum markers of cardiovascular disease risk: A systematic review. *Atherosclerosis*, *189*, 19–30.

14. Scarmeas, N., Luchsinger, J. A., Schupf, N., et al. (2009). Physical activity, diet, and risk of Alzheimer's disease. *Journal of the American Medical Association*, *302*, 627–637.

15. AARP (2007). *Complementary and alternative medicine: What people 50 and older are using and discussing with their physicians*. Washington, DC: AARP and NCCAM.

16. Mayo Clinic Staff (2010, Sept. 10). *Erectile dysfunction herbs: A natural treatment for ED?* Rochester, MN: Mayo Foundation for Medical Education and Research (MFMER).

17. AARP and National Center for Complementary and Alternative Medicine (2007). *Complementary and alternative medicine: What people 50 and older are using and discussing with their physicians*. Washington, DC: AARP.

18. Miller, L. G. (1998). Herbal medicinals: Selected clinical considerations focusing on known or potential drug-herb interactions. *Archives of Internal Medicine*, *158*, 2200–2211. Izzo, A. A., & Ernst, E. (2001). Interactions between herbal medicines and prescribed drugs: A systematic review. *Drugs*, *61*, 2163–2175.

19. National Center for Complementary and Alternative Medicine, National Institutes of Health (2008, Oct.). *Tips for talking with your health care providers about CAM*. Bethesda, MD: NCCAM, Document D417.

20. Koster, B. C., & Waskowiak, A. (2006). *The reflexology atlas*. New York: Healing Arts Press.

21. Keet, L. (2009). *The reflexology bible: The definitive guide to pressure point healing*. New York: Sterling.

22. Cheung, C. K., Wyman, J. F., & Halcon, L. L. (2007). Use of complementary and alternative therapies in community-dwelling older adults. *Journal of Alternative and Complementary Medicine*, *13*, 997–1006. McLaughlin, D., Adams, J., Sibbritt, D., et al. (2012). Sex differences in use of complementary and alternative medicine in older men and

women. *Australasian Journal on Ageing*, *31*, 78–82. Sharpe, P. A., Williams, H. G., Granner, M. L., et al. (2007). A randomized study of the effects of massage therapy compared to guided relaxation on well-being and stress perception among older adults. *Complementary Therapies in Medicine*, *15*, 157–163.

23. Lawrence, D. J., & Meeker, W. C. (2007). Chiropractic and CAM utilization: A descriptive review. *Chiropractic & Ostephathy*, 15. Released ahead of print, doi:10.1186/1746-1340-15-2.

24. Eisenberg, D. M., Kessler, R. C., Foster, C., et al. (1993). Unconventional medicine in the United States: Prevalence, costs, and patterns of use. *New England Journal of Medicine*, *328*, 246–252.

25. Dougherty, P. E., Hawk, C., Weiner, D. K., et al. (2012). The role of chiropractic care in older adults. *Chiropractic & Manual Therapies*, *20* (3). Released ahead of print, doi:10.1186/2045-709X-20-3.

26. Miles, P., & True, G. (2003). Reiki—review of a biofield therapy. History, theory, practice and research. *Alternative Therapies*, *9* (2), 62–72.

27. McCormack, G. (2009). The effects of non-contact therapeutic touch on pain in the elderly. *International Journal of Occupational Therapy*, *16* (1), 44–56.

28. Cohen, K. (n.d.). *What is qigong?* Nederland, CO: Qigong Research and Practice Center.

29. Saucier, K. (1996). Medical applications of qigong. *Alternative Therapies*, *2* (1), 40–46.

30. Komagata, S. & Newton, R. (2003). The effectiveness of Tai Chi on improving balance in older adults: An evidence-based review. *Journal of Geriatric Physical Therapy*, *26* (2), 9–16. Sancier, K. M., & Holman, D. (2004). Multifaceted health benefits of medical Qigong. *Journal of Alternative and Complementary Medicine*, *10*, 163–166.

31. Wieland, G. D. (2012). *Acupuncture.* Health in Aging. New York: American Geriatrics Society.

32. Berman, B., Lao, L., Langenberg, P., et al. (2004). Effectiveness of acupuncture as adjunctive therapy in osteoarthritis of the knee: A randomized, controlled trial. *Annals of Internal Medicine*, *141*, 901–910.

33. Huebscher, R., & Shuler, P. (2003). *Natural, alternative and complementary health care practices.* St. Louis, MO: Mosby.

34. Ibid.

35. Ullman, R., & Reichenberg-Ullman, J. (1997). Homeopathic self-care: The quick and easy guide for the whole family. New York: Three Rivers Press, p. 9.

36. National Center for Complementary and Alternative Medicine (2009). *Ayurvedic medicine: An introduction*. Bethesda, MD: NCCAM.

37. Chopra, A., & Doiphode, V. V. (2002). Ayurvedic medicine—core concept, therapeutic principles, and current relevance. *Medical Clinics of North America*, *86*, 75–88. Mishra, L., Singh, B. B., & Dagenais, S. (2001). Healthcare and disease management in Ayurveda. *Alternative Therapies in Health and Medicine*, *7* (2), 44–50.

38. National Center for Complementary and Alternative Medicine (2009). *Ayurvedic medicine: An introduction*. Bethesda, MD: NCCAM.

CHAPTER 12. HEART HEALTH

1. Heron, M. P., Hoyert, D. L., Murphy, S. L., et al. (2009). Deaths: Final data for 2006. *National Vital Statistics Reports*, *57* (14). Hyattsville, MD: National Center for Health Statistics.

2. Buckland, G., Gonzales, C. A., Agudo, A., et al. (2009). Adherence to the Mediterranean diet and risk of coronary heart disease in the Spanish EPIC cohort study. *American Journal of Epidemiology, 170,* 1518–1529.

3. Roger, V. L. (2009). Lifestyle and cardiovascular health. *JAMA, 302,* 437–439.

4. Mesas, A. E., Leon-Munoz, L. M., Rodriquez-Artalejo, F., et al. (2011). The effect of coffee on blood pressure and cardiovascular disease in hypertensive individuals: A systematic review and meta-analysis. *American Journal of Clinical Nutrition, 94,* 1113–1126.

5. Jassen, I. (2007). Physical activity and reducing the risk of cardiovascular morbidity and mortality in older men and women: Lessons learned in 2006. *Current Cardiovascular Risk Reports, 1,* 265–269. Smith, T. C., Wingard, D. L., Smith, B., et al. (2007). Walking decreased risk of cardiovascular disease mortality in older adults with diabetes. *Journal of Clinical Epidemiology, 60,* 309–317.

6. Djousse, L., Driver, J. A., & Gaziano, J. M. (2009). Relation between modifiable lifestyle factors and lifetime risk of heart failure. *JAMA, 302,* 394–400. Chiuve, S. E., McCullough, M. L., Sacks, F. M., et al. (2006). Healthy lifestyle factors in the primary prevention of coronary heart disease among men: Benefits among users and nonusers of lipid-lowering and antihypertensive medications. *Circulation, 114,* 160–167.

7. Lloyd-Jones, D. M., Leip, E. P., Larson, M. G., et al. (2006). Prediction of lifetime risk of cardiovascular disease by risk factor burden at age 50. *Circulation, 113,* 791–798.

8. Pearson, T. A., Blair, S. N., Daniels, S. P., et al. (2002). AHA guidelines for primary prevention of cardiovascular disease and stroke: 2002 update. *Circulation, 106,* 388–391.

9. Mitchell, B. D., McArdle, P. F., Shen, J., et al. (2008). The genetic response to short-term interventions affecting cardiovascular function: Rationale and design of the HAPI Heart Study. *American Heart Journal, 155,* 823–828. Greenland, P., Knoll, M. D., Stamler, J., et al. (2003). Major risk factors as antecedents of fatal and nonfatal coronary heart disease events. *JAMA, 290,* 891–897.

10. Helgeson, V. S. (1990). The role of masculinity in a prognostic predictor of heart attack severity. *Sex Roles, 22,* 755–774.

11. Siegman, A. W., Townsend, S. T., Civelek, A. C., et al. (2001). Antagonistic behavior, dominance, hostility, and coronary heart disease. *Psychosomatic Medicine, 62,* 248–257. Davidson, K., Hall, P., & McGregor, M. (1999). Gender differences in the relation between interview-based hostility scores and resting blood pressure. *Journal of Behavioral Medicine, 19,* 185–201.

12. Riska, E. (2004). *Masculinity and men's health: Coronary heart disease in medical and public discourse.* New York: Rowman & Littlefield.

13. Hunt, K., Lewars, J., Emslie, C., et al. (2007). Decreased risk of death from coronary heart disease amongst men with higher "femininity" scores. *International Journal of Epidemiology, 36,* 612–620.

14. Springer, K. W., & Mouzan, D. M. (2006). Masculinity and health care seeking among midlife men: Variation by context. Paper presented at the annual meeting of the American Sociological Association, San Francisco.

15. Galdas, P., Cheater, F., & Marshall, P. (2007). What is the role of masculinity in white and South Asian men's decisions to seek medical help for cardiac chest pain? *Journal of Health Services Research and Policy, 12,* 233–239.

16. Angus, J., Rukholm, E., St. Onge, R., et al. (2007). Habitus, stress, and the body: The everyday production of health and cardiovascular risk. *Qualitative Health Research, 17,* 1088–1102.

17. Crawford, M. B. (2009). *Shop class as soul craft: An inquiry into the value of work.* New York: Penguin.

18. Winkleby, M. (1997). Accelerating cardiovascular risk factor change in ethnic minority and low socioeconomic groups. *Annals of Epidemiology, 7* (suppl. 1), S96–S103. Kaplan, G. A., & Keil, J. (1993). Socioeconomic factors and cardiovascular disease: A review of the literature. *Circulation, 88,* 1973–1998.

19. Clark, A. M., Duncan, M. A., Trevoy, J. E., et al. (2010). Healthy diet in Canadians of low socioeconomic status with coronary heart disease: Not just a matter of knowledge and choice. *Heart & Lung: The Journal of Acute and Critical Care.* doi.org/10.1016/j.hrtlng .2010.01.007. Marmot, M. G., Shipley, M. J., & Rose, G. (1984). Inequalities in death: Specific explanations of a general pattern? *Lancet, 1,* 1003–1006.

20. Cohen, B., Vittinghoff, E., & Whooley, M. (2008). Association of socioeconomic status and exercise capacity in adults with coronary heart disease (from the Heart and Soul Study). *American Journal of Cardiology, 101,* 462–466. Marmot, M. (2005). *The status syndrome: How social standing affects our health and longevity.* New York: Holt.

21. Sacker, A., Head, J., & Bartley, M. (2008). Impact of coronary heart disease on health function in an aging population: Are there differences according to socioeconomic position? *Psychosomatic Medicine, 70,* 133–140.

22. Jones-Webb, R., Yu, X., O'Brien, J., et al. (2004). Does socioeconomic position moderate the effects of race on cardiovascular disease mortality? *Ethnicity & Disease, 14,* 489–496.

23. Marx, J. (2002). Pharmacogenetics: Gene mutation may boost risk of heart arrhythmias. *Science, 297,* 1252.

24. Rhodes, D. A., Welty, T. K., Wang, W., et al. (2007). Aging and the prevalence of cardiovascular disease risk factors in older American Indians: The Strong Heart Study. *Journal of the American Geriatrics Society, 55,* 87–94.

25. Starr, J. M., Inch, S., Cross, S., et al. (1998). Blood pressure and ageing: Longitudinal cohort study. *British Medical Journal, 317,* 513–514.

26. Bonora, E., & Mugger, M. (2001). Postprandial blood glucose as a risk factor for cardiovascular disease in Type II diabetes: The epidemiological evidence. *Diabetologia, 44,* 2107–2144.

27. Bonora, E., Kiechl S., Willeit, J., et al. (1999). Plasma glucose within the normal range is not associated with carotid atherosclerosis: prospective results in subjects with normal glucose tolerance from the Bruneck Study. *Diabetes Care, 22,* 1339–1346. Desouza, C., Raghaven, V. A., & Fonseca, V. A. (2010). The enigma of glucose and cardiovascular disease. *Heart, 96,* 649–651.

28. Doll, R., Peto, R., Boreham, J., et al. (2004). Mortality in relation to smoking: 50 years' observations on male British doctors. *British Medical Journal, 328,* 1519–1528.

29. Lloyd-Jones, D., Adams, R. J., Brown, T. M., et al. (2010). Heart disease and stroke statistics 2010 update: A report from the American Heart Association. *Circulation, 121,* e46–e215.

30. Gunzerath, L., Faden, V., Zakhari, S., et al. (2004). National Institute on Alcohol Abuse and Alcoholism report on moderate drinking. *Alcoholism: Clinical and Experimental Research, 28,* 829–847. Rimm, E. (2000). Alcohol and cardiovascular disease. *Current Atherosclerosis Reports, 2,* 529–535.

31. Ehrenreich, B. (1987). *The hearts of men: American dreams and the flight from commitment.* New York: Anchor Books.

32. Chandola, T., Brunner, E., & Marmot, M. (2006). Chronic stress at work and the metabolic syndrome: Prospective study. *British Medical Journal, 332,* 521–525. Marmot, M. (2005). *The status syndrome: How social standing affects our health and longevity.* New York: Holt.

33. Blumenthal, J. A., Sherwood, A., Babyak, M. A., et al. (2005). Effects of exercise and stress management training on markers of cardiovascular risk in patients with ischemic heart disease. *JAMA, 293,* 1626–1634.

34. Brindle, J. T., Antti, H., Holmes, E., et al. (2002). Rapid and noninvasive diagnosis of the presence and severity of coronary heart disease using H-NMR-based metabonomics. *Nature Medicine, 8,* 1439–1445.

35. Klocke, F. J., Baird, M. G., Lorell, B. H., et al. (2003). ACC/AHA/ASNC guidelines for the clinical use of cardiac radionuclide imaging—executive summary. *Journal of American College of Cardiology, 42,* 1318–1333.

36. Nissen, S. E., Tuzcu, E. M., Schoenhagen, P., et al. (2004). Effect of intensive compared to moderate lipid-lowering therapy on progression of coronary atherosclerosis. *JAMA, 291,* 1071–1080.

37. Blumenthal, J. A., Sherwood, A., Babyak, M. A., et al. (2005). Effects of exercise and stress management training on markers of cardiovascular risk in patients with ischemic heart disease. *JAMA, 293,* 1626–1634.

38. Stelle, C. (2008, Feb. 20). Dr. Chris discovers he has a life threatening heart condition. TheFamilyGP.com. Retrieved Sept. 1, 2010, from www.thefamilygp.com/dr-chris-cardiac-journey.htm.

39. Two other major types of diuretics are loop diuretics (such as Lasix, Diuril, and Bumex) and potassium-sparing diuretics (such as Inspra, Dyrenium, and Aldactone); however, only the thiazide diuretics are used to treat hypertension.

40. Cannon, C. P. (1998). Time to treatment of acute myocardial infarction revisited. *Current Opinion in Cardiology, 13,* 254–266. Cannon, C. P., Gibson, C. M., Lambrew, C. T., et al. (2000). Relationship of symptom-onset-to-balloon time and door-to-balloon time with mortality in patients undergoing angioplasty for acute myocardial infarction. *JAMA, 283,* 2941–2947.

41. Lewis, D. L., Davis, J. W., Archibald, D. G., et al. (1983). Protective effects of aspirin against acute myocardial infarction and death in men with unstable angina: Results of a Veterans Administration Cooperative study. *New England Journal of Medicine, 309,* 396–403.

42. Feldman, M., & Cryer, B. (1999). Aspirin absorption rates and platelet inhibition times with 325-mg buffered aspirin tablets (chewed or swallowed intact) and with buffered aspirin solution. *American Journal of Cardiology, 84,* 404–409.

43. Hyman, H. T., & Fenichel, N. M. (1932). The management of the decompensated cardiac invalid. *American Journal of Medical Sciences, 183,* 748–752.

44. Monterio, L. A. (1979). *Cardiac patient rehabilitation: Social aspects of recovery.* New York: Springer.

45. Sacco, R. L., Kargman, D. E., Gu, Q., et al. (1995). Race-ethnicity and determinants of intracranial cerebral infarction. *Stroke, 26,* 14–20.

46. National Institute of Neurologic Disorders and Stroke (2009). *Stroke: Challenges, progress, promise.* Washington, DC: U.S. Department of Health and Human Services.

47. Singh, K., Bonaa, K. H., Jacobsen, B. K., et al. (2001). Prevalence of and risk factors for abdominal aortic aneurysms in a population-based study. *American Journal of Epidemiology, 154,* 236–244.

48. Reilly, J. M., & Tilson, M. D. (1989). Incidence and etiology of abdominal aortic aneurysms. *Surgical Clinics of North America, 69,* 705–711.

49. Ailawadi, G., Eliason, J. L., & Upchurch, G. R. (2003). Current concepts in the pathogenesis of abdominal aortic aneurysm. *Journal of Vascular Surgery, 38,* 584–588. Fleisher, A. S., Patton, J. M., & Tindall, G. T. (1975). Cerebral aneurysms of traumatic origin. *Surgical Neurology, 4,* 233–239.

50. Coeytaux, R. R., Williams, J. W., Gray, R. N., et al. (2010, Aug. 2). Narrative review: Percutaneous heart valve replacement for aortic stenosis: State of the evidence. *Annals of Internal Medicine*. Epub.

51. Olsson, M., Janfjall, H., Orth-Gomer, K., et al. (1996). Quality of life in octogenarians after valve replacement due to aortic stenosis. *European Heart Journal*, *17*, 583–589.

52. Lemon, S. C., Olendzki, B., Magner, R., et al. (2010). The dietary quality of persons with heart failure in NHANES 1999–2006. *Journal of General Internal Medicine*, *25*, 135–140.

CHAPTER 13. COGNITIVE HEALTH: MEMORY AND MEMORY LOSS

1. Ardila, A. (2007). Normal aging increases cognitive heterogeneity: Analysis of dispersion in WAIS-II scores across age. *Archives of Clinical Neuropsychology*, *22*, 1003–1011. Caserta, M. T., Bannon, Y., Fernandez, F., et al. (2009). Normal brain aging: Clinical, immunological, neuropsychological, and neuroimaging features. *International Review of Neurobiology*, *84*, 1–19.

2. Anderson, N. D., Iidaka, T., Cabeza, R., et al. (2000). The effects of divided attention on encoding- and retrieval-related brain activity: A PET study of younger and older adults. *Journal of Cognitive Neuroscience*, *12*, 775–792.

3. Friedman, D., Nessler, D., & Johnson, R., Jr. 2007. Memory encoding and retrieval in the aging brain. *Clinical EEG and Neuroscience*, *38*, 2–7. Duverne, S., Motamedinia, S., & Rugg, M. D. (2009). Effects of age on retrieval cue processing revealed by ERPs in recognition and source memory tasks. *Journal of Cognitive Neuroscience*, *21*, 1–17.

4. Kang, S. (2010). Coverage of Alzheimer's disease from 1983 to 2008 in television news and information talk shows in the United States: An analysis of news framing. *American Journal of Alzheimer's Disease & Other Dementias*, *25*, 687–697.

5. Seidler, V. J. (1994). *Unreasonable men: Masculinity and social theory*. New York: Routledge.

6. Kopelman, M. D. (2002). Disorders of memory. *Brain*, *125*, 2152–2190.

7. Small, G. W., Silverman, D. J. S., Siddarth, P., et al. (2006). Effects of a 14-day healthy longevity lifestyle program on cognition and brain function. *American Journal of Geriatric Psychiatry*, *14*, 538–545.

8. Fillit, H. M., Butler, R. N., O'Connell, A. W., et al. (2002). Achieving and maintaining cognitive vitality with aging. *Mayo Clinic Proceedings*, *77*, 681–696.

9. Geda, Y. E., Roberts, R. O., Knopman, D. S., et al. (2010). Physical exercise, aging, and mild cognitive impairment. *Archives of Neurology*, *67*, 80–86. Colcombe, S. J., Erickson, K. I., Scalf, P. E., et al. (2006). Aerobic exercise training increases brain volume in aging humans. *Journal of Gerontology: Medical Sciences*, *61A*, 1166–1170.

10. Erickson, K. I., Voss, M. W., Prakash, R. S., et al. (2011). Exercise training increases size of hippocampus and improves memory. *Proceedings of the National Academy of Sciences*, *108*, 3017–3022. Fabre, C., Chamari, K., Mucci, P., et al. (2002). Improvement of cognitive function by mental and/or individualized aerobic training in healthy elderly subjects. *International Journal of Sports Medicine*, *23*, 415–421.

11. Larson, E. B., Wang, L., Bowen, J. D., et al. (2006). Exercise is associated with reduced risk for incident dementia among persons 65 years of age and older. *Annals of Internal Medicine*, *144*, 73–81. Abbott, R. D., White, L. R., Ross, G. W., et al. (2004). Walking and dementia in physically capable elderly men. *Journal of the American Medical Association*, *292*, 1447–1453. Wilson, R. S., de Leon, C. F. M., Barnes, L. L., et al. (2002).

Participation in cognitively stimulating activities and risk of incident Alzheimer's disease. *Journal of the American Medical Association*, *287*, 742–748.

12. Wilson, R. S., Segawa, E., Boyle, P. A., et al. (2012). Influence of late-life cognitive activity on cognitive health. *Neurology*, *78*, 1123–1129.

13. Verghese, J., Lipton, R. B., Katz, M. J., et al. (2003). Leisure activities and the risk of dementia in the elderly. *New England Journal of Medicine*, *348*, 2508–2516. Wilson, R. S., de Leon, C. F. M., Barnes, L. L., et al. (2002). Participation in cognitively stimulating activities and risk of incident Alzheimer's disease. *Journal of the American Medical Association*, *287*, 742–748.

14. Beard, R. L., Fetterman, D. L., Wu, B., et al. (2009). The two voices of Alzheimer's: Attitudes toward brain health by diagnosed individuals and support persons. *Gerontologist*, *49* (suppl.), S43–S49.

15. Scarmeas, N., Stern, Y., Mayeux, R., et al. (2009). Mediterranean diet and mild cognitive impairment. *Archives of Neurology*, *66*, 216–225. Gardener, H., Scarmeas, N., Gu, Y., et al. (2012). Mediterranean diet and white matter hyperintensity volume in the Northern Manhattan Study. *Archives of Neurology*, *69*, 251–256.

16. Shikitt-Hale, B. (2012). Blueberries and neuronal aging. *Gerontology*. Epub ahead of print, doi:10.1159/000341101.

17. Harrison, Y., & Horne, J. A. (2000). The impact of sleep deprivation on decision making: A review. *Journal of Experimental Psychology: Applied*, *6*, 236–249. Cooke, J. R., & Ancoli-Israel, S. (2006). Sleep and its disorders in older adults. *Psychiatric Clinics of North America*, *29*, 1077–1093.

18. Roberts, R. O., Roberts, L. A., Geda, Y. E., et al. (2012, July). Relative intake of macronutrients impacts risk of mild cognitive impairment or dementia. *Journal of Alzheimer's Disease*. Epub ahead of print, doi:10.3233/JAD-2012-120862.

19. Roberts, R. O., Geda, Y. E., Knopman, D. S., et al. (2012). The incidence of MCI differs by subtype and is higher in men: The Mayo Clinic Study of Aging. *Neurology*, *78*, 342–351.

20. Richard, E., Moll van Charante, E. P., & van Gool, W. A. (2012, Aug.). Vascular risk factors as treatment target to prevent cognitive decline. *Journal of Alzheimer's Disease*. doi:10.3233/JAD-2012-120772. Ghosh, D., Mishra, M. K., Das, S., et al. (2009). Tobacco carcinogen induces microglial activation and subsequent neuronal damage. *Journal of Neurochemistry*, *110*, 307–314.

21. Sapolsky R. (1994). Glucocorticoids, stress and exacerbation of excitotoxic neuron death. *Seminars in Neuroscience*, *6*, 323–331. Friedman, A., Kaufer, D., Shemer, J., et al. (1996). Pyridostigmine brain penetration under stress enhances neuronal excitability and induces early immediate transcriptional response. *Nature Medicine*, *2*, 1382–1385.

22. Grewal, R. P., & Finch, C. E. (1997). Normal brain aging and Alzheimer's disease pathology. In J. D. Brioni & M. W. Decker (eds.), *Pharmacological treatment of Alzheimer's disease: Molecular and neurobiological foundations* (pp. 179–192). New York: Wiley-Liss.

23. Williams, M. E. (1995). *The American Geriatrics Society's complete guide to aging and health*. New York: Harmony Books.

24. The term *working memory* refers to a brain system that provides temporary storage and ability to manipulate the information required for complex cognitive tasks such as language comprehension and reasoning. Baddeley, A. (1992). Working memory. *Science*, *255*, 556–559.

25. Haroutuniam, V., Purohit, D. P., Perl, D. P., et al. (1999). Neurofibrillary tangles in nondemented elderly subjects and mild Alzheimer disease. *Archives of Neurology*, *56*, 713–718.

26. Guillozet, A. L., Weintraub, S., Mash, D. C., et al. (2003). Neurofibrillary tangles, amyloid, and memory in aging and mild cognitive impairment. *Archives of Neurology*, *60*, 729–736.

27. Reuter-Lorenz, P. (2002). New visions of the aging mind and brain. *Trends in Cognitive Sciences*, *6*, 394–400. Morcom, A. M., Good, C. D., Francowiak, R. S. J., et al. (2002). Age effects of neural correlates of successful memory encoding. *Brain*, *126*, 213–229.

28. Verhaeghen, P., Geraerts, N., & Marcoen, A. (1999). Memory complaints, coping, and well-being in old age: A systematic approach. *Gerontologist*, *40*, 540–548.

29. Gilmore, J. A., & Huntington, A. D. (2005). Finding the balance: Living with memory loss. *International Journal of Nursing Practice*, *11*, 118–124.

30. Solfrizzi, V., D'Introno, A., Colacicco, A. M., et al. (2007). Alcohol consumption, mild cognitive impairment, and progression to dementia. *Neurology*, *68*, 1790–1799.

31. Spencer, R. L., & Hutchinson, K. E. (1999). Alcohol, aging, and the stress response. *Alcohol Research and Health*, *23*, 272–283.

32. Petersen, R. C., Parisi, J. E., Dickson, D. W., et al. (2006). Neuropathological features of amnestic mild cognitive impairment. *Archives of Neurology*, *63*, 665–672.

33. Petersen, R. C., Roberts, R. O., Knopman, D. S., et al. (2010). Prevalence of mild cognitive impairment is higher in men. *Neurology*, *75*, 889–897.

34. Beard, R. L. (2004). In their voices: Identity preservation and experiences of Alzheimer's disease. *Journal of Aging Studies*, *18*, 415–423.

35. Plassman, B. L., Langa, K. M., Fisher, G. G., et al. (2007). Prevalence of dementia in the United States: The Aging, Demographics, and Memory Study. *Neuroepidemiology*, *29*, 125–132.

36. Riley, K. P., Snowdon, D. A., & Markesbery, W. R. (2002). Alzheimer's neurofibrillary pathology and the spectrum of cognitive function: Findings from the Nun Study. *Annals of Neurology*, *51*, 567–577.

37. Series, H., & Degano, P. (2005). Hypersexuality in dementia. *Advances in Psychiatric Treatment*, *11*, 424–431.

38. van den Eeden, S. K., Tanner, C. M., Bernstein, A. L., et al. (2003). Incidence of Parkinson's disease: Variation by age, gender, race/ethnicity. *American Journal of Epidemiology*, *157*, 1015–1022.

39. Moore, O., Kreitler, S., Ehrenfeld, M., et al. (2005). Quality of life and gender identity in Parkinson's disease. *Journal of Neural Transmission*, *112*, 1511–1522.

40. Solimeo, S. (2008). Sex and gender in older adults' experience of Parkinson's disease. *Journal of Gerontology: Social Sciences*, *63*, S42–S48.

41. Hatcher, G. (2010). *You probably have Parkinson's: A light hearted look at a very serious subject*. Salisbury, Australia: Boolarong Press, p. 38.

42. Emre, M., Aarsland, D., Albanese, A., et al. (2004). Rivastigmine for dementia associated with Parkinson's disease. *New England Journal of Medicine*, *351*, 2508–2518.

CHAPTER 14. MEN AND DIABETES

1. Liburd, L. C., Namageyo-Fuma, A., Jack, L., et al. (2004). Views from within and beyond: Illness narratives of African-American men with type 2 diabetes. *Diabetes Spectrum*, *17*, 219–224, p. 222.

2. Fortier, J. M. (director, producer) (2008). Bad sugar. Episode 4, in *Unnatural causes: Is inequality making us sick?* California Newsreel. Bennett, P. H. (1999). Type 2 diabetes

among the Pima Indians of Arizona: An epidemic attributable to environmental change? *Nutrition Reviews*, *57* (5), 51–54.

3. Centers for Disease Control and Prevention (2011). *National diabetes fact sheet: National estimates and general information on diabetes and prediabetes in the United States, 2011*. Atlanta: U.S. Department of Health and Human Services, Centers for Disease Control and Prevention.

4. Weiler, D. M., & Crist, J. D. (2009). Diabetes self-management in a Latino social environment. *Diabetes Educator*, *35*, 285–292. Tessaro, I., Smith, S. L., & Rye, S. (2005, Apr.). Knowledge and perceptions of diabetes in an Appalachian population. *Preventing Chronic Disease*. Retrieved Apr. 25, 2011, from www.cdc.gov/pcd/issues/2005/apr/04_0098.htm.

5. Liburd, L. C., Namageyo-Fuma, A., & Jack, L. (2007). Understanding "masculinity" and the challenges of managing type-2 diabetes among African-American men. *Journal of the National Medical Association*, *99*, 550–558. Rees, C. A., Karter, A. J., & Young, B. A. (2010). Race/ethnicity, social support, and associations with diabetes self-care and clinical outcomes in NHANES. *Diabetes Educator*, *36*, 435–445.

6. Choi, S. E. (2009). Diet-specific family support and glucose control among Korean immigrants with type 2 diabetes. *Diabetes Educator*, *35*, 978–985.

7. Weiler, D. M., & Crist, J. D. (2009). Diabetes self-management in a Latino social environment. *Diabetes Educator*, *35*, 285–292.

8. Zellner, D. A., Saito, S., & Gonzalez, J. (2007). The effect of stress on men's food selection. *Appetite*, *49*, 696–699. Laugero, K. D., Falcon, L. M., & Tucker, K. L. (2011). Relationships between perceived stress and dietary and activity patterns in older adults participating in the Boston Puerto Rican Health Study. *Appetite*, *56*, 194–204.

9. Seematter, G., Binnert, C., & Tappy, L. (2005). Stress and metabolism. *Metabolic Syndrome and Related Disorders*, *3*, 8–13.

10. Chesla, C. A., & Chun, K. M. (2005). Accommodating type 2 diabetes in the Chinese American family. *Qualitative Health Research*, *15*, 240–255.

11. Chesla, C. A., & Chun, K. M. (2005). Accommodating type 2 diabetes in the Chinese American family. *Qualitative Health Research*, *15*, 240–255, p. 247.

12. Lanting, L. C., Joung, I. M., Mackenbach, J. P., et al. (2005). Ethnic differences in mortality, end-stage complications, and quality of care among diabetic patients: A review. *Diabetes Care*, *28*, 2280–2288.

13. Liburd, L. C., Namageyo-Fuma, A., & Jack, L. (2007). Understanding "masculinity" and the challenges of managing type-2 diabetes among African-American men. *Journal of the National Medical Association*, *99*, 550–558.

14. Penson, D. F., & Wessells, J. (2004). Erectile dysfunction in diabetic patients. *Diabetes Spectrum*, *17*, 225–230.

15. Polonsky, W. H., Fisher, L., Guzman, S., et al. (2010). Are patients' initial experiences at the diagnosis of type 2 diabetes associated with attitudes and self-management over time? *Diabetes Educator*, *36*, 828–834.

16. Harvard Medical School (2004). *Diabetes: A plan for living*. Cambridge, MA: Harvard Medical School.

17. Consumer Reports Health Best Buy Drugs (2012, Dec.). The oral diabetes drugs: Treating type 2 diabetes. Retrieved Jan. 15, 2013, from http://www.consumerreports.org/health/best-buy-drugs/best-buy-drugs/diabetes-medications/index.htm.

18. IMS Institute for Healthcare Informatics (2011, Nov.). The use of medicines in the United States: Review of 2010. Norwalk, VA: IMS Institute for Healthcare Informatics. www.imshealth.com/deployedfiles/imshealth/Global/Content/IMS%20Institute/Static%20File/IHII_UseOfMed_report.pdf.

19. Brod, M., Kongso, J. H., Lessard, S., et al. (2009). Psychological insulin resistance: Patient beliefs and implications for diabetes management. *Quality of Life Research*, *18*, 23–32.

20. Polonsky, W., & Jackson, R. A. (2004). What's so tough about taking insulin? Addressing the problem of psychological insulin resistance in type 2 diabetes. *Clinical Diabetes*, *22*, 147–150.

21. Bogatean, M. P., & Hâncu, N. (2004). People with type 2 diabetes facing the reality of starting insulin therapy: Factors involved in psychological insulin resistance. *Practical Diabetes International*, *21*, 247–252.

22. Wei, X., Schneider, J. G., Shenouda, S. M., et al. (2011). De novo lipogenesis maintains vascular homeostasis through endothelial nitric-oxide synthase (eNOS) palmitoylation. *Journal of Biological Chemistry*, *286*, 2933–2945.

23. Frykberg, R. G. (2003). An evidence-based approach to diabetic foot infections. *American Journal of Surgery*, *186*, 44S–55S.

24. Young, B. A., Maynard, C., Reiber, G., et al. (2003). Effects of ethnicity and nephropathy on lower-extremity amputation risk among diabetic veterans. *Diabetes Care*, *26*, 495–501.

25. Haroun, M. K., Jaar, B. G., Hoffman, S. C., et al. (2003). Risk factors for chronic kidney disease: A prospective study of 23,534 men and women in Washington County, Maryland. *Journal of the American Society of Nephrology*, *14*, 2934–2941.

26. Selvin, E., Burnett, A. L., & Platz, E. A. (2007). Prevalence and risk factors for erectile dysfunction in the U.S. *American Journal of Medicine*, *120*, 151–157.

27. Penson, D. F., Latini, D. M., Lubeck, D. P., et al. (2003). Do impotent men with diabetes have more severe erectile dysfunction and worse quality of life than the general population of impotent patients? Results from the Exploratory Comprehensive Evaluation of Erectile Dysfunction (ExCEED) database. *Diabetes Care*, *26*, 1093–1099.

28. Rance, J., Phillips, C., Davies, S., et al. (2003). How much of a priority is treating erectile dysfunction? A study of patients' perceptions. *Diabetic Medicine*, *20*, 205–209.

29. Fisher, L., Laurencin, G., Chesla, C. A., et al. (2004). Depressive affect among four ethnic groups of male patients with type 2 diabetes. *Diabetes Spectrum*, *17*, 215–219.

30. Fisher, L., Mullan, J. T., Arean, P., et al. (2010). Diabetes distress but not clinical depression or depressive symptoms is associated with glycemic control in both cross-sectional and longitudinal analyses. *Diabetes Care*, *33*, 23–28.

31. Mezuk, B., Eaton, W. W., Albrecht, S., et al. (2008). Depression and type 2 diabetes over the lifespan: A meta-analysis. *Diabetes Care*, *31*, 2383–2390.

CHAPTER 15. GENITOURINARY MATTERS AND SEXUAL HEALTH

1. Bloom, A. (2004). Prostate cancer and masculinity in Australian society: A case of stolen identity? *International Journal of Men's Health*, *3*, 73–91.

2. Collins, M. M., Stafford, R. S., O'Leary, M. P., et al. (1998). How common is prostatitis? A national survey of physician visits. *Journal of Urology*, *159*, 1224–1228.

3. Nickel, J. C., Tripp, D. A., Chuai, S., et al. (2008). Psychosocial variables affect the quality of life of men diagnosed with chronic prostatitis / chronic pelvic pain syndrome. *BJU International*, *101*, 59–64.

4. De Marzo, A. M., Coffey, D. S., & Nelson, W. G. (1999). New concepts in tissue specificity for prostate cancer and benign prostatic hyperplasia. *Urology*, *53* (suppl. 3a), 29–39.

5. American Urological Association (2003). Guideline on the management of benign prostatic hyperplasia: Chapter 1: Diagnosis and treatment recommendations. *Journal of Urology*, *170*, 530–537.

6. Becher, E., Roehrborn, C. G., Siami, P., et al. (2009). The effects of dutasteride, tamsulosin, and the combination on storage and voiding in men with benign prostatic hyperplasia and prostatic enlargement: 2-year results from the Combination of Avodart and Tamsulosin study. *Prostate Cancer and Prostate Disease*, *12*, 369–374.

7. McCullough, A. R., Hellstrom, W. G., Want, R., et al. (2010). Recovery of erectile function after nerve sparing radical prostatectomy and penile rehabilitation with nightly intraurethral alprostadil versus sildenafil citrate. *Journal of Urology*, *183*, 2451–2456.

8. Coe, F. L., Evan, A., & Worcester, E. (2005). Kidney stone disease. *Journal of Clinical Investigation*, *115*, 2598–2608.

9. Scales, C. D., Curtis, L. H., Norris, R. D., et al. (2007). Changing gender prevalence of stone disease. *Journal of Urology*, *177*, 979–982.

10. Curhan, G. C., Willett, W. C., Rimm, E. B., et al. (1998). Body size and risk of kidney stones. *Journal of the American Society of Nephrology*, *9*, 1645–1652.

11. Hirvonen, T., Pietinen, P., Virtanen, M., et al. (1999). Nutrient intake and use of beverages and the risk of kidney stones among male smokers. *American Journal of Epidemiology*, *150*, 187–194.

12. Wierzalis, E. A., Barret, B., Pope, M., et al. (2006). Gay men and aging: Sex and intimacy. In D. Kimmel, T. Rose, & S. David (eds.), *Lesbian, gay, bisexual, and transgendered aging: Research and clinical perspectives* (pp. 91–109). New York: Columbia University Press. Lindau, S. T., & Gavrilova, N. (2010). Sex, health, and years of sexually active life gained due to good health: Evidence from two US population based cross sectional surveys of aging. *British Medical Journal*, *340*. Epub ahead of print, doi:10.1136/bmj.c810.

13. Marshall, B. L. (2008). Old men and sexual health: Post-Viagra views of changes in function. *Generations*, *32* (1), 21–27. Marshall, B. L., & Katz, S. (2002). Forever functional: Sexual fitness and the ageing male body. *Body & Society*, *8*, 43–70.

14. Harvard Health Publications (2004, Jan.). Are they better than Viagra? Two new drugs for erectile dysfunction work like Viagra and carry similar risks and benefits. *Harvard Health Letter*, *29* (3), 3.

15. Beckman, N., Waern, M., Gustafson, D., et al. (2008). Secular trends in self reported sexual activity and satisfaction in Swedish 70 year olds: cross sectional survey of four populations, 1971–2001. *British Medical Journal*, *337*. Epub ahead of print, doi:10.1136/bmj.a279. American Association of Retired Persons (2010). Sex, romance, and relationships: AARP survey of midlife and older adults. Washington, DC: AARP.

16. DeLamater, J. D., & Sill, M. (2005). Sexual desire in later life. *Journal of Sex Research*, *42*, 138–149.

17. Waite, L. J., Laumann, E. O., Das, A., et al. (2009). Sexuality: Measures of partnerships, practices, attitudes, and problems in the National Social Life, Health, and Aging Study. *Journal of Gerontology: Psychological Sciences & Social Sciences*, *64B* (suppl. 1), i56–i66. DeLamater, J. D., & Moorman, S. M. (2007). Sexual behavior in later life. *Journal of Aging & Health*, *19*, 921–945.

18. Koskimaki, J., Shiri, R., Tammela, T., et al. (2008). Regular intercourse protects against erectile dysfunction: Tampere Aging Male Urologic Study. *American Journal of Medicine*, *121*, 592–596.

19. Rosen, R. C., Cappelleri, J. C., Smith, M. D., et al. (1999). Development and evaluation of an abridged, 5-item version of the International Index of Erectile Function (IIEF-5) as a diagnostic tool for erectile dysfunction. *International Journal of Impotence Research*, *11*, 319–326. Cappelleri, J. C., & Rosen, R. C. (2005). The Sexual Health Inventory

for Men (SHIM): A 5-year review of research and clinical experience. *International Journal of Impotence Research*, *17*, 307–319.

20. Chew, K., & Jamrozik, K. (2009). Sex life after 65: How does erectile dysfunction affect aging and elderly men? *Aging Male*, *12* (2/3), 41–46.

21. Goldstein, I. (2004). Epidemiology of erectile dysfunction. *Sexuality and Disability*, *22*, 113–120. American Association of Retired Persons (2010). Sex, romance, and relationships: AARP survey of midlife and older adults. Washington, DC: AARP.

22. Feldman, H. A., Johannes, C. B., Derby, C. A., et al. (2000). Erectile dysfunction and coronary risk factors: Prospective results from the Massachusetts male aging study. *Preventive Medicine*, *30*, 328–338.

23. Tomlinson, J., & Wright, D. (2004). Impact of erectile dysfunction and its subsequent treatment with sildenafil: Qualitative study. *British Medical Journal*, *328*, 1037. Epub ahead of print, doi:10.1136/bmj.38044.662176.EE.

24. Marshall, B. L., & Katz, S. (2002). Forever functional: Sexual fitness and the ageing male body. *Body & Society*, *8*, 43–70.

25. Rosen, D. (2008, Sept. 20). One billion pills later. *CounterPunch*. Retrieved Feb. 20, 2010, from www.counterpunch.org/rosen09202008.html.

26. Kupelain, V., Link, C. L., & McKinlay, J. B. (2007). Association between smoking, passive smoking, and erectile dysfunction: Results from the Boston Area Community Health (BACH) Study. *European Urology*, *52*, 416–422. McVary, K. T., Carrier, S., Wessells, H., et al. (2001). Smoking and erectile dysfunction: Evidenced based analysis. *Journal of Urology*, *166*, 1624–1632.

27. Tostes, R. S., Carneiro, F. S., Lee, A. J., et al. (2008). Cigarette smoking and erectile dysfunction: Focus on NO bioavailability and ROS generation. *Journal of Sexual Medicine*, *5*, 1284–1295. Gades, N. M., Nehra, A., Jacobson, D. J., et al. (2005). Association between smoking and erectile dysfunction: A population based study. *American Journal of Epidemiology*, *161*, 346–351.

28. Jiang, H., Reynolds, K., Chen, J., et al. (2007). Cigarette smoking and erectile dysfunction among Chinese men without clinical vascular disease. *American Journal of Epidemiology*, *166*, 803–809.

29. Potts, A., Grace, V. M., Vares, T., et al. (2006). "Sex for life"? Men's counter-stories on "erectile dysfunction," male sexuality and ageing. *Sociology of Health & Illness*, *28*, 306–329. Potts, A., Gavey, N., Grace, V. M., et al. (2003). The downside of Viagra: Women's experiences and concerns. *Sociology of Health & Illness*, *23*, 697–719.

30. Seftel, A. D., Buvat, J., Althof, S. E., et al. (2009). Improvements in confidence, sexual relationship and satisfaction measures: Results of a randomized trial of Tadalafil 5 mg taken once daily. *International Journal of Impotence Research*, *21*, 240–248. Fisher, W. A., Rosen, R. C., Eardley, I., et al. (2005). Sexual experience of female partners of men with erectile dysfunction: The Female Experience of Men's Attitudes to Life Events and Sexuality (FEMALES) study. *Journal of Sexual Medicine*, *2*, 675–684.

31. Bodley-Tickell, A. T., Olowokure, B., Bhaduri, S., et al. (2008). Trends in sexually transmitted infections (other than HIV) in older people: Analysis of data from an enhanced surveillance system. *Sexually Transmitted Infections*, *84*, 312–317. Centers for Disease Control and Protection (2011). Sexually transmitted disease surveillance annual report 2004 and 2010. Atlanta: U.S. Department of Health and Human Services, Centers for Disease Control and Prevention.

32. Reece, M., Herbenick, D., Schick, V., et al. (2010). Condom use rates in a national probability sample of males and females ages 14 to 94 in the United States. *Journal of Sexual Medicine*, *7*, 266–276.

33. Jena, A. B., Goldman, D. P., Kamdar, A., et al. (2010). Sexually transmitted diseases

among users of erectile dysfunction drugs: Analysis of claims data. *Annals of Internal Medicine, 153*, 1–7.

34. Smith, K. P., & Christakis, M. A. (2009). Association between widowhood and risk of diagnosis with a sexually transmitted disease in older adults. *American Journal of Public Health, 99*, 2055–2062.

35. Chandra, A., Mosher, W. D., Copen, C., et al. (2011). Sexual behavior, sexual attraction, and sexual identity in the United States: Data from the 2006–2008 National Survey of Family Growth. National Health Statistics Reports, no. 36. Hyattsville, MD: National Center for Health Statistics.

36. Liu, C. (2000). A theory of marital sexual life. *Journal of Marriage and Family, 62*, 363–374.

37. Waite, L. J., Laumann, E. O., Das, A., et al. (2009). Sexuality: Measures of partnerships, practices, attitudes, and problems in the National Social Life, Health, and Aging Study. *Journal of Gerontology: Psychological Sciences & Social Sciences, 64B* (suppl. 1), i56–i66.

38. American Association of Retired Persons (2010). Sex, romance, and relationships: AARP survey of midlife and older adults. Washington, DC: AARP.

39. Treas, J., & Giesen, D. (2000). Sexual infidelity among married and cohabiting Americans. *Journal of Marriage and Family, 62*, 48–60.

40. Reece, M., Herbenick, D., Schick, V., et al. (2010). Condom use rates in a national probability sample of males and females ages 14 to 94 in the United States. *Journal of Sexual Medicine, 7*, 266–276.

41. American Association of Retired Persons (2010). Sex, romance, and relationships: AARP survey of midlife and older adults. Washington, DC: AARP.

42. Centers for Disease Control and Prevention (2007). *HIV/AIDS surveillance report, 2005* (rev. ed.). Atlanta: U.S. Department of Health and Human Services, Centers for Disease Control and Prevention.

43. Lindau, S. T., Schumm, M. A., Laumann, E. O., et al. (2007). A study of sexuality and health among older adults in the United States. *New England Journal of Medicine, 357*, 762–774.

44. Centers for Disease Control and Prevention (2007). *HIV/AIDS surveillance report, 2005* (rev. ed.). Atlanta: U.S. Department of Health and Human Services, Centers for Disease Control and Prevention.

45. Centers for Disease Control and Prevention (2007). Syphilis and MSM—CDC fact sheet. Atlanta: U.S. Department of Health and Human Services, Centers for Disease Control and Prevention, Document CS115145.

46. Padian, N. S., Shiboski, S. C., Glass, S. O., et al. (1997). Heterosexual transmission of human immunodeficiency virus (HIV) in northern California: Results from a ten-year study. *American Journal of Epidemiology, 146*, 350–357.

CHAPTER 16. BONE, JOINT, AND MUSCLE HEALTH

1. Singh, H. (2005). Senescent changes in the human musculoskeletal system. In K. P. Speer (ed.), *Injury prevention and rehabilitation for active older adults* (pp. 3–17). Raleigh, NC: Human Kinetic, p. 5.

2. Ibid., p. 11.

3. Chenot, J., Becker, A., Leonhardt, C., et al. (2008). Sex differences in presentation, course, and management of low back pain in primary care. *Clinical Journal of Pain, 24*, 578–584. Schneider, S., Randoll, D., & Buchner, M. (2006). Why do women have back pain

more than men? A representative prevalence study in the Federal Republic of Germany. *Clinical Journal of Pain*, *22*, 738–747.

4. Harvard Health Publications (2012). *Low back pain: Healing your aching back*. Cambridge, MA: Harvard Medical School.

5. Griffith, H. W. (2004). *Complete guide to sports injuries: How to treat fractures, bruises, sprains, strains, dislocations, head injuries* (3rd ed.). New York: Body Press / Perigee.

6. Mayo Foundation (2011, Sept. 24). *Bursitis*. Rochester, MN: Mayo Foundation for Medical Education and Research.

7. Garrick, J. G., & Webb, D. R. (1990). *Sports injuries: Diagnosis and management* (2nd ed.). Philadelphia: W. B. Saunders.

8. Singh, H. (2005). Senescent changes in the human musculoskeletal system. In K. P. Speer (ed.), *Injury prevention and rehabilitation for active older adults* (pp. 3–17). Raleigh, NC: Human Kinetics.

9. Griffith, H. W. (2004). *Complete guide to sports injuries: How to treat fractures, bruises, sprains, strains, dislocations, head injuries* (3rd ed.). New York: Body Press / Perigee.

10. Clarke, B. (2008). Normal bone anatomy and physiology. *Clinical Journal of the American Society of Nephrology*, *3* (suppl. 3), S131–S139. National Institute of Arthritis and Musculoskeletal and Skin Diseases, a division of the National Institutes of Health (2009). *Osteoporosis in men*. Bethesda, MD: National Institutes of Health.

11. Mauck, K. F., & Clarke, B. L. (2006). Diagnosis, screening, prevention, and treatment of osteoporosis. *Mayo Clinic Proceedings*, *81* (5), 662–672.

12. National Osteoporosis Foundation (2008). *BMD testing*. Washington, DC: National Osteoporosis Foundation.

13. Harvard Mental Health (2009). The male face of osteoporosis. *Harvard Mental Health Letter*, *35* (1), 3.

14. Qaseen, A., Snow, V., Shekelle, P., et al. (2008). Screen for osteoporosis in men: A clinical practice guideline from the American College of Physicians. *Annals of Internal Medicine*, *148*, 680–684.

15. Nielsen, D. S., Brixen, K., & Huniche, L. (2011). Men's experiences of living with osteoporosis: Focus group interviews. *American Journal of Men's Health*, *5*, 166–176.

16. National Institutes of Health (2008). *Medline plus: Osteoporosis*. Bethesda, MD: National Institutes of Health.

17. Ibid.

18. Foundation for Osteoporosis Research and Education (2002). *Osteoporosis: Guidelines for the physician* (4th ed.). Oakland, CA: Foundation for Osteoporosis Research and Education.

19. Nelson, M. E., Fiatarone, M. A., Morganti, C. M., et al. (1994). Effects of high-intensity strength training on multiple risk factors for osteoporotic fractures: A randomized controlled trial. *Journal of the American Medical Association*, *272*, 1909–1914.

20. Francis, R. M. (1999). The effects of testosterone on osteoporosis in men. *Clinical Endocrinology*, *50*, 411–414.

21. Mehta, N. M., Malootian, A., & Gilligan, J. P. (2003). Calcitonin for osteoporosis and bone pain. *Current Pharmaceutical Design*, *9*, 2659–2676.

22. Centers for Disease Control and Prevention (n.d.). *Arthritis basics*. Atlanta: Centers for Disease Control and Prevention.

23. Centers for Disease Control and Prevention (2012, Apr.). *Arthritis: Meeting the challenge of living well*. Atlanta: Centers for Disease Control and Prevention. Publication CS231086-C.

24. Theis, K. A., Helmick, C. G., & Hootman, J. M. (2007). Arthritis burden and impact

are greater among U.S. women than men: Intervention opportunities. *J Women's Health*, *16* (4), 441–453. Cheng Y. J., Hootman, J. M., Murphy, L. B., et al. (2010). Prevalence of doctor-diagnosed arthritis and arthritis-attributable activity limitation—United States, 2007-2009. *MMWR*, *59* (39), 1261–1265. Hootman, J. M., & Helmick, C. G. (2006). Projections of U.S. prevalence of arthritis and associated activity limitations. *Arthritis Atlanta, GA: Rheum*, *54* (1), 226–229.

25. Arthritis Foundation (2007). *Disease center*. Atlanta: Arthritis Foundation.

26. Miltiades, H., & Kaye, L. W. (2006). Older adults with orthopedic and mobility limitations. In B Berkman (ed.), *Handbook of social work in health and aging*. New York: Oxford University Press.

27. Lindsay, K., Gow, P., Vanderply, J., et al. (2011). The experience and impact of living with gout: A study of men with chronic gout using a qualitative grounded theory approach. *Journal of Clinical Rheumatology*, *17*, 1–6.

28. Harrold, L. R., Mazor, K. M., Velten, S., et al. (2010). Patients and providers view gout differently: A qualitative study. *Chronic Illness*, *6*, 263–271.

29. Praemer, A., Furner, S., & Rice, D. P. (1999). *Musculoskeletal conditions in the United States* (2nd ed.). Rosemont, IL: American Academy of Orthopedic Surgeons.

30. Bureau of Labor Statistics (2009). Physical therapists. *Occupational Outlook Handbook, 2008–09 Edition*. Washington, DC: Bureau of Labor Statistics.

31. Stevens, J. A. (2005). Falls among older adults—risk factors and prevention strategies. NCOA falls free: Promoting a national falls prevention action plan. Research Review Papers. Washington, DC: National Council on the Aging. National Council on Aging (2010, Feb.). Fall prevention. Washington, DC: National Council on Aging.

32. Samaras, N., Chevalley, T., Samaras, D., et al. (2010). Older patients in the emergency department: A review. *Annals of Emergency Medicine*, *56*, 261–269.

33. Pietschmann, P., Rauner, M., Sipos, W., et al. (2009). Osteoporosis: An age-related and gender-specific disease—a mini-review. *Gerontology*, *55*, 3–12. Stevens, J. A., & Sogolow, E. D. (2005). Gender differences for non-fatal unintentional fall related injuries among older adults. *Injury Prevention*, *11*, 115–119.

34. National Institute on Aging Information Center, U.S. Department of Health and Human Services, Public Health Service, National Institutes of Health (2010, Aug.). Osteoporosis: The bone thief. *Age Page*. Bethesda, MD: National Institute on Aging.

35. National Center for Injury Prevention and Control (2012). What you can do to prevent falls. Atlanta: Centers for Disease Control and Prevention. National Institute on Aging Information Center, U.S. Department of Health and Human Services, Public Health Service, National Institutes of Health (2009, May). Falls and fractures. *Age Page*. Bethesda, MD: National Institute on Aging.

36. U.S. Department of Health and Human Services, National Institutes of Health (2009, May). Falls and fractures. *Age Page*. Bethesda, MD: National Institute on Aging.

37. Delbaere, K., Close, J. C., Brodaty, H., et al. (2010). Determinants of disparities between perceived and physiological risk of falling among elderly people: Cohort study. *British Medical Journal*, *341*. Epub ahead of print, doi:10.1136/bmj.c4165.

38. Peterson, E., & Clemson, L. (2008). Understanding the role of occupational therapy in fall prevention for community-dwelling older adults. *OT Practice*, *13* (3), CE-1–CE-8. Tennstedt, S., Howland, J., Lachman, M., et al. (1998). A randomized, controlled trial of a group intervention to reduce fear of falling and associated activity restriction in older adults. *Journal of Gerontology: Psychological Sciences*, *53B* (6), P383–P392.

CHAPTER 17. DENTAL AND ORAL HEALTH

1. The Access Project (2009). *The costs of dental care and the impact of dental insurance coverage*. Boston: Access Project.

2. Campaign for Oral Health Parity (2003). *Keep America smiling: The oral health America national grading project 2003*. Chicago: Oral Health America.

3. U.S. General Accounting Office (2000). *Report of Congressional requestors: Oral health in low-income populations* (GAO/HEHS-00–72). Washington, DC: U.S. General Accounting Office.

4. U.S. Department of Health and Human Services (2000). *Oral health in America: A report of the Surgeon General*. Rockville, MD: U.S. Department of Health and Human Services, National Institute of Dental and Craniofacial Research, National Institutes of Health.

5. Centers for Disease Control and Prevention (2010). National oral health surveillance system, 2008. Retrieved Sept. 7, 2010, from www.cdc.gov/nohss/.

6. Gatchell, R. J., Ingersoll, B. D., Bowman, L., et al. (1982). The prevalence of dental fear and avoidance: A recent survey study. *Journal of the American Dental Association, 107,* 609–610.

7. Borreani, E., Jones, K., Scambler, S., et al. (2010). Informing the debate on oral health care for older people: A qualitative study of older people's views on oral health and oral health care. *Gerodontology, 27,* 11–18.

8. Exley, C. (2009). Bridging a gap: The (lack of a) sociology of oral health and health-care. *Sociology of Health and Illness, 31,* 1093–1108.

9. Kressin, N., Spiro, A., Bosse, R., et al. (1996). Assessing oral health-related quality of life: Findings from the Normative Aging Study. *Medical Care, 34,* 416–427.

10. Karhunen, V., Forss, H., Goebeler, S., et al. (2006). Radiographic assessment of dental health in middle-age men following sudden cardiac death. *Journal of Dental Research, 85,* 89–93. Friedewald, V. E., Kornman, K. S., Beck, J. D., et al. (2009). The American Journal of Cardiology and Journal of Periodontology editors' consensus: Periodontitis and atherosclerotic cardiovascular disease. *Journal of Periodontology, 80,* 1021–1032.

11. Academy of General Dentistry (2007, Mar. 30). Men: Looking for a better job? Start by visiting the dentist. Oral Health Resources. Retrieved Sept. 8, 2010, from www .agd.org/support/articles/?ArtID=1265.

12. Manski, R. J., Goodman, H. S., Reid, B. C., et al. (2004). Dental insurance visits and expenditures among older adults. *American Journal of Public Health, 94,* 759–764. Phipps, K. R., Chan, B. K., Jennings-Holt, M., et al. (2009). Periodontal health of older men: The MrOS Study. *Gerodontology, 26,* 122–129.

13. Segelnick, S. L. (2004). A survey of floss frequency, habit and technique in a hospital dental clinic and private periodontal practice. *New York State Dental Journal, 70* (5), 28–33.

14. Reddy, M. S. (2001). Osteoporosis and periodontitis: Discussion, conclusions, and recommendations. *Annals of Peridontology, 6,* 214–217. Kaye, E. K. (2007). Bone health and oral health. *Journal of the American Dental Association, 138,* 616–619.

15. Krall, E. A. (2006). Calcium and oral health. In C. M. Weaver & R. P. Heaney (eds.), *Calcium and human health* (pp. 319–325). Tutowa, NJ: Humana Press.

16. Ma, J., Johns, R. A., & Stafford, R. S. (2007). Americans are not meeting current calcium recommendations. *American Journal of Clinical Nutrition, 85,* 1361–1366.

17. Friedman, P. K., & Isfeld, D. (2008). Xerostomia: The "invisible" oral health condition. *Journal of the Massachusetts Dental Society, 57* (3), 42–44.

18. Baum, B. J. (1989). Salivary gland fluid secretion during aging. *Journal of the American Geriatrics Society, 37,* 453–458.

19. Butt, G. M. (1991). Drug-induced xerostomia. *Journal of the Canadian Dental Association, 57,* 391–393.

20. Atkinson, J. C., Grisius, M., & Massey, W. (2004). Salivary hypofunction and xerostomia: Diagnosis and treatment. *Dental Clinics of North America, 49,* 309–326.

21. Borrell, L. N., Burt, B. A., & Taylor, G. W. (2005). Prevalence and trends in periodontitis in the USA: From the NHANES III to the NHANES, 1988–2000. *Journal of Dental Research, 84,* 924–930.

22. Borrell, L. N., & Crawford, N. D. (2008). Social disparities in periodontitis among United States adults, 1999–2004. *Community Dentistry and Oral Epidemiology, 36,* 383–391.

23. Craig, R. G., Yip, J. K., Mijares, D. Q., et al. (2003). Progression of destructive periodontal diseases in three urban minority populations: Role of clinical and demographic factors. *Journal of Clinical Periodontology, 30,* 1075–1083.

24. Cunha-Cruz, J., Hujoel, P. P., & Kressin, N. R. (2007). Oral health-related quality of life for periodontal patients. *Journal of Periodontal Research, 42,* 169–176.

25. Burke, F. M., & Samarawixkrama, D. Y. D. (1995). Progressive changes in the pulpo-dentinal complex and their clinical consequences. *Gerodontology, 12,* 57–66.

26. Jones, J. A., Orner, M. B., Spiro, A., et al. (2003). Tooth loss and dentures: Patients' perspectives. *International Dental Journal, 53* (suppl.), 327–334. Steele, J. G., Sanders, A. E., Slade, G. D., et al. (2004). How do age and tooth loss affect oral health impacts and quality of life? A study comparing two national samples. *Community Dentistry and Oral Epidemiology, 32,* 107–114.

27. Miller, C. S., & Johnstone, B. M. (2001). Human papillomavirus as a risk factor for oral squamous cell carcinoma: A meta-analysis, 1982–1997. *Oral Surgery, Oral Medicine, Oral Pathology, Oral Radiology & Endodontics, 91,* 622–635.

CHAPTER 18. VISION AND HEARING

1. Vitale, S., Ellwein, L., Cotch, M. F., et al. (2008). Prevalence of refractive error in the United States, 1999–2004. *Archives of Ophthalmology, 126,* 1111–1119.

2. O'Neill, G., Summer, L., & Shirey, L. (1999). Hearing loss: A growing problem that affects quality of life. Second profile in the Challenges for the 21st Century series. Washington, DC: National Academy on an Aging Society.

3. Kannel, W. B., & Gordon, T., eds. (1973). The Framingham Heart Study: An epidemiologic investigation of cardiovascular disease (NIH Publ. No 74–478). Leibowitz, H. M., Krueger, D. E., Maunder, L. R., et al. (1980). The Framingham Eye Study monograph: An ophthalmological and epidemiological study of cataract, glaucoma, diabetic retinopathy, macular degeneration, and visual acuity in a general population of 2631 adults, 1973–1975. *Survey of Ophthalmology, 24* (suppl.), 335–610.

4. Stuen, C., & Faye, E. E. (2003). Vision loss: Normal and not normal changes among older adults. *Generations, 27,* 8–14.

5. Age-related Study Research Group (2001). A randomized, placebo-controlled clinical trial of high-dose supplementation with vitamins C and E, beta carotene, and zinc for age-related macular degeneration and vision loss.

6. Fujita, M., Igarashi, T., Kurai, T., et al. (2005). Correlation between dry eye and rheumatoid arthritis activity. *American Journal of Ophthalmology, 140,* 808–813.

7. Biousee, V., Skibell, B. C., Watts, R. L., et al. (2004). Ophthalmologic features of Parkinson's disease. *Neurology, 62*, 177–180.

8. National Eye Institute (2012). Facts about dry eye. Retrieved Jan. 28, 2013, from www.nei.nih.gov/health/dryeye/dryeye.asp.

9. Asbell, P. A., Dualan, I., Mindel, J., et al. (2005). Age-related cataract. *Lancet, 365*, 599–609.

10. Fine, S. L., Beerger, J. W., Maguire, M. G., et al. (2000). Age-related macular degeneration. *New England Journal of Medicine, 342*, 483–492. Stuen, C., & Faye, E. E. (2003). Vision loss: Normal and not normal changes among older adults. *Generations, 27*, 8–14.

11. Kempen, J. J., O'Colmain, B. J., Leske, M. C., et al. (2004). The prevalence of diabetic retinopathy among adults in the United States. *Archives of Ophthalmology, 122*, 552–563.

12. Wong, T. Y., Mwamburi, M., Klein, R., et al. (2009). Rates of progression in diabetic retinopathy during different time periods. *Diabetes Care, 32*, 2307–2313. Stuen, C., & Faye, E. E. (2003). Vision loss: Normal and not normal changes among older adults. *Generations, 27*, 8–14.

13. Brennan, M. B., Horowitz, A., & Su, Y. (2005). Dual sensory loss and its impact on everyday competence. *Gerontologist, 45*, 337–346. Campbell, V. A., Crews, J. E., Moriarty, D. G., et al. (1999). Surveillance for sensory impairment, activity limitation, and health-related quality of life among older adults, United States, 1993–1997. *MMWR Morbidity Mortal Weekly Report, 48*, SS-8, 131–157. Ivers, R. Q., Norton, R., Cumming, R. G., et al. (2000). Visual impairment and risk of hip fracture. *American Journal of Epidemiology, 152*, 633–639.

14. Crews, J. E., & Campbell, V. A. (2001). Health conditions, activity limitations, and participation restrictions among older people with visual impairments. *Journal of Visual Impairment and Blindness, 95*, 453–468.

15. Horowitz, A., Reinhardt, J. P., & Kennedy, G. (2005). Major and subthreshold depression among older adults seeking vision rehabilitation services. *American Journal of Geriatric Psychiatry, 13*, 180–187.

16. Spafford, M. M., Laliberte Rudman, D., Lipert, B. D., et al. (2010). When self-presentation trumps access: Why older adults with low vision go without low-vision services. *Journal of Applied Gerontology, 14*, 579–602, p. 592.

17. Horowitz A., & Reinhardt, J. P. (2000). Mental health issues in visual impairment: Research in depression, disability and rehabilitation. In B. M. Silverstone, M. Lang, B. Rosenthal, et al. (eds.), *The Lighthouse handbook on vision impairment and vision rehabilitation*, vol. 2. New York: Oxford University Press. Rovner, B. W., & Casten, R. J. (2002). Activity loss and depression in age-related macular degeneration. *American Journal of Geriatric Psychiatry, 10*, 305–310.

18. Stuen, C. (1999). *Family involvement: Maximizing rehabilitation outcomes for older adults with a disability*. New York: Lighthouse International.

19. Horowitz, A., Teresi, J. E., & Cassels, L. A. (1991). Development of a vision screening questionnaire for older people. *Journal of Gerontological Social Work, 17* (3/4), 37–56.

20. Dewane, C. (2010). Hearing loss in older adults—its effect on mental health. *Social Work Today, 10* (4), 18–22.

21. Agrawal, Y., Platz, E. A., & Niparko, J. K. (2008). Prevalence of hearing loss and differences by demographic characteristics among U.S. adults: Data from the National Health and Nutrition Examination Survey, 1999–2004. *Archives of Internal Medicine, 168*, 1522–1530.

22. Lin, F. R., Thorpe, R., Gordon-Salant, S., et al. (2011). Hearing loss prevalence

and risk factors among older adults in the United States. *Journal of Gerontology: Medical Sciences*, *66A*, 582–590. Hawkins, K., Bottone, F. G., Ozminkowski, R. J., et al. (2011, Oct. 7). The prevalence of hearing impairment and its burden on the quality of life among adults with Medicare supplement insurance. *Quality of Life Research*. Epub ahead of print, doi:10.1007/s11136-011-0028z.

23. Image from National Aeronautics and Space Administration (NASA). The effects of space flight on the human vestibular system, EB-2002-09-011-KSC.

24. Gordon-Salant, S. (2005). Hearing loss and aging: New research findings and clinical implications. *Journal of Rehabilitation Research and Development*, *42*, 9–24.

25. Weinstein, B. (2003). A primer on hearing loss in the elderly. *Generations*, *27*, 15–19.

26. Curhan, S. G., Eavey, R., Shargorodsky, J., et al. (2010). Analgesic use and the risk of hearing loss in men. *American Journal of Medicine*, *123*, 231–237.

27. McGwin, G. (2010). Phosphodiesterase type-5 inhibitor use and hearing impairment. *Archives of Otolaryngology—Head & Neck Surgery*, *136*, 488–492.

28. National Academy on an Aging Society (1999, Dec.). Hearing loss: A growing problem that affects quality of life. *Challenges for the 21st Century: Chronic and Disabling Conditions*, *2*, 1–6. Kochkin, S. (1999). "Baby Boomers" spur growth in potential market, but penetration rate declines. *Hearing Journal*, *52*, 33–48. Staehelin, K., Bertoli, S., Probst, R., et al. (2011). Gender and hearing aids: Patterns of use and determinants of nonregular use. *Ear and Hearing*, *32*, 26–37.

29. Crews, J. E., & Campbell, V. A. (2004). Vision impairment and hearing loss among community-dwelling older Americans: Implications for health and functioning. *American Journal of Public Health*, *94*, 823–829. Brennan, M., Horowitz, A., & Su, Y. (2005). Dual sensory loss and its impact on everyday competence. *Gerontologist*, *45*, 337–346. Campbell, V. A., Crews, J. E., Moriarty, D. G., et al. (1999). Surveillance for sensory impairment, activity limitation, and health-related quality of life among older adults—United States, 1993–1997. *MMWR Morbidity and Mortality Weekly Report*, *48*, SS-8, 131–157.

30. Brennan, M., & Bally, S. J. (2007). Psychosocial adaptations to dual sensory loss in middle and late adulthood. *Trends in Amplification*, *11*, 281–300.

CHAPTER 19. THE CANCERS

1. Karami, S., Young, H. A., & Henson, D. E. (2007). Earlier age at diagnosis: Another dimension in cancer disparity. *Cancer Epidemiology*, *31*, 29–34.

2. American Cancer Society (2012). *Cancer facts & figures 2012*. Atlanta: American Cancer Society.

3. Centers for Disease Control and Prevention (2002). Annual smoking-attributable mortality, years of potential life lost, and productivity losses—United States, 1995–1999. *Morbidity and Mortality Weekly Report*, *51* (14), 300–303.

4. Cleveland Clinic (n.d.). Smoking and heart disease. Retrieved Mar. 4, 2010, from http://my.clevelandclinic.org/heart/prevention/smoking/smoking_hrtds.aspx.

5. Antonelli, J. A., Jones, L. W., Bañez, L. L., et al. (2009). Exercise and prostate cancer risk in a cohort of veterans undergoing prostate needle biopsy. *Journal of Urology*, *182*, 2226–2231.

6. Murphy, T. K., Calle, E. E., Rodriguez, C., et al. (2000). Body mass index and colon cancer mortality in a large prospective study. *American Journal of Epidemiology*, *152*, 847–854.

7. Shavers, V. L., Fagan, P., Jones, D., et al. (2012). The state of research on racial/

ethnic discrimination in the receipt of health care. *American Journal of Public Health, 102,* 953–966. Hammond, W. P. (2010). Psychosocial correlates of medical mistrust among African American men. *American Journal of Community Psychology, 45,* 87–106. Ngo-Metzger, Q., Legedza, A. T. R., & Phillips, R. S. (2004). Asian Americans' reports of their health care experiences. *Journal of General Internal Medicine, 19,* 111–119.

8. Deandrea, S., Montanari, M., Moja, L., et al. (2008). Prevalence of undertreatment in cancer pain. A review of published literature. *Annals of Oncology, 19,* 1985–1991.

9. Portenoy, R. K. (2011). Treatment of cancer pain. *Lancet, 377,* 2236–2247.

10. Levy, M. H. (1996). Pharmacological treatment of cancer pain. *New England Journal of Medicine, 335,* 1124–1132. Zaza, C., Sellick, S. M., Willan, A., et al. (1999). Health care professionals' familiarity with non-pharmacological strategies for managing cancer pain. *Psycho-Oncology, 8,* 99–111.

11. Oliffe, J. L., Ogrodniczuk, J., Bottorff, J. L., et al. (2009). Connecting humor, health, and masculinities at prostate cancer support groups. *Psycho-Oncology, 18,* 916–926.

12. Gray, R. E., Fitch, M., Phillips, C., et al. (2000). To tell or not to tell: Patterns of disclosure among men with prostate cancer. *Psycho-Oncology, 9,* 273–282.

13. Else-Quest, N. M., LoConte, N. K., Schiller, J. H., et al. (2009). Perceived stigma, self-blame, and adjustment among lung, breast, and prostate cancer patients. *Psychology & Health, 24,* 949–964.

14. Gray, R. E., Fitch, M., Phillips, C., et al. (2000). To tell or not to tell: Patterns of disclosure among men with prostate cancer. *Psycho-Oncology, 9,* 273–282.

15. American Cancer Society (2012). *Cancer facts & figures 2012.* Atlanta: American Cancer Society. Retrieved June 20, 2011.

16. Postow, M. A., Callahan, M. K., Barker, C. A., et al. (2012). Immunologic correlates of the abscopal effect in a patient with melanoma. *New England Journal of Medicine, 366,* 925–931.

17. American Cancer Society (2012). *Cancer facts & figures 2012.* Atlanta: American Cancer Society.

18. Stemmermann, G. N., Nomura, A. M., Chyou, P. H., et al. (1992). A prospective comparison of prostate cancer at autopsy and as a clinical event: The Hawaii Japanese experience. *Cancer Epidemiology, Biomarkers, & Prevention, 1,* 189–192. Sakr, W. A., Haas, G. P., Cassin, B. F., et al. (1993). The frequency of carcinoma and intraepithelial neoplasia of the prostate in young male patients. *Journal of Urology, 150,* 379–385.

19. Oliffe, J. (2009). Health behaviors, prostate cancer, and masculinities: A life course perspective. *Men and Masculinities, 11,* 346–366.

20. De Marzo, A. M., Coffey, D. S., & Nelson, W. G. (1999). New concepts in tissue specificity for prostate cancer and benign prostatic hyperplasia. *Urology, 53* (suppl. 3a), 29–39.

21. Platz, E. A., Rimm, E. B., Willett, W. C., et al. (2000). Racial variation in prostate cancer incidence in the hormonal system markers among male health professionals. *Journal of the National Cancer Institute, 92,* 2009–2017.

22. Bloom, A. (2004). Prostate cancer and masculinity in Australian society: A case of stolen identity? *International Journal of Men's Health, 3,* 73–91.

23. D'Amico, A. V., Chen, M., Roehl, K. A., et al. (2004). Preoperative PSA velocity and the risk of death from prostate cancer after radical prostatectomy. *New England Journal of Medicine, 351,* 125–135.

24. Smith, D. S., Humphrey, P. A., & Catalona, W. J. (1997). The early detection of prostate carcinoma with prostate specific antigen: The Washington University experience. *Cancer, 80,* 1853–1856.

25. Ouyang, B., Bracken, B., Burke, B., et al. (2009). A duplex quantitative polymerase chain reaction assay based on quantification of α-Methylacyl-CoA Racemase transcripts and *Prostate Cancer Antigen 3* in urine sediments improved diagnostic accuracy for prostate cancer. *Journal of Urology, 181,* 2508–2514.

26. Kelsey, S. G., Owens, J., & White, A. (2004). The experience of radiotherapy for localized prostate cancer: The men's perspective. *European Journal of Cancer, 13,* 272–278.

27. Hu, J. C., Gu, X., Lipsitz, S. R., et al. (2009). Comparative effectiveness of minimally invasive vs open radical prostatectomy. *Journal of the American Medical Association, 302,* 1557–1564.

28. Menon, M., Shrivastava, A., Kaul, S., et al. (2007). Vattikuti Institute prostatectomy: Contemporary technique and analysis of results. *European Urology, 51,* 648–658. Menon, M., Kaul, S., Bhandari, A., et al. (2005). Potency following robotic radical prostatectomy: A questionnaire-based analysis of outcomes after conventional nerve sparing and prostatic fascia sparing techniques. *Journal of Urology, 174,* 2351–2355.

29. Walsh, P. C., Marschke, P., Ricker, D., et al. (2000). Patient-reported urinary continence and sexual function after anatomic radical prostatectomy. *Urology, 55,* 58–61.

30. Weber, B. A., Roberts, B. L., Mills, T. L., et al. (2008). Physical and emotional predictors of depression after radical prostatectomy. *American Journal of Men's Health, 2,* 165–171. Blank, T. O. (2008). The challenge of prostate cancer: "Half a man or a man and a half." *Generations, 32* (1), 68–72.

31. Maliski, S. L., Rivera, S., Conner, S., et al. (2008). Renegotiating masculine identity after prostate cancer treatment. *Qualitative Health Research, 18,* 1609–1620.

32. Alterowitz, R., & Alterowitz, B. (2004). *Intimacy with impotence: The couple's guide to better sex after prostate disease.* New York: DaCapo. Laken, V., & Laken, K. (2002). *Making love again: Hope for couples facing loss of sexual intimacy.* Sandwich, MA: Ant Hill Press.

33. Cornfield, J., Haenszel, W., Hammond, E. C., et al. (2009). Smoking and lung cancer: Recent evidence and a discussion of some questions. *International Journal of Epidemiology, 38,* 1175–1191.

34. Alberg, A. J., & Samet, J. M. (2003). Epidemiology of lung cancer. *Chest, 123* (suppl.), 21S–49S.

35. Cepeda, O. A., & Gammack, J. K. (2006). Cancer in older men: A gender-based review. *Aging Male, 9,* 149–158.

36. Humphrey, L. L., Teutsch, S., & Johnson, M. S. (2004). Lung cancer screening with sputum cytologic examination, chest radiography, and computed tomography: An update for the U.S. Preventive Services Task Force. *Annals of Internal Medicine, 140,* 740–753.

37. American Cancer Society (2012). *Cancer facts & figures 2012.* Atlanta: American Cancer Society.

38. Tseng, H. F., Morgenstern, H., Mack, T. M., & Peters, R. K. (2003). Risk factors for anal cancer: Results of a population-based case-control study. *Cancer Causes & Control, 14,* 837–846.

39. Centers for Disease Control and Prevention (2011). HPV and men—CDC fact sheet. Atlanta: U.S. Department of Health and Human Services, Centers for Disease Control and Prevention, Document CS228547A.

40. Daling, J. R., Madeleine, M. M., Johnson, L. G., et al. (2004). Human papillomavirus, smoking, and sexual practices in the etiology of anal cancer. *Cancer, 101,* 270–280.

41. Daling, J. R., Sherman, K. J., Hislop, T. G., et al. (1992). Cigarette smoking and the risk of anogenital cancer. *American Journal of Epidemiology, 135,* 180–198.

42. Thompson, E. H., & Leichthammer, A. S. (2010). "You gotta be kidding me!": Male

breast cancer. Paper presented at the annual meeting of the American Psychological Association, San Diego.

43. Brennan, P., Bogillot, O., Cordier, S., et al. (2000). Cigarette smoking and bladder cancer in men: A pooled analysis of 11 case-control studies. *International Journal of Cancer*, *86*, 289–294.

44. Band, P. R., Le, N., MacArthur, A. C., et al. (2005). Identification of occupational cancer risks in British Columbia: A population-based case-controlled study of 1129 cases of bladder cancer. *Journal of Occupational and Environmental Medicine*, *47*, 854–858.

45. American Cancer Society (2012). *Cancer facts & figures 2012*. Atlanta: American Cancer Society.

46. Temel, J. S., Greer, J. A., Muzikansky, A., et al. (2010). Early palliative care for patients with metastatic non-small-cell lung cancer. *New England Journal of Medicine*, *363*, 733–742.

CHAPTER 20. SEXUAL INTIMACY

1. McClone, K. P. (2009). Intimacy and healthy affective maturity. *Human Development*, *30* (4), 5–13.

2. De Rougemont, D. (1940). *Love in the Western world*. New York: Harcourt, Brace.

3. Ryan, C., & Jetha, C. (2010). *Sex at dawn: The prehistoric origins of modern sexuality*. New York: HarperCollins.

4. Carstensen, L. L., Isaacowitc, D. M., & Charles, S. T. (1999). Taking time seriously: A theory of socioemotional selectivity. *American Psychologist*, *54*, 165–181.

5. Gray, J. (1992). *Men are from Mars, women are from Venus: The classical guide to understanding the opposite sex*. New York: HarperCollins.

6. Guttman, D., & Huyck, M. H. (1991). Development and pathology in postparental men: A community study. In E. H. Thompson (ed.), *Older men's lives* (pp. 65–84). Thousand Oaks, CA: Sage.

7. Segal, L. (2007). *Slow motion: Changing masculinities, changing men* (3rd ed.). Hampshire: Palgrave MacMillan.

8. Thompson, P., Itzin, C., & Abendstern, M. (1990). *I don't feel old: The experience of later life*. New York: Oxford University Press. Featherstone, M., & Hepworth, M. (1990). Images of ageing. In J. Bond & P. Coleman (eds.), *Ageing in society: An introduction to social gerontology* (pp. 304–332). London: Sage.

9. Zilbergeld, B. (1999). *The new male sexuality: The truth about men, sex, and pleasure* (rev. ed.). New York: Bantam.

10. Levant, R. F., & Brooks, G. R. (1997). *Men and sex: New psychological perspectives*. New York: Wiley & Sons. Connell, R. W., & Messerschmidt, J. W. (2005). Hegemonic masculinity: Rethinking the concept. *Gender & Society*, *19* (6), 829–859.

11. Bergling, T. (2004). *Reeling in the years: Gay men's perspectives on age and ageism*. Binghamton, NY: Harrington Park. Slevin, K. F., & Linneman, T. J. (2010). Old gay men's bodies and masculinities. *Men and Masculinities*, *12*, 483–507.

12. Cancian, F. (1986). Gender politics: Love and power in private and public spheres. In A. Skolnick & J. Skolnick (eds.), *Family in transition* (pp. 193–200). Boston: Little, Brown. Coontz, S. (1992). *The way we never were: American families and the nostalgia trap*. New York: Basic Books.

13. Tanner, D. (1990). *You just don't understand: Women and men in conversation*. New York: Ballantine Books.

14. MacGeorge, E. L., Graves, A. R., Feng, B., et al. (2004). The myth of gender cultures: Similarities outweigh differences in men's and women's provision of and responses to supportive communication. *Sex Roles, 50*, 143–174.

15. Swain, S. O. (1989). Covert intimacy: Closeness in men's friendships. In B. J. Risman & P. Schwartz (eds.), *Gender in intimate relationships: A microstructural approach* (pp. 71–86). Belmont, CA: Wadsworth. Slavin, S. (2009). "Instinctively, I'm not just a sexual beast": The complexity of intimacy among Australian gay men. *Sexualities, 12*, 79–96.

16. Mortensen, C. D. (1994). *Problematic communication: The construction of invisible walls*. Westport, CT: Praeger.

17. Buscaglia, L. (1996). *Love: What life is all about*. New York: Ballantine Books.

18. Wong, G. (1981). Typologies of intimacy. *Psychology of Women Quarterly, 5* (3), 435–443.

19. Amato, P. R. & Booth, A. (1991). Consequences of parental divorce and marital unhappiness for adult well-being. *Social Forces, 69*, 895–914. Christensen, T. M., & Brooks, M. C. (2001). Adult children of divorce and intimate relationships: A review of the literature. *Family Journal, 9*, 289–294. Feng, D., Giarrusso, R., Bengtson, V. L., et al. (1999). Intergenerational transmission of marital quality and marital instability. *Journal of Marriage and the Family, 61*, 451–464.

20. Amato, P. R., & Booth, A. (2001). The legacy of parents' marital discord: Consequences of children's marital quality. *Journal of Personality and Social Psychology, 81*, 627–638.

21. Butler, R. N., & Lewis, M. I. (1988). *The new love and sex after 60*. New York: Ballantine Books.

22. Barusch, A. S. (2008). *Love stories of later life: A narrative approach to understanding romance*. New York: Oxford University Press.

23. Gorchoff, S. M., John, O. P., & Helson, R. (2008). Contextualizing change in marital satisfaction during middle age: An 18-year longitudinal study. *Psychological Science, 19*, 1194–1200.

24. Saltz, G. (2011, Mar./Apr.). An empty nest means better sex. *AARP Magazine*. Washington, DC: AARP.

25. Schwartz, P. (2009, Oct.). Taking your job home with you? Does your job deflate your sex drive? *AARP Magazine*. Washington, DC: AARP.

26. Lloyd, E. A. (2005). *The case of the female orgasm: Bias in the science of evolution*. Boston, MA: Harvard University Press.

27. Duncan, D., & Dowsett, G. W. (2010). "There's no teleology to it; it's just about the spirit of play": Men, intimacy, and "late" modernity. *Journal of Men's Studies, 18*, 45–62.

28. Barusch, A. S. (2008). *Love stories of later life: A narrative approach to understanding romance*. New York: Oxford University Press.

29. Zilbergeld, B. (1999). *The new male sexuality: The truth about men, sex, and pleasure* (rev. ed.). New York: Bantam.

30. Barusch, A. S. (2008). *Love stories of later life: A narrative approach to understanding romance*. New York: Oxford University Press.

31. Heiman, J. R., Long, J. S., Smith, S. N., et al. (2011). Sexual satisfaction and relationship happiness in midlife and older couples in five countries. *Archives of Sexual Behavior, 40*, 741–753.

32. Lindau, S. T., Schumm, L. P., Laumann, E. O., et al. (2007). A study of sexuality and health among older adults in the United States. *New England Journal of Medicine, 357*, 762–774.

33. Roughan, P. A., Kaiser, F. E., & Morley, J. E. (1993). Sexuality and the older woman. *Clinical Geriatric Medicine, 9*, 87–106.

34. Lindau, S. T., Schumm, L. P., Laumann, E. O., et al. (2007). A study of sexuality and health among older adults in the United States. *New England Journal of Medicine, 357,* 762–774.

35. Zeiss, A. M., & Kasl-Godley, J. (2001). Sexuality in older adults' relationships. *Generations, 25* (2), 18–25.

36. American Association of Retired Persons (2005). *Sexuality at midlife and beyond.* Washington, DC: AARP.

37. Nicolosi, A., Laumann, E. O., Glasser, D. B., et al. (2004). Sexual behavior and sexual problems after the age of 40: The global study of sexual attitudes and behaviors. *Urology, 64,* 991–997.

38. Rosen, D. (2008, Sept. 20). One billion pills later. *CounterPunch.*

39. Barusch, A. S. (2008). *Love stories of later life: A narrative approach to understanding romance.* New York: Oxford University Press.

40. Sinclair Institute (n.d.). About Sinclair Intimacy Institute. Retrieved Nov. 15, 2010, from www.bettersex.com/t-absi-companyinfo.aspx.

41. Birditt, K. S., & Fingerman, K. L. (2005). Do we get better at picking our battles? Age group differences in descriptions of behavior reactions to interpersonal tensions. *Journal of Gerontology: Psychological Sciences, 60B* (3), P121–138.

42. Carstensen, L. L., Isaacowitc, D. M., & Charles, S. T. (1999). Taking time seriously: A theory of socioemotional selectivity. *American Psychologist, 54,* 165–181.

43. Patrick, S., & Bechenbach, J. (2009). Male perceptions of intimacy: A qualitative study. *Journal of Men's Studies, 17,* 47–56.

44. Emlet, C. (2004). HIV/AIDS and aging: A diverse population of vulnerable older adults. *Journal of Human Behavior in the Social Environment, 9* (4), 45–63. Emlet, C. (2006). "You're awfully old to have this disease": Experiences of stigma and ageism in adults 50 years and older living with HIV/AIDS. *Gerontologist, 46,* 781–790. Bodley-Tickell, A. T., Olowokure, B., Bhaduri, S., et al. (2008). Trends in sexually transmitted infections (other than HIV) in older people: Analysis of data from an enhanced surveillance system. *Sexually Transmitted Infections, 84,* 312–317.

45. The Mayo Clinic Staff (2011). *Health issues for gay men: Prevention first.* Rochester, MN: Mayo Foundation for Medical Education and Research.

46. Chew, K., Bremner, A., Stuckey, B., et al. (2009). Sex life after 65: How does erectile dysfunction affect aging and elderly men? *Aging Male, 12* (2/3), 41–46. Feldman, H. A., Johannes, C. B., Derby, C. A., et al. (2000). Erectile dysfunction and coronary risk factors: Prospective results from the Massachusetts male aging study. *Preventive Medicine, 30,* 328–338. Harvard Men's Health Watch (2006, Mar.). Life after 50: A new Harvard study of male sexuality. *Harvard Men's Health Watch, 10* (8), 1–3.

47. Goldstein, I. (2004). Epidemiology of erectile dysfunction. *Sexuality and Disability, 22,* 113–120.

48. Selvin, E., Burnett, A. L., & Platz, E. A. (2007). Prevalence and risk factors for erectile dysfunction in the U.S. *American Journal of Medicine, 120,* 151–157.

49. Pangman, V. C., & Seguire, M. (2000). Sexuality and the chronically ill older adult: A social justice issue. *Sexuality and Disability, 18,* 49–59.

50. Cahill, S., & South, K. (2002). Policy issues affecting lesbian, gay, bisexual and transgender people in retirement. *Generations, 26* (2), 49–54. Reingold, D., & Burros, N. (2004). Sexuality in the nursing home. *Journal of Gerontological Social Work, 43* (2/3), 175–186. Miles, S. H., & Parker, K. (1999). Sexuality in the nursing home: Iatrogenic loneliness. *Generations, 23* (1), 36–43. Fairchild, S. K., Carrino, G. E., & Ramirez, M. (1996). Social workers' perceptions of staff attitudes toward resident sexuality in a random sample

of New York state nursing homes: A pilot study. *Journal of Gerontological Social Work*, *26* (1/2), 153–169.

51. Henneberger, M. (2010). An affair to remember. Retrieved Nov. 16, 2010, from www.slate.com/id/2192178/.

52. Fairchild, S. K., Carrino, G. E., & Ramirez, M. (1996). Social workers' perceptions of staff attitudes toward resident sexuality in a random sample of New York state nursing homes: A pilot study. *Journal of Gerontological Social Work*, *26* (1/2), 153–169.

53. Dooghe, G., Vanderleyden L., & Van Loon, F. (1980). Social adjustment of the elderly residing in institutional homes: A multivariate analysis. *International Journal of Aging and Human Development*, *11*, 163–176.

54. American Medical Directors Association (2002). AMDA model care facility: Medical staff policies and procedures. Policy Number: Clin.CLI.13. Subject: Privacy and Sexuality. Retrieved Nov. 16, 2010, from www.amda.com/tools/library/policymanual /cli-13.cfm.

55. Kamble, P., Chen, H., Sherer, J. T., et al. (2009). Use of antipsychotics among elderly nursing home residents with dementia in the US: An analysis of National Survey Data. *Drugs and Aging*, *26*, 483–92.

CHAPTER 21. RETIREMENT

1. Costa, D. L. (1998). *The evolution of retirement: An American economic history, 1880–1990*. Chicago: University of Chicago Press.

2. Fullerton, H. N. (1999). Labor force participation: 75 years of change, 1950–1998 and 1998–2025. *Monthly Labor Review*, *122* (12), 3–12.

3. Savishinsky, J. S. (2000). *Breaking the watch: The meanings of retirement in America*. Ithaca, NY: Cornell University Press, p. 12.

4. Atchley, R. C. (1976). *The sociology of retirement*. New York: Schenkman.

5. Clarke, M. (2007). Choices and constraints: Individual perceptions of the voluntary redundancy experience. *Human Resource Management Journal*, *17*, 76–93.

6. Hardy, M. A., & Quadagno, J. (1995). Satisfaction with early retirement: Making choices in the auto industry. *Journal of Gerontology: Social Sciences*, *50*, S217–S228.

7. Ekerdt, D. J. (1986). The busy ethic: Moral continuity between work and retirement. *Gerontologist*, *26*, 239–244, p. 239.

8. Ekerdt, D. J., Hackney, J., Kosloski, K., et al. (2001). Eddies in the stream: The prevalence of uncertain plans for retirement. *Journal of Gerontology: Social Sciences*, *56B*, S162–S170, p. S169.

9. Ameriprise Financial (2010). *New Retirement Mindscape II study*. Minneapolis, MN: Ameriprise Financial Center. Retrieved Aug. 11, 2011, from http://newsroom.ameriprise .com/images/20018/Mindscape%20II%20Report%201.pdf.

10. Henretta, J. C. (1992). Uniformity and diversity: Life course institutionalization and late-life work exit. *Sociological Quarterly*, *33*, 265–279.

11. Munnell, A. H., & Sass, S. A. (2009). *Working longer: The solution to the retirement income challenge*. New York: Brookings Institution Press.

12. Phua, V. C., & McNally, J. W. (2008). Men planning for retirement: Changing meanings of preretirement planning. *Journal of Applied Gerontology*, *27*, 588–608, p. 602.

13. Transamerica Center for Retirement Studies (2011). *The new retirement: Working*. 12th Annual Transamerica Retirement Survey. Los Angeles: Transamerica Center for Retirement Studies. Retrieved Aug. 10, 2011, from www.transamericacenter.org/resources /TCRS12thAnnual%20WorkerNewRetirementFINAL05162011.pdf.

14. Employee Benefit Research Institute (2012). *2012 Retirement confidence survey: Fact Sheet #1*. Washington, DC: Employee Benefit Research Institute. Retrieved Jan. 14, 2013, from www.ebri.org/pdf/surveys/rcs/2012/fs-01-rcs-12-fs1-conf.pdf.

15. Johnson, R. W. (2005). Working longer to enhance retirement. *Retirement Project Brief No. 1*. Washington, DC: Urban Institute.

16. Phua, V. C., & McNally, J. W. (2008). Men planning for retirement: Changing meanings of preretirement planning. *Journal of Applied Gerontology*, 27, 588–608, p. 599.

17. Jones, I. R., Leontowitsch, M., & Higgs, P. (2010). The experience of retirement in second modernity: Generational habitus among retired senior managers. *Sociology*, 44, 103–120, p. 110.

18. Weiss, R. S. (2005). *The experience of retirement*. Ithaca: ILR Press, p. 25.

19. U.S. Census Bureau (2011). *Statistical abstract of the United States, 2011*. Washington, DC: U.S. Census Bureau, p. 384. Retrieved July 28, 2011, from www.census.gov/prod/www/abs/statab2011_2015.html.

20. Munnell, A. H., Webb, A., & Golub-Sass, F. (2009). The national retirement risk index: After the crash. Document Number 9–22. Boston, MA: Center for Retirement Research at Boston College. Retrieved Aug. 10, 2011, from www.oecd.org/dataoecd/2/27/46263009.pdf.

21. Weiss, R. S. (1990). *Staying the course: The emotional and social lives of men who have done well at work*. New York: Free Press.

22. Weiss, R. S. (2005). *The experience of retirement*. Ithaca: ILR Press, p. 116.

23. Ibid., p. 118.

24. Cahill, K., Giandrea, M., & Quinn, J. (2006). Retirement patterns from career employment. *Gerontologist*, 46, 514–523.

25. Giandrea, M. D., Cahill, K. E., & Quinn, J. F. (2009). Bridge jobs: A comparison across cohorts. *Research on Aging*, 31, 549–576.

26. Freeman, M. (2007). *Encore: Finding work that matters in the second half of life*. San Francisco: PublicAffairs.

27. Savishinsky, J. S. (2000). *Breaking the watch: The meanings of retirement in America*. Ithaca, NY: Cornell University Press, p. 66–84.

28. Ameriprise Financial (2010). *New Retirement Mindscape II study*. Minneapolis, MN: Ameriprise Financial Center. Retrieved Aug. 11, 2011, from http://newsroom.ameriprise.com/images/20018/Mindscape%20II%20Report%201.pdf.

29. Pinquart, M., & Schindler, I. (2007). Changes in life satisfaction in the transition to retirement: A latent-class approach. *Psychology and Aging*, 22, 442–455.

30. Boeninger, D. K., Shiraishi, R. W., Aldwin, C. M., et al. (2009). Why do older men report low stress ratings? Findings from the Veterans Affairs Normative Aging Study. *International Journal of Aging and Human Development*, 68, 149–170.

31. Weiss, R. S. (2005). *The experience of retirement*. Ithaca: ILR Press, p. 68.

32. Ameriprise Financial (2010). *New Retirement Mindscape II study*. Minneapolis, MN: Ameriprise Financial Center, p. 8. Retrieved Aug. 11, 2011, from http://newsroom.ameriprise.com/images/20018/Mindscape%20II%20Report%201.pdf.

33. Patterson, M. (2011, Jan. 27). 4 radical strategies to retire sooner. *U.S. News and World Report*.

34. Mein, G., Higgs, P., Ferrie, J., et al. (1998). Paradigms of retirement: The importance of health and ageing in the Whitehall II Study. *Social Science & Medicine*, 47, 535–545, p. 540.

CHAPTER 22. CAREGIVING: HELPING OTHERS THROUGH DIFFICULT TIMES

1. MetLife Mature Market Institute (2006). *The MetLife study of Alzheimer's disease: The caregiving experience.* New York: Metlife. Alzheimer's Association and National Alliance for Caregiving (2004). *Families care: Alzheimer's caregiving in the United States.* Chicago: Alzheimer's Association and National Alliance for Caregiving. National Alliance for Caregiving and AARP (2009). *Caregiving in the U.S.* Washington, DC: AARP and NAC.

2. National Alliance for Caregiving and AARP (2009). *Caregiving in the U.S.* Washington, DC: AARP and NAC, p. 4.

3. Metlife Mature Market Institute (2011). *Caregiving costs to working caregivers: Double jeopardy for baby boomers caring for their parents.* Westport, CT: Metlife Mature Market Institute.

4. Alzheimer's Association and National Alliance for Caregiving (2004). *Families care: Alzheimer's caregiving in the United States.* Chicago: Alzheimer's Association and National Alliance for Caregiving.

5. Schulz, F., & Martire, L. M. (2004). Family caregiving of persons with dementia: Prevalence, health effects, and support strategies. *American Journal of Geriatric Psychiatry*, *12*, 240–249. Alzheimer's Association and National Alliance for Caregiving (2004). *Families care: Alzheimer's caregiving in the United States.* Chicago: Alzheimer's Association and National Alliance for Caregiving.

6. Hayes, J., Zimmerman, M. K., & Boylstein, C. (2010). Responding to symptoms of Alzheimer's disease: Husbands, wives, and the gendered dynamics of recognition and disclosure. *Qualitative Health Research*, *20*, 1101–1115.

7. Hepburn, K., Lewis, M. L., Narayan, S., et al. (2002). Discourse-derived perspectives: Differentiating among spouses' experiences of caregiving. *American Journal of Alzheimer's Disease and Other Dementias*, *17*, 213–226. Russell, R., (2001). A man's gotta do what a man's gotta do: Husbands as caregivers to their demented wives: A discourse analytic approach. *Journal of Aging Studies*, *14*, 153–169. Alzheimer's Association (2012). *Alzheimer's disease facts and figures.* Chicago: Alzheimer's Association.

8. National Alliance for Caregiving and AARP (2009). *Caregiving in the U.S.* Washington, DC: AARP and NAC.

9. Ginzler, E. (2010, July). Caregiving: It's different for men: They're fewer in numbers, but equal in dedication. Washington, DC: AARP.

10. Thompson, E. H. (2002). What's unique about men's caregiving. In B. J. Kramer & E. H. Thompson (eds.), *Men as caregivers: Theory, research, and service implications* (pp. 20–47). New York: Springer. Kaye, L. W., & Applegate, J. A. (1990). *Men as caregivers to the elderly: Understanding and aiding unrecognized family support.* Lexington, MA: Lexington Books.

11. Thompson, E. H. (2000). The gendered caregiving of husbands and sons. In E. Markson & L. Hollings (eds.), *Intersections of aging: Readings in social gerontology* (pp. 333–344). Los Angeles: Roxbury.

12. National Alliance for Caregiving and AARP (2009). *Caregiving in the U.S.* Washington, DC: AARP and NAC.

13. Metlife Mature Market Institute (2010). *Working caregivers and employer health care costs.* New York: Metlife.

14. Kaye, L. W. (1997). Informal caregiving by older men. In J. I. Kosberg & L. W. Kaye (eds.), *Elderly men: Special problems and professional challenges* (pp. 231–249). New York: Springer. Carpenter, E. H., & Miller, B. H. (2002). Psychosocial challenges and rewards experienced by caregiving men: A review of the literature and an empirical case example.

In B. J. Kramer & E. H. Thompson (eds.), *Men as caregivers: Theory, research, and service implications* (pp. 99–126). New York: Springer. Adler, K. A., Patterson, T. L., & Grant, I. (2002). Physiological challenges associated with caregiving among men. In B. J. Kramer & E. H. Thompson (eds.), *Men as caregivers: Theory, research, and service implications* (pp. 127–150). New York: Springer.

15. Anderson, S. A. (2011, Mar. 3). Mickey Rooney tells Congress of abuse. Associated Press.

16. Russell, R. (2007). The work of elderly men caregivers: From public careers to an unseen world. *Men and Masculinities, 9,* 298–314.

17. Coe, M., & Neufeld, A. (1999). Male caregivers' use of formal support. *Western Journal of Nursing Research, 21,* 568–588. Delgado, M., & Tennstedt, S. (1997). Puerto Rican sons as primary caregivers of elderly parents. *Social Work, 42,* 125–134.

18. Russell, R. (2004). Social networks among elder men caregivers. *Journal of Men's Studies, 13,* 121–142.

19. National Institute on Aging (2010, Aug.). *So far away: Twenty questions and answers about long-distance caregiving* (NIH Publication No. 10–5496).

20. Moseley, P. W., Davies, H. D., & Priddy, J. M. (1988). Support groups for male caregivers of Alzheimer's patients: A follow-up. *Clinical Gerontologist, 7* (3/4), 127–136. Kaye, L. W. & Applegate, J. S. (1993). Family support groups for male caregivers: Benefits of participation. *Journal of Gerontological Social Work, 20* (3/4), 167–185.

21. National Alliance for Caregiving and AARP (2009). *Caregiving in the U.S.* Washington, DC: AARP and NAC.

22. Tergesen, A. (2011, Feb. 12). Caregiver tax breaks. *Wall Street Journal.*

23. Ibid.

24. Muraco, A., & Fredriksen-Goldsen, K. (2011). "That's what friends do": Informal caregiving for chronically ill midlife and older lesbian, gay, and bisexual adults. *Journal of Social and Personal Relationships, 28,* 1073–1092. Brotman, S., Ryan, B., Collins, S., et al. (2007). Coming out to care: Caregivers of gay and lesbian seniors in Canada. *Gerontologist, 47,* 490–503.

25. Sipes, C. S. (2002). The experiences and relationships of gay male caregivers who provide care for their partners with AIDS. In B. J. Kramer & E. H. Thompson (eds.), *Men as caregivers: Theory, research, and service implications* (pp. 151–189). New York: Springer. Hash, K. (2006). Caregiving and post-caregiving experiences of midlife and older gay men and lesbians. *Journal of Gerontological Social Work, 47,* 121–138. Leppel, K. (2008). The relationship between hours worked and partner's disability in opposite- and same-sex couples. *Culture, Health & Sexuality, 10,* 773–785.

26. Greenberg, J. S. (2002). Differences between fathers and mothers in the care of their children with mental illness. In B. J. Kramer & E. H. Thompson (eds.), *Men as caregivers: Theory, research, and service implications* (pp. 269–293). New York: Springer.

27. U.S. Bureau of the Census (2011, Aug. 26). *Facts for features: Grandparents as caregivers.* Washington, DC: U.S. Census Bureau. CB11–FF.17.

28. Letiecq, B., Bailey, S., & Kurtz, M. (2008). Depression among rural Native American and European American grandparents rearing their grandchildren. *Journal of Family Issues, 29* (3), 334–356.

29. Kaye, L. W., & Applegate, J. A. (1990). *Men as caregivers to the elderly: Understanding and aiding unrecognized family support.* Lexington, MA: Lexington Books. Kaye, L. W., & Applegate, J. A. (1994). Older men and the family caregiving orientation. In E. H. Thompson Jr. (ed.), *Older men's lives* (pp. 218–236). Thousand Oaks, CA: Sage.

30. National Alliance for Caregiving and AARP (2009). *Caregiving in the U.S.: A focused*

look at those caring for someone age 50 or older. Washington, DC: AARP and NAC. Document D19236(1209).

31. Colbert, L. G. (2011, Jan.–Feb.). Taking care of mom: A son's journey. *Aging Today*, *32* (1), 7, 10.

CHAPTER 23. END-OF-LIFE MATTERS

1. Heyland, D. K., Dodek, P., Rocker, G., et al. (2006). What matters most in end-of-life care: Perceptions of seriously ill patients and their family members. *Canadian Medical Association Journal*, *174*, 627–633.

2. Fagerlin, A., & Schneider, C. E. (2004). Enough: The failure of the living will. *Hastings Center Report*, *34* (2), 30–42. Perkins, H. S. (2007). Controlling death: The false promise of advance directives. *Annals of Internal Medicine*, *147*, 51–57.

3. Silveira, M. J., Kim, S. Y. H., & Langa, K. M. (2010). Advance directives and outcomes of surrogate decision making before death. *New England Journal of Medicine*, *362*, 1211–1218.

4. Hickman, S. E., Hammes, B. J., Moss, A. H., et al. (2005). Hope for the future: Achieving the original intent of advance directives. *Hastings Center Report*, *35* (spec. no.), S26–S30.

5. U.S. Department of Health and Human Services (2008). National Clearinghouse for long-term care information: Own your future. Retrieved Sept. 30, 2010, from www .longtermcare.gov/LTC/Main_Site/Planning/Importance/Examples.aspx.

6. Genworth Financial (2010, Apr.). Genworth 2010 Cost of Care Survey. Retrieved Sept. 30, 2010, from www.genworth.com/content/etc/medialib/genworth_v2/pdf/ltc _cost_of_care.Par.14625.File.dat/2010_Cost_of_Care_Survey_Full_Report.pdf.

7. U.S. Department of Health and Human Services (2010). Planning for long-term care. Retrieved Sept. 30, 2010, from www.longtermcare.gov/LTC/Main_Site/Paying/Costs /Index.aspx.

8. Temel, J. S., Greer, J. A., Muzikansky, A., et al. (2010). Early palliative care for patients with metastatic non-small-cell lung cancer. *New England Journal of Medicine*, *363*, 733–742.

9. Fadul, N., Elsayem, A., Palmer, J. L., et al. (2009). Supportive versus palliative care: What's in a name? A survey of medical oncologists and midlevel providers at a comprehensive cancer center. *Cancer*, *115*, 2013–2021.

10. Jennings, B., Rundes, T., D'Onofrio, C., et al. (2003). Access to hospice care: Expanding boundaries, overcoming barriers. *Hastings Center Report*, *33* (2), S3–S7.

11. Steinhauser, K. E., Clipp, E. C., McNeilly, M., et al. (2000). In search of a good death: Observations of patients, families, and providers. *Annals of Internal Medicine*, *132*, 825–832.

12. Kapo, J., Harrold, J., Carroll, J. T., et al. (2005). Are we referring patients to hospice too late? Patients' and families' opinions. *Journal of Palliative Medicine*, *8*, 521–527.

Contributors

Alison Ashley, LMSW, earned her MSW from the University of Maine in 2011 and BA from Husson University in 2003, obtained a Certificate in Leadership in Rural Gerontological Social Work Practice during her studies at UMaine, and is currently a clinician / clinical supervisor at Care & Comfort, a Maine agency providing home health and mental health services.

Kaitlyn Barnes, BA, completed her undergraduate work at College of the Holy Cross in 2010, worked as a Clinical Research Coordinator at the Diabetes Research Center at Massachusetts General Hospital for 2 years, and currently is a PhD candidate in sociology at Case Western Reserve University studying medical sociology and aging.

Amanda Barusch, PhD, is Professor and Director of the PhD Program, College of Social Work, University of Utah, and since June 2007 she has held an appointment as Professor of Gerontology at the University of Otago in Dunedin, New Zealand, where she continues to serve on a part-time basis.

Elizabeth Conner, BA, earned her undergraduate degree in sociology from College of the Holy Cross in 2010, graduated with honors, worked throughout her undergraduate career as a model, and is now in New York employed by the Bella Agency, New York; Maggie, Inc., Boston; and several other distinguished agencies.

Jennifer A. Crittenden, MSW, earned her BA in psychology from the University of Maine in 2003 and her MSW in 2005 also from the University of Maine. She is currently the Fiscal and Administrative Officer at the University of Maine Center on Aging, where she oversees the daily administration of a variety of education, research, and community service projects in gerontology.

Lindsay J. Day, LMSW-CC, earned her BASW from the University of Maine in 2004 and her MSW in 2012 also from the University of Maine. She is currently the Social Services Director at Collier's Rehab and Nursing Facility in Ellsworth, Maine.

Elisha M. Foss, LMSW-CC, CADC, earned her BS in Mental Health and Human Services from the University of Maine at Augusta in 2009 and her MSW in 2012 from the University of Maine. She is currently the ICS School-Based Clinician for Old Town Elementary and Middle School.

Katherine Guardino, BA, received an Undergraduate Research Fellowship in summer 2008 from College of the Holy Cross to investigate older men's heart health, graduated with honors in 2010, moved to England for 2 years, and is currently working as the Coordinator of the Coastal Georgia Combined Federal Campaign.

Kristianna Hall, MSW, MHRTC, earned her MSW from the University of Maine in 2010, is currently working toward independent licensure in social work, and works in adult mental health case management with Catholic Charities Support & Recovery Services in Portland, Maine.

Elizabeth Kayajian, BA, completed her Women's and Gender Studies Capstone in 2010 investigating men's dietary behavior; graduated with honors from College of the Holy Cross; currently works as the Program Coordinator at Faith House, a residential treatment facility for women with substance use disorders; and has an eye on beginning a joint MSW/MPH graduate program.

Alexandra Leichthammer, BA, while an undergraduate at College of the Holy Cross, was awarded the Gerisch Summer Research Fellowship in Sociology in 2009 to study male breast cancer; later worked at the Brigham and Women's Hospital in an administrative role in grant management; and is now with the Office of Gift Planning, Harvard University.

Bethany O'Dell, BA, then a sociology undergraduate and captain of the NCAA Division 1 College of the Holy Cross women's varsity basketball team, diligently investigated men's dental health and is now a U.S. Associate Marketing Manager for Reebok International.

Clifford M. Singer, MD, is Chief, Division of Geriatric Mental Health and Neuropsychiatry at Acadia Hospital and Eastern Maine Medical Center in Bangor, and an Adjunct Professor at the University of Maine. Earlier, he was Associate Professor of Psychiatry and Neurology, University of Vermont College of Medicine.

Cynthia Stuen, DSW, PhD, is the former Senior Vice President of Policy and Evaluation and Chief Professional Affairs Officer at Lighthouse International in New York

City, a Fellow with the New York Academy of Medicine, and previous Chair of the Board of Directors, American Society on Aging.

Kristen Sutherland, MSW, received her BS and MSW at the University of Maine in 2008 and 2010, respectively, and recently served as the Director of My Friends Place, a nonprofit adult social program in Bangor, Maine.

Stefanie Tedesco, while an undergraduate at College of the Holy Cross, received the Rosalie S. Wolf Gerontology Award in 2010 and graduated with honors, later worked as a Guardianship Case Manager at the Jewish Family Services of Worcester, and is currently a Juris Doctoral candidate at the Boston College Law School and staff writer for the *Boston College Law Review*.

David C. Wihry, MPA, is a Research Associate at the University of Maine Center on Aging. He graduated from the University of Maine in 2008 with a BA in philosophy and received his Master of Public Administration from the University of Delaware in 2010.

Reviewers

Linda Bandini, PhD
Clinical Professor, Department of Health
 Sciences
College of Health & Rehabilitation Services
Boston University
Boston, MA 02215

Renee Beard, PhD
Assistant Professor, Department of
 Sociology and Anthropology
College of the Holy Cross
Worcester, MA 01610

Kate M. Bennett, PhD
Professor, Behavioural Health Sciences
School of Psychology
University of Liverpool
Liverpool L69 7ZA
UK

Silvia Corvera, MD
Professor, Program in Molecular Medicine
University of Massachusetts Medical
 School
55 Lake Avenue North
Worcester, MA 01655

Kate Davidson, PhD
Emeritus Professor, Centre for Research
 on Ageing and Gender
University of Surrey
Guildford GU2 7XH
UK

George W. Dowdall, PhD
Professor, Department of Sociology
Saint Joseph's University
Philadelphia, PA 19131

David J. Ekerdt, PhD
Director, Gerontology Center
Professor of Sociology
University of Kansas
1000 Sunnyside Avenue, Room 3090
Lawrence, KS 66045-7561

Daniel Fanselow, DC, DACNB
Clinical Chiropractor
Family Chiropractic of Westboro
Westboro, MA 01581

Richard A. Grossman, OD
Optometry Associates
488 Pleasant Street
Worcester, MA 01609

Anita Hoffer, PhD, EdD
Sexuality Educator and Counselor
President, Hoffer Associates
Brookline, MA 02445

Ellen L. Idler, PhD
Director, Religion and Public Health
 Collaborative
Department of Sociology, Emory College
Department of Epidemiology, Rollins
 School of Public Health
Emory University
Atlanta, GA 30322

Sarah H. Matthews, PhD
Emeritus Professor, Department of
 Sociology
Cleveland State University
Cleveland, OH 44115

Terrance F. McGovern, DDS
Private Practice
715 Pleasant Street
Worcester, MA 01602

Jennifer D. McNulty
Adjunct Professor, Kinesiology and
 Physical Education
College of Education and Human
 Development
University of Maine
Orono, ME 04469

Robert Meadows, PhD
Lecturer, Department of Sociology
University of Surrey
Guildford GU2 7XH
UK

Alinde J. Moore, PhD
Professor, Department of Psychology
Ashland University
Ashland, OH 44805

Katharine Munn, DDS
Clinical Periodontist
Periodontics in Fitchburg and Worcester
64 Whalon Street
Fitchburg, MA 01420

Ira S. Ockene, MD
Professor, Cardiovascular Medicine
University of Massachusetts Medical
    School
55 Lake Avenue North
Worcester, MA 01605

John Oliff, RN
Associate Professor, School of Nursing
University of British Columbia
Vancouver, BC V6T 1Z3
Canada

James M. O'Neil, PhD
Professor, Department of Educational
    Psychology
Neag School of Education
University of Connecticut
Storrs, CT 06269-2064

Alan G. Rosmarin, MD
Chief, Division of Hematology/Oncology
Co-Director, Cancer Center of Excellence
University of Massachusetts Medical
    School
55 Lake Avenue North
Worcester, MA 01655

Richard Russell, PhD, LMSW
Associate Professor of Social Work
Greater Rochester Collaborative MSW
    Program
55 St. Paul Street
Rochester, NY 14604

Jeanne Tolomeo, CMC
Geriatric Care Manager, Paralegal
Fletcher Tilton, PC
370 Main Street, Suite 1200
Worcester, MA 01608

Dyan Walsh, MSW
Director of Community Services
Eastern Area Agency on Aging
450 Essex Street
Bangor, ME 04401

Amy R. Wolfson, PhD
Professor, and Associate Dean for Faculty
    Development
College of the Holy Cross
Worcester, MA 01610

Michael R. Wollin, MD
Clinical Associate Professor of Surgery
University of Massachusetts Medical
    School
Worcester Urological Associates
25 Oak Avenue
Worcester, MA 01605

Index

AARP (American Association of Retired Persons), 5, 98, 106, 194, 306, 425, 459

abdomen: colostomy and, 406–7; size of, 33, 147–48. *See also* belly

abdominal obesity, 80, 221, 385, 405; metabolic syndrome and, 211

accidents: drug misuse and, 180; end-of-life-care and, 469; posttraumatic stress and, 87; sleep deprivation and, 122

ACE inhibitors, 228–29

acetaminophen: alcohol and, 172; hearing loss and, 373; for pain, 314, 332

acetylcholine, 254, 259

acid reflux, 386; osteoporosis and, 323

activity: aerobic, 17; anaerobic, 21; angina and, 223; maintaining, 10–25, 111; meaningful and enjoyable, 61–63, 64, 91–92, 96, 167, 243, 450; metabolism and, 12, 15, 20; recommended level of, 15–18, 275–76, 331; sleep and, 131–32; spiritual, 161, 163. *See also* exercise; physical activity; sexual activity

acupressure, 198

acupuncture, 84, 188, 199, 201–3, 312, 332, 390

adaptability, 50–52, 56, 58, 59, 70, 94; brain and, 51; psychological loss and, 61, 69–71; sexual aging and, 426; stress and, 76–77; vision loss and, 367. *See also* resilience

addiction, 175–76; drug and alcohol, 177, 182–83; tobacco, 383. *See also* alcoholism, treatment for

adrenal glands, 77

adrenaline, 78

adrenocorticotropin (ACTH), 77

advance directives, 463, 465–70

Advil, 253, 254, 314, 326

aerobic activity, 17; vs. anaerobic, 21; benefits of, 20, 72, 131, 244, 276–77, 327

affair, sexual. *See* sexual relations, nonexclusive

ageism, 4–6, 419, 421, 425, 429–30

age-related macular degeneration (AMD), 362–64; prevention of, 190, 359–60, 369; treatment for, 178

age spots, 134, 142, 144

aging, intrinsic (or chronologic), 7, 10, 12, 15, 45

AIDS, 309; caregiving and, 110, 458; experimental treatments for, 179; sexual intimacy and, 428–29. *See also* safer sex

alcohol, 168–71, 172; cognition and, 253–54; dependence on, 173–74; effects of, 41–42, 173; health benefits of, 170; health risks of, 48, 171–72, 173, 211, 222, 244, 323, 361, 381 (*see also* belly; erectile problems; sleep apnea, obstructive); insomnia and, 124–25; light and moderate use of, 169–70; medications and, 172, 177, 183; nutrition and, 45; prostate and, 286, 295; tolerance of, 170, 174

alcohol abuse, 174–75; comorbidities and, 67, 178, 302, 323–24, 381; risks of, 56, 62; screening tests for, 185–86

alcoholism, treatment for, 182–83, 183–85

allergies, 30, 290; medication side effects, 125, 253, 339, 340, 361

alopecia, androgenic, 135. *See also* male pattern hair loss

alopecia areata, 137

alpha blockers, 229, 292

Alzheimer's disease, 249–50, 255–57, 259–63; caring for, 446–47, 451, 456; fear of, 242; lowering risk of, 12, 192; symptoms of, 66, 260, 340; wives with, 103–4

anal cancer, 407–8

androgens, 135, 292. *See also* testosterone

anesthesia, 149, 294, 295, 298, 395

aneurysm, 237–38

anger: causes of, 60, 85, 272, 368, 379; dealing with, 160, 206, 272, 391, 452; and depression, 62–63; and distress, 82; as grouchiness, 61; health risks of, 215

angina, 215, 223, 233; atherosclerosis and, 225–26; bradyarrhythmia and, 230; exercise and, 235; heart medication and, 229, 429

angiography, 224, 234, 237

angioplasty, 234